Pathology
of the Prostate

OTHER MONOGRAPHS IN THE SERIES
MAJOR PROBLEMS IN PATHOLOGY

VIRGINIA A. LiVOLSI, M.D.
Series Editor

Published

Forthcoming

MPP

34

CHRISTOPHER S. FOSTER, M.D., Ph.D., FRCPath

Professor and Director of Cellular and Molecular Pathology
Department of Pathology
Royal Liverpool University Hospital
Liverpool, United Kingdom

DAVID G. BOSTWICK, M.D.

Professor of Pathology
Department of Pathology and Laboratory Medicine
Mayo Medical School
Consultant in Pathology
Mayo Clinic
Rochester, Minnesota

Pathology of the Prostate

Volume 34 in the Series
MAJOR PROBLEMS IN PATHOLOGY

W.B. SAUNDERS COMPANY
A Division of Harcourt Brace & Company
PHILADELPHIA LONDON TORONTO MONTREAL SYDNEY TOKYO

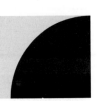

W.B. SAUNDERS COMPANY

A Division of Harcourt Brace & Company

The Curtis Center
Independence Square West
Philadelphia, Pennsylvania 19106

Library of Congress Cataloging-in-Publication Data

Pathology of the prostate / [edited by] Christopher S. Foster, David G. Bostwick

p.   cm.—(Major problems in pathology v. 34)

ISBN 0–7216–6951–4

1. Prostate—Cancer—Histopathology.   2. Prostate—Cancer—Cytopathology.
    I. Foster, Christopher S.   II. Bostwick, David G.   III. Series.
    [DNLM: 1. Prostatic Neoplasms—pathology.   2. Prostate—pathology.
    W1 MA492X v. 34 1998 / WJ 752 P2973 1998]

RC280.P7P372   1998

616.99′463—dc20

DNLM/DLC   96-23370

PATHOLOGY OF THE PROSTATE   ISBN 0–7216–6951–4

Printed in the United States of America.

Last digit is the print number: 9   8   7   6   5   4   3   2   1

To my wife, Joan, for your enduring loyalty; and to Katharine and Alexander for allowing me those rare but necessary moments of peace and quiet in the turmoil of daily life that have enabled me to concentrate on producing this book.

Christopher S. Foster

To my wife, Elizabeth, for your boundless patience, support, and encouragement.

David G. Bostwick

Contributors

WILLIAM C. ALLSBROOK, Jr, M.D.

Associate Professor, Department of Pathology, School of Medicine, Medical College of Georgia, Augusta, Georgia
Histochemistry of the Prostate

MAHUL AMIN, M.D.

Associate Professor of Pathology, Case Western Reserve University, Cleveland, Ohio; Senior Staff Pathologist, Senior Staff, Bone and Joint Center, and Associate Director, Immunohistochemistry Laboratory, Henry Ford Medical Center, Detroit, Michigan
Small Glandular Patterns in the Prostate Gland: The Differential Diagnosis of Small Acinar Carcinoma

GERHARD AUMÜLLER, Prof. Dr. med.

Professor of Anatomy, Klinikum der Philipps-Universität, Institut für Anatomie und Zellbiologie, Marburg, Germany
Embryology and Postnatal Development of the Prostate

MARGRIT AUMÜLLER, Dr. med.

Scientific Assistant, Klinikum der Philipps-Universität, Institut für Anatomie und Zellbiologie, Marburg, Germany
Embryology and Postnatal Development of the Prostate

DAVID G. BOSTWICK, M.D.

Professor of Pathology, Department of Pathology and Laboratory Medicine, Mayo Medical School; Consultant in Pathology, Mayo Clinic, Rochester, Minnesota
Prostatic Intraepithelial Neoplasia; Basal Cell Proliferations and Tumors of the Prostate; Examination of Radical Prostatectomy Specimens: Therapeutic and Prognostic Significance

MICHAEL K. BRAWER, M.D.

Professor, Department of Urology, Adjunct Professor, Department of Pathology, University of Washington, Seattle; Chief, Section of Urology, VA Puget Sound Health Care System, Seattle, Washington
Significance of Neovascularity in Tumor Prostate Carcinoma

PETER N. BRAWN, M.D.

Department of Pathology, University of Michigan School of Medicine, Ann Arbor; Department of Pathology, Veterans Administration Medical Center, Ann Arbor, Michigan
Histologic Features of Metastatic Prostate Cancer

MARTIN BULLOCK, M.D.

Lecturer, University of Toronto, Toronto; Pathologist, Women's College Hospital, Toronto, Ontario, Canada
Small Glandular Patterns in the Prostate Gland: The Differential Diagnosis of Small Acinar Carcinoma

ARLINE D. DEITCH, Ph.D.

Emeritus Professor, Department of Urology, University of California, Davis, Sacramento, California
DNA Flow Cytometry and Immunohistochemistry of p53 Pathway Genes as Predictive Modalities in Localized Prostate Cancer

NAYNEETA DESHMUKH, M.D., MRCPath

Registrar in Histopathology, Department of Pathology, The Royal Liverpool University Hospital, Liverpool, United Kingdom
Grading Prostate Cancer

LEENA T. DEVARAJ, M.D.

Department of Laboratory Medicine and Pathology, Mayo Clinic, Rochester, Minnesota
Basal Cell Proliferations and Tumors of the Prostate

P. ANTHONY DI SANT'AGNESE, M.D.

Professor of Pathology and Laboratory Medicine, University of Rochester School of Medicine, Rochester; Director of Surgical Pathology, Strong Memorial Hospital, Rochester, New York
Identification and Pathologic Significance of Neuroendocrine Differentiation in Human Prostate Carcinoma

JONATHAN I. EPSTEIN, M.D.

Professor of Pathology, Urology, and Oncology, Johns Hopkins University School of Medicine, Baltimore; Associate Director of Surgical Pathology, Johns Hopkins Hospital, Baltimore, Maryland
Pathologic Features That Predict Progression of Disease Following Radical Prostatectomy

CHRISTOPHER S. FOSTER, M.D., Ph.D., FRCPath

Professor and Director of Cellular and Molecular Pathology, Department of Pathology, Royal Liverpool University Hospital, Liverpool, United Kingdom
Examination of Radical Prostatectomy Specimens: Therapeutic and Prognostic Significance; Grading Prostate Cancer

STEPHANIE GROOS, Dr. med.

Scientific Assistant, Klinikum der Philipps-Universität, Institut für Anatomie und Zellbiologie, Marburg, Germany
Embryology and Postnatal Development of the Prostate

BURKHARD HELPAP, M.D.

Professor and Director of Pathology, Institut of Pathology, Hegar-Klinkum, Singen, Germany
Benign Prostatic Hyperplasia

PETER A. HUMPHREY, M.D., Ph.D.

Associate Professor of Pathology, Washington University School of Medicine, St. Louis; Attending Surgical Pathologist, Barnes–Jewish Hospital at Washington University Medical Center, St. Louis, Missouri
Relationships Between Serum Prostate-Specific Antigen and Histopathologic Appearances of Prostate Carcinoma

EDWARD C. JONES, M.D., FRCPC

Clinical Professor, Faculty of Medicine, University of British Columbia, Vancouver; Consultant Pathologist, Department of Pathology, Vancouver Hospital and Health Sciences Center, Vancouver, British Columbia, Canada
Differential Diagnosis of Prostatic Intraglandular Proliferative Lesions

ELAINE KAY, M.D., M.A., FRCSI, MRCPath

Senior Lecturer, Royal College of Surgeons, Dublin; Consultant Histopathologist, Beaumont Hospital, Dublin, Ireland
Soft Tissue Neoplasms and Other Unusual Tumors of Prostate, Including Uncommon Carcinomas

MITSURU KINJO, M.D., Ph.D.

Chief of Clinical Pathology, Harasanshin Hospital, Fukuoka, Japan
Critical Assessment of Inflammatory Lesions of the Prostate, Including Cytopathologic Appearances and Diagnosis

LUTZ KONRAD, Dr. rer. nat.

Scientific Assistant, Klinikum der Philipps-Universität, Institut für Anatomie und Zellbiologie, Marburg, Germany
Embryology and Postnatal Development of the Prostate

JOICHI KUMAZAWA, M.D., Ph.D.

Professor, Faculty of Medicine, Department of Urology, Kyushu University, Fukuoka, Japan
Critical Assessment of Inflammatory Lesions of the Prostate, Including Cytopathologic Appearances and Diagnosis

MARY LEADER, M.D., FRCPath, FRCPI, DCH

Professor of Pathology, Royal College of Surgeons, Dublin; Consultant Histopathologist, Beaumont Hospital, Dublin, Ireland
Soft Tissue Neoplasms and Other Unusual Tumors of Prostate, Including Uncommon Carcinomas

FRED LEE, M.D.

Director of Research, Crittenton Hospital, Rochester, Minnesota
Diagnosis of Prostate Cancer Altered by Ionizing Radiation With and Without Neoadjuvant Antiandrogen Hormonal Ablation

JOHN A. MAKSEM, M.D.

Chief Pathologist, Mercy Hospital Medical Center, Des Moines, Iowa
Aspiration Biopsy and Prostate Cytology

TETSURO MATSUMOTO, M.D., Ph.D.

Associate Professor, Faculty of Medicine, Department of Urology, Kyushu University, Fukuoka, Japan
Critical Assessment of Inflammatory Lesions of the Prostate, Including Cytopathologic Appearances and Diagnosis

DANIEL M. MAYMAN, B.G.S.

Research Assistant, St. Joseph Mercy Hospital, Ann Arbor, Minnesota
Diagnosis of Prostate Cancer Altered by Ionizing Radiation With and Without Neoadjuvant Antiandrogen Hormonal Ablation

JOHN E. McNEAL, M.D.

Clinical Professor, Department of Urology, Stanford University Medical School, Stanford, California
Anatomy and Normal Histology of the Human Prostate

OSAMU MOCHIDA, M.D.

Faculty of Medicine, Department of Urology, Kyushu University, Fukuoka, Japan
Critical Assessment of Inflammatory Lesions of the Prostate, Including Cytopathologic Appearances and Diagnosis

ERIC A. PFEIFER, M.D.

Senior Resident, Department of Pathology, Medical College of Georgia, School of Medicine, Augusta, Georgia
Histochemistry of the Prostate

HEINER RENNEBERG, Dipl. Biol.

Scientific Assistant, Klinikum der Philipps-Universität, Institut für Anatomie und Zellbiologie, Marburg, Germany
Embryology and Postnatal Development of the Prostate

MATTHEW D. RIFKIN, M.D.

Professor and Director of Radiology, Department of Radiology, The Albany Medical College, Albany, New York
Ultrasonography in the Diagnosis of Prostate Cancer

JEFFREY S. ROSS, M.D.

Professor and Chairman, Department of Pathology, The Albany Medical College, Albany, New York
Ultrasonography in the Diagnosis of Prostate Cancer

KAZUYUKI SAGIYAMA, M.D., Ph.D.

Chief of Urology Department, Harasanshin Hospital, Fukuoka, Japan
Critical Assessment of Inflammatory Lesions of the Prostate, Including Cytopathologic Appearances and Diagnosis

WAEL SAKR, M.D.

Associate Professor of Pathology, Wayne State University, School of Medicine, and the Barbara Ann Karmanos Cancer Institute, Detroit; Director, Immunohistochemistry Laboratory, Harper Hospital, Detroit, Michigan
Prostatic Intraepithelial Neoplasia

AVERY A. SANDBERG, M.D., D.Sc.

Senior Clinical Lecturer in Medicine, University of Arizona Medical School, Tucson; Adjunct Professor, Arizona State University, Department of Microbiology, Tempe; Senior Medical Director, Genzyme Genetics, Scottsdale; Vice President and Research Director, Southwest Biomedical Research Institute, Scottsdale, Arizona
Chromosomal Abnormalities in Human Prostate Cancer: Their Detection and Pathologic Significance

DOUGLAS B. SIDERS, M.D.

Associate Pathologist, Department of Pathology, St. Joseph Mercy Hospital, Ann Arbor, Michigan
Diagnosis of Prostate Cancer Altered by Ionizing Radiation With and Without Neoadjuvant Antiandrogen Hormonal Ablation

JUSTIN A. SIEGAL, B.S.

Research Associate, VA Puget Sound Health Care System, Seattle, Washington
Significance of Neovascularity in Human Prostate Carcinoma

JOHN R. SRIGLEY, M.D., FRCPC

Associate Professor, Department of Laboratory Medicine and Pathobiology, University of Toronto, Toronto, Ontario; Associate Professor, Department of Pathology, McMaster University, Hamilton, Ontario; Chief of Laboratory Medicine, The Credit Valley Hospital, Mississauga, Ontario, Canada
Small Glandular Patterns in the Prostate Gland: The Differential Diagnosis of Small Acinar Carcinoma

ROBIN T. VOLLMER, M.D., M.S.

Clinical Assistant Professor, Department of Pathology, Duke University School of Medicine, Durham; Chief, Surgical Pathology, Veterans Administration Medical Center, Durham, North Carolina
Relationships Between Serum Prostate-Specific Antigen and Histopathologic Appearances of Prostate Carcinoma

CAITRIONA BARRY WALSH, M.B., FRCPath

Senior Lecturer, Royal College of Surgeons, Dublin; Consultant Histopathologist, Beaumont Hospital, Dublin, Ireland
Soft Tissue Neoplasms and Other Unusual Tumors of Prostate, Including Uncommon Carcinomas

VICTOR WALUCH, M.D., Ph.D.

Clinical Professor of Radiology, University of Southern California, Los Angeles; Director, Magnetic Resonance Imaging Unit, St. Vincent Medical Center, Los Angeles, California
Magnetic Resonance Imaging of Prostate Carcinoma

RALPH W. DE VERE WHITE, M.B., B.Ch., B.A.O., FRCSEd

Professor and Chairman, Department of Urology, University of California, Davis, Sacramento; Director, Cancer Center, University of California, Davis Medical Center, Sacramento, California
DNA Flow Cytometry and Immunohistochemistry of p53 Pathway Genes as Predictive Modalities in Localized Prostate Cancer

ROBERT H. YOUNG, M.D., FRCPath

Associate Professor, Harvard Medical School, Boston; Associate Professor of Pathology, Director of Surgical Pathology, Massachusetts General Hospital, Boston, Massachusetts
Differential Diagnosis of Prostatic Intraglandular Proliferative Lesions

Preface

Prostatic disease, benign and malignant, is collectively responsible for significant morbidity and mortality in men throughout the world. Accurate diagnosis of prostatic disease is not facile, frequently requiring simultaneous data from clinical chemistry, radiology, urology, and, ultimately, the surgical pathology laboratory. Even following detailed histopathologic examination of biopsy tissues taken from precisely defined microanatomic sites within the prostate, informed opinions as to the diagnostic or prognostic significance of particular morphologic features frequently remain controversial, to the extent that distinction of benign from malignant neoplastic disease may not be possible. This is the current clinicopathologic context within which this book has been conceived and written.

The subject of prostatic disease, particularly prostate cancer, is complex and is fraught with doubts, uncertainties, and apparent contradictions. The natural biology of prostatic neoplasia, which has been poorly understood, is gradually becoming clearer, as those molecules and morphologic relationships that determine clinically important phenotypes are identified, assessed as prognostic indicators, and evaluated for their clinical relevance. Therefore, we have taken this opportunity to assemble a wide spectrum of expert, and occasionally divergent, opinions on those topics we consider to be of the greatest importance in understanding fundamental diagnostic problems in prostate pathology. The roots of this understanding are buried deep within the normal embryology, histology, and anatomy of the prostate gland and without which there cannot be a firm or reliable foundation on which to base sophisticated concepts of prostatic disease diagnosis, pathogenesis, or treatment. We have included detailed applications of magnetic resonance imaging and ultrasound to the tissue biopsy in formulating an initial histopathologic diagnosis, as well as in the evaluation of prostatic tissue following hormonal and irradiation therapy. Modern imaging techniques offer promise in accurately identifying intrinsic regions of benign and malignant disease and provide pathologists with tissues that, in the near future, will allow molecular-genetic mapping of different phenotypic and genotypic subtypes of prostatic cancer. We have also included a chapter detailing the current status of molecular genetics in prostate cancer. We anticipate rapid advances in this field with identification of nucleic acid sequences that, when employed as diagnostic probes, will reveal the emergence of behavioral (e.g., metastatic) or therapeutically responsive subtypes during progression of prostate cancer—not only refining diagnosis, but also influencing differential or selective approaches to the clinical management of individual patients.

Within the chapters dealing with strictly morphologic aspects of diagnostic prostatic histopathology, particularly prostatic neoplasia, there is intrinsic redundancy among selected parts of several of the contributions. This we not only accept as inevitable, particularly in the circumstance that there are no absolute or incontrovertible relationships between morphologic appearances and behavioral or prognostic phenotypes, but also we welcome as reinforcing those most important aspects of prostate histopathology. To evaluate the tissue diagnosis of prostatic disease, we have assembled a comprehensive collection of informed opinion on prostate pathology. Repetition among authors should signify enlightened agreement, rather than unquestioning acceptance of current dogma. In contrast, apparent conflict between opinions emphasizes real differences of interpretation among experienced diagnostic pathologists, and hence highlights the most important problems yet to be answered in the diagnostic surgical pathology of the human prostate. We anticipate that the current rate at which the field of human prostatic neoplasia is evolving will ensure rapid resolution of many of these important and fundamental issues within the foreseeable future.

CHRISTOPHER S. FOSTER
DAVID G. BOSTWICK

Contents

Chapter

EMBRYOLOGY AND POSTNATAL DEVELOPMENT OF THE PROSTATE

GERHARD AUMÜLLER, STEPHANIE GROOS, HEINER RENNEBERG, LUTZ KONRAD, and MARGRIT AUMÜLLER

GENERAL CONSIDERATIONS

The prostate has a dual functional commitment in that it is both a urethral gland (vestiges of which being present also in the female urethra[1]) and an accessory sex gland. This ambiguous functional commitment is reflected by its relatively short period of intact morphologic organization. The prostate reaches its mature morphologic and functional structure usually only by age 18 to 20 years and retains this organization for approximately 10 years. Around age 30 years, initial signs of structural and functional disintegration occur, and the gland gradually loses its functionally organized structure. At this time stromal and parenchymal cells within the gland are proliferatively quiescent. However, some 15 to 20 years later, proliferative activity is resumed, following a changed hormonal environment, although under restricted regulatory conditions.[2]

The increase in proliferative disorders of the prostate in elderly men, now apparently inevitable, contrasts sharply with that of the adjacent sex gland, the seminal vesicle, and the urethral Cowper's gland. In these two glands carcinomas are very rarely reported. Both the prostate and the seminal vesicle are androgen target organs and are more (seminal vesicle) or less (prostate) intimately related to male reproductive functions. There are obvious differences in the comparative biology and natural history of both glands. The seminal vesicle is a derivative of the wolffian duct, requiring exclusively androgens for its embryonic development. The prostate, however, is derived from a composite area of the urogenital sinus, requiring both estrogens and androgens during organogenesis. It undergoes different phases of estrogen and androgen responsivity, perinatally and during puberty. During these imprinting steps, cell populations develop that have lost the characteristics of their simple-structured progenitor cells and that differ in their biologic determination or functional commitment along the prostatic ducts (surface protection, resorption, secretion, regeneration, apoptosis); however, they lack a clear-cut function-related characteristic structure. This means that, although morphologically homogeneous, these cells are functionally heterogeneous. In this respect they resemble the mammary gland cells in females.

EMBRYONIC DEVELOPMENT

During embryogenesis the developing urogenital system passes through several steps of cellular imprinting that are characterized by an initial ambisexual phase and a subsequent, committed sexual phase. During these stages

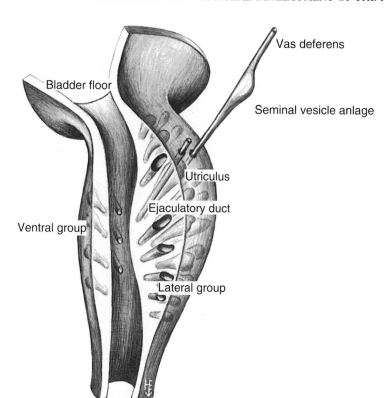

Figure 1–1. Schematic representation of the early development of the prostate and related structures.

different mechanisms of cell-to-cell communication are activated that influence the subsequent direction of maturation. A detailed review of these interactions was recently published by Cunha.[3]

Early Fetal Development of the Wolffian and Müllerian Ducts and the Urogenital Sinus

During the ambisexual phase of development, the gonads are morphologically undifferentiated. The mesonephric (wolffian) and the paramesonephric (müllerian) ducts and their openings into the urogenital sinus develop as precursors of the inner genital organs. For each of these precursor structures, the timing of sexual differentiation is slightly different. The gonads are the first structures to undergo sexual differentiation and the urogenital sinus is the last.

Wolffian Duct and Urogenital Sinus

Under the influence of the müllerian duct inhibitor, a member of the inhibin/activin/

transforming growth factor family, produced in the developing male gonad, the müllerian ducts undergo regression by apoptosis.[4] Their only distal remnant is the utriculus prostaticus close to their common opening on top of the müllerian hillock. The portion of the urogenital sinus where the müllerian and wolffian ducts enter its wall is equated with its upper border. The urogenital sinus is usually subdivided into a pelvic and a phallic part; the pelvic part being the site where the prostate develops. During its progressive enlargement, it drives the phallic part with its primitive urogenital ostium and the urethral plate forward.

The junction of the upper dorsal sinus wall with the wolffian and müllerian ducts has provoked many contradictory opinions (for discussion, see Aumüller[5]). Particularly, the contribution of the müllerian ducts to the cellular investment of this cranial portion of the urogenital sinus is not fully understood. According to Glenister,[6] the epithelium of this region has a composite origin, being derived from an admixture of endodermal urogenital sinus cells, mesodermal mesonephric or wolffian cells, and paramesonephric or müllerian cells. Most of the epithelium of this region, however, is derived from endoderm. It develops into the prostate, bulbourethral glands, urethra, and periurethral glands.[7]

The wolffian duct, whose epithelium is mesodermal in origin, develops into the epididymis, ductus deferens, seminal vesicle, and ejaculatory duct. The mesonephric tubules associated with the wolffian duct develop into the efferent ductules of the epididymis. Stabilization of the wolffian duct during development of the male genital system is achieved only by androgens, as has been clearly shown by experimental pharmacology using antiandrogens.[8, 9] The following steps are strictly androgen dependent:

1. Prevention of programmed cell death in the wolffian duct
2. Appearance and early morphogenesis of the seminal vesicle anlagen.
3. Emergence and initial branching of prostatic duct and Cowper's glandular anlagen.
4. Degeneration of male mammary epithelial anlagen.

In its proximal portion, the mesonephric duct gives rise to the seminal vesicle (Fig. 1–1). Brewster found the first sign of incipient seminal vesicle development in an embryo aged 12.5 weeks (65 mm crown-rump length [CRL]).[10] The formal development of these glands (Figs. 1–1 and 1–2) has been described in detail by Aumüller.[5]

Impact of Epithelial-Stromal Interactions

Most of our understanding of the complex and intricate interactions that occur during early induction of the male accessory sex glands is derived from the early studies of Lasnitzki and particularly the work of Cunha and his collaborators.[3, 11] These authors found out that the basic morphogenetic mechanisms during urogenital development are similar in different mammalian species and are highly conserved. Development requires the interaction between epithelium and mesenchyme (the latter inducing epithelial proliferation and specifying epithelial differentiation and functional activity). Concerning the androgen dependence of development, androgen-sensitive wild-type urogenital mesenchyme is the primary target (Fig. 1–3) and mediator of androgens as a morphogenetic signal that is operative during prostate development, in that it determines the expression of hormonal sensitivity of epithelial derivatives of the urogenital

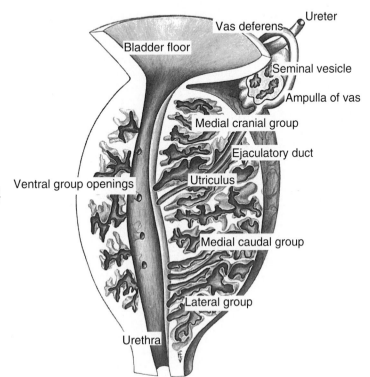

Figure 1–2. Schematic representation of prostate development at the end of the fetal period.

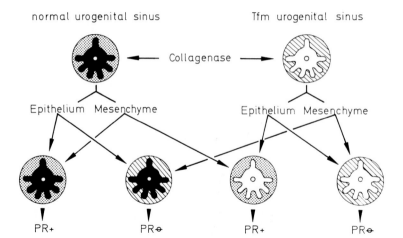

Figure 1–3. Recombination experiments of epithelium from wild-type *(black)* and androgen-insensitive (Tfm, *white*) urogenital sinus with mesenchyme from wild-type *(stippled)* and androgen-insensitive (Tfm, *hatched*) urogenital sinus; prostate development occurs only by induction through androgen-competent urogenital mesenchyme. (From Cienha GR: Role of mesenchymal-epithelial interaction of male urogenital glands. *In* Riva A, Testa Riva F, Motta PM (eds): Ultrastructure of the Male Urogenital Glands. Boston: Kluwer Academic, 1994.)

sinus. Mesenchyme displays its inductive capacity not only during embryonic and neonatal development, but it can partly reprogram the differentiated state of adult epithelium (see Cunha et al.[12]). For the fetal prostate, Cunha and his collaborators have shown in a number of very elegant recombination experiments that urogenital sinus mesenchyme induces ductal morphogenesis and that the expression of epithelial androgen receptors regulates epithelial proliferation and specifies the expression of prostatic secretory proteins.[3, 13–17] The prune belly syndrome (PBS) is a congenital defect associated with prostatic aplasia, especially the primary absence of prostatic smooth muscle, that causes weakness of the prostate wall with resultant sacculation of the prostatic urethra, bladder distension, and, eventually, hydronephrosis.[18] It also points to the decisive role of the mesenchyme in inducing prostatic epithelium.

Growth factors (GFs) have been postulated to be the decisive modulators of epithelial differentiation during epithelial-stromal interaction, the most significant being insulin-like GFs, platelet-derived GF (PDGF), nerve GFs (NGFs), epidermal GF (EGF), the transforming GF family, and the heparin-binding GF family, including the keratinocyte GF (KGF). Most effects of growth factors in the prostate have been studied *in vitro* using highly artificial and reductive systems, especially when human prostate cancer cell lines are used as a substitute for reliable intact and normal human prostatic epithelial cell lines. This type of study has been widely used owing to the fact that the adult prostate contains an unusually ample variety of GFs and their respective receptors.[2, 3] As was recently stressed by Cunha, "It is now timely to focus attention on the *in vivo* biologic relevance of growth factors in the growing or developing male urogenital tract."[3]

Endocrine and Experimental Studies

Development and growth of the prostate are clearly androgen dependent. Ablation of fetal testes in rodents during the ambisexual period of sex differentiation when testes start to produce androgens inhibits masculine development.[19] Similarly, administration of antiandrogens to pregnant females suppresses masculine development of internal and external genitalia (in a species- and a dose-dependent manner).[8, 9] As 5α-dihydrotestosterone is the essential androgen both in the developing and in the mature prostate, inhibition of 5α-reductase (the enzyme responsible for testosterone reduction, which is present in the urogenital sinus, wolffian ducts, and neonatal accessory sex glands) blocks masculinization of the external genitalia and urethra and partially inhibits prostatic morphogenesis in rats.[20] The development of a rudimentary prostate in the case of 5α-reductase deficiency or in the presence of 5α-reductase inhibitors suggests that the developing prostate may be responsive to exceedingly low levels of dihydrotestosterone (DHT) or other androgens. Androgen receptors, responsible for signal transduction of androgens into the respective cells, have been detected in the fetal urogenital anlage (of rodents). They are present in the mesenchyme of urogenital rudiments during the ambisexual stage but are not detectable until later in the epithelium of the developing male urogenital tract.[21]

Development of the Prostatic Anlagen Until Birth

Formal Development of the Human Prostate

The prostate gland is formed from the upper part of the definitive urogenital sinus in the region into which the mesonephric and paramesonephric ducts open. At 7 weeks, male embryos develop a colliculus seminalis in the cranial part of the urethra. The epithelium of the urethra is composed of two or three cell layers. By the ninth week, the epithelium covering the colliculus has been transformed into a monolayer of columnar epithelial cells. The early embryonic development of the human prostate has been carefully studied by Kellokumpu-Lehtinen and colleagues in embryos measuring CRLs from 43 to 130 mm (corresponding to an age of 9 to 17 weeks).[22] Human fetal prostatic differentiation begins with mesenchymal proliferation in the urogenital sinus. In 10-week-old embryos the cellular density of the urethral mesenchyme has considerably increased with differentiation into three concentric zones.[23] The inner zone consists of elongated fibroblastic cells with a well-developed endoplasmic reticulum. The intermediate zone is composed of primitive mesenchymal cells. In the outer zone, myoblasts can be seen and the amount of intercellular collagen has increased. Differentiation of the mesenchyme adjacent to the epithelium of the urethra is taken as the first ultrastructural sign of incipient prostate development.

At age 10 weeks, when the verumontanum has developed, histologic differentiation begins close to the openings of the mesonephric ducts by outgrowth of several buds of the urethral epithelium into the surrounding mesenchyme. The location, number, and proliferation of prostate gland buds vary significantly between individuals. Usually, one or two gland buds per side grow laterad and caudad to the openings of the wolffian and müllerian ducts. Somewhat later, similar buds develop laterally, cranially, and ventrally (see Fig. 1–1).

Lowsley has grouped prostatic glandular anlagen into five different portions[24]: an anterior group (budding from the ventral urethral wall and receding later completely), a lateral group on either side (from the lateral wall), a middle group (from the posterior urethral wall craniad to the openings of the wolffian ducts), and a posterior group (caudal to the openings of the wolffian ducts). The epithelium of these outgrowths resembles that of the neighboring stratified urethral epithelium. The cells rest on an undulating or serrate continuous basement membrane (Figs. 1–4C, and 1–5A, C), which separates the epithelium from the surrounding mesenchyme. The initially solid buds acquire a lumen at their terminal or central portions by the end of the eleventh week. Immunohistochemically, the nuclei of these urethral outgrowths contain 5α-reductase isoenzyme 1, whereas only scant amounts of 5α-reductase isoenzyme 2 have been found (see Fig. 1–8A, unpublished observations and Table 1–2). The urethral cells at that time do not show 5α-reductase 1 immunoreactivity.

Between weeks 11 and 14, when the number of epithelial outgrowths increases, the lumen-containing buds transform into tubuloacinar anlagen. The formation of the lumen is accompanied by the appearance of adluminal immunoreactivity of the so-called 100-kd antigen, a prostate-specific membrane marker (see Fig. 1–8B, unpublished observations). The epithelium of the primitive glands consists of layers of three to five cells, most of which are round and apolar (Fig. 1–4C, D). They have numerous slender cytoplasmic processes extending into wide intercellular spaces. Some apical cells have become columnar and polarized apicobasally with a large elongate to oval nucleus in the center of the cell; very few contain apical granules. Even after the 13th week, some apical cells become polarized, displaying apical granules. These cells appear to be quiescent when compared with the secretory cells of the mature prostate.

During weeks 15 and 16, the height of the cellular cords decreases, perhaps under the influence of maternal estrogens, but otherwise the histologic organization and ultrastructure of the epithelium remain unchanged (Figs. 1–5 and 1–6). Triangular cells similar to the basal cells observed postnatally are seen in the basal portion of the epithelium. At the same time, cells with neuroendocrine characteristics have also appeared in the basal portions of the buds. They are particularly frequent and regularly arranged in the urethral epithelium covering the verumontanum. These cells display strong immunoreactivity for chromogranin A, serotonin, and/or calcitonin, but extremely rarely any to somatostatin.

According to Kellokumpu-Lehtinen (see Sinowatz et al.[23]), three characteristic processes can be observed in specimens of 120 to 190 mm CRL (i.e., 16 to 22 weeks' gestation): (1)

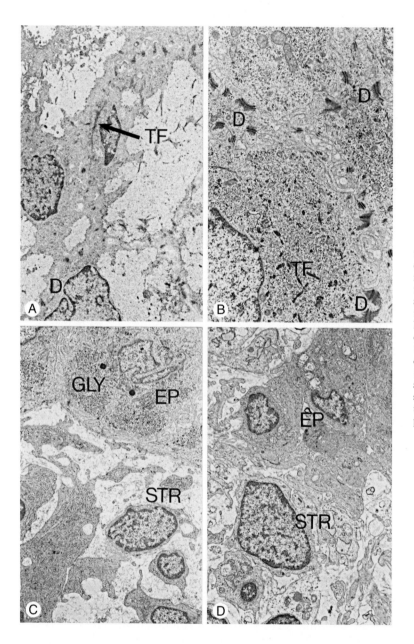

Figure 1–4. Ultrastructure of the prostate gland bud from an embryo of about 60 mm crown-rump length. *A,* Adluminal epithelial cell with desmosomes (D) and few tonofilaments (TF). *B,* In the intermediate layer, the epithelial buds consist of interdigitating cells with numerous desmosomes (D), some tonofilaments, and clusters of glycogen. *C,* Epithelium (EP) with glycogen-rich (GLY) cells and stroma (STR) in the same specimen. *D,* Epithelium (EP) at the tip of a sprouting gland bud piercing into the stroma (STR).

Figure 1–5. Epitheliostromal interface in the developing prostate. *A*, Basement membrane (BM) separating developing epithelium (EP) from stroma (STR). The stromal cell is a fibroblast. *B*, Immature myoblast from prostatic stroma shows aggregates of myofilaments (MF). *C*, Capillary (CAP) and nerve axon (AX) close to the basement membrane (BM) underneath the prostatic epithelium (EP) in an infantile rhesus monkey prostate. *D*, Mature smooth muscle cells (MYO) from the prostate of an infantile monkey.

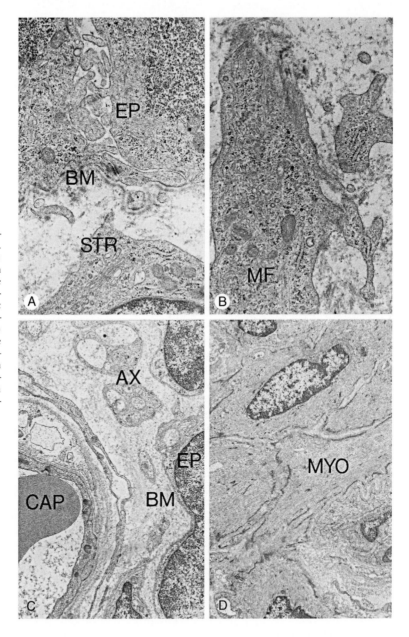

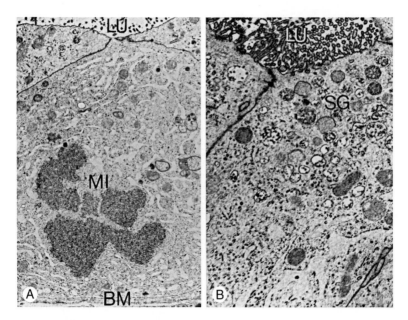

Figure 1–6. Proliferating epithelial cells in the ventral prostate of an 18-day-old rat. *A,* The mitotic cell (MI) reaches the glandular lumen (LU) and already contains secretory granules. *B,* Maturating secretion granules (SG) in a secretory cell of the immature rat prostate. Numerous microvilli project into the lumen (BM, basement membrane).

a reduction of the ventral glandular anlagen, (2) development of the utriculus prostaticus into a large cystic structure, and (3) incipient formation of a muscular capsule. At their urethral openings prostatic ducts are covered by a stratified columnar or squamous epithelium. Epithelial cells are connected by numerous desmosomes and junctional complexes. The surrounding prostatic stroma now consists of loosely arranged bundles of collagen fibers, numerous fibroblasts, and myoblasts, which form concentric layers around the epithelium. In the ventral portion of the prostatic urethra where only small immature prostatic anlagen remain, striated muscle cells derived from the sphincter urethrae muscle intermingle with myoblasts and fibroblasts. Here, large, wide and thin-walled veins are found. In the dorsolateral portion of the gland at the angle formed with the seminal vesicles, numerous arteries and thick bundles of unmyelinated nerve fibers and interspersed bi- or multinucleate nerve cells and several paraganglionic cells are encountered. Figure 1–2 is a schematic sketch of the structure of the prostate immediately before birth.

The complex contribution of different precursor structures in the formation of the prostatic urethra, the prostate, and the ejaculatory-vesicular-ampullary (EVA) organs renders this region prone to malformations and may result in the formation of cysts (müllerian, utricular, ejaculatory, ampullary, vesicular, prostatic; Fig. 1–7) that are of different origins and may compress the seminal pathways, depending on their location.

Histogenesis of Epithelial Cells

The epithelium of the early prostatic anlagen consists of apolar round to polyhedric cells connected to each other by numerous desmosomes. The cells have a large round or oval nucleus with smooth outlines, prominent nucleoli, and heterochromatin locally detached from the nuclear envelope. With the exception of rare Golgi complexes, cytoplasmic organelles (mitochondria, polysomes, some granular endoplasmic reticulum) are well-developed and usually are more prominent in the cells close to the urethral openings.

After the twelfth week of gestation, some apical cells surrounding the developing lumen become columnar and develop apicobasal polarization. These cells have a large elongate to oval nucleus in the center of the cell and a supranuclear Golgi apparatus. Kellokompu-Lehtinen and coworkers found enzyme-histochemically-detectable acid phosphatase in urethral and prostatic epithelium throughout the development period from week 8 to 14, when fetal androgen production begins and reaches its maximum, although estrogen is also present in large amounts.[25–27] In early developmental stages, acid phosphatase activity was predominantly localized in lysosomes and in the Golgi complex. Later, when some of the immature prostate cells became polarized and had increased amounts of rough endoplasmic reticulum and a larger Golgi apparatus, reaction products were also seen in the apical secretory complex.

In yet unpublished observations using specific antibodies against different acid phosphatase isoenzymes, we found that the enzyme histochemical method demonstrates the lysosomal isoenzyme, at least a nonsecretory androgen-independent form of acid phosphatase, in these immature glands. There is no immunoreactivity of secretory prostatic acid phosphatase (PAP) or of prostate-specific antigen (PSA) in the prenatal prostatic secretory cells. Most of the secretions of immature glands stain intensely with the PAS reaction and Alcian blue at pH 3.0, indicating the presence of neutral and acidic mucopolysaccharides (e.g., proteoglycans).

Stromal Differentiation

Mesenchymal cells underlying—and presumably inducing—development and (out)-growth of the epithelial cells appear as poorly differentiated multipolar cells containing a few scattered cytoplasmic organelles. Later in development, the basal lamina becomes discontinuous in a few places, according to Kello-

kumpu-Lehtinen and coworkers, and the outgrowing epithelium comes into contact with the underlying mesenchymal cells.[25] Specializations of the cell membrane to maintain close cell-to-cell contact have not been observed. The authors presume that the mesenchyme may regulate epithelial differentiation into secretory cells. This was not observed in our specimens (see Fig. 1–5).

Transformation of mesenchymal cells into myoblasts starts in the periphery of the gland, at the site of the future capsule, and proceeds into the interior of the organ. In the outer layer of concentric mesenchyme sheath surrounding the epithelial ducts, cells start to elongate and to develop filamentous structures that displace the cytoplasmic organelles into a perinuclear portion. This process ends at a layer of flattened fibroblasts that separates the myoblast layer from the epithelium. Myoblasts then arrange in a basketlike pattern surrounding the prostatic ducts (see Fig. 1–5D).

Significance of Steroid Hormone Receptors and Growth Factors

Based on the studies of morphogenesis of the duct system in the mouse prostate by Sugimura and associates, who presumed a difference in androgen sensitivity along a proximo-

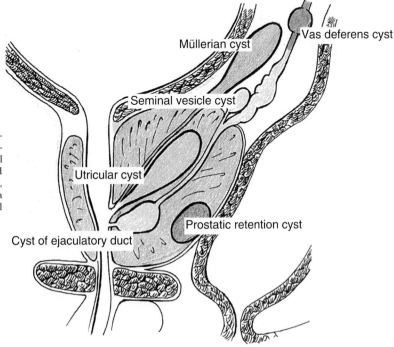

Figure 1–7. Schematic representation of different cysts in the prostate region and their potential embryonic precursors. (Adapted from van Poppel H, Vereecken P, de Geeter P, et al.: Hemospermia owing to utricular cyst. J Urol 129:608, 1983.)

Müllerian cyst

Vas deferens cyst

Seminal vesicle cyst

Uticular cyst

Prostatic retention cyst

Cyst of ejaculatory duct

distal gradient of the prostatic ducts, Prins and colleagues examined the androgen receptor (AR) levels and 5α-reductase activity along the proximodistal axis of ventral prostate ducts of young rats.[28, 29] The results revealed no discernible differences in androgen receptor levels. In the human fetal prostate we were unable to detect any AR immunoreactivity, whereas a positive signal was achieved by in situ hybridization, which was localized exclusively to the epithelium. There were, however, no obvious differences in signal intensity along the ducts. Using specific antibodies against 5α-reductase isoenzymes 1 and 2, respectively, we found nearly no immunoreaction with the antibody directed against isoenzyme 2, whereas a weak but specific nuclear (and slight cytoplasmic) reaction was achieved with the antibody against isoenzyme 1. No immunoreactivity was found in urethral cells; only the prostatic duct epithelium was homogeneously immunoreactive. Weak immunoreactivity was also found in stromal (fibroblastic and smooth muscle) cells. Among the different growth factors studied, basic fibroblast-growth factor (bFGF) immunoreactivity was the only one to be found in prenatal prostatic anlagen and it was restricted to the periductal stroma. No immunoreactivity was found for EGF or NGF or their respective receptors. Apparently, the preservation of antigens in these specimens was impaired, so no definite conclusions can be drawn from these observations.

Estrogens have been considered other potential regulators of prostate growth. Pylkkänen and associates studied the immunohistochemical distribution of estradiol–17β-hydroxysteroid oxidoreductase in the urogenital tracts of control and neonatally estrogenized male mice.[30] The epithelium of the urethra and the adjacent periurethral ducts were stained with an antibody prepared against human placental 17β-hydroxysteroid oxidoreductase. Immunohistochemical staining patterns were not significantly altered after neonatal estrogenization. According to Pylkkänen's group, it is possible that there are specific sites, preferentially in the prostatic urethra and collecting ducts, in which the changes in 17β-oxidoreduction of estrogen does play a role in the regulation of androgen action (see below).[30, 31] In our own immunohistochemical studies of the estrogen receptor in fetal and perinatal human prostates we did not observe specific nuclear staining of either epithelial or stromal cells (Table 1–1).

Table 1–1. Changes in Dimensions of the Prostate Gland During Postnatal Growth

Age (yr)	Weight (g)	Length (mm)	Width (mm)
Neonate	0.9	11–17	14
1	1.2	13	15
5	1.3	15	15
10	1.4	18	17
14	3.5	24	28
15	5.1	24	28
18	11.0–17.9	28	35
21–30	16.2 ± 0.9	34–78	32–47
61–70	23.3 ± 2.5	ave. 35.9	ave. 43
71–90	28.1 ± 1.7		

Metaplastic Changes During the Perinatal Period

The most common form of metaplasia observed in the perinatal prostate is a strong squamous metaplasia of the epithelium covering the large ducts. In addition, transitional cell metaplasia is sometimes seen. The relatively high frequency of periodic acid-Schiff (PAS)–positive mucus cells is not regarded as a sign of metaplasia; these cells are present in all prostate specimens until these have achieved full maturity. Cells containing acidic mucins are sometimes found in hyperplastic glands as well as in adenocarcinomas of the prostate.[32]

A perinatal increase in estrogen sensitivity of the prostatic anlagen is probably responsible for the strong squamous epithelial metaplasia, preferentially in the portions of the glandular ducts close to the verumontanum. There is a progressive decrease in the intensity of stratified squamous metaplasia in the larger periurethral ducts throughout infancy, but remnants may be present until the onset of puberty. The only exception is the prostatic utricle, which may retain foci of metaplastic epithelium that potentially develop into utricular cysts.[33, 34]

POSTNATAL DEVELOPMENT

General Considerations

During human prostate development, different cell types appear and disappear sequentially, especially in prostatic epithelium and to a lesser degree in prostatic stroma. Cells derived from urogenital sinus epithelium, containing characteristic aggregates of glycogen, transform into undifferentiated squamous epithelial cells. Immediately after lumen formation, adluminal cells develop into polarized columnar cells, whereas undifferentiated "pacemaker" cells reside in the basal layer and eventually form typical triangular basal cells and neuroendocrine cells. These are particularly numerous in the urethral portion of the developing ducts and later in peripheral gland buds; these findings may indicate in situ histogenesis. During perinatal development periurethral nests of squamous metaplastic epithelium are formed, which disappear shortly after birth. With the onset of puberty, the pseudostratified epithelium of the gland ducts is replaced by the terminally differentiated form (i.e., glandular cells, basal cells, and neuroendocrine cells). In rats the most frequently dividing cell type is the secretory cell (see Fig. 1–7), which often contains immature-looking secretion granules. Less frequently, mitoses of the basal cells are observed. The ultrastructural equivalents of secretory maturation of the prostate cells have been described in rats by Flickinger[35]: the amount and complexity of the rough endoplasmic reticulum and the size of the Golgi apparatus increase and secretory granules appear, which initially show a dense core surrounded by a halo and later achieve the typical floccular appearance observed in adult animals.

In the human prostate the shape of the acini becomes very complex, owing to development of papillary folds that contain fibroblasts, myocytes, and capillaries and protrude into the acinar lumen. Changes in the cell populations of prostatic epithelium during development are accompanied by chemical differentiation steps with or without apoptosis of the parental forms.

Postnatal development of the prostate is most appropriately divided into different phases[5, 36–38]:

1. A perinatal and subsequent regression phase (eighth month of pregnancy to second postnatal month)

2. An infantile resting period (second postnatal month to age 10 to 12 years)

3. The pubertal maturation period (age 14 to 18 years).

Postnatal Regression and Infantile Quiescent Period

The sometimes strong metaplasia observed in the prostatic urethra and the periurethral ducts is gradually lost after birth. New solid buds develop from the larger elongate ducts and sprout into the periphery. According to Stieve, throughout the postnatal period until the onset of puberty, new gland ducts develop from the urethral epithelium, some of which (mostly in the ventral part of the urethra) show abortive growth.[39] Three different portions can be distinguished in the prepubertal prostatic ducts: (1) a urethral portion containing a stratified epithelium with squamous metaplasia; (2) an intermediate portion with a well-developed lumen and a pseudostratified columnar epithelium (often with transitional epithelial features); and (3) a peripheral portion with solid buds gradually developing a lumen and showing signs of continuous growth and ramification. In some young (8 to 10 years old) specimens the intermediate duct portions show slight immunoreactivity for PSA or PAP. The luminal cell layer has plasma membranes immunoreactive for the 100-kd antigen (unpublished results). There is gradual transition from the postnatal regression period into the infantile quiescent period, during which most prostatic ducts are completely devoid of PSA immunoreactivity.

Prepubertal Growth Period

The onset of puberty is reflected in the prostate by a sudden increase in organ weight and size (see Table 1–1). There is much variation in the initiation of growth (and differentiation) among individuals. Sometimes, specimens from younger boys appear significantly more developed than those from older ones. The general pattern of development, however, is identical. In the periurethral portions of the gland ducts, height of the epithelium decreases and the usual pseudostratified two-layered appearance develops. Usually, the littoral epithelial cells become columnar in shape and typical basal cells appear (Fig. 1–8A, B). This transformation is accompanied by a change in immunoreactivity for intermediate filament proteins.[40] From the fetal period up to puberty, the immature epithelium of the prostate glands, the prostatic ducts, the ejaculatory ducts and seminal vesicles, and the urothelium of the prostatic urethra are strongly immunoreactive for (stratum corneum) keratins (e.g., keratin isoforms 7, 8, 18, and 19). The epithelium of the ejaculatory ducts and seminal vesicles in addition shows vimentin immunoreactivity, which is rare in immature prostatic epithelium. When during puberty the imma-

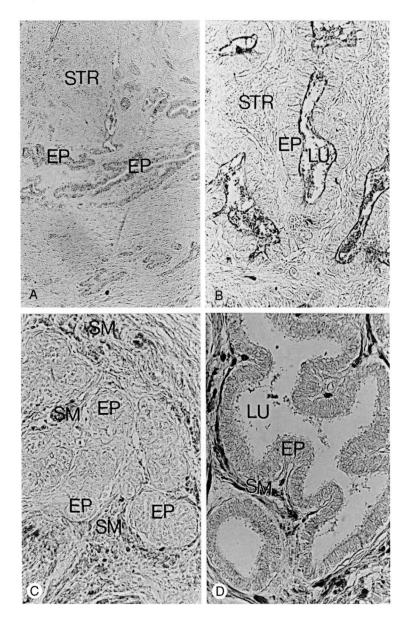

Figure 1–8. Immunohistochemistry of the developing human prostate. *A,* 5α-Reductase isoenzyme 1 in the epithelial cells (EP) of the prostate from a 4-year-old boy. Nuclei of the stromal cell (STR) are less clearly labeled. *B,* Same specimen. Labeling of the apical plasma membrane of epithelial (EP) cells surrounding a developing ductal lumen (LU). An antiserum against the prostate membrane–specific 100-kD antigen was used. Immunostaining of smooth muscle–specific actin in smooth muscle cells (SM) of the prostate from a 3-year-old *(C)* and an 8-year-old *(D)* boy. Epithelial cells (EP) surrounding a lumen (LU) are free of immunoreactivity.

ture prostatic epithelium differentiates into basal and secretory cells, keratin immunoreactivity also changes. Keratins from human stratum corneum are exclusively demonstrable in the basal cells, whereas keratins 8 and 18 are present only in prostatic secretory cells. For keratins 7 and 19 and a "pankeratin-antibody," both cell types are positive. Some mature secretory cells co-express keratin and vimentin. Contrary to that, the urothelium in the prostatic urethra and the proximal portions of the prostatic ducts is extensively positive for all keratins but negative for vimentin.[40]

In the intermediate portion of the gland ducts, where differentiation into secretory and epithelial cells started during the infantile quiescent period, signs of incipient secretion occur. Here, PAS-positive mucus cells are interspersed into nonreactive columnar cells and secretory cells that contain a small apical rim of material immunoreactive for all three essential prostatic secretory proteins (PAP, PSA, and β-microseminoprotein [β-MSP]).[41]

In the peripheral subcapsular portion numerous newly formed ramifications of the duct system appear that are initially solid, but rapidly develop a lumen. By this mechanism, clusters or lobules of glandular anlagen develop that are separated from each other by thick stromal septa containing densely packed smooth muscle cells (Fig. 1–8C, D).

Pubertal Differentiation Period and Maturation

The pubertal maturation period, starting about age 11 or 12 years, is characterized by the general development of pseudostratified epithelium with basal and secretory cells in all parts of the gland, an increase in the diameter of the lumen of the ducts (Fig. 1–9A, B), and the formation of secondary and tertiary rami-

fications of the glandular ducts, pushing the interstitial stroma aside. At the same time, any remnants of squamous metaplastic epithelium are removed and the number of PAS-positive cells decreases significantly. Chromogranin A–immunoreactive cells spread out through the whole gland, being concentrated in the periurethral portion and the peripheral ramifications of individual ducts.

Formation of Mature Acini

The formation of mature acini starts at about 15 to 16 years and can easily be traced by using specific immunohistochemical reac-

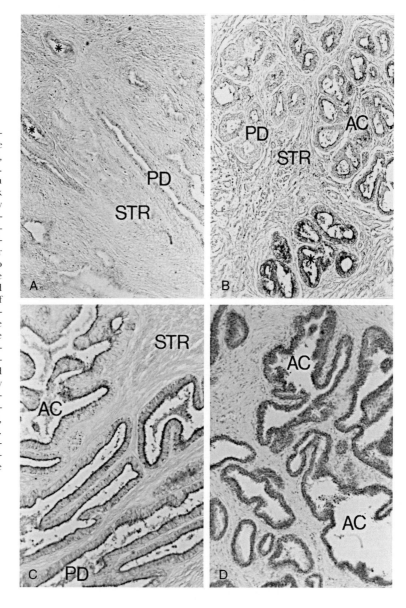

Figure 1–9. Immunohistochemistry of secretory proteins in the developing human prostate. *A*, Specimen from a 3-year-old boy. Prostatic ducts (PD) running in prostatic stroma (STR) show weak immunoreactivity for secretory acid phosphatase only in their distal portions (asterisks). *B*, Specimen from a 12-year-old boy. Prostatic ducts (PD) with rather narrow lumen contain nearly no immunoreactive material and are separated from more developed acini (AC) by thick strands of stroma (STR). More immunoreactive material is seen in clusterlike acini (AC), some of which are strongly immunoreactive (asterisk). *C*, Specimen from a 15-year-old boy. Prostatic ducts (PD) and acini (AC) regularly separated by stromal septa (STR) show homogeneous labeling of the apical portion of the epithelial cells. *D*, Specimen from a 17-year-old boy. Acini show a nearly mature outline and pattern. Immunoreactivity is less pronounced than in the younger specimen *(C)*.

tions (Fig. 1–9C, D). In the large periurethral ducts, which usually contain a multilayered epithelium, until the age of 15 to 16 years adluminal cells containing secretory material are interspersed with nonreactive cells. The intermediate duct portion forms secondary and tertiary ramifications that distend gradually, forming sacculations separated by papillae made of connective tissue and smooth muscle cells. The epithelium in these maturing acini consists of typical basal cells and adluminal columnar secretory cells displaying immunoreactivity for PSA, PAP, β-MSP, and the 100-kd antigen at the luminal border. In some cases the apical border of the cells bulges into the lumen, but mostly the supranuclear portion is rather small and immunoreactive material is constricted to the Golgi apparatus and the secretion granules (Fig. 1–9C). The peripheral subcapsular acini are small and round (or have few sacculations), and their epithelium consists of cells that are non-immunoreactive for secretory proteins. Some of these acini still contain cells that stain avidly with the PAS reaction. In three specimens from 18-year-old males, very few PAS-positive cells were yet seen in small, immature acini. Usually with the inception of secretion, prostatic calculi become visible in fully maturated acini.

Proliferation Patterns

In postnatal rats Prins and coworkers have examined the AR levels and 5α-reductase activity along the proximodistal axis of microdissected ventral prostatic ducts of 15-, 30-, and 100-day-old rats.[29] Their results revealed no discernible differences in AR levels, or binding activity in any cell type along the duct length in prepubertal, pubertal, or adult rats. In addition, 5α-reductase activity was the same in the distal and proximal regions. The authors therefore concluded that regional heterogeneity in prostatic growth and function is not the result of differences in levels of AR or 5α-reductase, but that perhaps other region-specific structural or intracellular, or even paracrine factors may be responsible for the differences in androgen responsiveness along the duct.

In this regard the studies of Pylkkänen and coworkers require attention, who studied distribution of estradiol-17β hydroxysteroid oxidoreductase in the urogenital tract of controls and neonatally estrogenized male mice.[30] They found the highest ratios of NADPH-dependent

³H-estrogen reduction-to-oxidation ratio in cell-free homogenates from coagulating gland and seminal vesicle, as well as from the prostatic and lower intrapelvic urethra, which are considered the most estrogen-sensitive parts of the male urogenital system. The epithelium of the prostatic urethra, as well as the periurethral collecting ducts, was stained with an antibody against human placental 17β-hydroxysteroid oxidoreductase. Staining patterns were not significantly altered after neonatal estrogenization. The authors therefore conclude that these areas represent sites where estrogens play a role in the regulation of androgen action. This interpretation is consistent with the reported localization of estrogen receptors in the stroma underlying urethral epithelium and surrounding periurethral collecting ducts in monkey and mouse prostates.[42] In our own series of human specimens, estrogen receptor (ER) immunoreactivity was only weak in prostatic and periurethral stroma (for age-dependent receptor distribution, Table 1–2).

Prins observed permanently altered prostatic growth in neonatally estrogenized rats and lobe-specific changes in AR expression in the adult gland.[43] Immunohistochemistry revealed a marked reduction or absence of epithelial AR in the ventral or dorsal prostate of estrogenized rats, whereas the epithelial cells of the lateral prostate expressed AR similar to controls. The incidence of AR-positive fibroblastic stroma cells increased in lateral prostates from 5% in controls to about 25% in estrogenized rats. These alterations in AR distribution may partially explain the aberrant growth responses observed in these tissues.

In summary, the heterogeneity in estrogen sensitivity within the prostatic duct system, along with the homogeneous androgen sensitivity of epithelium in the proximodistal axis of prostatic ducts may be regarded as essential prerequisites to the different functional behavior of prostatic cells, which in addition may be under the influence of local paracrine modulators in stroma (myocytes, fibroblasts?) or epithelium (neuroendocrine cells?)

We have scrutinized prostatic epithelium of 8- to 19-year-old boys and found a number of mitoses in different compartments of the gland. Nuclei of secretory or other cells were only exceptionally immunoreactive for the Ki-67 antigen. Before the onset of puberty (age 8 years), 1% mitotic cells were found in periurethral glandular ducts; the corresponding figure in peripheral ducts was 0.7%. During

Table 1–2. Steroid Hormone Receptors and 5α-Reductase Isoenzymes in the Developing Human Prostate

	AR		ER	5αR-1	5αR-2
	IHC	*ISH*			
Fetal Glands					
19 WG	−	nd	−	+	(+)
26 WG	+met e	nd	−	+ +	(+)
34 WG	+met e	nd	−	+	(+)
Infantile Glands					
3.5 mo:	+met e	+	+str	+	(+)
3 yr:	−	+	(+)	+	+
5 yr:	(+) ducts	+	(+)	+ e, + +str	+
8 yr:	(+)	+	(+)	+ +e, + +str	+
Pubertal Glands					
16 yr	+/−	+	+	+	(+)
17 yr	−	+	+	+	+
18 yr	+/−	+	(+)	+	+
Adult Glands					
23 yr	+	+	(+)	+	+
BPH	+ +	+	+/+ +	+ +	+

Key: AR, androgen receptor; ER, estrogen receptor; 5αR-1(-2), 5α-reductase isoenzymes 1(2); −, negative; +/−, partly negative, partly positive; (+), weakly positive; +, positive; + +, strongly positive; nd, not determined; IHC, immunohistochemistry; ISH, in situ hybridization; e, epithelium; met e, metaplastic epithelium; str, stroma; WG, weeks' gestation.

puberty (age 12 to 19 years) the periurethral glands contained about 1.6% mitotic cells and the peripheral glands around 2.1%.

Proliferative activity in the prostate rapidly increases by two- to three-fold during the initial years of puberty (age 13 to 15 years), remains elevated for an additional 3 to 4 years, and then gradually decreases. After several divisions, cells more and more resemble typical prostate cells, unlike the dividing immature cells in the embryonic and pubertal prostate, which usually cannot be identified as secretory or basal cells, but, instead, as apical intermediate and basal cells. With regard to this situation the formerly coined term "embryological re-awakening of the prostate" (during the onset of benign prostatic hyperplasia) is a misnomer and should be replaced by "secondary pubertal proliferation."

Significance of Apoptosis During Prostatic Development

Apoptosis, or active cell death, is a process whereby cells die in response to specific physiologic signals.[44] The morphologic sequence of events appears to be common to most epithelial cells. Histologically, the process is characterized by cell shrinking to the extent that cells retract from neighboring cells and the basement membrane, undergoing both nuclear and cytoplasmic condensation. The latter results in the formation of the so-called apoptotic bodies, potentially under the cross-linking activity of a transglutaminase (TGase). Chromatin condensation is thought to result from activation of an endogenous calcium-dependent endonuclease (possibly DNAse I[45]). The resulting DNA fragments (180-bp multimers) can be visualized by means of the so-called terminal transferase reaction.[46]

We have compared proliferative and apoptotic events in both the embryonic and the pubertal prostate.[47] In embryonic specimens only few cells were labeled with the proliferation marker Ki-67, and, similarly, mitotic figures were rare. Concerning cellular regression, no indication for that was found in that transglutaminase and DNAse I immunoreactivities were in the background range. No labeling was obtained with the terminal transferase reaction. In infantile prostatic glands, transglutaminase and DNAse I immunoreactive cells were scattered throughout the gland and were somewhat concentrated in the periurethral zone. The terminal transferase reaction (Fig. 1–10C) and Ki-67 antigen labeling were very varied, labeling densities ranging from 0.1% through 1.0%. No correlation was found between steroid hormone receptor expression and apoptotic cells.

In our pubertal specimens (derived mainly from victims of fatal traffic accidents), tissue preservation was impaired, so immunoreactivities of the AR (see Fig. 1–10A, B, D) must be interpreted with great caution. In situ hybrid-

ization using a digoxigenin-labeled 714-bp riboprobe of the AR resulted in a rather homogeneous reaction of the epithelium in the specimens from 17- and 18-year-old boys, whereas specimens from younger children were unlabeled. In positively labeled specimens the staining was concentrated at the base of the epithelium and perinuclear portions of the stromal smooth muscle and vascular endothelial cells. Despite the rather homogeneous distribution of the AR and h5aR-1 and h5aR-2 immunoreactivities, some TGase and DNAse I immunoreactive areas and cells show-

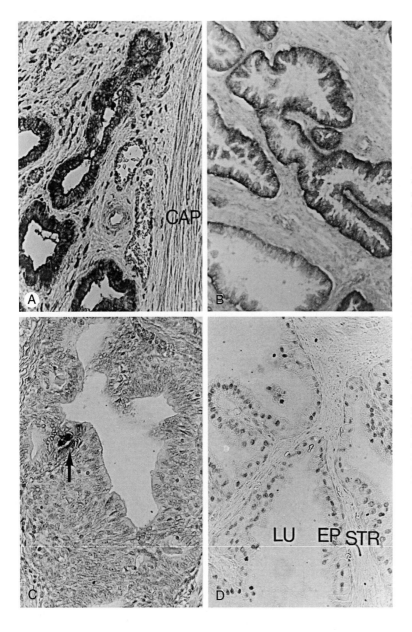

Figure 1–10. Androgen receptor and apoptosis in the developing prostate. *A,* Specimen from an 8-year-old. In situ hybridization of the androgen receptor using a 714-bp digoxigenin-labeled riboprobe; strong reaction of the epithelial cells and weak reaction of the stromal smooth muscles cells. In the capsule (CAP) no reactive cells are seen. *B,* In a 17-year-old's specimen the glandular epithelium shows mostly a moderate signal; only few acini are strongly reactive. *C,* Terminal transferase reaction in metaplastic epithelium of the periurethral portion in the prostate of a 3-year-old boy. Arrow points at one labeled (i.e., apoptotic) cell. *D,* Immunohistochemical demonstration of the androgen receptor in the prostate of a young man (19 years). Nuclei of secretory cells surrounding the acinar lumen (LU) are stained. Immunoreactivity is less pronounced in nuclei of basal cells in epithelium (EP) and stroma (STR).

ing a positive terminal transferase reaction were observed (not shown). There was, however, no correlation between these parameters in individual cells. TGase immunmoreactivity was very low and was restricted to a few randomly distributed cells. DNAse I immunoreactivity was visible at the bottom of the papillary foldings septating the large ducts, whereas the terminal transferase reaction was frequently positive in urethral epithelium. The latter showed positive AR and ER immunoreactivity. In the epithelium of the late pubertal prostate (age 16 to 19 years) there were fewer than 0.1% proliferating and apoptotic cells.

Broadly, whereas mitotic activity is high in cells of the pubertal prostate mostly within the secretory cell population, removal of excess cells is comparably low but is encountered more frequently in areas of morphologic plasticity, such as the papillary folds.

REFERENCES

1. Didio LJA, Correr S: (1994) Female prostatic glands: A comparative study. *In* Riva A, Testa Riva F, Motta PM (Eds): Ultrastructure of Male Urogenital Glands. Boston: Kluwer Academic, 1994, pp 113–122.
2. Aumüller G, Seitz J, Riva A: Functional morphology of prostate gland. *In* Riva A, Testa Riva F, Motta PM (eds): Ultrastructure of Male Urogenital Glands. Boston: Kluwer Academic, 1994, pp 61–112.
3. Cunha GR: Role of mesenchymal-epithelial interactions in normal and abnormal development of male urogenital glands. *In* Riva A, Testa Riva F, Motta PM (eds): Ultrastructure of the Male Urogenital Glands. Boston: Kluwer Academic, 1994, pp 14–34.
4. Josso N, Picard JY, Tran D: The anti-Müllerian hormone. Recent Progr Hormone Res 33:117–167, 1976.
5. Aumüller G: Prostate gland and seminal vesicles. In Oksche A, Vollrath L (eds): Handbuch der Mikroskopischen Anatomie, vol 7, pt 6. Berlin: Springer-Verlag, 1979.
6. Glenister TW: The development of the utricle and the so-called middle or median lobe of the human prostate. J Anat (Lond) 96:443–455, 1962.
7. Cunha GR: Development of the male urogenital tract. *In* Rajfer J (ed): Urologic Endocrinology. Philadelphia: WB Saunders, 1986, pp 6–16.
8. Elger W, Graf KJ, Steinbeck H, et al: Hormonal control of sexual development. Adv Biosci 13:41–69, 1974.
9. Neumann F, Graf KJ, Elger W: Hormone-induced disturbances in sexual differentiation. Adv Biosci 13:71–101, 1974.
10. Brewster SF: The development and differentiation of human seminal vesicles. J Anat (Lond) 143:45–55, 1985.
11. Lasnitzki I, Mizuno T: Role of the mesenchyme in the induction of the rat prostate gland by androgens in organ culture. J Endocrinol 82:171–178, 1979.
12. Cunha GR, Shannon JM, Neubauer BL, et al.: Mesenchymal-epithelial interactions in sex differentiation. Hum Genet 58:68–77, 1981.
13. Chung LWK, Cunha GR: Stromal-epithelial interactions. II. Regulation of prostatic growth by embryonic urogenital sinus mesenchyme. Prostate 4:503–511, 1983.
14. Cunha GR: Epithelio-mesenchymal interactions in primordial gland structures which become responsive to androgenic stimulation. Anat Rec 172:179–196, 1972.
15. Cunha GR: Epithelial-stromal interactions in development of the urogenital tract. Int Rev Cytol 47:137–194, 1976.
16. Cunha GR, Reese BA, Sekkingstad M: Induction of nuclear androgen-binding sites in epithelium of the embryonic urinary bladder by mesenchyme of the urogenital sinus of embryonic mice. Endocrinology 107:1767–1770, 1980.
17. Cunha GR, Chung LWK, Shannon JM, et al.: Hormone-induced morphogenesis and growth: Role of mesenchymal-epithelial interactions. Recent Progr Horm Res 39:559–598, 1983.
18. Moerman P, Fryns JP, Goddeeris P, et al.: Pathogenesis of the prune-belly syndrome: A functional urethral obstruction caused by prostatic hypoplasia. Pediatrics 73:470–475, 1984.
19. Jost A: Hormonal factors in the sex differentiation of the mammalian foetus. Philos Trans R Soc Lond [Biol] 259:119–130, 1970.
20. Imperato-McGinley J, Binienda Z, Arthus A, et al.: The development of a male pseudohermaphroditic rat using an inhibitor of the enzyme 5α-reductase. Endocrinology 116:807–812, 1985.
21. Husmann DA, McPhaul M, Wilson JD: Androgen receptor expression in the developing rat prostate is not altered by castration, flutamide, or suppression of the adrenal axis. Endocrinology 128:1902–1906, 1991.
22. Kellokumpu-Lehtinen P, Santti R, Pelliniemi LJ: Correlation of early cytodifferentiation of the human fetal prostate and Leydig cells. Anat Rec 196:263–273, 1980.
23. Sinowatz F, Kellokumpu-Lehtinen P, Amselgruber W: Normal and abnormal development of human male accessory sex glands. *In* Riva A, Testa Riva F, Motta PM (eds): Ultrastructure of the Male Urogenital Glands. Boston: Kluwer, 1994, pp 1–14.
24. Lowsley DS: The development of the human prostate gland with reference to the development of other structures at the neck of the urinary bladder. Am J Anat 13:299–349, 1912.
25. Kellokumpu-Lehtinen P, Santti R, Pelliniemi LJ: Development of human fetal prostate in culture. Urol Res 9:89–98, 1981.
26. Kellokumpu-Lehtinen P: Localization of acid phosphatase activity in testosterone-treated prostatic urethra of human fetuses. Prostate 4:265–270, 1983.
27. Zondek T, Mansfield MD, Attree SL, et al.: Hormone levels in the foetal and neonatal prostate. Acta Endocrinol 112:447–456, 1986.
28. Sugimura Y, Cunha GR, Donjacour AA: Morphogenesis of ductal networks in the mouse prostate. Biol Reprod 34:961–971, 1986.
29. Prins GS, Cooke PA, Birch L, et al.: Androgen receptor expression and 5α-reductase activity along the proximo-distal axis of the rat prostatic duct. Endocrinology 130:3066–3073, 1991.
30. Pylkkänen L, Santti R, Mäentausta O, et al.: Distribution of estradiol-17β hydroxysteroid oxidoreductase in the urogenital tract of control and neonatally estrogenized male mice: Immunohistochemical, enzyme histochemical, and biochemical study. Prostate 20:59–72, 1992.

31. Pylkkänen L, Santti R, Newbold R, et al.: Regional differences in the prostate of the neonatally estrogenized mouse. Prostate 18:117–129, 1991.

32. Epstein JI, Fynheer J: Acidic mucin in the prostate. Can it differentiate adenosis from adenocarcinoma? Hum Pathol 23:1321–1325, 1992.

33. Schuhrke TD, Kaplan GW: Prostatic utricle cysts (Müllerian duct cysts). J Urol 119:765–767, 1978.

34. van Poppel H, Vereecken P, de Geeter P, et al.: Hemospermia owing to utricular cyst: Embryological summary and surgical review. J Urol 129:608–609, 1983.

35. Flickinger CJ: Ultrastructural observations on the postnatal development of the rat prostate. Z Zellforsch 113:157–173, 1971.

36. Swyer GIM: Postnatal growth changes in the human prostate. J Anat (Lond) 78:130–145, 1944.

37. Andrews GS: The histology of the human foetal and prepubertal prostates. J Anat (Lond) 85:44–54, 1951.

38. Aumüller G, Seitz J, Bischof W: Immunohistochemical study on the initiation of acid phosphatase secretion in the human prostate. J Androl 4:183–191, 1983.

39. Stieve H: Die Vorsteherdrüse. In Möllendorff WV (ed): Handbuch der mikroskopischen Anatomie des Menschen. VII. Harn- und Geschlechtsapparat, 2. Männliche Genitalorgane. Berlin: Springer-Verlag, 1930, pp 246–272.

40. Wernert N, Seitz G, Achtstätter T: Immunohistochemical investigation of different cytokreatins and vimentin in the prostate from the fetal period up to adulthood and in prostate carcinoma. Pathol Res Pract 182:617–626, 1987.

41. Lilja H, Abrahamsson PA: Three predominant proteins secreted by the human prostate gland. Prostate 12:29–38, 1988.

42. Brenner RM, West N, McClellan M: Estrogen and progestin receptors in the reproductive tract of male and female primates. Biol Reprod 42:11–19, 1990.

43. Prins GS: Neonatal estrogen exposure induces lobespecific alterations in adult rat prostate androgen receptor expression. Endocrinology 130:3703–3714, 1992.

44. Bursch W, Oberhammer F, Schulte-Hermann R: Cell death by apoptosis and its protective role against disease. Trends Pharmacol Sci 13:245–251, 1992.

45. Peitsch MC, Mannherz HG, Tschopp J: The apoptotic endonucleases: Cleaning up after cell death? Trends Cell Biol 4:37–41, 1994.

46. Gavrieli Y, Sherman Y, Ben Sasson SA: Identification of programmed cell death in situ via specific labeling of nuclear DNA fragmentation. J Cell Biol 119:493–501, 1992.

47. Aumüller G, Holterhus PM, Eicheler W, et al.: Hormonal control of prostatic differentiation and morphogenesis: The impact of apoptosis and steroid hormone receptor expression. In Habenicht UF, Michna H, Tenniswood M (eds): Apoptosis in Hormone-Dependent Cancers. Berlin: Springer-Verlag, 1995, pp 1–33.

2

ANATOMY AND NORMAL HISTOLOGY OF THE HUMAN PROSTATE

JOHN E. MCNEAL

GENERAL RELATIONSHIPS

The Glandular Prostate

The human prostate gland is a composite organ, made up of several glandular and nonglandular components. These different tissues are tightly fused together within a common capsule so that gross dissection is difficult and unreliable. Anatomic features are best demonstrated by examination of sections cut in carefully selected planes.[1, 2] The *nonglandular tissue* of the prostate is concentrated anteromedially and is responsible for much of the anterior convexity of the organ. The contour of the *glandular prostate* approximates a disc with lateral wings that fold anteriorly to partially encircle the nonglandular tissue. Each of four distinct glandular regions arises from a different segment of the prostatic urethra.

The urethra is therefore a primary anatomic reference point whose relationships are best visualized in a sagittal plane of section (Fig. 2–1). The prostatic urethra is divided into proximal and distal segments of approximately equal length by an abrupt anterior angulation of its posterior wall at the midpoint between prostate apex and bladder neck.[3] The angle of deviation is roughly 35 degrees, but it is quite variable and is greater in men with nodular

Research supported in part by the Richard M. Lucas Foundation.

hyperplasia. The base of the verumontanum protrudes from the posterior urethral wall at the point of angulation. The verumontanum bulges into the urethral lumen along its posterior wall for about half the length of the distal segment and tapers distally to form the crista urethralis.

The *distal urethral segment* receives the ejaculatory ducts and the ducts of about 95% of the glandular prostate; it is, thus, the only segment that is primarily involved in ejaculatory function. The ejaculatory ducts extend proximally from the verumontanum to the base of the prostate, following a course that is nearly a direct extension of the long axis of the distal urethral segment, though usually offset a few millimeters posteriorly.

A coronal plane of section along the course of the ejaculatory ducts and distal urethral segment best demonstrates the anatomic relationships between the two major regions of the glandular prostate (Fig. 2–2).[4] The *peripheral zone* comprises about 70% of the mass of the normal glandular prostate. Its ducts exit from the posterolateral recesses of the urethral wall along a double row extending from the base of the verumontanum to the prostate apex. The ducts extend mainly laterally in the coronal plane, with major branches that curve anteriorly and minor branches that curve posteriorly (Fig. 2–3). The *central zone* comprises about 25% of the glandular prostate mass. Its ducts arise in a small focus on the convexity

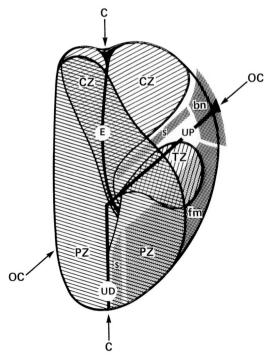

Figure 2–1. Sagittal diagram of distal prostatic urethral segment (UD), proximal urethral segment (UP), and ejaculatory ducts (E) shows their relationships to a sagittal section of the anteromedial nonglandular tissues—bladder neck (bn), anterior fibromuscular stroma (fm), preprostatic sphincter (s), distal striated sphincter (s). These structures are shown in relation to a three-dimensional representation of the glandular prostate—central zone (CZ), peripheral zone (PZ), transition zone (TZ). The coronal plane (C) of Figure 2–2 and the oblique coronal plane (OC) of Figure 2–3 are indicated by arrows.

zone consists of two independent small lobes whose ducts leave the posterolateral recesses of the urethral wall at a single point just proximal to the point of urethral angulation and at the lower border of the *preprostatic sphincter.* The sphincter is a sleeve of smooth muscle fibers surrounding the proximal urethral segment.[3, 5] The main ducts of the transition zone extend laterally around the distal border of the sphincter and curve sharply anteriorly, arborizing toward the bladder neck immediately external to the preprostatic sphincter. Main duct branches fan out laterally and also ventrally toward the apex but not dorsally above the plane of the urethra. The most medial ducts and acini of the transition zone curve medially to penetrate into the sphincter.

The *periurethral gland region* is only a fraction of the size of the transition zone. It consists of tiny ducts and abortive acinar systems scattered along the length of the proximal urethral segment and arborizing exclusively inside the confines of the preprostatic sphincter. These glands lie within the longitudinal periurethral smooth muscle stroma.

The peripheral zone is the most susceptible region to inflammation and is the site of origin

of the verumontanum and immediately surrounding the ejaculatory duct orifices. The ducts branch directly toward the base of the prostate along the course of the ejaculatory ducts, fanning out mainly in the coronal plane to form a conical structure that is flattened in its anteroposterior dimension. The base of the cone comprises almost the entire base of the prostate. The most lateral central zone ducts run parallel to the most proximal peripheral zone ducts, separated only by a narrow band of stroma.

The proximal segment of the prostatic urethra is best visualized in an oblique coronal plane of section running along its long axis from the base of the verumontanum to the bladder neck (Fig. 2–3). The *proximal urethral segment* is related to only about 5% of the prostatic glandular tissue, and almost all of this is represented by the *transition zone.*[5] This

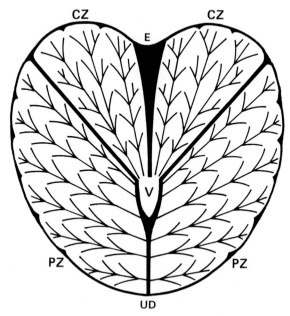

Figure 2–2. Coronal section diagram of prostate shows location of the central zone (CZ) and peripheral zone (PZ) in relation to the distal urethral segment (UD), verumontanum (V), and ejaculatory ducts (E). Branching pattern of prostatic ducts is indicated; subsidiary ducts provide uniform density of acini along entire main duct's course.

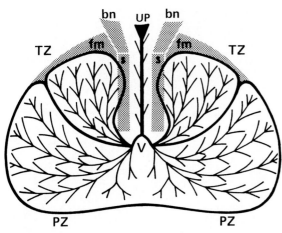

Figure 2–3. Oblique coronal section diagram of prostate shows the location of the peripheral zone (PZ) and transition zone (TZ) in relation to the proximal urethral segment (UP), verumontanum (V), preprostatic sphincter (S), bladder neck (bn), and periurethral region with periurethral glands. Branching pattern of prostatic ducts is indicated: the medial transition zone ducts penetrate into sphincter.

of most carcinomas.[4, 6] Some cancers arise in the transition zone, and most tumors found incidentally at transurethral resection of the prostate (TURP) represent this site of origin.[7, 8] The central zone is quite resistant to both carcinoma and inflammation.

The transition zone and periurethral region are the exclusive sites of origin of benign nodular hyperplasia (BPH).[5] Most cases consist almost entirely of transition zone enlargement—so-called lateral lobe hyperplasia. BPH in the periurethral region seldom attains significant mass, except occasionally as a midline dorsal nodule at the bladder neck protruding into the bladder lumen.

Nonglandular Tissue

The nonglandular tissues of the prostate are the preprostatic sphincter, striated sphincter, anterior fibromuscular stroma, and prostatic capsule. The nerves and vascular supply are also included in this section.

The *preprostatic sphincter* consists of precisely parallel, compact ring fibers that form a cylinder whose proximal end abuts the detrusor muscle surrounding the urethra at the bladder neck. The coarse interwoven, somewhat randomly arranged smooth muscle bundles of the detrusor contrast sharply with the uniform ar-

rangement of the sphincter fibers, but there is no boundary between the two structures.

The preprostatic sphincter is thought to function during ejaculation to prevent retrograde flow of seminal fluid from the distal urethral segment.[9] It may also have resting tone that maintains closure of the proximal urethral segment.[3] Dorsal to the urethra the sphincter is compact, but laterally its fibers spread apart and mingle with the small ducts and acini of the medial transition zone.[5] Anterior and ventral to the urethra its fibers do not form identifiable complete rings but blend with the tissue of the anterior fibromuscular stroma.

The *anterior fibromuscular stroma* is an apron of tissue that extends downward from the bladder neck over the anteromedial surface of the prostate, narrowing to join the urethra at the prostate apex (see Fig. 2–1).[5] Its lateral margins blend with the prostate capsule along the line where the capsule covers the most anteriorly projecting border of the peripheral zone (see Fig. 2–3). Its deep surface is in contact with the preprostatic sphincter and transition zone proximally and with the striated sphincter distally. It is composed of large, compact bundles of smooth muscle cells that are similar to those of the bladder neck and that blend with them at its proximal extent. The smooth muscle fibers are more random in orientation than those of the bladder neck, but they tend to be aligned more or less vertically. They are often separated by bands of dense fibrous tissue.

The anterior fibromuscular stroma is distinguished from the capsule of the prostate by its thickness, its coarse interwoven muscle bundles, and its rough external surface. Microscopically its external aspect shows interdigitation of the muscle bundles along its surface with the adipose tissue of the space of Retzius.

Between the verumontanum and the prostate apex is a sphincter of small, uniform, compactly arranged striated muscle fibers. It is best-developed near the apex and is continuous with the external sphincter below the prostate apex.[3, 10] The sphincter is incomplete posterolaterally, where its semicircular fibers anchor into the anterior glandular tissue of the peripheral zone rather than encircling the posterior aspect of the urethra. Its degree of development and precise anatomic relationships vary from man to man. Near the apex of some prostates, individual striated fibers may penetrate deeply into the glandular tissue of the peripheral zone. Consequently, most of the length of the prostatic urethra is provided with sphincter muscle. The distal striated sphincter is incomplete posteriorly, and the proximal smooth muscle sphincter is probably incomplete anteriorly.

The prostatic capsule envelops most of the external surface of the prostate, and the terminal acini of the central zone and the peripheral zone abut the capsule. The terminal acini of the transition zone abut the anterior fibromuscular stroma, and the periurethral glands never reach the prostate's surface.[5, 8] At the prostate apex, there is a defect in the capsule anteriorly and anterolaterally. Here, the most distal fibers of the anterior fibromuscular stroma and the striated sphincter often mingle with the prostatic glandular tissue anterolateral to the urethra, and the relative extent of these three tissue components can vary considerably between prostates. Thus, if carcinoma at the prostate apex invades anteriorly, it may be difficult or impossible to determine whether it has invaded beyond the boundary of the gland. However, around most of the circumference of the apex, the capsule is complete up to the border of the periurethral stroma, where the urethra penetrates the prostate's surface. Even with extensive BPH, a thin compressed rim of peripheral zone tissue enclosed by capsule usually still forms the apical prostate boundary, except anterior and anterolateral to the urethra.

Ideally, the capsule of the prostate consists of an inner layer of smooth muscle fibers, mainly oriented transversely, and an outer collagenous membrane; however, the relative and absolute amounts of fibrous and muscle tissue and their arrangement vary considerably from area to area (Fig. 2–4).[11, 12] At the inner capsular border transverse smooth muscle blends with periacinar smooth muscle, and clear separation between them cannot be identified either microscopically or by gross dissection. The distance from terminal acinus to prostate surface is variable, even between different regions of a single gland, and the proportion and arrangement of collagenous tissue are inconstant except in the most superficial layer, which appears to form a very thin continuous collagenous membrane over the prostate's surface. Consequently, the prostate capsule cannot be regarded as a well-defined anatomic structure with constant features, except for its external surface. In evaluating capsule penetration by prostatic carcinoma, there are no

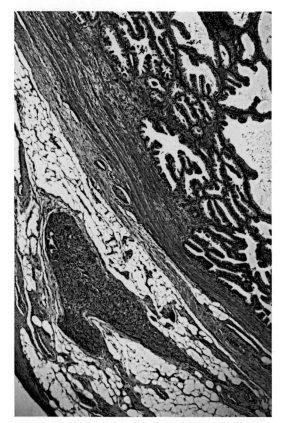

Figure 2–4. Prostate capsule over lateral aspect of peripheral zone near prostate base. Extraprostatic tissue consists of fat with nerve and ganglion. Capsule has layers of collagenous (pale) and smooth muscle (dark) tissue. Deepest smooth muscle blends with acinar smooth muscle, and there is no inner capsule boundary. Capsule thickness and composition vary between areas. (H&E× 35.)

reliable landmarks for determining the depth of capsule invasion; however, it has been proposed that only complete penetration with perforation through the capsule surface may be related to prognosis in prostatic carcinoma.[12, 13] Thus, penetration of cancer into the capsule without perforation has no clinical importance.

Over the medial half of the posterior (rectal) surface of the prostate, the thickness of the capsule is increased by its fusion to Denonvilliers' fascia (Fig. 2–5). This is a thin, compact collagenous membrane whose smooth posterior surface rests directly against the muscle of the rectal wall.[14] The capsule typically is fused to the fascia without any trace of its original surface except for occasional remnants of an interposed adipose layer that in embryonic life covered the anterior aspect of the fascia. In adults only scattered microscopic islands of fat remain, usually forming a layer only one adipose cell thick.

Smooth muscle fibers are found to a variable extent in Denonvilliers' fascia, but they usually course vertically, in contrast to the transverse muscle fibers of the adherent capsule. In some prostates, the smooth muscle of Denonvilliers' fascia is gathered into a thick, flattened vertical band at the midline, where it may easily be mistaken in a radical prostatectomy specimen for muscle of the rectal wall. This is an important distinction because carcinoma invading such a longitudinal muscle

bundle may still be confined within the prostate and should not be considered to have invaded the rectum. Wherever the capsule and fascia are fused, it is the surface of the fascia, rather than the capsule's surface, that presents a barrier to the spread of carcinoma.

Superiorly, Denonvilliers' fascia extends above the prostate to cover the posterior surface of the seminal vesicles, but it is only loosely adherent to them. Laterally the fascia leaves the posterior capsule at the point where the prostate surface begins to deviate anteriorly, and it continues in a coronal plane to anchor against the pelvic sidewalls. So the

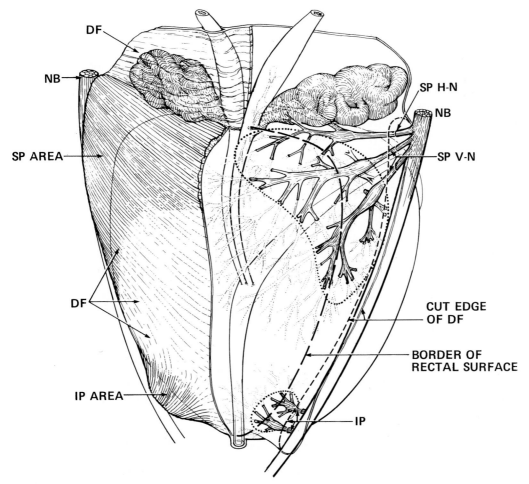

Figure 2–5. Distribution of nerve branches to prostate, right posterolateral view. Nerves within the neurovascular bundle (NB) branch to supply the prostate in a large superior pedicle (SP) at the prostate's base and a small inferior pedicle (IP) at its apex. Nerve branches leave the lateral pelvic fascia (not shown) to travel in Denonvilliers' fascia (DF), which has been cut away from the right half of the prostate. Nerve branches from the superior pedicle fan out over a large pedicle area. A small horizontal subdivision (H-N) crosses the base to midline; a very large vertical subdivision (V-N) fans out extensively over the prostate's surface as far distal as midprostate. Branches continue their course within the prostate after penetrating into the capsule within a large nerve penetration area *(dotted area)*. A small inferior pedicle has a limited ramification and nerve penetration area *(dotted area)*.

prostate and seminal vesicles are suspended along the anterior aspect of this fascial membrane as the uterus is suspended from the broad ligament in females. This can be demonstrated in the radical prostatectomy specimen after surgery for carcinoma. If the specimen is picked up at the right and left superior margins, its posterior aspect is a smooth-surfaced triangular membrane whose apex coincides with the prostate apex and whose base is a transverse line above the seminal vesicles (see Fig. 2–5). Any surgical defect in the fascia potentially compromises complete resection of the tumor, since tears in the fascia tend to extend through the adherent capsule and into the gland.

Where Denonvilliers' fascia separates from the prostate capsule posterolaterally the space between them is filled with adipose tissue in a thick layer between the anterior aspect of the fascia and the posterolateral capsular surface of the prostate. The autonomic nerves from the pelvic plexus to the seminal vesicles, prostate, and corpora cavernosa of the penis travel in this fatty layer. The nerves, along with the blood vessels to the prostate, originate from the paired *neurovascular bundles*, which course vertically along the pelvic sidewalls just anterior to the junction of Denonvilliers' fascia with the pelvis.[15] Most of the nerve branches to the prostate leave the neurovascular bundle at a single level just above the prostate base and course medially as the *superior pedicle.* These nerve branches fan out to penetrate the *superior pedicle insertion area* of the capsule (see Fig. 2–5), which is centered at the lateral aspect of the prostate base posteriorly.[15] The insertion area does not usually extend far onto the rectal surface but extends toward the prostate apex as far as the midprostate. Some nerve trunks travel medially across the prostate base, sending branches into the central zone, but the majority of nerve branches fan out distally and penetrate the capsule at a very oblique angle.

In most cases of capsule penetration by cancer, tumor extends through the capsule along perineural spaces.[16] Because of the oblique retrograde nerve pathway toward the prostate base, perforation through the capsule most commonly occurs near, or even above, the superior border of the cancer within the gland. Because of the boundaries of the superior pedicle insertion area plus the additional thickness of Denonvilliers' fascia overlying the capsule posteromedially, penetration of cancer

directly through the rectal surface of the prostate is uncommon.

Before supplying the corpora cavernosa, nerve branches leave the neurovascular bundle at the prostate apex in the very small *inferior pedicle* and penetrate the capsule directly in a small apical insertion area located laterally and posterolaterally.[16] Here the distance from neurovascular bundle to prostate capsule is narrowed to only a few millimeters. The prostate apex is the most common location for positive surgical margins at radical prostatectomy. This may result either from capsule penetration along inferior pedicle nerves by cancers that are located near the apex or from inadvertent surgical incision into the prostate. In this area the surgeon is most concerned with staying close to the prostate capsule to spare the nerves involved in erectile function.[17, 18]

Arterial branches follow the nerve branches from the neurovascular bundle; they spread over the prostate surface and penetrate the capsule to extend directly inward toward the distal urethral segment between the radiating duct systems of the central zone and peripheral zones.[19, 20] A major arterial branch enters the prostate at each side of the bladder neck and runs toward the verumontanum parallel to the course of the proximal urethral segment. It supplies the periurethral region and medial transition zone. TURP regularly obliterates this arterial branch and all the tissue it supplies.[19]

ARCHITECTURE OF THE GLANDULAR PROSTATE

The biologic role of the prostate calls for slow accumulation and occasional rapid expulsion of small volumes of fluid. These requirements are optimally met by a muscular organ having a large storage capacity and low secretory capacity. For such an organ the functionally different specialization of ducts and acini typical of organs of high secretory capacity (such as the pancreas) would appear to be of limited value. Accordingly, the prostatic ducts and acini are morphologically identical except for their geometry, and both appear to function as *distensible secretory reservoirs.* Within each prostate zone, the entire duct-acinar system (except for the main ducts near the urethra) is lined by columnar secretory cells of identical appearance in ducts and acini. Immunohistochemical staining for prostate-specific antigen (PSA) and prostatic acid phosphatase (PAP) shows uniform granular staining of all ductal and acinar cells. In view of these considerations, there is probably no functional duct-acinar distinction in the prostate, and it is unlikely that there is any morphologic or biologic distinction between carcinomas of ductal and of acinar origin.

The main ducts of the prostate originate at the urethra and terminate near the capsule, except for the main transition zone ducts, which terminate at the anterior fibromuscular stroma (see Figs. 2–2 and 2–3).[1, 4, 5] Because ducts and acini within each zone have comparable caliber, spacing, and histologic appearance, ducts and acini cannot reliably be distinguished microscopically except in sections cut along the ductal long axis. Thus, abnormalities of architectural pattern are identified in routine sections mainly by deviations from normal size and spacing of glandular units.

The main excretory ducts of the peripheral zone arise from the urethral wall about every 2 mm along a double lateral line extending the full 1.5-cm length of the distal urethral segment. Then, about every 2 mm along the course of each main excretory duct from urethra to capsule a cluster of three or four subsidiary ducts arises. They branch at angles of about 15 degrees and extend only a short distance, rebranching and giving rise to groups of acini (Fig. 2–6). Thus, acini tend to be distributed with nearly uniform density along the course of the main duct between urethra and capsule, except that no acini are found immediately adjacent to the urethra, and for a few millimeters below the capsule all glands are acinar. The architecture in the transition zone is similar to that of the peripheral zone; however, arborization is more extensive because the main ducts arise from the urethra in a small focus.

The duct origins of the transition zone and periurethral glands from the proximal urethral segment represent a proximal continuation of the double lateral line of the peripheral zone duct origins along the distal urethral segment; however, periurethral ducts also originate anteriorly and posteriorly. This accounts for the presentation of periurethral gland BPH as a dorsal midline bladder neck mass, while the lateral locations of transition zone BPH masses reflect the constant location of their main ducts.[5]

In the peripheral zone and transition zone,

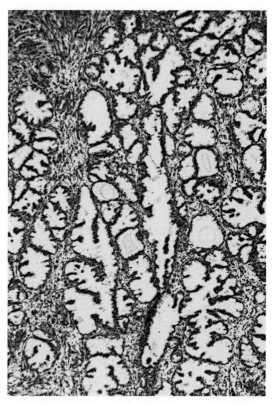

Figure 2–6. Subsidiary duct and branches in peripheral zone terminate in small, rounded acini with undulating borders. Ducts and acini have similar calibers and histologic appearances. (H&E × 35.)

ducts and acini are usually 0.15 to 0.3 mm in diameter and have simple rounded contours that are not perfectly circular because of prominent undulations of the epithelial border.[1, 21] The undulations mainly reflect the presence of corrugations of the wall, which presumably provide for expansion of the lumina as secretory reservoirs. An important criterion for the diagnosis of many highly differentiated prostate carcinomas is their tendency to form precisely round or oval glandular contours, reflecting a loss of reservoir function.[22]

Central zone ducts and acini are distinctly larger than those of the peripheral zone and transition zone—as much as 0.6 mm in diameter or larger (Fig. 2–7). In contrast to the peripheral zone, both ducts and acini of the central zone become progressively larger toward the capsule at the prostate base, where they often exceed 1 mm in diameter. There is also a gradient of increasing density of acini toward the base. Both gradients reflect the great expansion of central zone cross-sectional

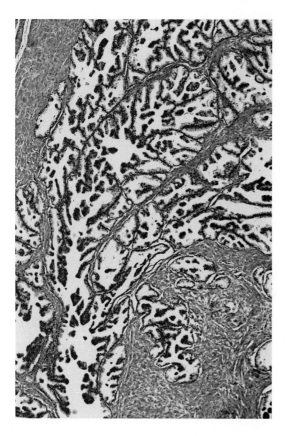

Figure 2–7. Subsidiary ducts and acini in the central zone form a compact lobule with flattened gland borders and prominent intraluminal ridges. (H&E × 35.)

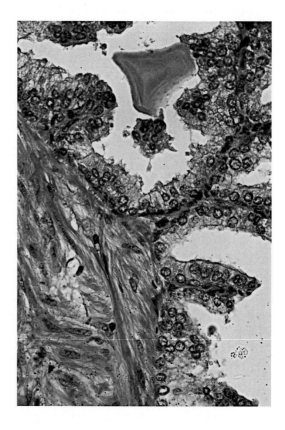

Figure 2–8. Central zone acini at lobule border surrounded by compact muscular stroma. Secretory cells are irregularly arranged with large nuclei at different levels and granular, variably dark cytoplasm. (H&E × 350.)

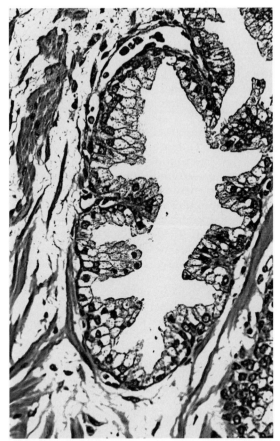

Figure 2–9. Peripheral zone acini set in loosely woven fibromuscular stroma. Secretory cells are more regular than in central zone, with smaller basal nuclei and pale cytoplasm. (H&E × 350.)

is roughly double that of the peripheral zone and transition zone. In the peripheral zone, the more abundant stroma is loosely woven, with randomly arranged muscle bundles separated by indistinct spaces containing loose, finely fibrillar collagenous tissue (Fig. 2–9). Between the glandular spaces in a given duct branch, stroma is as abundant as between different branches.

An abrupt contrast in stromal morphology delineates the boundary between central zone and peripheral zone and a similar one defines the peripheral zone and the transition zone (Fig. 2–10).[8] The transition zone stroma is composed of compact interlacing smooth muscle bundles (Fig. 2–11). This stromal density contrasts sharply with the adjacent loose peripheral zone stroma, but it blends with the stromata of the preprostatic sphincter and anterior fibromuscular stroma. Stromal distinctions are less evident in older prostates and may be obliterated by disease.

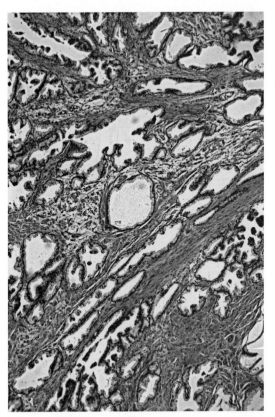

Figure 2–10. Border between the transition zone *(below)* and peripheral zone *(above left)* shows contrast in stromal texture plus band of smooth muscle at zone boundary. Glandular histology is similar between zones (H&E × 35.)

area from a small focus on the verumontanum to almost the entire prostate base. Near the urethra, the central zone ducts have few branches and lack distinctive histologic features. Thus, they may not be recognizable in transverse planes of section near the base of the verumontanum. Acini are clustered into lobules around a central subsidiary duct, which is distinguishable from the acini in cross section only by its central location. Ducts and acini are polygonal in contour. Many of the corrugations in their walls are exaggerated into distinctive intraluminal ridges with stromal cores, which partially subdivide acini.

Glandular subdivisions within a given duct branch in the central zone are separated by narrow bands of distinctively compact smooth muscle fibers (Fig. 2–8), whereas broader bands separate different branches. The normal overall ratio of epithelium to stroma here

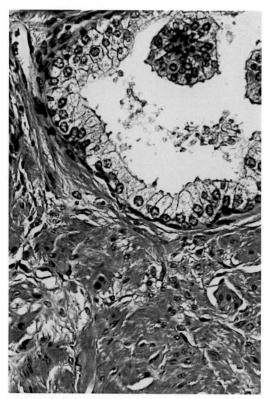

Figure 2–11. Transition zone acini set in a compact stroma composed of interlacing, coarse, smooth muscle bundles. Acinar histology is identical to that in peripheral zone. (H&E × 350.)

EPITHELIAL COMPARTMENTS

As in other glandular organs, the secretory cells throughout the prostate are separated from the basement membrane and stroma by a layer of *basal cells*. These cells are markedly elongated and flattened parallel to the basement membrane and have slender, filiform, dark nuclei and usually little or no discernible cytoplasm.[24] They are typically quite inconspicuous, and in routine preparations the basal cell envelope around individual ducts or acini may appear incomplete or even absent. However, immunohistochemical staining using basal cell–specific keratin 34β-E12 (see Chapter 15) usually shows the envelope to be complete, even where no basal cells are identified with routine stains.[25] This stain is consistently negative in the cells of invasive malignant glands.[26] In the central zone, basal cells are more numerous, and their nuclei usually appear larger than elsewhere in the prostate.

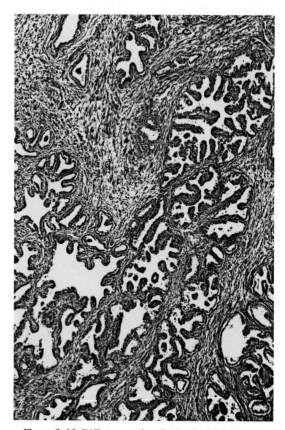

Figure 2–12. Diffuse atrophy of aging is visible in central zone with shrunken simplified glands and reduced luminal area. (H&E × 35.)

Atrophy in the prostate related to aging and presumably due to androgen withdrawal is a fairly consistent finding only after age 70 years, and then, still is not universal.[21, 23] There is no explanation for a great variation in rate of involution between individuals younger than 70, but severe debilitating disease can produce advanced atrophy even in young men.[4]

Characteristically, atrophy due to aging is diffuse. In advanced atrophy, reduced secretory cell volume is usually accompanied by markedly reduced or absent staining for PSA and PAP. Nuclei are small and stain densely, and cytoplasm is scant. In the central zone, architecture is dramatically altered. Intraluminal ridges are often lost, and the normally polygonal ducts and acini collapse into a stellate outline with reduced luminal area (Fig. 2–12). In the peripheral zone and transition zone there is no change in architecture, or gland lumina may be somewhat enlarged (Fig. 2–13).

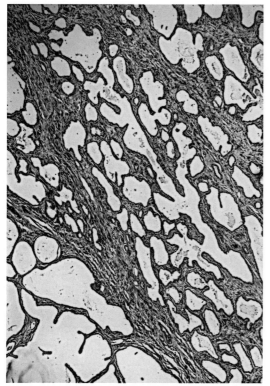

Figure 2–13. Advanced diffuse atrophy of aging is evident in peripheral zone with ducts and acini of normal caliber and markedly flattened epithelium. A focus of cystic atrophy is seen at lower left. (H&E × 35.)

Basal cells are not myoepithelial cells analogous to those of the breast, since by electron microscopy they do not contain muscle filaments.[24] Logically, myoepithelial cells would appear to be functionally superfluous in a muscular organ.[24] Basal cells have been found to be the proliferative compartment of the prostate epithelium, normally dividing and maturing into secretory cells.[27, 28]

In all zones of the prostate the epithelium contains a small population of isolated, randomly scattered *endocrine-paracrine cells* that are rich in serotonin-containing granules and contain neuron-specific enolase.[29, 30] Subpopulations of these cells also contain a variety of peptide hormones, such as somatostatin, calcitonin, and bombesin.[29, 31] They rest on the basal cell layer between secretory cells but typically do not appear to extend to the lumen, although they may send a narrow apical extension to the lumen. They often have laterally spreading dendritic processes (Fig. 2–14). They are not reliably identifiable microscopically except with immunohistochemical and

other special stains. Their specific role in prostate biology is unknown, but they presumably have paracrine function, perhaps in response to neural stimulation. Like similar cells in the lung and other organs, they occasionally give rise to small cell carcinomas, which do not contain PSA or PAP.[32] Not infrequently, however, small cell carcinoma arises as a variant morphologic pattern within adenocarcinomas that elsewhere contain PSA and PAP; peptide hormones are found only in the small cell component.[32] The status of these cells as an independent lineage in the prostate is doubtful.

The *secretory cells* of the prostate contribute a wide variety of products to the seminal plasma. PSA and PAP are produced by the secretory cells of the ducts and acini of all zones. Pepsinogen II and tissue plasminogen activator are normally produced only in the ducts and acini of the central zone.[33, 34] Lactoferrin is also exclusively a secretory product of

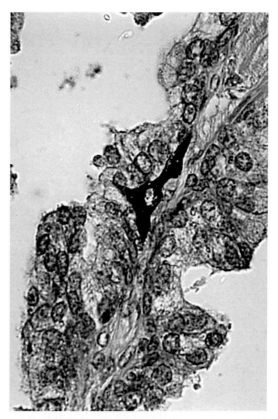

Figure 2–14. Cytologic features of serotonin-containing cells: their basal location between secretory cells and lateral dendritic processes with no apparent luminal contact. (Immunoperoxidase with serotonin antibody × 700.)

the central zone, except in areas of inflammation, where both the cells and secretions anywhere in the prostate may produce this substance.[35] Lectin staining for cell membrane carbohydrates also shows significant differences between the two zones.[36] It has been suggested that the central zone may be specialized for the production of enzymes whose substrates are secreted by the peripheral zone, but probable substrates have not been recognized.[34]

The distinctive biologic role of the central zone is paralleled by distinctive morphologic features.[4, 5, 21] The secretory cells of the central zone have a darker, more prominently granular cytoplasm than other prostate regions. The columnar cells appear crowded, with relatively large nuclei displaced to different levels in adjacent cells. The luminal epithelial border tends to be uneven, with individual cells protruding into the lumen (see Fig. 2–8). This protrusion is probably a marker for apocrine secretion. In the normally active central zone, small globules of cytoplasm may be prominent in luminal secretions, and their origin is apparent as shedding from the lining secretory cells.

Unique specialized secretory structures called *lacunae* are also common in the central zone.[35] These are tiny round lumina that appear to lie entirely within the epithelial cell layer, isolated from the main duct-acinar lumen system. A complete layer of flattened epithelial cells is seen to surround each lacuna, but these lacunar cells have no apparent contact with stroma. They only abut secretory cells. Lacunae are a specialized apparatus for lactoferrin production and storage, as demonstrated by immunohistochemical staining.

By contrast, the secretory cells of the peripheral zone, transition zone, periurethral glands, and BPH nodules have smaller nuclei in a more basal location but with modest variation between cells. Nuclei appear more evenly spaced, and cells are more uniformly columnar with a less irregular luminal border (see Figs. 2–9 and 2–11). These cells are very pale owing to the numerous clear vacuoles that fill the cytoplasm. Vacuoles are also present, but somewhat less abundantly, in central zone cells. This probably accounts for their denser cytoplasmic staining and may correlate with a higher concentration of secretory proteins. The apocrine secretion of the central zone lumina usually contains none of the cytoplasmic clear vacuoles and stains even more densely than the parent cytoplasm.

The central zone appears to represent a separate glandular organ within the prostate capsule. Aside from its unique morphologic features, its ducts arise from the urethra separately from the double lateral line of the remainder of the prostate. In addition, its ducts lie close to the ejaculatory ducts and seminal vesicles. It has been suggested that the central zone may arise embryonically as an intrusion of wolffian duct stroma around the ejaculatory ducts into an organ that is otherwise of urogenital sinus origin.[4] Pepsinogen II and lactoferrin are secreted by both central zone and seminal vesicle but are not normally found in peripheral zone or transition zone.[33, 35]

The *transitional epithelium,* which lines the prostatic urethra and extends for a variable distance into the main prostatic ducts, differs histologically from that which lines the bladder and is also distinguishable from the lining of the female urethra.[37] The transitional epithelial cells of the prostatic urethra and main ducts have scant cytoplasm with no evidence of maturation toward luminal umbrella cells. Instead, the luminal surface is lined by a single layer of columnar secretory cells that resemble the secretory epithelium of the peripheral zone (Fig. 2–15) and are positive with immunohistochemical stains for PSA and PAP. The extent of transitional epithelium lining the normal main prostatic ducts in proximity to the urethra is extremely variable; in occasional prostates it is nearly absent.

DEVIATIONS FROM NORMAL HISTOLOGY

After age 30 years many prostates begin to show a variety of focal deviations from normal morphology.[1, 4] Their prevalence, extent, and severity increase progressively with age so that by the seventh decade most prostates are quite heterogeneous in tissue composition. Though these deviant histologic patterns seldom have clinical significance, their distinction from adenocarcinoma or BPH is sometimes difficult.

Early morphologic studies concluded that focal atrophy of the prostate was a manifestation of aging and was seen as early as age 40 years. In fact, focal atrophy in the prostate is almost always the consequence of previous inflammation rather than aging.[1, 4, 23] The severity and extent of atrophic foci tend to increase with age, but their histologic appearance is identical to that of isolated foci found

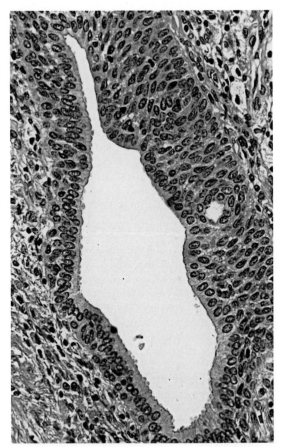

Figure 2–15. Epithelial lining of main peripheral zone duct near urethra is identical to lining of prostatic urethra. Multilayered transitional epithelium at right is surmounted by a single layer of luminal secretory cells. (H&E × 175.)

as early as age 30 years. The histologic features are identical to those produced by chronic bacterial prostatitis, but no pathogen has been identified in the vast majority of cases, most of which appear to be asymptomatic.

Postinflammatory atrophy is an extremely common lesion and is mainly a disease of the peripheral zone, where its distribution is sharply segmental along the ramifications of a duct branch.[1, 4, 9] It is characterized by marked shrinkage of ducts and acini with periglandular fibrosis and variable distortion of architecture (Figs. 2–16 and 2–17). Glandular units may be drawn together into clusters or spread out into a pattern that suggests invasive carcinoma. In addition to the presence of tiny distorted glands, the resemblance to cancer is further increased by the fact that nuclei may remain relatively large with occasional small nucleoli.

In contrast to carcinoma, cell cytoplasm is usually much reduced in volume, and evidence of the original duct-acinar architecture can often be detected. Furthermore, there is usually residual inflammation, with scattered round cells in the adjacent stroma. Finally, there is sometimes an admixture of glands showing the earlier active phase of the process, with prominent periductal and periacinar chronic inflammatory infiltrate and less prominent gland shrinkage.

Cystic atrophy is another common focal lesion that typically is found in the peripheral zone and is segmental in distribution. The markedly enlarged, nearly spherical acini with flattened epithelium and the segmental distribution suggest an obstructive cause (see Fig. 2–13); however, obstruction is not typically demonstrable and the cause is unknown.

The histologic hallmark of *benign prostatic hyperplasia* (BPH) is the expansile nodule (Fig.

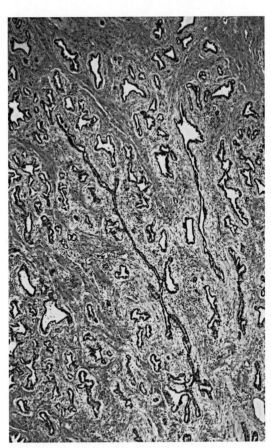

Figure 2–16. Focus of postinflammatory atrophy in peripheral zone. Duct acinar architecture is apparent but distorted by marked gland shrinkage, with reduced luminal area and perigland fibrosis. (H&E × 35.)

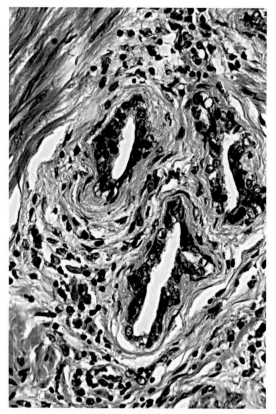

Figure 2–17. Tiny distorted glands of postinflammatory atrophy. Irregular contour and large nuclei mimic carcinoma, but cytoplasm is scant and there are periglandular collagenous rings. (H&E × 350.)

2–18) produced by the budding and branching of newly formed duct-acinar structures, by the focal proliferation of stroma, or by a combination of both elements.[1, 2, 5, 38] It mainly affects the transition zone, with occasional contributions from the periurethral region.

In TURP specimens weighing less than 50 g, nodules are usually small and widely scattered, representing only a small proportion of the tissue resected. The intervening tissue is indistinguishable histologically from normal transition zone tissue, although foci of atrophy, inflammation, or cystic change may be present. This intervening tissue represents diffuse enlargement of the transition zone, in which glands and stroma participate equally and normal architecture is preserved.[25] Some degree of diffuse transition zone enlargement is an almost universal accompaniment of aging. The weight of resected tissue reflects the amount of diffuse enlargement, but there are no features by which diffuse transition zone enlarge-

ment can be detected histologically in TURP samples. In TURP or enucleation specimens weighing more than 50 g, nodules are often the predominant tissue component, and individual nodules tend to be much larger than the nodules of smaller-volume resections.[25]

Basal cell hyperplasia is most often seen as a secondary change in BPH nodules or inflammatory foci.[7] The basal cells of ducts and acini become somewhat rounded and form a multilayered lining that stains for basal cell–specific keratin; this lining is surmounted by a single row of columnar secretory cells (Fig. 2–19) that stain for PSA and PAP. In BPH, basal cell hyperplasia is often found at the margin of nodule infarcts, where it presumably represents a reaction to ischemia. Consistent with this proposal is the finding of smooth muscle atrophy and replacement by fibroblastic stroma in these areas. Where basal cell hyperplasia is found in BPH nodules without infarcts it is almost always associated with a fibroblastic

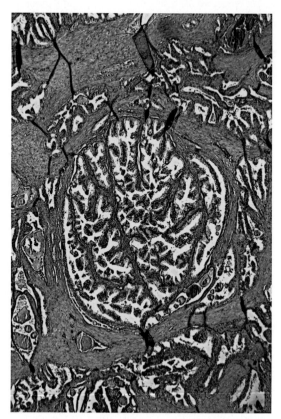

Figure 2–18. BPH nodule in transition zone showing new duct-acinar architecture, which branches inward from the nodule border. Glandular histology is identical to that of normal transition zone.

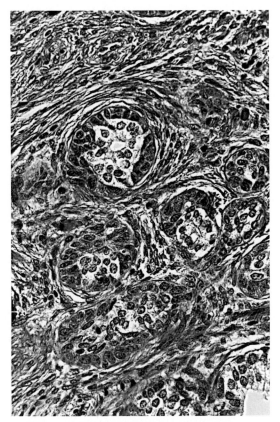

Figure 2–19. Basal cell hyperplasia. Tiny glands suggest carcinoma, but there are two distinct cell populations with central secretory cells even where no lumen is seen. Cellular fibrous stroma is oriented concentrically around glands.

stroma and smooth muscle atrophy, suggesting that, here also, ischemia may be the cause.

REFERENCES

1. McNeal JE, Stamey TA, Hodge KK: The prostate gland: Morphology, pathology, ultrasound anatomy. Monogr Urol 9:36–54, 1988.
2. McNeal JE: Anatomy of the prostate and morphogenesis of BPH. Prog Clin Biol Res 145:27–53, 1984.
3. McNeal JE: The prostate and prostatic urethra: A morphologic synthesis. J Urol 107:1008–1016, 1972.
4. McNeal JE: Regional morphology and pathology of the prostate. Am J Clin Pathol 49:347–357, 1968.
5. McNeal JE: Origin and evolution of benign prostatic enlargement. Invest Urol 15:340–345, 1978.
6. McNeal JE: Origin and development of carcinoma in the prostate. Cancer 23:24–34, 1969.
7. McNeal JE, Price H, Redwine EA, et al.: Stage A versus stage B adenocarcinoma of the prostate: Morphologic comparison and biologic significance. J Urol 139:61–65, 1988.
8. McNeal JE, Redwine EA, Freiha FS, et al.: Zonal distri-bution of prostatic adenocarcinoma: Correlation with histologic patterns and direction spread. Am J Surg Pathol 12:897–906, 1988.
9. Blacklock NJ: Anatomical factors in prostatitis. Br J Urol 46:47–54, 1947.
10. Myers RP, Goellner JR, Cahill DR: Prostate shape, external striated urethral sphincter and radical prostatectomy: The apical dissection. J Urol 138:543–550, 1987.
11. Ayala AG, Rae YR, Babaian R, et al.: The prostatic capsule: Does it exist?: Its importance in the staging and treatment of prostatic carcinoma. Am J Surg Pathol 13:21–27, 1989.
12. McNeal JE, Villers A, Redwine EA, et al.: Capsular penetration in prostate cancer: Significance for natural history and treatment. Am J Surg Pathol 14:240–247, 1990.
13. McNeal JE, Bostwick DG, Kindrachuk RA, et al.: Patterns of progression in prostate cancer. Lancet 1:60–63, 1986.
14. Villers A, McNeal EA, Freiha FS, et al.: Invasion of Denonvilliers' fascia in radical prostatectomy specimens. J Urol 149:793–798, 1993.
15. Lepor H, Gregerman M, Crosby R, et al.: Precise localization of the autonomic nerves from the pelvic plexus to the corpora cavernosa: A detailed anatomical study of the adult male prostate. J Urol 133:207–212, 1985.
16. Villers A, McNeal JE, Redwine EA, et al.: The role of perineural space invasion in the local spread of prostatic adenocarcinoma. J Urol 142:763–768, 1989.
17. Catalona WJ, Dresner SM: Nerve-sparing radical prostatectomy: Extraprostatic tumor extension and preservation of erectile function. J Urol 134:1149–1151, 1985.
18. Eggleston JC, Walsh PC: Radical prostatectomy with preservation of sexual function: Pathologic findings in the first 100 cases. J Urol 134:1146–1148, 1985.
19. Flocks RH: Arterial distribution within the prostate gland: Its role in transurethral prostatic resection. In Nesbit RM (ed): Transurethral Prostatectomy. Springfield, IL: Charles C Thomas, 1943, pp 3–11.
20. Clegg EV: The vascular arrangements within the human prostate gland. Br J Urol 28:428–435, 1956.
21. McNeal JE: Age-related changes in the prostatic epithelium associated with carcinoma. In Griffiths K, Pierrepoint CG (eds): Some Aspects of the Aetiology and Biochemistry of Prostatic Cancer. Cardiff: Tenovus Publications, 1970, pp 23–32.
22. Gleason DF: Histologic grading and staging of prostatic carcinoma. In Tannenbaum M (ed): Urologic Pathology: The Prostate. Philadelphia: Lea & Febiger, 1977, pp 171–197.
23. McNeal JE: Aging and the prostate. In Brocklehurst JC (ed): Urology in the Elderly. Edinburgh: Churchill Livingstone, 1984, pp 193–202.
24. Mao P, Angrist A: The fine structure of the basal cell of the human prostate. Lab Invest 15:1768–1782, 1966.
25. Brawer MK, Peehl DM, Stamey TA, et al.: Keratin immunoreactivity in the benign and neoplastic human prostate. Cancer Res 45:3663–3667, 1985.
26. Bostwick DG, Brawer MK: Prostatic intra-epithelial neoplasia and early invasion in prostate cancer. Cancer 59:788–794, 1987.
27. Dermer GB: Basal cell proliferation in benign prostatic hyperplasia. Cancer 41:1857–1862, 1978.
28. Cleary KR, Choi HY, Ayala AG: Basal cell hyperplasia of the prostate. Am J Clin Pathol 80:850–854, 1983.

29. Di Sant'Agnese PA, de Mesy Jensen KL: Somatostatin and/or somatostatin-like immunoreactive endocrine-paracrine cells in the human prostate gland. Arch Pathol Lab Med 108:693–696, 1984.

30. Di Sant'Agnese PA, de Mesy Jensen KL, Churkian CV: Human prostatic endocrine-paracrine (APUD) cells: Distributional analysis with a comparison of serotonin and neuron-specific enolase immunoreactivity and silver stains. Arch Pathol Lab Med 109:607–612, 1985.

31. DiSant'Agnese PA: Calcitonin-like immunoreactive and bombesin-like immunoreactive endocrine-paracrine cells of the human prostate. Arch Pathol Lab Med 110:412–415, 1986.

32. Ro JY, Tetu B, Ayala AG, et al.: Small cell carcinoma of the prostate: II. Immunohistochemical and electron microscopic studies of 18 cases. Cancer 59:977–982, 1987.

33. Reese JH, McNeal JE, Redwine EA, et al.: Differential distribution of pepsinogen II between the zones of the human prostate and the seminal vesicle. J Urol 136:1148–1152, 1986.

34. Reese JH, McNeal JE, Redwine EA, et al.: Tissue type plasminogen activator as a marker for functional zones within the human prostate gland. Prostate 12:47–53, 1988.

35. Reese JH, McNeal JE, Goldenberg L, et al.: Distribution of lacteroferrin in the normal and inflamed human prostate: an immunohistochemical study. Prostate 20:73–85, 1992.

36. McNeal JE, Leav I, Alroy J, et al.: Differential lectin staining of central and peripheral zones of the prostate and alterations in dysplasia. Am J Clin Pathol 89:41–48, 1988.

37. McNeal JE: Developmental and comparative anatomy of the prostate. *In* Grayhack J, Wilson J, Scherbenske M (eds): Benign Prostatic Hyperplasia. Washington, DC: Department of Health, Education and Welfare, 1976; DHEW#(NIH)76-1113:1–10.

38. Price H, McNeal JE, Stamey TA: Evolving patterns of tissue composition in benign prostatic hyperplasia as a function of specimen size. Hum Pathol 21:578–585, 1990.

Chapter

ASPIRATION BIOPSY
AND PROSTATE CYTOLOGY

3

John A. Maksem

In the United States, urologists perform prostate biopsies under transrectal ultrasound guidance with 18-gauge cutting needles using automated biopsy devices. Before automated needle biopsy was available, many pathologists regarded aspiration biopsy cytology as diagnostically difficult. Prostate aspiration biopsy remains, as Fox called it, the "Scandinavian curiosity."[1] In Scandinavian countries, a single physician examines the patient, performs the biopsy, and prepares and interprets the slides. Unlike transperineal or transrectal large-bore cutting-needle biopsy, transrectal automated needle biopsy facilitated the convergence of several forces: state-of-the-art histologic diagnosis that is understood by most pathologists, ease of biopsy performance for the operating physician, cost reduction for the payor, and patient acceptance. These factors have diminished the use of aspiration biopsy as a diagnostic method in the United States.

Prostatic biopsy provides pathologic correlation to a clinical finding. Aspiration biopsy is easily performed and well-accepted by the patient and may be processed reliably by the laboratory and interpreted confidently by the pathologist. Aspiration biopsy may be used to examine palpably abnormal prostate glands or palpably normal ones in patients with an elevated serum prostate-specific antigen (PSA) concentration. Cancer diagnosis and treatment planning are the goals of aspiration biopsy.[2] It may be used to evaluate the effects on prostate cancer of hormone or radiation therapy.[3–6] It has been used with computed

tomography (CT) for lymph node staging of localized prostate carcinoma, and some authors consider it efficient for this purpose.[7–9] Using the related method of touch preparation cytology, Bastacky and colleagues reported a combined technique of frozen section and lymph node biopsy touch preparation to identify small deposits of metastatic prostate carcinoma at the time of staging lymphadenectomy.[10]

Agatstein and coworkers proposed that aspiration biopsy be used to detect T1 (American Joint Committee on Cancer [AJCC] stage I; American Urological Association [AUA] stage A) prostate carcinoma prior to transurethral resection of the prostate (TURP).[11] In their study of 102 men with clinically benign prostates by rectal examination they performed four-quadrant aspiration biopsy before TURP. Nineteen men had T1 adenocarcinomas, seventeen of which were diagnosed by aspiration biopsy. After correcting for adequate diagnostic material, they found that aspiration biopsy identified all cases of T1b (AJCC stage I, AUA stage A2) prostate carcinoma but no cases of T1a (AJCC stage I, AUA stage A1) carcinoma, and, there were no false positive diagnoses. They concluded that pre-TURP aspiration biopsy increased the number of potentially curable patients with carcinoma and reduced the per capita cost of cancer detection. Juusela and associates examined case-matched specimens from 343 patients undergoing TURP for clinically benign obstructive disease.[12] Cytologic examination found 1 of 16 T1a carcinomas and 13 of 33 T1b carcinomas, 7 of which were considered "suspicious." Likewise, Honig and coworkers found that pre-TURP aspiration biopsy increased the detection of incidental prostate cancer only from 10% to 14%.[13] These findings support the observation of Hostetter and colleagues that aspiration biopsy underestimates the extent of tumor and the degree of differentiation.[14]

Benson recommended to the National Institutes of Health Consensus Development Panel on the Management of Clinically Localized Prostate Cancer that fine-needle aspiration biopsy be promoted as a standard part of the diagnostic armamentarium[15]; that it should be performed by urologists because the "learning curve" mandates that core biopsy be performed concurrently until proficiency is achieved; that the skills necessary to perform fine-needle aspiration be acquired by urology residents during their training; and, that pathology residents learn to interpret aspiration cytology specimens.

In this chapter we present contemporary observations on how the specimen should be collected, the cellular material prepared, and the slide interpreted. These opinions are based on personal experience with more than 20,000 prostate specimens examined by aspiration biopsy cytology over a period of 10 years. They are not meant to diminish the valuable experience of others who advocate other approaches to the procedure; rather, emphasis is placed on technical methods and interpretive algorithms with which the author has the greatest familiarity and success. The reader is referred to a recent review of this subject by Eble and Angermeier.[16]

PERFORMANCE AND PROCESSING

Aspiration biopsy may be performed with the patient in the dorsal lithotomy, knee-chest, or lateral supine position, or standing bent over an examining table. The dorsal lithotomy and knee-chest positions are particularly good. The prostate feels more conspicuous and the rectal examination is more exact with the knee-chest position because higher intra-abdominal pressures are created; with the prostate above the level of the patient's heart, varicocele blood pools are not mistaken for nodules and less blood is collected in the course of the biopsy. It is sometimes difficult

for elderly men to endure this position, and it is possible for unattended patients to fall from the examining table. Given these considerations, the dorsal lithotomy position, which requires a special examination table, may be safer.

The rectum contains no pain-sensitive nerves, so aspiration biopsy is performed without anesthesia and the patient feels no more discomfort than from rectal examination. Antibiotic prophylaxis is not required; however, as for many urologic procedures, untreated urinary tract infection, acute prostatitis, and acute infectious rectal disease are contraindications.[15]

A large portion of the epithelium that is obtained is available for examination, unlike histologic preparations for which representative cross sections of tissue are obtained. When the aspiration biopsy specimen consists of several discrete collections, sampling error is decreased. The needle is fully inserted into the prostate and withdrawn, as collection proceeds from deep to superficial while the operator performs a back-and-forth sawing movement and maintains low suction pressure. Cutting dislodges and aspiration harvests. In this manner, cell material is obtained that is minimally contaminated by blood, tissue fluid, rectal mucosa, or stool. The cell material is expelled into a liquid fixative capable of lysing red blood cells without precipitating serum proteins or tissue juices, allowing the operator to judge cellularity visually, repeat hypocellular collections, and ensure adequate sampling of suspicious lesions.

An illustrated account of these collection and processing methods has been published.[17, 18] Included herein are recent modifications that were made to streamline biopsy performance, directly judge the products of the collection, and standardize slide preparation.

Saline Anticoagulation of Syringes

Ten milliliters of sterile, bacteriostatic physiologic saline solution is added to a sterile Venoject test tube (Terumo Medical, Elkton, MO) containing powdered sodium heparin. About 2 mL are withdrawn into each of four 10-mL Luer-Lok syringes. The four preloaded syringes are set aside for use in sequential biopsy collections.

Fixative Tubes

Four screw-capped test tubes are filled with about 8 mL of CytoRich Red, an erythrocytolytic preservative for general cytology and fine-needle aspiration (AutoCyte, Inc., Elon College, NC). This is a good cytology liquid fixative that can also be used to rinse small tissue fragments to obtain cell samples from core biopsy specimens. Test tubes are positioned upright in a test tube rack at the site of the procedure, for convenience.

Needle Syringe Assembly

Biopsies are performed with a 20-cm long, 22-gauge needle through a sheath assembly attached to a gloved finger (fine-needle aspiration biopsy kit; Product number E-2084; Medtronic Interventional Radiology, Grand Rapids, MI).[18] Before the first biopsy collection, a small amount of heparinized saline solution from the first syringe is ejected forward into the biopsy needle to anticoagulate the needle. At the end of the biopsy collection (which usually consists of 25 to 50 back-and-forth cutting strokes or concludes when the hub of the syringe fills with bloody cellular material), the preloaded saline-filled syringe and the contents of the cutting needle and syringe hub are discharged into the pre-measured fixative. The needle is reseated on a clean, preloaded, saline-filled syringe and the process is performed four times. The operator's finger remains in the rectum throughout the procedure because constantly removing and replacing the digit is uncomfortable for the patient and does not allow for progression from one known site to another along the surface of the prostate, especially if its landmarks are subtle.

Immediate Sample Assessment

At the end of four collections the sample tubes are assessed visually by the operator. In the United States, aspiration biopsy is an office procedure, and immediate slide preparation and staining for adequacy assessment is not the norm. Since the fixative that we recommend lyses red blood cells and does not precipitate serum or tissue juice proteins, turbid fluid usually represents an adequate collection. If any sample tubes remain clear, additional collections may be performed to ensure sample adequacy. This strategy ensures uniformly fixed material, minimizes insufficient biopsies, and gives the pathology laboratory control of specimen processing, including slide preparation.

Sample Processing

Liquid fixation adds "steps" and "time" to specimen processing; however, it may be worthwhile to trade processing steps to ensure optimal fixation of all material that has been collected. Furthermore, timeliness is not an issue for a specimen that has spent 1 or 2 days traveling from the urologist's office to the laboratory. Collections are ready for processing after about 30 minutes in fixative and are stable for morphologic assessment for about 3 months in fixative. The cell sample is separated from the fixative solution by centrifugation, and the fixative is removed either by decanting or aspirating the supernatant. The cell sample is resuspended in 4 mL of CytoRich Yellow (AutoCyte, Inc., Elon College, NC), equilibrated with this solution for about 10 minutes, and prepared using a Hettich Universal cytocentrifuge (Hettich Zentrifugen, Gartenstr. 100, 7200 Tuttlingen, Germany). Glass slides are precoated with poly-L-lysine. Presoaking the glass slides in a weak (e.g., 0.01 normal) ammonium hydroxide solution for about 10 minutes before coating with poly-L-lysine solution allows the cell material to adhere better to the slide, and the slide may be stored longer.

CytoRich Yellow may act as a holding solution for as long as several weeks. Because samples are prefixed and the dispersal solution prevents specimen dehydration (which causes collapse of three-dimensional structures), the slides are air-dried for about 10 to 30 minutes and stained by the Papanicolaou method. Staining may be delayed as long as 2 days, but longer delay requires transfer of the prepared slides to 95% ethanol.

COMPLICATIONS

Infection is the most frequent complication of aspiration biopsy and occurs in fewer than 2% of cases. Esposti and colleagues reported the Karolinska Institute's experience with about 14,000 transrectal aspiration biopsies between 1966 and 1975.[19, 20] In a 1966 report, there were no noteworthy complications among 1430 biopsies. By 1968, the complication rate among 3002 cases was 0.4%, including epididymitis (two cases), transient hematuria (two cases), hemospermia (three cases), and febrile reactions (five cases). Among 14,000 biopsies reported in 1975 were four cases of *Escherichia coli* sepsis, one of which was fatal.

Rheumatic disease patients had the highest complication rate. Of 42 biopsies from 32 patients with chronic polyarthritis, 7.2% had complications, a considerably higher rate than the 1% observed among 508 biopsies from urology patients. These rheumatology patients were usually referred to establish prostatitis as the cause of polyarthritis. Four of five urology patients with complications had prostatitis. Because complications were associated with prostatitis, Esposti's group "ceased to perform [transrectal aspiration biopsy] of the prostate in order to reveal inflammatory reactions," noting, though, that "a history of prostatitis is not in itself a contraindication to [transrectal aspiration biopsy] of the prostate." Ten percent of patients with a clinical diagnosis of prostatitis had carcinoma.[19, 20] This rate was similar to the 14.1% and 17.5% frequencies reported by us.[21, 22]

Cohen and Ljung described the results among more than 350 patients and found no complications with aspiration biopsy.[23] By comparison, Desmond and associates reported on 607 transrectal ultrasound–guided 18-gauge cutting-needle biopsies[24]; complications included fever or prostatitis (0.6%, half requiring hospitalization); gross hematuria (0.6%, a quarter requiring cystoscopy and clot evacuation); vasovagal reaction (0.3%, half requiring hospitalization); and, hemospermia (0.7%). Webb and coworkers looked at ultrasound-guided transperineal 18-gauge cutting-needle biopsies in a prospective study of 171 patients, 150 of whom returned a questionnaire within 1 week of biopsy.[25] One patient required hospital admission for presumed septicemia, and one developed acute urinary retention. Minor complications included hematuria (42%), hemospermia (13%), and pain (31%); 18% of patients required analgesia. In our experience, only an occasional patient requires over-the-counter analgesia for pain or discomfort associated with aspiration biopsy. Gustafsson and colleagues reported the results of combined ultrasound-guided aspiration and 18-gauge automated cutting-needle biopsy in 145 pa-

tients.[26] Hemorrhage occurred in 98 patients, including 57 with hematuria, 66 hemospermia, and about a quarter of all patients with both. Bleeding was never a complication of aspiration biopsy. Nine patients had symptoms of urinary tract infection, with fever ranging from 38° to 40.3° Centigrade. Five required hospitalization and parenteral antibiotic therapy for 1 to 8 days.

Haddad and Somsin suggested that aspiration biopsy be used as an alternative to large-bore transperineal cutting-needle biopsy to avoid cancer seeding of the needle track.[27] Bastacky and coworkers reviewed 350 previously biopsied totally embedded clinical stage B radical prostatectomy specimens to identify the incidence of cutting-needle biopsy tumor tracking into periprostatic soft tissue.[28] They found eighteen reported cases of tumor tracking before their study, all due to large-bore transperineal needle biopsy and each presenting with a discrete nodule. They reported 2% prevalence of cutting-needle biopsy–associated tumor tracking; all were microscopic, and six of seven were connected with transrectal cutting-needle biopsy. In three of seven, tumor penetration was limited to the needle biopsy track; thus, the cancer was "upstaged" from pathologic stage T2 to T3. These findings were refuted in a large series by Bostwick and colleagues, who studied the sequelae of contemporary transrectal needle biopsy of the prostate and concluded that the 18-gauge needle induces a predictable inflammatory response in a narrow track and does not pose a risk of local cancer seeding.[29] Tumor seeding has not been reported with 22-gauge transrectal fine-needle aspiration biopsy.

BENIGN PROSTATE

The prostate is the largest male reproductive accessory gland. Its microscopic features include an enveloping fibrous capsule, a fibromuscular stroma, and duct-acinar glands (tubuloalveolar or tubuloacinar glands). Aspiration biopsy evaluates duct-acinar glands shaped by their development in the fibromuscular stroma from which they are mechanically extracted. In elderly men, the most likely candidates for aspiration biopsy, duct-acinar glands are inconstant in form, varying from narrow to wide, sometimes with cystic dilatation owing to prostatic hyperplasia. Prostatic ducts and acini are morphologically similar,

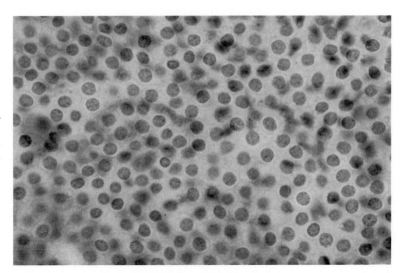

Figure 3–1. Secretory cells of prostate epithelium are seen with evenly distributed, round, regular nuclei. Cell borders form a hexagonal array.

and both function as distensible secretory reservoirs. There is probably no functional duct-acinar difference in the prostate, and there may be no morphologic or biologic difference between ductal and acinar carcinoma.[30]

The secretory cells of the prostate are separated from the basement membrane and stroma by a layer of basal cells (Figs. 3–1, 3–2).Basal cells are flattened cells with slender, elongate nuclei that lie parallel to the basement membrane and perpendicular to the overlying secretory cells. In cytologic preparations, basal cells form an open or basket-weave cytoplasmic pattern in a continuous jacket around benign duct-acinar glands and are conspicuously absent in malignancy (Fig. 3–3). They are the proliferative cells of the prostate

epithelium and divide and develop into secretory cells. They stain for basal cell–specific keratin (cytokeratins 5 and 14) but not for PSA or prostate-specific acid phosphatase.[30]

Basal cells are present in normal, atrophic, and hyperplastic epithelium. There are fewer basal cells in atrophic epithelium than in hyperplastic epithelium. They are conspicuous in reactive or reparative epithelium, where their nuclear contours appear enlarged and rounded (Fig. 3–4). Their numbers are reduced in atypical adenomatous hyperplasia (AAH) and prostatic intraepithelial neoplasia (PIN), where their density is (crudely) inversely proportional to the degree of secretory cell nuclear atypia.[18, 31, 32] Basal cells are absent in transitional cell and squamous cell metaplasia.

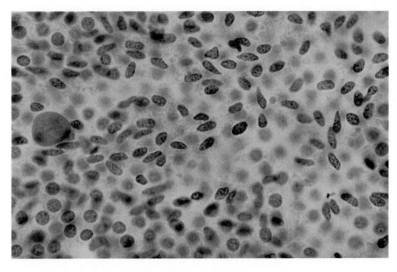

Figure 3–2. In the epithelial sheet seen in Figure 3–1 the plane of focus selects the basal cell layer. Nuclei of this layer are fusiform, perpendicular to the overlying secretory cell layer, discontinuous, and haphazardly distributed.

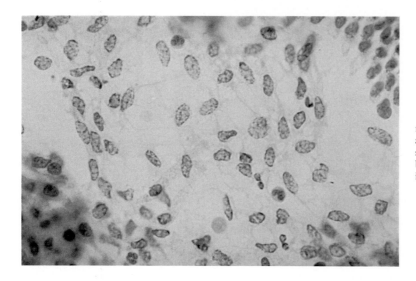

Figure 3–3. When basal cells are mechanically separated from their associated secretory cells, their slender cytoplasmic processes and basket-weave configuration are evident.

Benign prostatic ducts are regular, branching, tubular structures that consist of benign epithelial cells, rare endocrine cells, and a jacket of basal cells. Benign prostatic acini are small, regular, baglike structures that consist of cells identical to those in the ducts. Ducts gradually transform into acini, with intermediate-size structures between. Nuclei are similar in all benign epithelium. They are evenly distributed, monotonous, unilayered, round to oval, finely granular, and about the size of a red blood cell. Nucleoli are small to indistinct.[2, 18, 31, 32]

In cytologic preparations ducts are flat sheets of cells with an orderly configuration of nuclei because ducts are large and mechanically disrupted by aspiration biopsy (Figs. 3–5, 3–6). Conversely, acini are unaltered and intact because they are small (Figs. 3–7, 3–8). The cell borders of ducts and acini have a distinct, hexagonal, honeycomb or "chickenwire" configuration.[2, 18, 22, 32] In hyperplasia, epithelial cells are present above the plane of the epithelial cell sheet, forming hills, valleys, and clublike aggregates. In atrophy, cells are cuboidal, with sharp cell boundaries that lack scalloping of the apical cytoplasm. Hyperplasia and atrophy may coexist.[33]

The prostates of men younger than 40 years differ from those of older men. They contain a higher density of glands, more acinar glands than ductal glands, and a more uniform population of columnar cells, rather than a mixture of columnar and cuboidal cells. Age-related

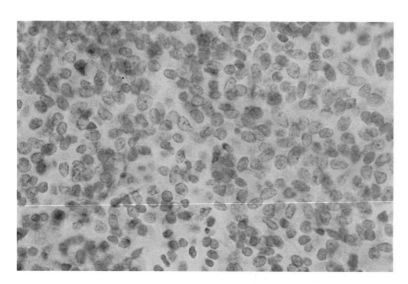

Figure 3–4. Basal cells are conspicuous in injury and repair reactions when their nuclear contours are enlarged and rounded.

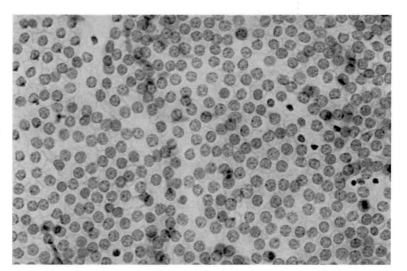

Figure 3–5. A flat sheet of prostate epithelial cells shows an orderly array of benign nuclei. The size of this aggregate suggests duct origin.

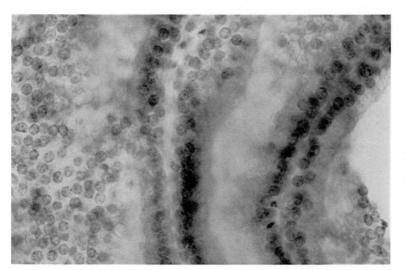

Figure 3–6. Ridges and valleys of prostate epithelial cells are seen above and below the plane of focus. The size and complexity of this aggregate suggest ductal origin.

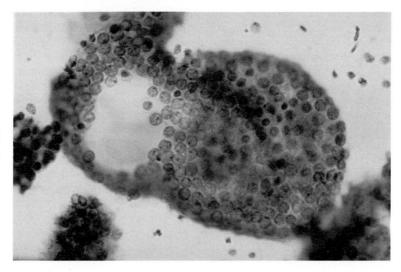

Figure 3–7. An intact prostate epithelial acinus. The plane of focus selects the epithelial cell layer.

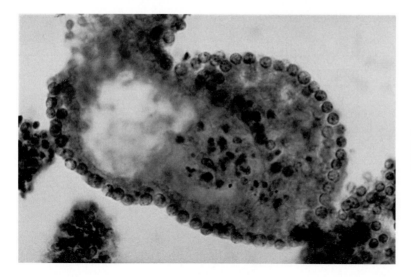

Figure 3–8. The same prostate acinus shown in Figure 3–7. The plane of focus selects the lumen, which contains a few inflammatory cells.

atrophy and cyst formation are absent, so the yield of small acinar glands is sizable.[34] Frequent small acinar glands are also the low-power hallmark of well-differentiated adenocarcinoma, but adenocarcinoma contains malignant nuclei without basal cells.

CYTOLOGIC ATYPIA

Cellular atypia is an important finding in aspiration specimens. Cases with atypia are equivocal and form a heterogeneous group composed of both benign and malignant proliferations in which repeat aspiration biopsy or cutting-needle biopsy may be necessary. Sources of atypical cells include injury or inflammation, seminal vesicle puncture, putative premalignant conditions (atypical adenomatous hyperplasia and PIN), and poorly sampled or small-volume prostate carcinoma. Follow-up of patients with atypia shows carcinoma in a considerable number of cases.[35–38] In an analysis of smears from twelve aspiration biopsies, including six from histologically proven benign disease and six from cancer, Layfield and Goldstein were unable to identify any cytomorphometric criteria that accurately subdivided cases into benign and malignant categories.[38] On the other hand, Bittinger and colleagues showed that using silver staining of nucleolar organizing regions in aspiration specimens improved the sensitivity of cancer diagnosis from 87% to 96%, making it a useful and inexpensive tool in routine practice.[39] Nonetheless, all patients with a diagnosis of atypia must be followed.

Changes of Injury or Inflammation

Prostatitis can produce a palpably abnormal prostate and alter the appearance of the prostatic epithelium. Koss and coworkers warned that carcinoma should be diagnosed with caution in the setting of prostatitis.[2] Atypia must be judged for whether it is due to injury or repair and whether it is proportional to the degree of inflammation or if its disproportionality is sufficient to permit a cancer diagnosis.[31, 40]

Acute prostatitis contains a substantial number of neutrophils. Scattered necrotic epithelial cell groups may be admixed with histiocytes, eosinophils, and bacteria. Collections are cellular, owing to abundant neutrophils. Epithelial cells occur as small aggregates admixed with the neutrophils. Epithelial cells are atypical and exhibit loss of distinct cell borders, slight to moderate anisonucleosis, nuclear crowding, overlapping, and indentation (Fig. 3–9). Small to intermediate-sized nucleoli may be present. Many neutrophils may also be observed in bloody collections, in the absence of bona fide prostatitis, in which the red blood cell component has been lysed. Here, platelets are present as granular corpuscles, often in clusters, usually in proportion to the number of neutrophils. Since entry of macrophages into inflammatory foci is time constant, the number of histiocytes is proportional to the duration of the process.

Histiocytes are the hallmark of chronic prostatitis (Fig. 3–10). They are round and plump, have finely granular cytoplasm, and often contain coarse, pigmented, irregular-shaped

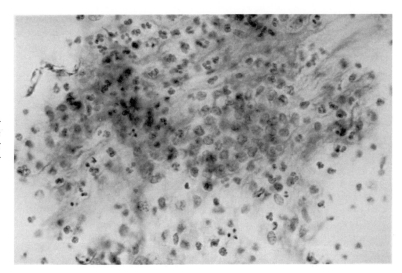

Figure 3–9. Neutrophils, necrotic debris, and small, dyshesive epithelial cell clusters with nuclear atypia may be seen in acute prostatitis.

phagocytic material. Neutrophils, eosinophils, lymphocytes, and plasma cells may be seen. Epithelial atypia is less severe than with acute prostatitis. Epithelial changes include complete or incomplete squamous and transitional cell metaplasia (which characteristically lacks basal cells), basal cell proliferation, and cells containing refractile golden brown pigment (coarse basophilic material in tetrachrome stains) representing "constipated" tertiary lysosomes. Microorganisms generally are not seen.

The hallmark of granulomatous prostatitis is the granuloma. Granulomas are ill-defined cellular aggregates of immobilized macrophages. We refer to them as "fibrohistiocytic aggregates" because of the dendritic borders, probably caused by juxtaposition to stromal cells (Fig. 3–11). Cytoplasmic fusion among adjacent histiocytes leads to the formation of giant cells with prominent dendritic processes. Amorphous necrotic debris is seen occasionally. Epithelial atypia is seen with granulomatous prostatitis. Epithelial cells show slight to moderate nuclear pleomorphism, small to medium-sized nucleoli, and finely granular chromatin. Epithelial atypia is less severe than that associated with acute prostatitis. Reactive epithelial changes include complete or incomplete squamous and transitional cell metaplasia, basal cell proliferation, and epithelial cell pigmentation. Special staining for acid-fast bacteria and fungi may be positive (as they are not in chronic prostatitis).

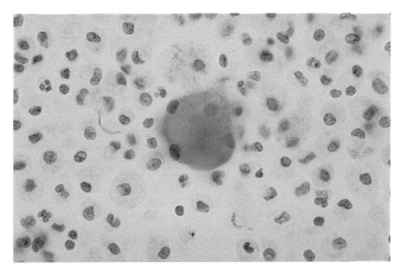

Figure 3–10. Histiocytes are the hallmark of chronic prostatitis. The relative histiocyte content of the inflammatory diathesis is crudely proportional to the chronicity of the inflammation.

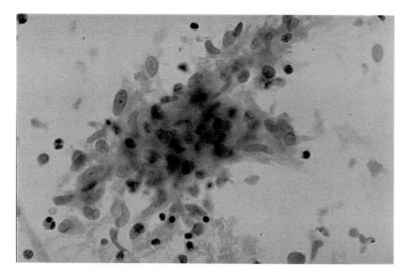

Figure 3–11. The "fibrohistiocytic aggregate" is the hallmark of granulomatous prostatitis, and it is characterized by tissue histiocytes closely juxtaposed with dendritic cytoplasmic borders formed by the cells' juxtaposition to prostate stroma.

Although lymphocytes are seen in chronic and granulomatous prostatitis, we have seen a case of lymphocytic prostatitis with well-formed germinal centers and debris-laden macrophages from a patient with rheumatoid arthritis. The cohesive germinal center cells and high content of other dyshesive activated lymphocytes mimicked undifferentiated carcinoma (Fig. 3–12). Staining for leukocyte common antigen was useful in demonstrating the lymphoid origin of the cohesive cell aggregates and dyshesive cells. We have seen several cases of small cell lymphoproliferative disorders such as chronic lymphocytic leukemia or lymphoma and mantle zone lymphoma involving the prostate secondarily and presenting with a homogeneous population of benign looking lymphocytes.

Seminal Vesicle Puncture

Seminal vesicle puncture may yield bizarre cells that can be misinterpreted as undifferentiated large cell malignant neoplasia (Fig. 3–13). Seminal vesicle epithelium has coarse golden pigment, and puncture often yields blobs and angulated aggregates of waxy eosinophilic material. Similar epithelium is present in the ejaculatory ducts, but amorphous secretory material is not seen and collections may be admixed with contaminant urothelial cells.[41]

Premalignant Conditions

Putative premalignant changes are separated into two categories: AAH, chiefly an aci-

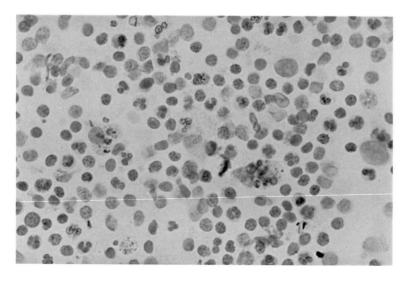

Figure 3–12. Lymphocyte-rich chronic prostatitis may be seen in patients with or without chronic systemic diseases such as rheumatoid arthritis. Lymphocytes are dyshesive and may be pleomorphic, especially when germinal centers are formed. They should not be confused with anaplastic small cell carcinoma of the prostate, which may also show dyshesive, pleomorphic cells (see Fig. 3–26).

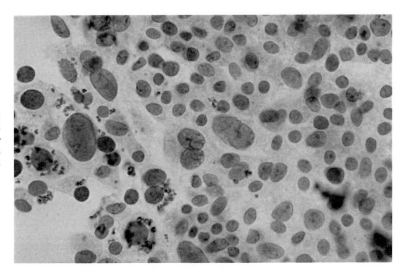

Figure 3–13. Seminal vesicle puncture yields bizarre cells and may be misinterpreted as anaplastic large cell carcinoma. Pigment constipation is a clue to seminal vesicle puncture.

nar lesion, and PIN, which is chiefly a ductal lesion.[42, 43]

AAH and so-called atypical small gland proliferation of undetermined significance are graded counterparts of acinar proliferations whose nuclei are not normal but are less atypical than those of frank carcinoma (Fig. 3–14). It is most difficult to distinguish AAH from carcinoma in lesions that contain nucleoli intermediate in size between those of benign and malignant cells, and to accommodate the uncertainty of this borderline group of lesions, Bostwick's group "... recommend the noncommittal term 'atypical small acinar proliferation of undetermined significance, not further classified.' "[44] These lesions contain infrequent prostatic crystalloids (which can be seen

on cytologic examination; Fig. 3–15) lack basophilic mucin (which can be seen cytologically and is actually "orangeophilic" with the Papanicolaou stain), and do not have the disorganization of high-grade acinar carcinoma. The acini are small, regular, histologically clustered structures with smooth and round borders; although clustering cannot be appreciated cytologically, regularity of gland shape can. Destructive tissue invasion is not seen with AAH, but the absence of invasion cannot be appreciated cytologically. Basal cells are retained and may occasionally be demonstrated by immunohistochemical staining for basal cell–specific keratin; basal cells *can* be appreciated cytologically, especially with the aid of immunohistochemistry; however, the key to the diagnosis

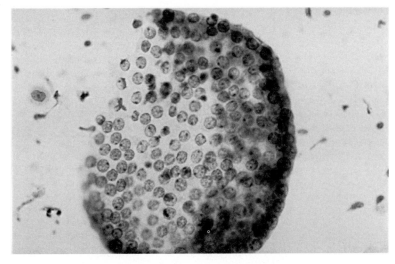

Figure 3–14. Acinar proliferations with low-grade nuclear atypia and smooth borders most frequently correspond to atypical adenomatous hyperplasia in matched tissue material.

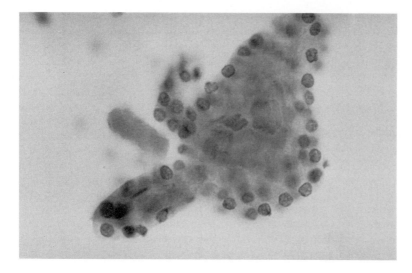

Figure 3–15. Acinar proliferations interpreted as atypical adenomatous hyperplasia may contain prostatic crystalloids.

relies not so much on demonstrating the presence of basal cells as on ensuring the absence of frank cancer nuclei.

PIN encompasses lesions in which epithelial proliferation occurs within preformed spaces. PIN is easy to identify in aspiration biopsy specimens because ducts are seen as sheets of several hundred nuclei laid side to side en face. This arrangement exposes aberrations among large numbers of juxtaposed nuclei in which the benign epithelium provides excellent internal control material to which the eye is exquisitely sensitive (Figs. 3–16 through 3–18). Basal cells are retained and may be demonstrated in routinely stained cytologic preparations or, in difficult cases, by staining for basal cell–specific keratin. Their presence

is important in distinguishing PIN from carcinoma because the nuclear atypia of PIN is more pronounced than that of AAH.

How can the two lesions, AAH and PIN, be reconciled with a "single-epithelium model" of prostatic neoplasia? Is there a fundamental difference between the acinus and the duct other than the epithelium? The difference may be in the interplay of glands and stroma, such as tissue resistance, which probably accounts for tumor invasion of the perineurium, the path of least resistance.[45] PIN occurs within preexisting ducts because there is little resistance to cell growth at this site. Anaplasia outpaces tissue invasion, and invasion usually occurs after the cell has acquired the biologic potential of moderately or poorly differenti-

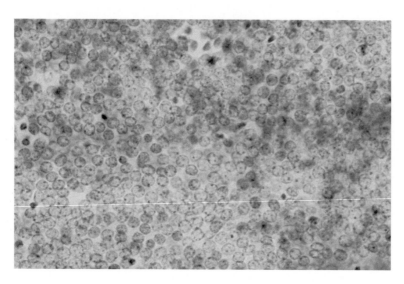

Figure 3–16. A flat sheet of prostate epithelial cells shows a disordered array of atypical nuclei. The size of this structure suggests ductal origin, and it is interpreted as low-grade PIN.

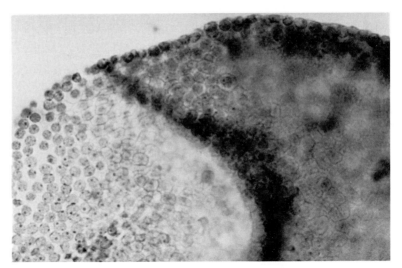

Figure 3–17. A large three-dimensional structure whose size and complexity suggests ductal origin. Nuclei are atypical with prominent nucleoli, but the register of epithelial cells is regular. This structure is interpreted as representing high-grade PIN (PIN 2).

ated adenocarcinoma. Conversely, the epithelial proliferation of AAH does not occur within pre-existing structures because small acini offer significant resistance to inward cell growth. Acini grow outward into the stroma, but the proliferation remains in check and is first recognized as AAH. If tissue invasion outpaces nuclear anaplasia invasion occurs before the cancer cell has acquired the biologic potential of moderately differentiated adenocarcinoma. This hypothesis explains why Gleason pattern 1 and 2 carcinomas are of the acinar-gland type; show ordered expansive growth; are biologically indolent; and may be associated with PIN and why there is no well-differentiated biologically indolent ductal carcinoma of the prostate.

Poorly Sampled or Small Amounts of Prostate Carcinoma

Excluding technical limitations of liquid-phase fixation, the main reasons that cancer is not diagnosed are (1) that the sample is hypocellular, or (2) the lesion is small and not sampled, or (3) the tumor is well-differentiated and difficult to distinguish from AAH, or (4) the cytologic changes are obscured by inflammation. An aspiration biopsy may be technically satisfactory and contain cell groupings ordinarily considered diagnostic for well-differentiated adenocarcinoma, but the diagnosis of cancer requires a minimum amount of tumor. The diagnosis ''highly suspicious for carcinoma'' may be used in cases with less

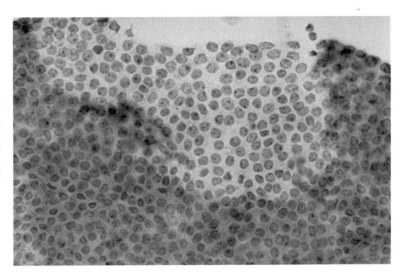

Figure 3–18. A large three-dimensional structure whose size and complexity suggests ductal origin. Nuclei are atypical with prominent nucleoli, and the register of epithelial cells is irregular. This structure is interpreted as representing high-grade PIN (PIN 3).

than three cancer cell groupings (well-differentiated adenocarcinoma) per slide on one or two slides. Well-differentiated adenocarcinoma is a medium-sized acinar phenomenon that may be mistaken for AAH, and a total of six cell groupings or fewer may be too few to confirm the absence of a basal cell component or to judge the extent of nuclear anaplasia. This approach should avoid a false positive diagnosis of cancer. Similarly, when a few small sheets, pseudopapillae, or papillae with malignant nuclei are present and the cell groupings are too small and too few to confirm the absence of a basal cell component (to differentiate PIN from ductal adenocarcinoma), repeat biopsy is indicated.[46]

It is essential that the cytopathologist be aware of a history of therapy for prostate cancer. Radiation and hormone therapy may cause downgrading or disappearance of cancer in biopsy specimens. The cytologic findings after therapy include cancer cell shrinkage (nuclei and cytoplasm) and reduction or apparent loss of nuclei. Other effects of therapy include squamous and/or glycogenic metaplasia, especially after hormone therapy.[3–6, 47]

Erroneous diagnosis of cancer is avoided if the following conditions are satisfied: the sample is adequately cellular and demonstrates several diagnostic cancer cell groupings, especially for Gleason pattern 1 and 2 carcinoma or pattern 3 ductal carcinoma; malignant nuclei are present and basal cells are absent in cancer cell groupings; cancer patterns (intermediate to small acini, attenuated glands, papillary-cribriform glands, solid or dyshesive epithelial aggregates) are seen among the cell groupings; and conditions such as inflammation, infarction, and seminal vesicle puncture that may cause pseudoneoplastic cell groupings are excluded.

CARCINOMA

The histopathologist observes prostatic acini and ducts in a fibromuscular tissue matrix, and the cytopathologist observes them after extraction from the matrix. Glands retain a substantial part of their three-dimensional structure when fixed in a liquid suspension. In tissue, the patterns of cancer include intermediate to small acini, attenuated angulated glands, papillary-cribriform glands, and solid or dyshesive epithelial cell groupings.[48] In cytologic preparations the same patterns are pres-

ent, but the degree of gland crowding and the presence of stromal invasion cannot be assessed.[17, 22]

The cytologic diagnosis of cancer requires the presence of malignant nuclei characterized by variation in nuclear shape and contour (poikilonucleosis), variation in nuclear size (anisonucleosis), increased staining (hyperchromasia), and nucleolar enlargement. If three of four features are present the nucleus is malignant. For example, enlarged nucleoli may be hidden by cell folds, angulation, or hyperchromasia.

Historically, cytologic grading of carcinoma relied on the degree of nuclear anaplasia, with two exceptions: the recognition of microadenomatous complexes in well-differentiated carcinoma and cellular dyshesion in poorly differentiated carcinoma. The worst grade determines the final diagnosis.[49] If this method is used to compare cytology and histology specimens, histologic grading should also consider nuclear features in addition to the tendency of cancer cells to form acini, or complex or solid structures, or to infiltrate tissue as small tumor cell clusters; also, the worst grade should determine the final diagnosis.[50]

The microadenomatous complex is diagnostic of well-differentiated adenocarcinoma in aspiration biopsy specimens prepared by smear techniques and air-dried or alcohol-fixed.[2, 6, 19, 51]

This complex is a rosette of five to ten tumor cell nuclei organized about a central space. Liquid-fixed preparations show these complexes in the walls of tumor acini and ducts. It is uncertain just what this structure is, but it may represent a branch point in the epithelial sheet. Microadenomatous complexes are readily distinguished from three-dimensional cribriform formations by their lack of depth in liquid-fixed preparations.

The cytomorphology of prostate cancer depends on the degree of differentiation (how closely tumor resembles benign epithelium) and the degree of nuclear anaplasia (deviation of tumor nuclei from normal nuclei). Lesser degrees of differentiation accompany greater degrees of anaplasia. Cytologic grading of prostate carcinoma is similar to breast cancer grading using the system of Bloom and Richardson in which architectural, nuclear, and proliferative features are separately evaluated.[52] Abundant mitoses are not characteristic of prostate cancer, but poorly differentiated cancers may show DNA aneuploidy and an increase in the S-phase fraction.

Acinus size is useful in determining Gleason pattern. Large acini often correspond to ductal carcinoma (Gleason patterns 3 and 4), whereas small to intermediate-sized acini correspond to Gleason patterns 1 and 2, small acini to pattern 3, and very small or abortive acini to pattern 4. The Gleason system does not recognize a well-differentiated ductal lesion. Undifferentiated carcinoma (Gleason pattern 5) appears as either solid clusters of cells or dissociated single cells.[17, 18, 31, 32, 40, 48] In all, the diagnosis of cancer requires absence of basal cells and the presence of frankly malignant nuclei. The degree of nuclear anaplasia may vary among the patterns of cancer, but at least some degree of anaplasia must be present.

The small or intermediate-sized acini of well-differentiated cancer appear as sheets or as intact structures because the aspiration needle slices off portions of larger glands and dislodges intact smaller glands. As gland size decreases, the likelihood of harvesting unaltered acinar structures increases. Because high-grade AAH is morphologically similar to well-differentiated carcinoma, we limit the diagnosis of well-differentiated carcinoma to tumor glands with smooth contours, which implies the maintenance of an orderly interplay between the glands and stroma (Fig. 3–19). The separation of patterns 1 and 2 is not realistic in cytology preparations because the regularity of the gland-to-gland arrangement cannot be assessed. Also, because of this restriction, pattern 3 may be "undercalled" because the infiltration of malignant glands between preformed benign glands cannot be assessed.

Ductal carcinoma typically has a pseudopapillary pattern but occasionally may be mixed with flat sheets of tumor cells. The flat sheet part of ductal carcinoma is usually interrupted because pseudopapillae and true papillae cause clumping and protrusion of cancer nuclei among such sheets; conversely, well-differentiated carcinoma with intermediate-sized acini appears as an uninterrupted monolayer of cancer cells. At low magnifications, it may be difficult to distinguish well-differentiated carcinoma from normal prostatic epithelium or AAH; consequently, it may be necessary to use high magnification to evaluate such specimens, especially when basal cells are not readily apparent and nuclear anaplasia is low.

Small or highly attenuated glands with straight or jagged contours, with or without branching, correspond to Gleason patterns 3 and 4. Smaller, more irregular, more branched or fused structures usually indicate Gleason pattern 4. Nuclear anaplasia is conspicuous and is roughly proportional to the degree of architectural distortion [Figs. 3–20, 3–21]. Anaplasia includes irregular, hyperchromatic nuclei in which nucleoli may be difficult to see. Recognition of irregular, small, attenuated glands is never a problem, and the presence of even small amounts of such glands is diagnostic of cancer.

Cribriform carcinoma is either regular or irregular (Fig. 3–22). The regular variety shows smooth, uniform arborization of lumina punctuating a solid core of epithelial cells, usually with a smooth, even external surface. The irregular variety shows angulated arborization of variably sized lumens punctuating an epithelial

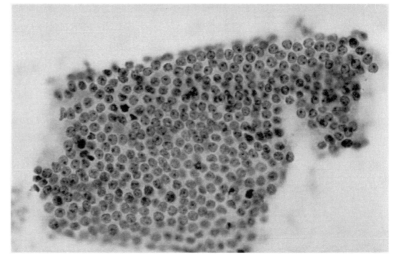

Figure 3–19. Well-differentiated adenocarcinoma with tubuloacinar features. The borders of this structure are smooth; there are malignant nuclei, no basal cells, and an uninterrupted monolayer of cancer cells. The margins of this structure are out of focus because it is three dimensional and tubelike, and this level of focus shows only the roof, not the lumen.

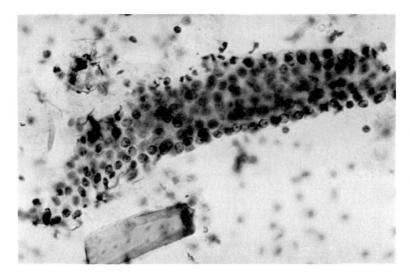

Figure 3–20. Moderately differentiated adenocarcinoma with tubuloacinar features. There are malignant nuclei, no basal cells, and an uninterrupted monolayer of cancer cells. The margins of this structure are in focus because it is three dimensional and tube-like, and this level of focus shows the lumen. Note the highly refractive prostatic crystalloid.

Figure 3–21. Poorly differentiated adenocarcinoma with tubuloacinar features. There are malignant nuclei with a high degree of anaplasia and prominent nucleoli, no basal cells, and an uninterrupted monolayer of cancer cells about a highly attenuated lumen. Figures 3–19 through 3–21 show that there is crude inverse proportionality between the degree of differentiation and nuclear anaplasia.

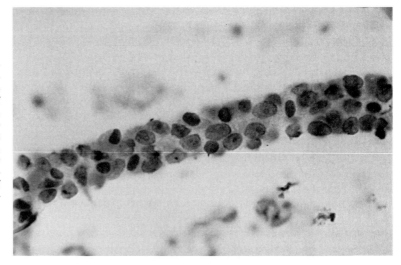

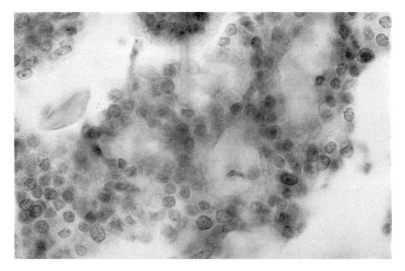

Figure 3–22. Cribriform carcinoma shows arborizing lumens punctuating a solid core of epithelial cells.

cell core with an uneven external surface. Occasionally, structures measuring about the size of intermediate-size acini have a smooth external surface and a complex internal cribriform structure. These are considered the irregular variety of cribriform carcinoma and correspond to the fused glands of Gleason pattern 4. Nuclear anaplasia of cribriform carcinoma is roughly proportional to the degree of architectural distortion.

Sheets of neoplastic cells with papillary or pseudopapillary fronds and a cribriform pattern may originate in the ducts of the prostate.[33] Cribriform patterns may coexist with pseudopapillae that consist of clubbed aggregates of tumor cells whose cytoplasm is scalloped over the luminal aspect of the epithelium (Fig. 3–23). Isolated pseudopapillae of cancer cannot be differentiated from high-grade PIN. When they occur in the absence of other obvious cancer patterns or without large tumor cell sheets (so that the lack of basal cells can be satisfactorily evaluated) they should be interpreted with caution, and the differential diagnosis of "carcinoma versus high-grade PIN" should be offered. Regular cribriform structures and pseudopapillary aggregates usually correspond to Gleason pattern 3 carcinoma. Irregular cribriform structures, with or without hypernephroid clear cells, correspond to Gleason pattern 4 carcinoma.

Endometrioid (ductal) carcinoma of the prostate appears as papillae and clusters of malignant cells that have lost polarity and cohesion with crowded, overlapping, hyperchromatic nuclei and prominent nucleoli. A novel finding is the presence of grooved nuclei in a minority of tumor cells.[53] We have seen several post-cystoscopy urine cytologic preparations with cell clusters showing papillary structures, grooved nuclei, and nuclear pseudoinclusions. The nuclei showed moderate anisopoikilonucleosis, but there was only slight hyperchromasia and nucleolar enlargement. Benign cells with these features are present beneath the secretory cell layer in the region of the prostatic utricle and may be present in association with benign secretory epithelium in prostatitis. The cells are located immediately beneath the secretory cell layer, and the enlarged, atypical grooved cells are probably basal cells with proliferative features (Figs. 3–24, 3–25). The significance of grooved nuclei for the diagnosis of endometrioid (ductal) carcinoma is unresolved.

Undifferentiated carcinoma appears as solid tumor clusters or dissociated single tumor cells, corresponding to Gleason pattern 5 carcinoma (Fig. 3–26). Poorly differentiated invasive transitional cell cancer may be mistaken for these lesions, as may anaplastic large cell lymphoma. High mitotic activity is less likely in undifferentiated prostate cancer than in its mimicks. Immunohistochemical stains that are useful in differentiating tumor types include leukocyte common antigen and Ki-1 (positive in certain large cell lymphomas), neuron-specific enolase, chromogranin, prostate-specific acid phosphatase, PSA, keratin (positive in small cell carcinoma of prostate), and carcinoembryonic antigen (CEA; to support the diagnosis of extraprostatic neoplasm, including transitional cell carcinoma). Prostate carcinoma may be weakly positive for CEA in liquid-

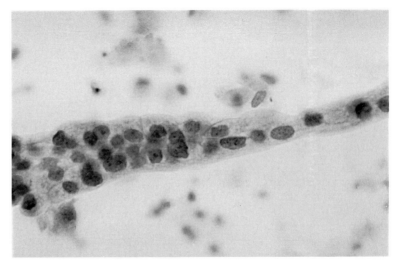

Figure 3–23. Pseudopapillae are clubbed aggregates of neoplastic cells whose apical cytoplasm is scalloped over their external surface. They should not be confused with highly attenuated tubuloacinar glands (compare Fig. 3–21).

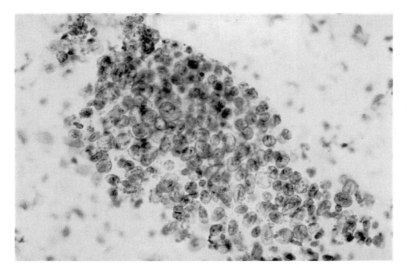

Figure 3–24. Atypical cells with a high degree of anisopoikilonucleosis and nuclear grooves, similar in appearance to those described by Masood and coworkers in their case of endometrioid carcinoma of prostate.[53] The cells in this photomicrograph are interpreted as highly atypical basal cells, and they are intimately associated with overlying benign-looking secretory epithelium (see Fig. 3–25).

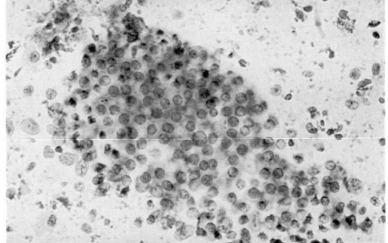

Figure 3–25. Benign-looking secretory epithelial cells seen in a different plane of focus of Fig. 3–24.

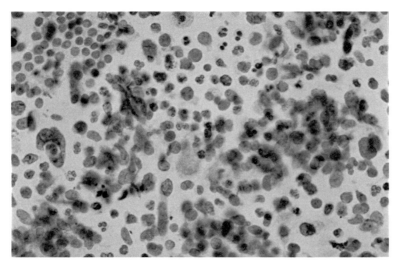

Figure 3–26. Undifferentiated prostate carcinoma shows a high degree of dyshesion and complete loss of polarity among tumor cells. Nuclei are highly anaplastic, but mitotic activity is not marked.

fixed preparations, but strong reactivity for this antigen is not the rule. Seminal vesicle punctures may yield bizarre cells that can be misinterpreted as undifferentiated large cell malignant neoplasm.

With the help of Dr. Donald Gleason we determined the predictive accuracy of pattern grading in cytology using 50 cases with matched tissue biopsy specimens. Cases were chosen from the files of Aspiration Biopsy Laboratory, Inc. (now, OncoDiagnostics Laboratory, Inc., Cleveland, OH). Cases were included in which transrectal core biopsy and aspiration biopsy specimens were obtained simultaneously, transrectal core biopsy was obtained by ultrasound-guided automated cutting needle, a defined lesion was detected either by ultrasound or digital rectal examination (as recorded on test requisition forms originally submitted with the specimens), and four-quadrant biopsies were obtained with both methods. Fifty-three patients with cancer were identified, and 50 had cancer in both core biopsy and aspiration biopsy material.

The Gleason score predicted from cytology material and the tissue Gleason score were not statistically different. The modal Gleason score of tissue specimens was 6 and 7, whereas the modal score of cytology specimens was 6. In three cases, the tissue biopsy was negative and the cytology was positive. Other findings that were more frequent in cytology specimens included, in decreasing order, papillary type PIN, AAH, and cribriform type PIN.

COMPLEMENTARY TECHNIQUES

When an appropriate number of samples is obtained from palpably abnormal prostates, the cancer detection rate is the same for aspiration and core biopsies. Among experienced teams of urologists and pathologists both methods have equal sensitivity and specificity, and false positives are rare or nonexistent.[16, 54–56] We studied 228 aspiration quadrant biopsies and matched ultrasound-guided quadrant core biopsies. Overall, 90 prostatic adenocarcinomas were detected, including 84 by core biopsy, 86 by aspiration biopsy, and 80 by both techniques. Directed sampling of palpable or impalpable lesions by ultrasound-guided core biopsy is complemented by sampling of palpable lesions and the remainder of the prostate by aspiration biopsy.[57]

Aspiration biopsy is a nondestructive

method. Adolfsson and Tribukait evaluated tumor progression by repeated aspiration biopsies in 84 patients with untreated prostate cancer followed for at least 2 years.[58] They showed that modal DNA values of tumors increased (became aneuploid) in 17 patients, whereas cytologic differentiation decreased in 18. Stege and coworkers used aspiration biopsy in 133 patients to measure DNA ploidy, quantitate cellular prostatic acid phosphatase (PAP) and PSA antigen, and grade tumors.[59] They showed that a decrease in PAP and PSA correlated with higher-grade malignancy and more advanced tumor stage and a shift from diploid to aneuploid. They also performed quantitative estimation of tissue PSA, DNA ploidy, and cytologic grading in aspiration biopsies of 67 cancer patients treated with androgen deprivation.[60] Cytology and tissue PSA were the most important factors in determining cancer progression. Oomens and associates studied aspiration biopsies from nine patients receiving endocrine or radiation therapy for cancer and found interval decreases in the Ki-67 index of 58%, 27%, and 7%, respectively, at 1-, 2-, and 3-month intervals.[61]

Galang and Park studied 1198 core biopsies and their matched washings using cytocentrifugation to capture the cell sample shed from core biopsies during transit to laboratory (CF Galang, CH Park, personal communication). In cancer cases, core biopsy washings were diagnostic in 96% and biopsies were diagnostic in 97%. Thirteen cases of cancer were diagnosed from core washings in the absence of a tissue diagnosis of cancer. Because of the small size of the core biopsy and its inherent delicateness, information loss occurs when it is fixed and processed. This loss is lessened by salvaging exfoliated cells that would otherwise be discarded. The value of studying the cytology of core biopsy washings includes the possibility of confirming the diagnosis of cancer in borderline tissue samplings, salvaging "exploded" or "dispersed" specimens, performing quality assurance of histologic diagnoses, and procuring material for special studies such as DNA ploidy analysis or in situ hybridization without "sectioned partial nucleus" artifact and without destruction or further diminution of the tissue block.

Perhaps the greatest merit of core biopsy washings is that their study allows pathologists the opportunity to learn prostate cytology. Gleason observed, "... Cytologic diagnosis and grading are performed better in Europe, not because American pathologists are stubborn or uninformed, but because of medico-politico-socioeconomic differences.[62] Europe has many large, often nationalized, central medical centers that can support a few expert cytologists to develop and maintain their expertise with large numbers of referred patients and material. In our pluralistic United States medical system patient material is divided among many good, smaller hospitals that simply cannot have enough material to train, maintain, and pay for expert cytologists."[62] The cellular component that is spontaneously shed from prostate core biopsies and discarded provides pathologists invaluable material from which to learn prostate cytology. By correlating tissue sections with cytology slides pathologists could face the challenges and reap the rewards of prostatic aspiration biopsy.

REFERENCES

1. Fox CH: Innovation in medical diagnosis—the Scandinavian curiosity. Lancet 1:1387, 1979.
2. Koss LG, Woyke S, Schreiber K, et al.: Thin-needle aspiration biopsy of the prostate. Urol Clin North Am 11:237–251, 1984.
3. Das DK, Hedlund PO, Lowhagen T, et al.: Squamous-metaplasia in hormonally treated prostatic cancer. Significance during follow-up. Urology 38:70–75, 1991.
4. Esposti PL: Cytologic malignancy grading of prostatic carcinoma by transrectal aspiration biopsy. A five-year follow-up study of 469 hormone-treated patients. Scand J Urol Nephrol 5:199–209, 1971.
5. Faul P, Schmiedt E, Kern R: Prognostic significance of cytological differentiation grading in estrogen-treated prostatic carcinoma diagnosed by fine-needle aspiration biopsy (five-year follow-up of 496 patients). Int J Urol Nephrol 12:347–54, 1980.
6. Leistenschneider W, Nagel R: Atlas of Prostatic Cytology: Techniques and Diagnosis. New York: Springer-Verlag, 1985.
7. Oyen RH, Van Poppel HP, Ameye FE, et al.: Lymph node staging of localized prostatic carcinoma with CT and CT-guided fine-needle aspiration biopsy: Prospective study of 285 patients. Radiology 190:315–322, 1994.
8. Van Poppel H, Ameye F, Oyen R, et al.: Accuracy of combined computerized tomography and fine needle aspiration cytology in lymph node staging of localized prostatic carcinoma. J Urol 151:1324–1325, 1994.
9. Wolf JS, Cher M, Dall'era M, et al.: The use and accuracy of cross-sectional imaging and fine needle aspiration cytology for detection of pelvic lymph node metastases before radical prostatectomy. J Urol 153:993–999, 1995.
10. Bastacky SS, Silver SA, Epstein JI: Composite cytological smears of pelvic lymph nodes at the time of radical prostatectomy to identify nodal metastases. Hum Pathol 25:1352–1359, 1994.
11. Agatstein EH, Hernandez FJ, Layfield LJ, et al.: Use of needle aspiration for detection of stage A prostatic carcinoma before transurethral resection of the prostate: A clinical trial. J Urol 138:551–553, 1987.
12. Juusela H, Ruutu M, Permi J, et al.: Can fine needle aspiration biopsy detect incidental prostatic carcinoma (T1) prior to TUR? Eur Urol 21:131–133, 1992.
13. Honig SC, Stilmant MM, Klavans MS, et al.: The role of fine-needle aspiration biopsy of the prostate in staging adenocarcinoma. Cancer 69:2978–2982, 1992.
14. Hostetter AL, Pedersen KV, Gustafsson BL, et al.: Diagnosis and localization of prostate carcinoma by fine-needle aspiration cytology and correlation with histologic whole-organ sections after radical prostatectomy. Am J Clin Pathol 94:693–697, 1990.
15. Benson MC: Fine-needle aspiration of the prostate. NCI Monogr 7:19–24, 1988.
16. Eble JN, Angermeier PA: The roles of fine needle aspiration and needle core biopsies in the diagnosis of primary prostatic cancer. Hum Pathol 23:249–257, 1992.
17. Maksem JA, Resnik MI, Johenning PW: Can a cytological grading system be predictive of Gleason's scores in aspiration biopsy cytology specimens of prostate carcinoma? World J Urol 5:99–102, 1987.
18. Maksem JA, Galang CF, Johenning PW, et al.: Aspiration biopsy of the prostate gland: A brief review of collection, fixation, and pattern recognition with special attention to benign and malignant prostatic epithelium. Diagn Cytopathol 6:258–266, 1990.
19. Esposti PL: Aspiration Biopsy Cytology in the Diagnosis and Management of Prostatic Carcinoma. Stockholm: Stoal & Accidenstryck, 1974.
20. Esposti PL, Elman A, Norlen H: Complications of transrectal aspiration biopsy of prostate. Scand J Urol Nephrol 9:208–213, 1975.
21. Maksem JA, Johenning PW: Prostatitis and aspiration biopsy cytology of the prostate. Urology 32:263–268, 1988.
22. Maksem JA, Johenning PW, Park CH, et al.: Prostatitis and aspiration biopsy of the prostate gland. ASCP check sample. Cytopathology 16, 1988.
23. Cohen MB, Ljung B-ME: Fine-needle aspiration biopsy of the prostate. Pathol Annu 26(2):89–108, 1991.
24. Desmond PM, Clark J, Thompson IM, et al.: Morbidity with contemporary prostate biopsy. J Urol 150(5 Pt 1):1425–1426, 1993.
25. Webb JA, Shanmuganathan K, McLean A: Complications of ultrasound-guided transperineal prostate biopsy. A prospective study. Br J Urol 72:775–777, 1993.
26. Gustafsson O, Norming U, Nyman CR, et al.: Complications following combined transrectal aspiration and core biopsy of the prostate. Scand J Urol Nephrol 24:249–251, 1990.
27. Haddad FS, Somsin AA: Seeding and perineal implantation of prostatic cancer in the tract of the biopsy needle: Three case reports and a review of the literature. J Surg Oncol 335:184–191, 1987.
28. Bastacky SS, Walsh PC, Epstein JI: Needle biopsy associated tumor tracking of adenocarcinoma of the prostate. J Urol 145:1003–1007, 1991.
29. Bostwick DG, Vonk JB, Picado A: Pathologic changes in the prostate following contemporary 18-gauge needle biopsy: No apparent risk of local cancer seeding. J Urol Pathol 2:203–211, 1994.
30. McNeal JE: Prostate. In Sternberg SS (ed): Histology for Pathologists. New York: Raven Press, 1992, pp. 749–763.
31. Maksem JA, Park CH, Johenning PW, et al.: Aspiration biopsy of the prostate gland. Urol Clin North Am 15:555–575, 1988.

32. Maksem JA, Galang CF, Johenning PW, et al.: Aspiration biopsy cytology of the prostate. In Bostwick D (ed): Pathology of the Prostate. New York: Churchill Livingstone, 1990, pp 161–191.

33. Miller GJ: An atlas of prostatic biopsies: Dilemmas of morphologic variance. Progr Surg Pathol 8:81–112, 1988.

34. Howell LP, Amott TR, de Vere-White R: Aspiration biopsy cytology of the prostate in young adult men. Diagn Cytopathol 6:89–94, 1990.

35. Chodak GW, Smith FL, Bibbo M, et al.: The role of transrectal aspiration biopsy in the diagnosis of carcinoma of the prostate. Progr Clin Biol Res 269:11–20, 1988.

36. Smith FL, Bibbo M, Schoenberg HW, et al.: Transrectal aspiration biopsy of the prostate: The importance of atypia. J Urol 140:766–768, 1988.

37. Ritchie AWS, Layfield LJ, Turcillo P, et al.: The significance of atypia in fine needle aspiration cytology of the prostate. J Urol 140:761–765, 1988.

38. Layfield LJ, Goldstein NS: Morphometric analysis of borderline atypia in prostatic aspiration biopsy specimens. Analyt Quant Cytol Histol 13:288–292, 1991.

39. Bittinger A, von Keitz A, Ruschoff J, et al.: Silver staining nucleolar organizer region in prostate cytology. Zentralbl Pathol 140:103–106, 1994.

40. Maksem JA, Johenning PW: Is cytology capable of adequately grading prostate carcinoma? Matched series of 50 cases comparing cytologic and histologic pattern diagnosis. Urology 31:437–444, 1988.

41. Mesonero CE, Oertel YC: Cells from ejaculatory ducts and seminal vesicles and diagnostic difficulties in prostatic aspirates. Modern Pathol 4:723–726, 1991.

42. McNeal JE: Morphogenesis of prostatic carcinoma. Cancer 18:1659–1666, 1965.

43. Jones EC, Young RH: The differential diagnosis of prostatic carcinoma. Its distinction from premalignant and pseudocarcinomatous lesions of the prostate gland. Am J Clin Pathol 101:48–64, 1994.

44. Bostwick DG, Srigley J, Grignon D, et al.: Atypical adenomatous hyperplasia of the prostate: Morphologic criteria for its distinction from well-differentiated carcinoma. Hum Pathol 24:819–832, 1993.

45. Hassan MO, Maksem J: The prostatic perineural space and its relation to tumor spread: An ultrastructural study. Am J Surg Pathol 4:143–148, 1980.

46. Bostwick DG: High grade prostatic intraepithelial neoplasia. The most likely precursor of prostate cancer. Cancer 75:1823–1836, 1995.

47. Tomic R, Bergman B, Hietala SO, et al.: Prognostic significance of transrectal fine-needle aspiration biopsy findings after orchiectomy for carcinoma of the prostate. Eur Urol 11:378–381, 1985.

48. Gleason DF, Mellinger GT: The Veterans Administration Cooperative Urological Research Group: Prediction of prognosis for prostatic adenocarcinoma by combined histological grading and clinical staging. J Urol 111:58–64, 1974.

49. Waisman J, Lowhagen T: Fine Needle Aspiration of the Prostate Gland. Tutorials of Cytology, International Academy of Cytology, 1640 E 50th St., #20-B Chicago, IL, 1984.

50. Mott LJM, Waisman J, Boxer RJ, et al.: Significant microscopic features of prostate adenocarcinoma with a comparison of current methods of grading (Abstract). Lab Invest 40:274, 1979.

51. Kline TS: Guides to Clinical Aspiration Biopsy: Prostate. New York: Igaku-Shoin, 1985.

52. Bloom HJG, Richardson WW: Histological grading and prognosis in breast cancer: A study of 1,409 cases of which 359 have been followed for 15 years. Br J Cancer 11:359–377, 1957.

53. Masood S, Swartz DA, Meneses M, et al.: Fine needle aspiration cytology of papillary endometrioid carcinoma of the prostate: The grooved nucleus as a cytologic marker. Acta Cytol 35:451–455, 1991.

54. Brenner DW, Ladaga LE, Fillion MB, et al.: Comparison of transrectal fine-needle aspiration cytology and core needle biopsy in diagnosis of prostate cancer. Urology 35:381–384, 1990.

55. Waisman J, Adolfsson J, Lowhagen T, et al.: Comparison of transrectal prostate digital aspiration and ultrasound-guided core biopsies in 99 men. Urology 37:301–307, 1991.

56. Engelstein D, Mukamel E, Cytron S, et al.: A comparison between digitally-guided fine needle aspiration and ultrasound-guided transperineal core needle biopsy of the prostate for the detection of prostate cancer. Br J Urol 74:210–213, 1994.

57. Maksem JA: Ultrasound assisted core and aspiration biopsy of the prostate gland—their complementary function in prostate cancer diagnosis. *In* Resnick M, Watanabe H, Karr JP (eds): Diagnostic Ultrasound of the Prostate: Proceedings of the First International Workshop on Diagnostic Ultrasound of the Prostate. New York: Elsevier, c1989, pp 183–185.

58. Adolfsson J, Tribukait B: Modal DNA values in prostate cancer with deferred therapy or endocrine therapy. Acta Oncol (Sweden) 30:209–210, 1991.

59. Stege R, Tribukait B, Pousette A, et al.: Deoxyribonucleic acid ploidy and the direct assay of prostatic acid phosphatase and prostate specific antigen in fine needle aspiration biopsies as diagnostic methods in prostatic carcinoma. J Urol 144:299–302, 1990.

60. Stege R, Tribukait B, Lundh B, et al.: Quantitative estimation of tissue prostate specific antigen, deoxyribonucleic acid ploidy and cytological grade in fine needle aspiration biopsies for prognosis of hormonally treated prostatic carcinoma. J Urol 148:833–837, 1992.

61. Oomens EH, van Steenbrugge GJ, van der Kwast TH, et al.: Application of the monoclonal antibody Ki-67 on prostate biopsies to assess the fraction of human prostatic carcinoma. J Urol 145:81–85, 1991.

62. Gleason DF: Re: The natural course of prostatic carcinoma in relation to initial cytological grade [letter; comment on: J. Urol. 1988;140:1452–4]. J Urol 142: 831–832, 1989.

4

CRITICAL ASSESSMENT OF INFLAMMATORY LESIONS OF THE PROSTATE, INCLUDING CYTOPATHOLOGIC APPEARANCES AND DIAGNOSIS

TETSURO MATSUMOTO, OSAMU MOCHIDA, JOICHI KUMAZAWA, MITSURU KINJO, and KAZUYUKI SAGIYAMA

CLINICAL FEATURES OF INFLAMMATORY LESIONS OF THE PROSTATE

Prostatitis syndromes include not only infectious and inflammatory disorders but also noninfectious and noninflammatory conditions.[1] Clinically, prostatitis has been subdivided into four conditions based on a modification of the classification proposed by Meares and Stamey, which is based on the four-specimen technique: acute bacterial prostatitis, chronic bacterial prostatitis, nonbacterial prostatitis, and prostatodynia (Table 4–1).[2] Other inflammatory conditions, such as specific and nonspecific granulomas, need to be differentiated from prostatic cancer.

Acute Bacterial Prostatitis

Acute bacterial prostatitis is characterized by sudden onset of fever, obstructive and irritating symptoms on voiding, and perineal pain that is frequently associated with malaise, arthralgia, and myalgia. Samples of midstream urine (VB$_2$), of expressed prostatic secretion (EPS), or of voided urine after prostatic massage (VB$_3$) show a significant number of white blood cells (WBC) (10 or more per high-power field) and the presence of bacteria (at least 10^3 cfu/mL gram-negative bacteria [GNB] or at least 10^4 cfu/mL gram-positive cocci [GPC]). Prostatic massage should be avoided when acute bacterial prostatitis is suspected as vigorous manipulation may cause bacteremia. Antimicrobial therapy is the standard treatment for acute bacterial prostatitis. Analysis of a VB$_2$, EPS, or VB$_3$ sample usually shows the presence of gram-negative organisms such as *Escherichia coli, Klebsiella pneumoniae,* or other Enterobacteriaceae.

Chronic Bacterial Prostatitis

Chronic bacterial prostatitis causes perineal, low-back, or suprapubic pain. Symptoms are

Table 4–1. Common and Uncommon Types of Prostatitis

Common types
   Acute bacterial prostatitis
   Chronic bacterial prostatitis
   Chronic bacterial prostatitis with infected calculi
   Nonbacterial prostatitis
   Prostatodynia
Uncommon types
   Gonococcal prostatitis
   Tuberculous prostatitis
   Parasitic prostatitis
   Mycotic prostatitis
   Nonspecific granulomatous prostatitis
      Noneosinophilic variety
      Eosinophilic variety
Suspected but unproved types
   Prostatitis due to ureaplasmas (mycoplasmas)
   Prostatitis due to *Chlamydia trachomatis*
   Prostatitis due to viruses

generally mild or subtle. Transrectal massage should be performed to obtain an EPS or VB_3 sample. The presence of a significant number of WBC and of bacteria is typical of chronic bacterial prostatitis. *E. coli* and other Enterobacteriaceae organisms are the most common causes of chronic bacterial prostatitis. The role of GPC is controversial, although some investigators have suggested that some, especially enterococci, *Staphylococcus aureus, Staphylococcus saprophyticus,* and *Staphylococcus epidermidis,* play important roles.[3–9] Stones in the prostate (prostatic calculi) are frequently detected by transrectal ultrasound in patients with chronic bacterial prostatitis.[10–12] Chronic bacterial prostatitis is also treated with antimicrobial therapy. Nickel and coworkers reported that chronic bacterial prostatitis, particularly in refractory cases, may be associated with the formation of a bacterial biofilm in the prostatic ducts.[13, 14]

Nonbacterial Prostatitis

Nonbacterial prostatitis, the most common type of prostatitis, has the same characteristics as chronic bacterial prostatitis, except that no infective organism is detected by conventional culture methods. Microscopic examination of an EPS or VB_3 sample shows a significant number of WBCs, indicating the presence of inflammation. Although some studies have suggested that a number of organisms, including *Chlamydia trachomatis, Ureaplasma urealyticum,* and *Trichomonas vaginalis,* are involved in nonbacterial prostatitis, their roles are still contro-

versial.[15–18] A study using newer microbiologic probes did not consistently find these organisms to be responsible for nonbacterial prostatitis.[19]

Chlamydial elementary bodies have been detected in EPS samples by direct immunofluorescence, and chlamydia-specific immunoglobulin A (IgA) and IgG responses have been observed in EPS and seminal fluid samples[20, 21]; however, it was impossible to avoid completely contamination by colonized organisms in the urethra when samples of EPS and VB_3 or specimens of transrectal biopsy and transurethral resection were obtained.

U. urealyticum is part of the normal flora of the male urethra. Comparison of the *U. urealyticum* counts in first voided urine (VB_1) samples and VB_3 samples may provide useful diagnostic information. Counts of fewer than 10^3 cfu/mL in a VB_1 sample are considered normal urethral colonization.[22] Some investigators have observed a correlation between an increase in the number of leukocytes and high counts of GNB, GPB, or *U. urealyticum.*[23, 24] Nonbacterial prostatitis is usually treated with an antimicrobial agent effective against these controversial organisms.

Prostatodynia

Although prostatodynia is considered the other specific entity of prostatitis, it is actually a symptom complex of unknown cause that may reflect various pelvic disorders. The symptoms of prostatodynia resemble those of prostatitis, but no objective findings indicated that such symptoms arise in the prostate. Patients may have perineal, pelvic, or low back pain or discomfort or other symptoms that suggest prostatitis yet exhibit no inflammation of the prostate gland. Another characteristic is the presence of increased tension of the musculature of the pelvic floor. Stress and emotional problems are potential contributors in patients with prostatodynia.[10]

Other Inflammatory Lesions

Granulomatous prostatitis, a unique form of chronic prostatitis, is usually diagnosed by histologic examination to differentiate it from prostatic cancer. This condition has been classified into four categories by Epstein and Hutchins: specific, nonspecific, post-transurethral resection (TURP), and allergic.[25]

Specific Granulomas of the Prostate

Tuberculous Infection

Tuberculous infection of the prostate is uncommon and is usually associated with a more obvious infection elsewhere in the genitourinary tract, such as kidney or bladder. It sometimes is a prostatitic manifestation of miliary tuberculosis due to blood-borne infection.[26] Most patients have no prostate symptoms, and infection is documented by culture or histologic examination. Granulomatous prostatitis, like tuberculous prostatitis, is also induced by bacillus Calmette-Guérin (BCG) treatment for superficial transitional cell carcinoma of the bladder.[27, 28]

Others

Histoplasmosis, blastomycosis, and fungal (cryptococcal, actinomycotic, nocardial) and viral prostatitis are rare manifestations in the prostate and are also prostatic manifestations of general infection.[29–31]

Nonspecific Granuloma

Nonspecific Granulomatous Prostatitis

The etiology of nonspecific granulomatous prostatitis, which is distinct from specific granulomas due to causes such as tuberculosis, syphilis, brucellosis, viruses, and fungi, is unknown. Spillage of prostatic fluid due to rupture of ducts and acini is proposed as a possible mechanism.[32, 33] The patient's clinical history frequently suggests a lower urinary tract infection (UTI): symptoms include fever, urgency, burning on urination, and symptoms of minimal to moderate prostatic obstruction. Transrectal palpation and ultrasound examination of the prostate yield findings that suggest carcinoma in almost all patients.[34]

Eosinophilic granulomatous prostatitis and Wegener's granulomatosis are included in the category of allergic granulomatous prostatitis.[35, 36] This classification is now widely accepted.

Malakoplakia

Malakoplakia is a rare condition that tends to occur in the urinary tract. The bladder is the most common site, and prostatic involvement is extremely rare.[37] Malakoplakia of the prostate is a form of chronic bacterial prostatitis in which bacteria are phagocytosed but incompletely digested by histiocytes.[38, 39] *E. coli* is the most common infectious organism. A defect in the host's lysosomal response has been cited as a possible cause, but the exact mechanism is unclear. Rectal examination typically demonstrates an enlarged, firm, and frequently nodular prostate gland, strongly suggestive of carcinoma.

PATHOLOGIC AND CYTOLOGIC FEATURES OF INFLAMMATORY LESIONS OF THE PROSTATE

Acute Prostatitis

Biopsy specimens are seldom obtained from patients with acute prostatitis. Acute prostatitis

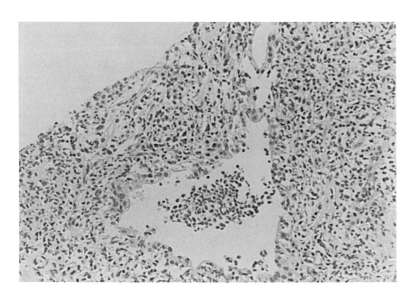

Figure 4–1. Histologic appearance of acute prostatitis. Needle biopsy specimen shows dense accumulation of neutrophils, macrophages, and lymphocytes. Inflammatory exudate is also observed in the prostatic duct. (H& E ×200.)

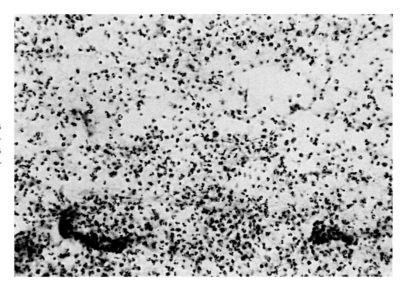

Figure 4–2. Cytologic findings of acute prostatitis. Diffuse and voluminous neutrophil infiltration is observed in the specimen. (Papanicolaou ×20.)

has occasionally been detected in prostate tissue samples obtained from patients with benign prostatic hyperplasia (BPH). Inflammation begins in the prostatic ducts and glands, where a large number of leukocytes are present. Acute prostatitis may remain localized or may result in diffuse disease. The ducts and acini are eventually destroyed, and the infection spreads to the surrounding parenchyma, leading to edema, hyperemia, and diffuse infiltration of leukocytes. Infiltrating cells include polymorphonuclear leukocytes (PMN), lymphocytes, and/or plasma cells, depending on the infection phase. Further necrosis and liquefaction may result in the development of an abscess (Fig. 4–1).[40, 41] Cytologic examination of specimens shows diffuse accumulation

of neutrophils within the epithelial compartment of ducts and acini (Fig. 4–2).

Chronic Prostatitis

The histologic characteristics of chronic bacterial and nonbacterial prostatitis are identical. Focal infiltration of plasma cells, histiocytes, and lymphocytes is seen mainly in the tissue surrounding ducts and acini. Small foci of lymphocytes are frequently observed in the parenchyma (Fig. 4–3). There are a few differences between the cytologic findings in chronic bacterial and nonbacterial prostatitis. The number of inflammatory cells, especially leukocytes, observed in chronic nonbacterial prostatitis is

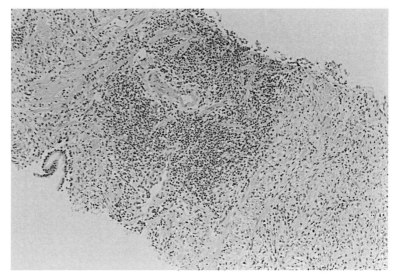

Figure 4–3. Histologic appearance of chronic bacterial prostatitis. Focal infiltration of chronic inflammatory cells is observed in the prostate. (H&E ×100.)

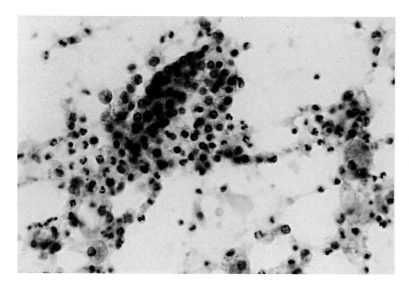

Figure 4–4. Cytologic finding of chronic bacterial prostatitis. Clusters of neutrophils, macrophages, and lymphocytes are observed in the specimen. (Giemsa ×20.)

smaller than the number present in chronic bacterial prostatitis. Clusters of neutrophils, histiocytes, lymphocytes, and plasma cells are observed in specimens from patients with chronic bacterial prostatitis (Fig. 4–4). Histiocytes, lymphocytes, and plasma cells, but not neutrophils, are often observed in specimens obtained from patients with chronic nonbacterial prostatitis (Fig. 4–5).

Other Types of Prostatitis

Specific Granulomatous Prostatitis

Tuberculosis

Tuberculous infection of the prostate produces caseating granulomas that may be grossly visible as zones of liquefied, central necrosis with a "cheesy" appearance. Microscopically, tuberculous infection is characterized by infiltrates of epithelioid, often multinucleate, histiocytes (Fig. 4–6). Because infectious and noninfectious processes may produce similar microscopic findings, definitive diagnosis requires culture, identification of acid-fast organisms, or new microbiologic methods such as the use of DNA probes or polymerase chain reaction (PCR) (Fig. 4–7). Histologic features of BCG-induced granulomatous prostatitis are also similar to those of tuberculous prostatitis.[42] A few Langhans' giant cells are always detected by cytologic examination. The most distinctive feature of tuberculosis is the presence of granular eosinophilic

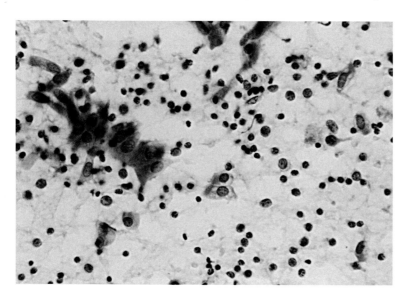

Figure 4–5. Cytologic finding of chronic nonbacterial prostatitis. Infiltration consisted of lymphocytes and histiocytes, but no neutrophils are observed. (Giemsa ×20.)

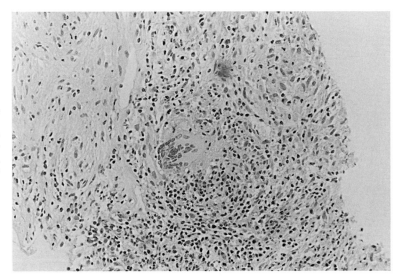

Figure 4–6. Histologic appearance of tuberculous prostatitis. Many epithelioid granulomas containing Langerhans' giant cells associated with caseous necrosis and mild chronic inflammatory infiltrate are observed. (H&E ×200.)

material and cellular debris, indicating the presence of caseous necrosis.[43]

Nonspecific Granulomatous Prostatitis

Microscopically, nonspecific granulomatous prostatitis is characterized by nodular granulomatous infiltrates that replace the prostatic acini and stroma. Ruptured ducts and acini with leakage of secretions into the surrounding stroma are common, and multinucleate histiocytes are invariably present (Fig. 4–8).[44] In some instances, large numbers of

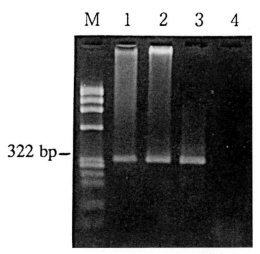

322 bp—

Figure 4–7. Polymerase chain reaction (PCR) of prostatic tuberculosis. Two different DNA primers specific for *Mycobacterium tuberculosis* were used for nested PCR. PCR products of 322 bp were detected in three samples obtained from patients with tuberculous prostatitis.

histiocytes have foamy or xanthogranulomatous cytoplasm owing to phagocytosis of lipids. Xanthogranulomatous prostatitis is a variant of nonspecific granulomatous prostatitis.[45] The center of large granulomas may contain liquefactive necrosis, but caseous necrosis like that seen in tuberculous infection is absent. The stroma surrounding the granulomas may be fibrotic or show muscular hyperplasia (Fig. 4–9).[46] Eosinophic fluid contains polymorphonuclear leukocytes, abundant histiocytes, corpora amylacea, and clusters of benign prostatic epithelial cells.[47]

Focal epithelial cellular atypia characterized by slightly larger nuclei with a vesicular appearance, punctate nuclear chromatin, and inconspicuous nucleoli is observed in cytologic preparations of urine. These changes represent reactive atypia, which is probably caused by the inflammatory process.[48] Epithelioid cells, singly and in small or large groups, are also detected by cytologic examination. Multinucleate giant cells are often present. The individual nuclei of the multinucleate giant cells closely resemble the nuclei of the epithelioid cells. Their cytoplasm contains different types of phagocytic material, such as degenerating granulocytes, laminated bodies, and amorphous prostatic secretions. The large nuclei of the epithelioid cells and irregular clustering of nuclei may suggest carcinoma (Fig. 4–10).[49]

Malakoplakia of the Prostate

Microscopy shows dense, inflammatory infiltrates replacing the prostate glands and

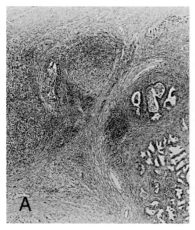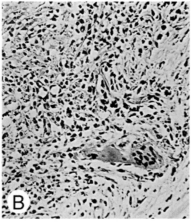

Figure 4–8. Histologic appearance of nonspecific granulomatous prostatitis. Specimen obtained by TUR of prostate shows granulose lesions associated with glandular and fibromuscular hyperplasia of the prostate. (H&E ×25[A], × 100[B].)

Figure 4–9. Histologic appearance of xanthogranulomatous prostatitis. Transrectal needle biopsy specimen shows xanthogranulomatous prostatitis, with main cellular component being foamy histiocytes. (H&E ×60[A], ×100[B].)

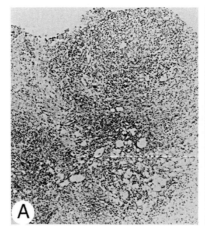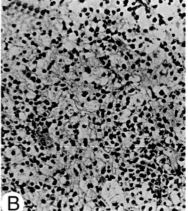

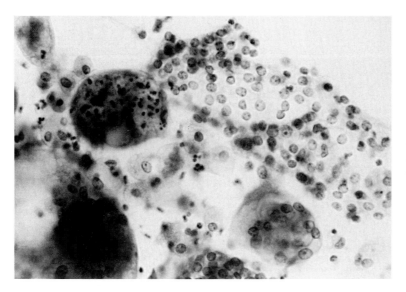

Figure 4–10. Cytologic finding of nonspecific granulomatous prostatitis. Clusters of histiocytes and multinucleate cells are observed in the specimen. (Giemsa ×20.)

stroma. Large, epithelioid, typically mononuclear histiocytes with abundant eosinophilic or vacuolated cytoplasm are predominant. Eosinophilic inclusions known as Michaelis-Gutmann bodies, which represent mineralized remnants of bacterial cell walls, are present in the cytoplasm of scattered histiocytes. These bodies are easily visualized with periodic acid-Schiff (PAS) stain (Fig. 4–11).[50, 51]

Postsurgical Necrobiotic Prostatic Granuloma

Postsurgical granulomas are often observed after transurethral resection of the prostate (TURP) or prostatectomy, and occasionally after needle biopsy. These lesions are not grossly visible. A central, circular, or irregular-shaped zone of fibrinoid necrosis is surrounded by a rim of palisading epithelioid histiocytes. Its appearance is indistinguishable from that of a rheumatoid nodule. Minimal inflammation of the surrounding stroma, consisting of lymphocytes and plasma cells, is observed. Scattered eosinophils may be present, and in some patients may be numerous, if a subsequent biopsy or operation is performed shortly after the initial biopsy. Multinucleate histiocytes may also be present in the stroma.[52–54]

Allergic Eosinophilic Granulomatous Prostatitis

Allergic granulomatous prostatitis occasionally is observed in patients with allergic vasculitis, bronchial asthma, or Wegener's granulomatosis.[55] It is characterized by yellowish white small nodules in resected tissue. Histologically, allergic granulomatous prostatitis is characterized by central fibrinoid necrosis associated with histiocytic granulomas and massive infiltration of eosinophils. Many eosinophils are associated with small clusters of epithelioid cells, and on cytologic examination no giant cells are observed.[56]

USEFULNESS OF CYTOLOGIC EXAMINATION OF PROSTATIC INFLAMMATORY LESIONS

Cytologic techniques are available for examination of urine or of fine-needle aspiration specimens. Interstitial cystitis, carcinoma in situ, and invasive bladder cancers may cause complaints similar to those of prostatitis. De la Rossette and colleagues reported that 20.4% of urine samples from patients with prostatitis syndrome showed slight or moderate atypia and that 6.3% showed severe atypia.[57] Malignancies were found in almost 50% of the patients whose specimens exhibited severe atypia. The investigators suggested that the usefulness of the cytologic screening in patients with prostatic syndrome depends on the knowledge and the experience of the examining cytopathologist.

Fine-needle aspiration of the prostate is widely used to detect cancer cells and has been suggested as a means of assessing the inflam-

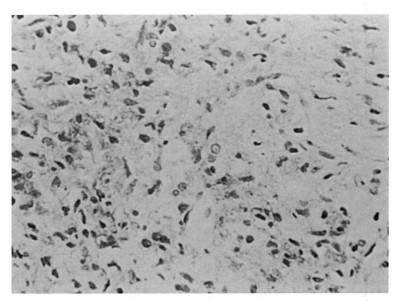

Figure 4–11. Histologic appearance of malakoplakia. Histiocytes in the lesion contain the PAS-positive granules of Michaelis-Gutmann bodies. (PAS ×650.)

Table 4–2. Inflammatory Indices of Prostatic Aspirates

Diagnosis	PMN	Lymphocyte	Macrophage	Total Index
Chronic bacterial prostatitis (n = 8)	2.00 ± 0.76	1.19 ± 0.53	1.00 ± 0.53	4.19 ± 1.31 ⎤* ⎤
Nonbacterial prostatitis (n = 20)	1.50 ± 0.60	1.16 ± 0.58	0.40 ± 0.45	3.15 ± 1.03 ⎦ ⎤*
Prostatodynia (n = 3)	0.67 ± 0.29	1.33 ± 0.58	0.17 ± 0.29	2.17 ± 0.76 ⎦
Nonprostatitis (n = 12)				
BPH or prostatic cancer	1.79 ± 0.78	1.00 ± 0	0.54 ± 0.89	3.33 ± 1.05

* $P < 0.05$
Inflammatory index: 0 : 0–4 cells/hpf   0.5 : 5–9 cells/hpf
                    1 : 10–29 cells/hpf   2 : ≧30 cells/hpf

matory response in the prostate gland and of detecting the presence of microorganisms.[58] Miralless and coworkers suggested that fine-needle aspiration cytology may be one of the best means of obtaining a morphologic diagnosis and of distinguishing inflammation from carcinoma in subacute, chronic, or granulomatous prostatitis whenever the clinical picture is unclear.[48] Matsumoto and colleagues tried to detect inflammatory cells in prostatic aspirates obtained from patients with chronic bacterial prostatitis, chronic nonbacterial prostatitis, prostatodynia, and other conditions such as BPH and prostate cancer.[59] A large number of neutrophils and macrophages were detected in cytologic specimens obtained from patients with chronic bacterial prostatitis but not in those obtained from patients with chronic nonbacterial prostatitis, prostatodynia, or other conditions (Table 4–2). Infiltration of inflammatory cells in prostate tissue is increased in patients with chronic bacterial prostatitis as compared with patients with chronic nonbacterial prostatitis or prostatodynia, suggesting that chemotactic stimulation of the prostate may be more severe in chronic bacterial prostatitis than in chronic nonbacterial prostatitis or prostatodynia.

REFERENCES

1. Meares EM: Prostatitis. Med Clin North Am 75:405–424, 1991.
2. Meares EM, Stamey TA: Bacteriologic localization patterns in bacterial prostatitis and urethritis. Invest Urol 5:492–518, 1968.
3. Meares EM: Prostatitis syndromes: New perspectives about old woes. J Urol 123:141–147, 1980.
4. Leigh DA: Prostatitis: An increasing clinical problem for diagnosis and management. J Antimicrob Chemother 32(Suppl A):1–9, 1993.
5. Childs SJ: Ciprofloxacin in treatment of chronic bacterial prostatitis. Urology 35(Suppl):15–18, 1990.
6. Drach GW: Problems in diagnosis of bacterial prostatitis: Gram-negative, gram-positive and mixed infections. J Urol 111:630–636, 1974.
7. Carson CC, McGraw VD, Zwadyk P: Bacterial prostatitis caused by *Staphylococcus saprophyticus*. Urology 19:576–578, 1982.
8. Bergman B, Wedren H, Holm SE: *Staphylococcus saprophyticus* in males with symptoms of chronic prostatitis. Urology 34:241–245, 1989.
9. Wedren H: On chronic prostatitis with special studies of *Staphylococcus epidermidis*. Scand J Urol Nephrol 123(Suppl):1–36, 1989.
10. Moul JW: Prostatitis. Sorting out the different causes. Postgrad Med 94:191–194, 1994.
11. Eykyn S, Bultitude MI, Mays ME, et al.: Prostatic calculi as a source of recurrent bacteriuria in the male. Br J Urol 46:527–532, 1974.
12. Ludwig M, Weidner W, Schroeder-Printzen I, et al.: Transrectal prostatic sonography as a useful diagnostic means for patients with chronic prostatitis or prostatodynia. Br J Urol 73:664–668, 1994.
13. Nickel JC, Costerton JW: Bacterial localization in antibiotic-refractory chronic bacterial prostatitis. Prostate 23:107–114, 1993.
14. Nickel JC, Costerton JW, McLean RJC, et al.: Bacterial biofilm: Influence on the pathogenesis, diagnosis and treatment of urinary tract infections. J Antimicrob Chemother 33(Suppl A):31–41, 1994.
15. Ohkawa M, Yamaguchi S, Tokunaga T, et al.: *Ureaplasma urealyticum* in the urogenital tract of patients with chronic prostatitis or related symptomatology. Br J Urol 72:918–921, 1993.
16. Brunner H, Weidner W, Schiefer HG: Studies on the role of *Ureaplasma urealyticum* and *Mycoplasma hominis* in prostatitis. J Infect Dis 147:807–813, 1983.
17. Weidner W, Brunner H, Krauss W: Quantitative culture of *Ureaplasma urealyticum* in patients with chronic prostatitis. J Urol 124:622–625, 1980.
18. Poletti P, Medici MC, Alinovi A, et al.: Isolation of *Chlamydia trachomatis* from the prostatic cells in patients affected by nonacute abacterial prostatitis. J Urol 134:691–693, 1985.
19. Shortliffe LMD, Sellers RG, Schachter J: The characterization of nonbacterial prostatitis: Search for an etiology. J Urol 148:1461–1466, 1992.
20. Weidner W, Schiefer HG, Krauss H, et al.: Chronic prostatitis: A thorough search for etiologically involved microorganisms in 1461 patients. Infection 19(Suppl 3):119–125, 1991.
21. Tsunekawa T, Kumamoto Y: *Chlamydia trachomatis* Ig-A. J Jpn Soc Infect Dis 63:130–137, 1989.
22. Berger RE, Krieger JN, Kessler D, et al.: Case control study of men with suspected chronic idiopathic prostatitis. J Urol 141:328–331, 1989.

23. Anderson RU, Weller CH: Prostatic secretion leukocyte studies in non-bacterial prostatitis (prostatosis). J Urol 121:292–294, 1979.
24. Schaeffer AJ, Wendel EF, Dunn JK, et al.: Prevalence and significance of prostatic inflammation. J Urol 125:215–219, 1981.
25. Epstein JI, Hutchins GM: Granulomatous prostatitis: Distinction among allergic, non-specific, and post-transurethral resection lesions. Hum Pathol 15:818–825, 1984.
26. Sporer A, Auerback MD: Tuberculosis of the prostate. Urology 11:362–365, 1978.
27. Oates RD, Stilmant MM, Freedlund MC, et al.: Granulomatous prostatitis following bacillus Calmette-Guérin immunotherapy of bladder cancer. J Urol 140:751–754, 1988.
28. Lamm DL, Stogdill VD, Stogdill BK, et al.: Complications of bacillus Calmette-Guérin immunotherapy in 1278 patients with bladder cancer. J Urol 135:272–274, 1986.
29. Kelalis PP, Reene LF, Weed LA: Brucellosis of the urogenital tract: A mimic of tuberculosis. J Urol 88:347–354, 1962.
30. Hinchey WW, Someren A: Cryptococcal prostatitis. Am J Clin Pathol 75:257–260, 1981.
31. Benson PJ, Smith CS: Cytomegalovirus prostatitis. Urology 40:165–167, 1992.
32. Tanner FH, McDonald JR: Granulomatous prostatitis. A histologic study of a group of granulomatous lesions collected from prostate glands. Arch Pathol 36:358–370, 1943.
33. Bryan RL, Newman J, Campbell A, et al.: Granulomatous prostatitis: A clinicopathological study. Histopathology 19:453–457, 1991.
34. Clements R, Thomas KG, Griffiths GJ, et al.: Transrectal ultrasound appearances of granulomatous prostatitis. Clin Radiol 47:174–176, 1993.
35. Stillwell TJ, Engen DE, Farrow GM: The clinical spectrum of granulomatous prostatitis: A report of 200 cases. J Urol 138:320–323, 1987.
36. Stillwell TJ, DeRemee RA, McDonald TJ, et al.: Prostatic involvement in Wegener's granulomatosis. J Urol 138:1251–1253, 1987.
37. Smith BH: Malakoplakia of the urinary tract: A study of twenty four cases. Am J Clin Pathol 43:409–417, 1965.
38. Lewin KJ, Harell GS, Lee AS, et al.: Malakoplakia: An electron-microscopic study; demonstration of bacilliform organisms in malakoplakic macrophages. Gastroenterology 66:28–45, 1974.
39. Mackay EH: Malakoplakia in ulcerative colitis. Arch Pathol Lab Med 102:140–145, 1978.
40. Orland SM, Hanno PW, Wein AJ: Prostatitis, prostatosis, and prostatodynia. Urology 25:439–459, 1985.
41. Meares EM: Bacterial prostatitis vs "prostatosis," a clinical and bacteriological study. JAMA 224:1372–1375, 1973.
42. Miyashita H, Troncoso P, Babaian RJ: BCG-induced granulomatous prostatitis: A comparative ultrasound pathologic study. Urology 39:364–367, 1992.
43. Stilmant M, Siroky MB, Johnson KB: Fine needle aspiration cytology of granulomatous prostatitis induced by BCG immunotherapy of bladder cancer. Acta Cytol 29:961–966, 1985.
44. O'Dea MJ, Hunting DB, Greene CF: Non-specific granulomatous prostatitis. J Urol 118:58, 1977.
45. Weiss MA, Mills SE: Nonspecific granulomatous prostatitis. In: Weiss MA, Mills SE (eds): Genitourinary Tract Pathology. New York: Bower Medical, 1993, pp 134–136.
46. Matsumoto T, Sakamoto N, Kimiya K, et al.: Nonspecific granulomatous prostatitis. Urology 39:420–423, 1992.
47. Towfighi J, Sadeghee S, Wheeler JE, et al.: Granulomatous prostatitis with emphasis on the eosinophilic variety. Am J Clin Pathol 58:630–641, 1972.
48. Miralles TG, Gosalbez F, Menendez P, et al.: Fine needle aspiration cytology of granulomatous prostatitis. Acta Cytol 34:57–62, 1990.
49. Presti B, Weidner N: Granulomatous prostatitis and poorly differentiated prostate carcinoma. Am J Clin Pathol 95:330–334, 1991.
50. Matsumoto T, Ih H, Yamada Y, et al.: Prostatic malakoplakia. Urol Int 40:10–12, 1985.
51. Hansemann D: Malakoplakie der Harnblase. Virchows Arch [A] 173:302–308, 1903.
52. Eyre RC, Aaronson AG, Weinstein BJ: Palisading granulomas of the prostate associated with prior prostatic surgery. J Urol 136:121–122, 1986.
53. Lee G, Shepherd N: Necrotising granulomata in prostatic resection specimens—a sequel to previous operation. J Clin Pathol 36:1067–1070, 1983.
54. Mies C, Balogh K, Stadecker M: Palisading prostate granulomas following surgery. Am J Surg Pathol 8:217–221, 1984.
55. Stanley MW, Horwitz CA, Sharer W, et al.: Granulomatous prostatitis: A spectrum including nonspecific, infectious, and spindle cell lesions. Diagn Cytopathol 7:508–512, 1991.
56. Middleton G, Karp D, Lee E, et al.: Wegener's granulomatosis presenting as lower back pain with prostatitis and ureteral obstruction. J Rheumatol 21:566–569, 1994.
57. de la Rossette J, Hubregste MR, Wiersma AM, et al.: Value of urine cytology in screening patients with prostatitis syndromes. Acta Cytol 37:710–712, 1993.
58. Cytron S, Weinberger M, Servadio C, et al.: Per-rectal ultrasonography plus transperineal fine-needle aspiration in the diagnosis and treatment of prostatic infection. In: Kass EH, Svanborg-Eden C (eds): Host-Parasite Interaction in Urinary Tract Infection. Chicago: University of Chicago Press, 1989, pp 315–316.
59. Matsumoto T, Soejima T, Tanaka M, et al.: Cytologic findings of fine needle aspirates in chronic prostatitis. Int Urol Nephrol 24:43–47, 1992.

5

BENIGN PROSTATIC HYPERPLASIA

BURKHARD HELPAP

Benign, nodular, paraurethral hyperplasia of the prostate (BPH) is one of the most common diseases of elderly men. Eighty percent of all men older than 40 years suffer from urodynamic consequences of BPH. The usual therapy in advanced stages with obstructive symptoms is surgical treatment, most often transurethral resection of the prostate (TURP). More recently, conservative drug therapies are also being discussed subsequent to obtaining novel data on the likely cause and pathogenesis of BPH. Based on the idea that prostatitis might induce the process or occur as an intercurrent phenomenon, treatments directed against contributing inflammatory or congestive processes have been suggested. Also significant in BPH are growth factors, hormone imbalances, and immune-mediated reactions—for example, the stromal infiltration of T lymphocytes and activation of tissue antigens. In this context, histopathologic and anatomic findings, recent immunohistochemical and cell kinetic studies, and complicating associated phenomena in patients with typical BPH are discussed.

ANATOMY

The outer/peripheral and inner/central zones of the prostate are subdivided according to new anatomic studies into three zones:[1, 2] 1. A dorsocranially located *central zone* with wide lumina and a high cylindrical epithelium. The glands show papillary folding. The cellu-

lar cytoplasm is light and granular; the stroma, loose. 2. A *transition zone* is located mediolateral to the urethra. This zone is characterized by narrow glands and a very tight stroma. 3. A *peripheral zone,* with loose stroma and glands, is similar to the transition zone. In all three zones, glandular acini and ducts with basal and secretory cells are found with interspersed endocrine cellular elements that clearly show chromogranin-A and/or B and Grimelius-positive staining.[3] Prostatic hyperplasia develops in the inner/central and transition zones, whereas in 70% to 80% of cases prostate carcinoma develops in the outer/dorsoperipheral zone. Only 20% of all carcinomas are found in the anterocentral (transition) zone, and these are usually highly differentiated incidental carcinomas.

PATHOGENESIS

Hormonal (Dys-)Regulation

Paraurethral hyperplasia of the prostate does not develop after prepubertal castration, and the regression of fully developed disease can be achieved by castration with increase of smooth muscle by a factor of 2.5 and fibrous stroma by a factor of 4.[4] This indicates a hormonal cause for nodular prostatic hyperplasia, combined with aging processes. Studies have shown that the effective androgen in the prostate is dihydrotestosterone (DHT), derived from testosterone via reduction by the enzyme

5α-reductase. DHT is bound to receptor proteins and accumulates in the nuclei of the glandular epithelium. Synthesis of RNA, DNA, and protein is thus activated. Further catabolism proceeds via 3α-androstanediol, which exerts strong androgen effects. Both normal prostate and nodular hyperplastic prostate contain DHT, which accumulates by a factor of 4 to 6 in the latter. 3α-Androstanediol is also significantly increased, especially in the glandular parts of nodular hyperplasia. Furthermore, estrogens seem to play an important role: in dogs, which frequently develop prostatic hyperplasia similar to that of humans, elevated plasma estrogen levels were found; however the growth-inducing, synergistic estrogen effect is due only to 3α-androstanediol and apparently does not influence the activity of 5α-reductase. Prolactin is also presumed to play some role in the development of prostatic hyperplasia. According to current knowledge, however, the androgenic regulation of normal and hyperplastic prostate is the dominating factor. Recent analyses of the effects of the enzyme 5α-reductase indicate that the development of prostatic hyperplasia is linked to continuous age-dependent changes in androgen metabolism. Whereas the stromal DHT production rate remains constant at all ages, with increasing age the epithelium looses its ability to produce DHT from testosterone. This dissociation of DHT formation rates with age leads to a relative predominance of stromal DHT production. Therefore, aging should not be omitted as a factor in prostatic hyperplasia.[4, 5]

Growth Factors

BPH can be the result of hormonal imbalance (altered estrogen-testosterone ratio) as well as stimulation by testosterone, dihydrotestosterone, or estrogen. Growth factors may play an important role in regulating activities of epithelial and stromal cells in BPH.[4, 6] Among the various growth factors in the prostate gland, epidermal growth factor (EGF), basic fibroblastic growth factor (bFGF), and transforming growth factors (TGF-α and TGF-β) play important roles (Table 5–1). EGF and TGF-α are very similar and share a receptor.[4, 7, 8] EGF stimulates epithelial cell proliferation. TGF-α is an autocrine and paracrine growth factor that was found first in prostate carcinoma and then in BPH tissue. TGF increases in correlation with the grade of malignancy of the prostate carcinoma.[7, 8] The TGF receptor is expressed by basal cells of BPH but is lacking in prostatic carcinoma because there are no basal cells. TGF-receptor expression underlies androgenic control. Since androgens downregulate EGF receptor, the EGF receptor number is high if the androgen level is low, but owing to the low EGF level, involution of epithelial cells results. In contrast to EGF-α, with stimulating activity, TGF-β1 inhibits a growth of epithelial cells and fibroblasts. TGF-β1 and EGF are antagonistic on prostatic epithelium cells. EGF has a stimulatory effect, while TGF-β is inhibitory. The two factors interact to achieve prostatic homeostasis. Recent results have shown that prostatic epithelial cells proliferate in the presence of EGF alone but that proliferation is suppressed when TGF-β is added in the presence of EGF.[9] In the absence of EGF, TGF-β induces cell death in prostate epithelium (apoptosis). Furthermore, the interaction of TGF-β1 and basic fibroblast growth factor (bFGF) has been studied. The level of bFGF is elevated in BPH as compared with normal prostate. Basic FGF is a mitogen for cultured human prostate-derived fibroblasts. Human prostate-derived fibroblasts also synthesize bFGF. Therefore bFGF appears to

Table 5–1. Growth Factors and Receptors in Prostate Tissue

Protein	Molecular Weight (kD)	Protein Receptor	Molecular Weight (kD)
Epidermal growth factor (EGF)	6	EGF-(TGF-α) receptors	170
Transforming growth factor-alpha (TGF-α)	6	TGF-β receptor	65 (Type I)
Transforming growth factor-beta (TGF-β)	25		
Platelet-derived growth factor (PDGF)	14–15	PDGF receptors	Unknown
Acidic fibroblast growth factor (a-FGF)	18	FGF receptors	1125/145
Basic fibroblast growth factor (bFGF)	17		
Prostate stromal growth factor (PmodS)	50–60		
Prostate stromal growth factor	10		

Modified from Aumüller G: Benign prostatic hyperplasia: Mechanisms and hypotheses. Urologe A 31:159–165, 1992. Copyright Springer-Verlag.

play a role in this disease of the prostate, and growth of human prostate-derived fibroblasts may be under autocrine control. In contrast, TGF-β1 inhibits proliferation of human prostate-derived fibroblasts, which is controlled by the interaction of two different growth factors. It is possible that bFGF/TGF-β imbalance in favor of cell proliferation promotes prostatic stromal hyperplasia in BPH.[4, 10] In addition, nerve growth factor (NGF) receptor may also be involved in the development of BPH. NGF-like protein is localized to the stroma and may contribute to the paracrine-stimulated growth of epithelial cells of the prostate. Platelet-derived growth factor (PDGF) and its receptor have been demonstrated in the prostate. The release of PDGF in inflammation suggests that PDGF may participate in the development of BPH.[11] A significant role has also been attributed to prostate stromal growth factors, which have mitogenic and nonmitogenic effects on prostatic epithelium as well as on neuronal and nonneuronal cells.[12–15] The stroma of the hyperplastic prostate is infiltrated by lymphocytes. These lymphocytes are T cells with a high proportion of T helper cells. It has been suggested that these lymphocytes recognize and/or react with antigens of BPH, which may initiate cell proliferation.[16, 17]

MORPHOLOGIC PATHOGENESIS

Nodular hyperplasia of the prostate is the result of proliferation of the mesenchymal-stromal and glandular-epithelial compartments. This proliferation begins to appear in the stroma. Proliferation of the glandular epithelium is induced secondarily; secretory glandular activity being slightly reduced when compared with unaltered prostate. In the pathomorphogenesis of hyperplasia, the role of the stroma—especially of the activated smooth muscle cells—is more important: in relation to cytoplasmic volume, there is a significant increase in smooth muscle cell organelles accompanied by an increase of the protein synthesis of the extracellular matrix.[20, 21] The peripheral prostate is compressed to a capsule-like shape by the hyperplastic paraurethral process. Glandular hyperplasia develops from an orderly, slow glandular proliferation with an intact epithelial/stromal relationship. Together with increased glandular proliferation, incompletely differentiated glands can develop that show activated basal cells, re-

sulting in immature nodular hyperplasia. Basal cells are activated, and incompletely matured glands result. Immature (basal) cell hyperplasia is the final result of this process. Characteristics of atypical hyperplasia include a disturbed epithelial-stromal relationship and increased cellular proliferative activity in the glands with the formation of atypical epithelial complexes, but distinctly confined stroma. Secondary epithelial proliferation in microalveolar as well as atrophic cystic glands is called secondary (postatrophic) hyperplasia. If the epithelial stromal unit is disturbed, in the case of increased cellular proliferation with inversion of the proliferation compartment and shift to secretory luminal cells,[29] atypical glandular adenomatous hyperplasia or intraglandular/intraductal cribriform atypia may develop. If this occurs in the central part of the gland it is called *atypical adenomatous hyperplasia* (AAH); in the peripheral parts it is termed *prostatic intraepithelial neoplasia* (PIN), with different grades of atypia.[18, 19]

MACROSCOPIC ANATOMY

The weight of the prostate in BPH ranges between 40 and 400 g (mean 60 g). The relation of the absolute weights (in grams) of the stromal, glandular, and luminal parts of normal human prostate are 11:5:8 and in cases of BPH, 45:9:21.[20, 21] The hyperplastic prostate is nodular and exhibits a partially solid and par-

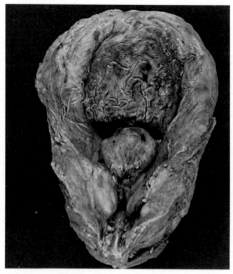

Figure 5–1. Benign prostatic hyperplasia with chronic urocystitis and bladder trabeculation.

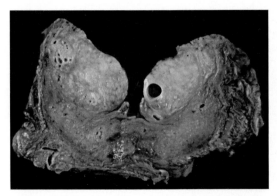

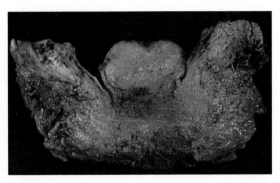

Figure 5–3. Benign prostatic hyperplasia with enlargement of the median lobe.

Figure 5–2. Benign prostatic hyperplasia with hyperplastic lateral lobes.

tially micro- or macrocystic pattern. An exclusive hyperplasia of the lateral lobes or an isolated enlargement of the median lobe may result (Figs. 5–1 to 5–3). In most cases a combination of both is present. Obstruction of urine flow induces development of so-called bladder trabeculation, often combined with chronic cystitis. Consistency of the hyperplastic prostate is influenced by the predominance of either the glandular-cystic or the fibromuscular portions (Figs. 5–2 and 5–3). In a macro- or micronodular hyperplastic prostate small focal carcinomas, particularly those arising in the anterocentral area, cannot be detected with the naked eye. Exact histomorphologic examination of enucleated glands or TURP specimens is therefore mandatory (Fig. 5–4).

MICROSCOPIC ANATOMY

The hyperplastic prostate may consist of purely fibroleiomyomatous nodules or of purely glandular or glandular-atrophic-cystic areas (Figs. 5–5 to 5–7). Often, however, these structures are intermingled. The precise content of smooth muscle fibers is variable, particularly when concomitant chronic inflammatory processes are present. If, after TURP in a recurrent hyperplastic gland, chronic TUR prostatitis develops, the fibromatous portion increases with little or no nodule formation. Vascularization and cell content also change. Mitotic activity often is not measurable.

Stroma

Franks distinguished (1) stromal, (2) fibromuscular, and (3) muscular nodules from fibroadenomatous and fibromyoadenomatous ones.[22] The classification proposed by Vogel and coworkers is (1) embryonal-mesenchymal, (2) fibroblastic, (3) fibromuscular, and (4)

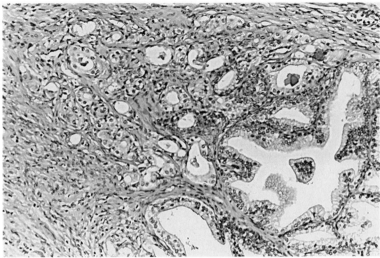

Figure 5–4. Benign prostatic hyperplasia with small focal glandular carcinoma.

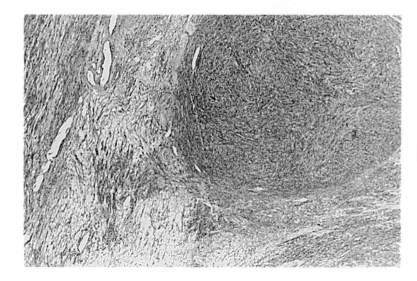

Figure 5–5. Benign prostatic hyperplasia with fibroleiomyomatous nodule.

smooth muscle nodules and their transitional forms (Table 5–2).[23, 24] All types of stromal nodules can be observed simultaneously in the prostate (Fig. 5–8).

Stromal nodules are localized predominantly in the transition zone. The majority occur in the central periurethral regions although they are also encountered in the intermediate and subcapsular regions. Embryonal mesenchymal nodules arise exclusively in the periurethral zone. Fibroblastic and fibromuscular nodules appear in all regions, whereas the smooth muscle nodules are detected only in the intermediate and subcapsular regions. The stromal nodules contain thin-walled capil-

lary-like vascular channels and thick-walled vessels in proportions that change with each morphologic type of nodule (Fig. 5–9).[24, 25]

Embryonal-mesenchymal nodules are composed of a loose homogeneous network of spindle-like cells with sparse cytoplasm and loose chromatin. Strong Alcian blue positivity indicates a high concentration of matrix substances. The embryonal and immature mesenchyme-like cells do not express either vimentin or smooth muscle actin (see Table 5–2).

Fibroblastic nodules are characterized by a predominantly bundle-like arrangement and higher density of fibroblastic spindle-like fibers with a more compact cytoplasm and some

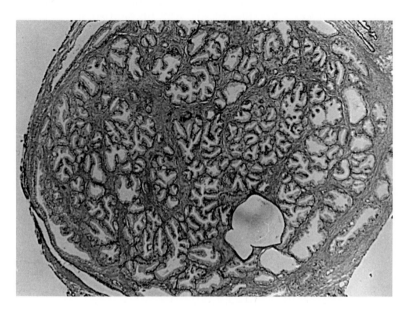

Figure 5–6. Benign prostatic hyperplasia with glandular nodule.

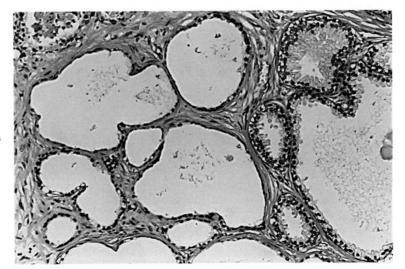

Figure 5–7. Glandular-cystic area in benign prostatic hyperplasia.

Table 5–2. Immunohistochemical Pattern of Prostatic Stromal Nodules

Histochemical Reaction/ Antibody	Nodule Type			
	Embryonal-Mesenchymal	Fibroblastic	Fibromuscular	Smooth Muscle
Alcian blue	+ + +	+	+	−
Vimentin	−	+ +	+ +	−
Desmin	−	−	+ +	+ + +
Actin	−	−	+ +	+ + +
S-100 protein	+ +	+ +	+ + +	+ +
Neuron-specific enolase (NSE)	+	+ +	+ + +	+
Progesterone receptor (PR)	+ + +	+ +	+ +	(+)
Estrogen receptor (ER)	+ +	+ +	+	(+)
T lymphocytes (T4)	+	+ + +	+ + +	+ +
B lymphocytes	−	+	+ (+)	+ + +
Ki-67/PCNA	+ +	+	(+)	−
AgNOR	+ +	+ +	+	(+)

Staining intensity defined in the range − (absent) to + + + (strong).

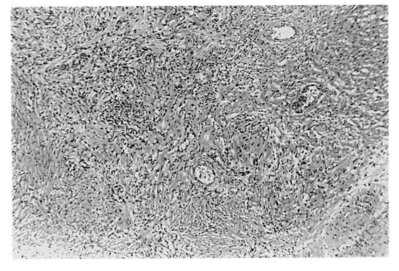

Figure 5–8. Prostatic stromal nodule of fibromuscular mixed type.

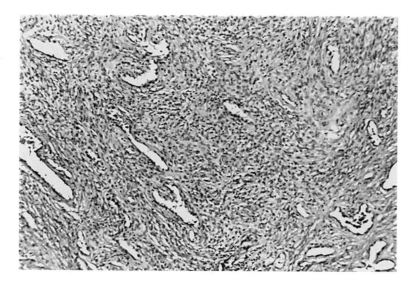

Figure 5–9. Stromal nodule of benign prostatic hyperplasia with thin- and thick-walled capillaries.

smaller nuclei. Alcian blue staining is less strong, indicating sparse matrix substances. The cytoplasm of these cells is positive for vimentin but does not express smooth muscle actin (see Table 5–2).[24, 25]

Mixed fibromuscular nodules present a balanced distribution of fibers of the fibroblastic and smooth muscle types with concomitant expression of both smooth muscle actin and vimentin.

Smooth muscle nodules are composed of smooth muscle cells arranged in intermingled bundles. The cytoplasm is eosinophilic, and the small nuclei show rather dense chromatin. No elastic fibers are found in any type of nodule, in contrast to the diffuse hyperplastic stroma. Beyond these four morphologically well-defined types of stromal nodules, transitional forms with a changing mixture of either (1) embryonal-mesenchymal and fibroblastic or (2) fibroblastic and smooth muscle cells exist (see Table 5–2).[24, 25]

The number of S-100–protein and neuron-specific enolase (NSE)–positive cells is greater in nodules than in the surrounding stroma. The lowest values are found in the embryonal-mesenchymal nodules, the highest ones in the fibromuscular nodules (see Table 5–2).

Stromal nodules of BPH are infiltrated by lymphocytes. The lymphocytic infiltrates are much more dense than in the surrounding diffuse hyperplastic stroma. Embryonal-mesenchymal–like nodules contain significantly less dense lymphocytic infiltrates than more differentiated types of stromal nodules. Immunohistochemistry has identified the lymphocytes

mainly as T lymphocytes with a high constant mean incidence (65%) of helper T cells before the immigration of neuroendocrine and neural elements.[24] Expression of progesterone receptor (PR) is inverse, since high PR values may be found in immature embryonal mesenchymal nodules and low values in differentiated smooth muscle nodules (see Table 5–2).

The fact that immature embryonal-mesenchymal nodes contain significantly fewer T lymphocytes than more mature nodes is suggestive of immigration of T lymphocytes during maturation of stromal nodules (see Table 5–2). The possibility that T lymphocytes—and especially helper T cells, neuroendocrine cells, and expression of growth factors—may influence proliferation and differentiation of the stromal nodules has to be considered.[24]

Stromal nodules of predominantly fibroblastic and fibromuscular types can be infiltrated by glands like fibroadenomas in the breast. Glandular nodules in BPH often contain a fibroblastic and fibromuscular stroma and not the usual periglandular stroma with smooth muscle cells. Glandular infiltration of stromal nodules is consistent with the assumption of close epithelial-stromal interaction combined with an inductive potency of the stroma for epithelial proliferation. In the stromal-epithelial interaction, steroid hormones and their receptors, metabolizing enzymes such as 5α-dihydrotestosterone reductase are involved together with matrix substances including growth factors, their receptors, and growth-inhibiting factors. The complex interdependence of epithelial and stromal factors in the prostate leads to

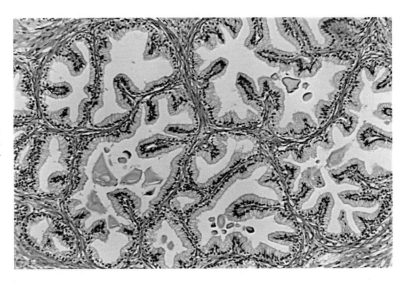

Figure 5–10. Hyperplastic glands with luminal/secretory and basal cells of benign prostatic hyperplasia.

the concept of the functional unit of the prostate.[1, 4, 6] The immature embryonal-mesenchymal stromal nodule around the urethra could represent the first functional prostatic unit and the initial step toward prostate hyperplasia. The sequence of stromal differentiation in this latter process includes phenomena similar to the development of prostatic stroma during ontogenesis.

Glands

The hyperplastic glandular component resembles the normal prostate. The glands have basal cell layers and an intraluminal zone of secretory epithelial cells. Depending on the grade of hyperplasia, intraglandular papillae form, containing a narrow stromal center with capillary blood supplies. The epithelium, however, may also flatten or form a cribriform pattern (Figs. 5–10 and 5–11). The mitotic activity of the glandular epithelium is very low: usually 1 or 2 mitotic figures per 5000 to 10,000 cells. In basal cell hyperplasia of the prostate, slightly increased numbers of mitotic figures are observed (Table 5–3).

IMMUNOHISTOCHEMISTRY AND CELL KINETICS

The fibroleiomyomatous parts of BPH exhibit a strong reaction with antibodies against

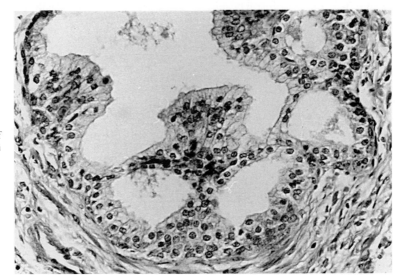

Figure 5–11. Glandular area of benign prostatic hyperplasia with cribriform pattern.

Table 5–3. Cell Kinetic Findings in Prostate Tissue

Histology	Autoradiography ^{3}H-Thymidine (%)	Immunohistochemistry		DNA Cytometry	Apoptosis (%)
		AgNOR (N/nucleus)	PCNA Ki-67 MIB 1 (%)		
BPH	0.49 ± 0.04	1.7–2.6	0.6–3.2	Euploid	0.26 ± 0.03
Secretory cells		2.2	1.62 ± 0.17	Euploid	0.09 ± 0.04
Basal cells		3.3	3.16 ± 0.31	Euploid	0.56 ± 0.07
Stroma		2.1	0.015 ± 0.008	Euploid	———
Prostatrophic hyperplasia	1.6 ± 0.8	———	0.21 ± 0.04	Euploid	———
Atrophy	0.24 ± 0.08	———	0.56 ± 0.09	Euploid	———
Squamous metaplasia	4.3 ± 2.2	———	———	Euploid	———
BPH with inflammation	0.66 ± 0.04	2.3–4.3	———	Euploid	———
Nonbacterial prostatitis	1.5 ± 0.08	5.1	———	Euploid	———
Granulomatous prostatitis	2.1 ± 0.3	6.2	———	Euploid	———
AAH	0.66	2.1–3.7	———	(An)Euploid	———
PIN	0.8–1.5	4.3–6.8	6.0–13.8	(An)Euploid	0.47–1.00

Table 5–4. Histologic and Immunohistochemical Characteristics of BPH With and Without Chronic Bacterial Prostatitis

Histologic Appearance	n	Stromal Reaction		
		Lymphocytes	Vimentin	Desmin/Actin
Normal	10	−	+	+
BPH without inflammation	12	+	+	+
BPH with mild inflammation	4	+	+	+
BPH with strong inflammation	6	+ + +	+	+
BPH with stromal nodules, predominantly fibrous	4	+ (T)	+ + +	+
BPH with stromal nodules, predominantly leiomyomatous	6	+	+	+

Staining intensity defined in the range − (absent) to + + + (strong).

Table 5–5. Immunohistochemistry of Normal and Hyperplastic Epithelia of the Prostate Gland

Antibodies	Secretory Cells	Basal Cells	Neuro-endocrine Cells	Antibodies	Secretory Cells	Basal Cells	Neuro-endocrine Cells
PSA	+	−	(+)	Antichymotrypsin	+	−	
PAP	+	−	(+)	Vimentin	(+)	−	
Cytokeratin				SMA (actin)	−	−/(+)	
5, 10, 11	−	+	−	Desmin	−	−	−
13, 14, 16	−	+	−	Serotonin	−	−	+
19	+	+	−	S-100-protein	−	−/(+)	
7, 8, 18	+	−	−	NSE	−	−	+
CEA	+	−	−	Chromogranin A	−	−	+
ABO blood groups	(+)	(+)	−	Calcitonin	−	−	+
Receptors				Somatostatin	−	−	(+)
Androgen	+	(+)	(+)	TSH	−	−	(+)
Estrogen	−	+					
Progesterone	−	+					
Lectins (PNA)	+	+					

Staining intensity defined in the range − (absent) to + (present).
From Helpap B: Atlas der Pathologie Urologischer Tumoren. Berlin: Springer-Verlag, 1993.

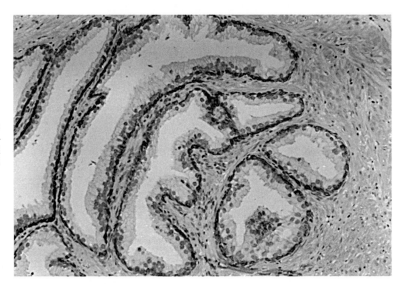

Figure 5–12. Hyperplastic glands of benign prostatic hyperplasia with basal cells labeled by cytokeratin 34β-E12. (ABC method.)

vimentin, desmin, and actin but with indifferent distribution (Table 5–4; see also Table 5–2). The embryonal mesenchymal type does not express any specific antigen but does reveal a strong reaction with Alcian blue. The fibroblastic and fibromuscular types exhibit a positive reaction for vimentin, and the muscular parts of nodules are strongly positive for desmin and actin. S-100 protein and NSE, as well as progesterone and estrogen receptors, are positive in all types of nodules.

The basal cell layer can be delineated by the cytokeratin of high molecular weight (34β-E12) (Fig. 5–12).[26] The expression of prostate-specific antigen (PSA) and prostate-specific acid phosphatase (PAP) is negative in the basal cell layer. The secretory cells exhibit an inverse pattern of PSA and PAP showing strong staining (Fig. 5–13).

Occasionally chromogranin-A– and chromogranin-B–positive neuroendocrine cells are detected between the hyperplastic secretory glandular epithelium. The reaction of cytokeratin of high molecular weight is negative (Table 5–5; Fig. 5–14).[3]

The staining of the basal cell layer by the Cytokeratin 34β-E12 reaction has been found to be an important differential diagnostic index distinguishing between typical hyperplasia (BPH) and atypical adenomatous hyperplasia (AAH) as well as between prostatic intraepithelial neoplasia (PIN) of moderate and severe

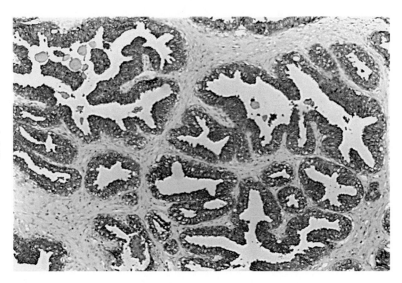

Figure 5–13. Hyperplastic PSA-positive secretory cells of benign prostatic hyperplasia (ABC method.)

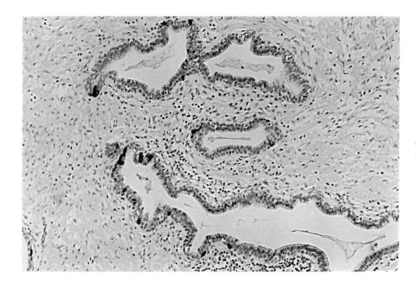

Figure 5–14. Neuroendocrine cells in hyperplastic glands of benign prostatic hyperplasia. (Chromogranin A, ABC method.)

grade and glandular prostate carcinoma (see Chapters 6, 7, and 9). The expression pattern of basal cell cytokeratin becomes more and more patchy with increasing atypia and finally disappears, corresponding to the dissolution of the basal cell layer and the loss of this layer in the case of carcinoma (Figs. 5–15 to 5–17). Basal cell prostatic hyperplasia is characterized by strong cytokeratin expression 34β-E12 with a lack of PSA or PAP staining (see Table 5–5).[26]

Intranuclear estrogen and progesterone receptors (ER, PR) are not found in secretory cells; however, basal cells in hyperplastic prostate may express these receptors. The receptors are found mainly in the periglandular stromal cells.[27] The androgen receptor (AR) is found in the secretory cells and in some basal cells. Neuroendocrine cells are negative for AR (see Table 5–5).[28]

The basal cells are the proliferative compartment of normal and hyperplastic prostatic epithelium (Figs. 5–18 and 5–19; see Table 5–3). Proliferative activity decreases from basal to apical. The basal cells are more heterogeneous than the secretory cells. They express different steroid receptors (e.g., ER, PR, AR), and they may show intermediate forms of differentiation toward AR-responsive secretory cells and AR-negative neuroendocrine cells.[28, 29] Regeneration of secretory cells depends on the presence of responsive progenitor cells in the basal cell layer (stem cells).[29]

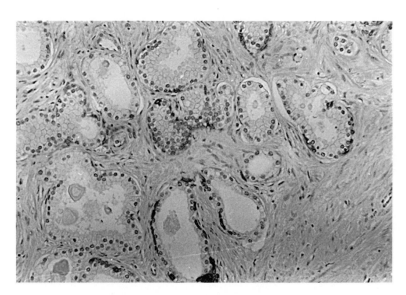

Figure 5–15. Spotted expression of cytokeratin of high molecular weight (34β-E12) in basal cells of atypical adenomatous hyperplasia of the prostate. (ABC method.)

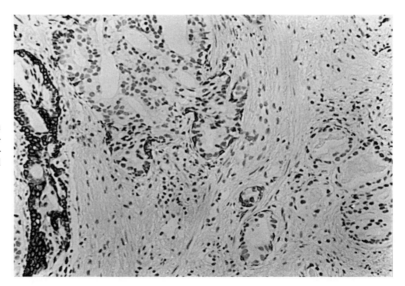

Figure 5–16. Distinct reduction of basal cell staining by cytokeratin of high molecular weight (34β-E12) in prostatic intraepithelial neoplasia. (ABC method.)

Accordingly, abnormal growth of the secretory epithelium in BPH may be related to an increase in the total number of androgenresponsive basal cells. By utilizing the proliferation marker Ki-67 (MIB 1) and/or proliferation cell nuclear antigen (PCNA), proliferating cells can be demonstrated in the basal cell layer of BPH and in basal cell hyperplasia (see Fig. 5–19 and Table 5–3). The range of labeled cells is 0.5% to 4.0%. No MIB 1 or PCNA-positive cells are found in the lumina of ducts or acini. The frequency of apoptotic bodies (cell loss) is very low in epithelial cell layers of the normal and hyperplastic prostate (0.09%–0.6%); however, in BPH after hormonal treatment the frequency of apoptotic bodies is in-creased, in contrast to a decrease of PCNA-positive nuclei of the epithelia.[30] The mitotic activity of basal and secretory cells is very low. The mitotic index increases to values of 0.03% only in glandular cells stimulated by surrounding inflammation. DNA labeling by in vitro incorporation techniques using ^{3}H-thymidine shows labeling indices of cells in hyperplastic glands without inflammation between 0.3% and 0.8%, predominantly among basal cells. In cases of periglandular inflammation as well as in nonbacterial and granulomatous prostatitis, these indices increase up to 0.7%–2.1%. In cases of basal cell hyperplasia, particularly in the postatrophic hyperplasia, the index may rise to 1.6% labeled cells (Fig. 5–20;

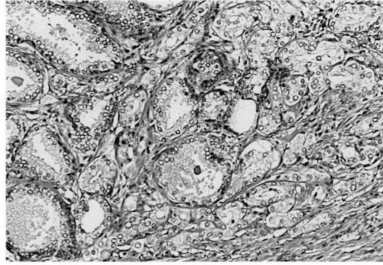

Figure 5–17. Lack of basal cells in highly differentiated glandular carcinoma of the prostate.

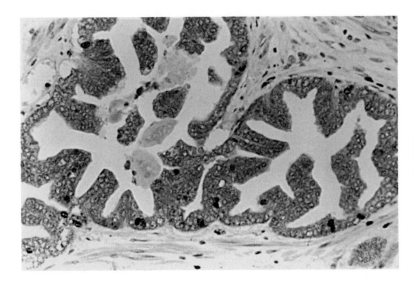

Figure 5–18. Basal cell proliferation labeled by Ki-67/MIB 1 in hyperplastic glands of the prostate with cribriform pattern. (ABC method.)

see Fig. 5–19 and Table 5–3). The stromal cells show no mitotic activity. In immature cell-rich stromal nodules few labeled cells can be demonstrated by Ki-67 antigen. This correlates well with cell kinetic autoradiographic results with ^{3}H-thymidine. Radioactively labeled stromal cells show a labeling index of less than 0.02%.

This pattern does not change significantly in the so-called florid mesenchymal nodule formation (see Fig. 5–19 and Table 5–3).

In the analysis of silver-stained nucleolar organizer regions (AgNOR), the number of AgNORs in glandular epithelium in BPH is higher than in normal prostate tissue (1.7:2.6);

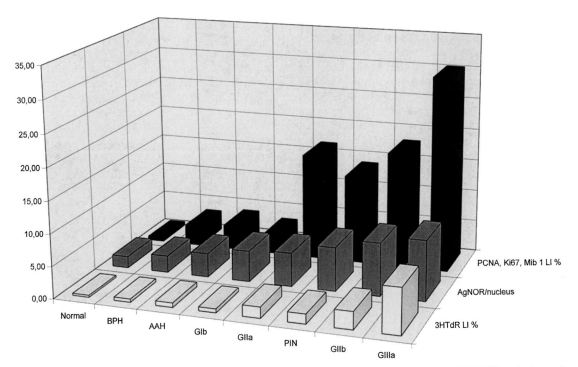

Figure 5–19. Different cell kinetic analyses with autoradiography, immunohistochemistry, and AgNOR technique of normal and hyperplastic prostate tissue, preneoplasias, and carcinomas. PCNA, proliferation cell nuclear antigen labeling index; Ki 67/Mib 1, cell proliferation labeling index; AgNOR, silver stained nuclear organizer region; 3HTdR, tritiated thymidine labeling index; BPH, benign prostatic hyperplasia; AAH, atypical adenomatous hyperplasia; PIN, prostatic intraepithelial neoplasia; GI-GIII; prostatic carcinomas grade of malignancy I-III (WHO). Gleason 1-5.

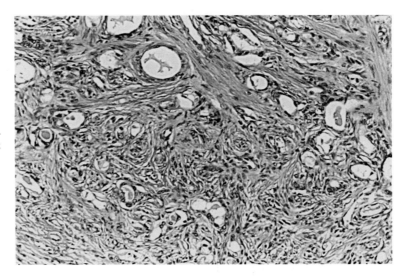

Figure 5–20. Sclerosing adenosis of the prostate with distinct
stromal sclerosis.

(Fig. 5–21). Similar differences exist in the
AgNOR values between normal and hyperplastic stromal cells (1.5:2.1). AgNOR values of
stromal cells in BPH with leiomyomatous and
fibrous nodules are 1.5:2.3. So-called juvenile
nodules are characterized by higher values of
AgNOR. Thus, there is still slightly increased
proliferative activity (see Fig. 5–19 and Table
5–3).

SPECIAL FORMS OF BENIGN
PROSTATIC HYPERPLASIA

Clear Cell and/or
Cribriform Hyperplasia

An abnormal architectural pattern without
cytologic atypia commonly occurs at the base

of the prostate with cribriform formations. If
these abnormal formations lack significant cytologic atypia, they are of no clinical significance since they are frequently seen in entirely
benign prostate glands. Clear cell cribriform
hyperplasia is a pattern that does not appear
to be associated with carcinoma. It is composed of glands with abundant clear cytoplasm
and a nodular growth pattern. The feature of
clear cell cribriform hyperplasia that distinguishes it from carcinoma is a well-defined
basal cell layer in many of the glands. Most
cribriform carcinomas contain nuclear atypia
and are accompanied by small glands of infiltrating cancer, whereas clear cell cribriform
hyperplasia lacks both of these findings (Fig.
5–22).

In some cases of cribriform carcinoma, the

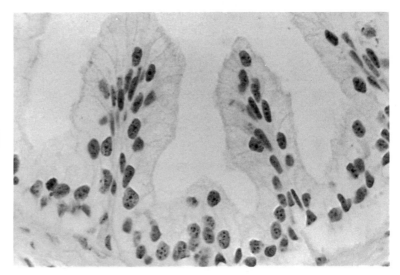

Figure 5–21. AgNOR in nuclei
of basal cells and luminal cells of
BPH. (AgNOR staining.)

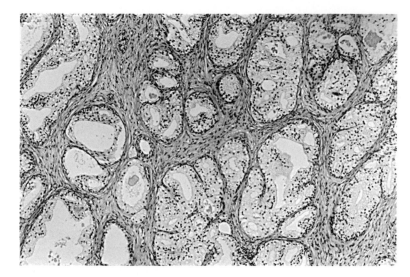

Figure 5–22. Clear cell cribriform hyperplasia of the prostate.

differential diagnosis is very difficult. In the intraductal spreading form of cribriform cancer, the basal cell layer within the ducts may be intact and then the immunohistochemical reaction of 34β-E12 cytokeratin is positive, as in normal or hyperplastic glands with the cribriform pattern (Table 5–6; see Chapters 11 and 15).

Sclerosing Adenosis

A rare variant of adenosis termed "sclerosing adenosis" with infiltrating cords may be mistaken for glandular carcinoma of the prostate (Fig. 5–23; see also Fig. 5–20). Sclerosing adenosis is characterized by irregular-shaped small acinar components with proliferation of glands, compressed tubules, and small round epithelioid cells scattered in loose edematous stromal components within the transition zone. Histologically the lesion resembles an invasive glandular carcinoma, but in contrast a poorly differentiated carcinoma would tend to be much more infiltrative. In sclerosing adenosis, however, the glandular areas with basal cell layers merge with cells without recognizable lumina to solid cords. The nuclear and cytoplasmic features of these cords of cells are cytologically identical to the same features in the cells within the glandular component of sclerosing adenosis. In sclerosing adenosis there is a peculiar stromoglandular relation distinct from that seen in carcinoma. The benign nature of sclerosing adenosis can be verified by immunohistochemistry for cytokeratin. In addition to the presence of cytokeratin (34β-E12) immunoreactivity within the basal cells of the glandular component of sclerosing adenosis, there is also immunoreactivity within the sclerosed tubules of adenosis. Even the spindle cell/epithelioid cell component is pos-

Table 5–6. Prostate Lesions with Cribriform Pattern

| Cribriform Pattern | Immunohistochemistry | | Nucleolar Status | |
	PSA	Cytokeratin 34β-E12	Size	Position Within the Nucleus
BPH	+	+	small	central
Basal cell hyperplasia				
Without atypia	–	+	small	central
With atypia	–	+	moderate	central/eccentric
PIN	+	(+)	prominent solitary	central/eccentric
Carcinoma	+	–	prominent multiple	eccentric

Staining intensity defined in the range − (absent) to + (present).

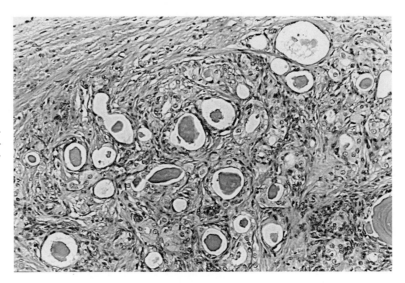

Figure 5–23. Sclerosing adenosis with PAS-positive intraglandular secrete and basal cells and luminal/secretory cells.

itive for cytokeratin 34β-E12, S-100 protein and in some cases even for PSA. This differs from non-neoplastic prostate glands and BPH, in which basal cells lack myoepithelial differentiation. Prostatic glandular carcinomas show no immunoreactivity with cytokeratin 34β-E12, a feature in contrast to the glands containing positive basal cells in sclerosing adenosis (Table 5–7).[31]

Basal Cell Hyperplasia

Small foci of hyperplastic basal cells often occur within hyperplastic acini. Large areas of basal cell hyperplasia appear as closely packed nests and often suggest putative malignancy, especially in the florid stage (Fig. 5–24).[32] Frequently, prominent nucleoli are found within basal cell nuclei. Basal cell hyperplasia is negative with PSA, but the reaction with cytokeratin of high molecular weight (34β-E12) is positive (see Tables 5–5 to 5–7). In contrast to most cases of transition cell metaplasia, basal cell hyperplasia occurs in terminal ducts and acini of peripheral glands. In addition to distinctive antigen expression, basal cell hyperplasia can be differentiated from glandular prostate carcinoma by the uniform configuration of the

Table 5–7. Immunohistochemical Antibody Patterns of Prostate Lesions

Diagnosis/ Cell Type	Cytokeratin Molecular Weight Low M902	Cytokeratin Molecular Weight High 34β-E12	S-100 Protein	SMA	PSA
BPH					
Secretory cells	+ + +	−	−	−	+ + +
Basal cells	+ + +	+ +	−	−	−
BCH	+ + +	+ + +	(+)	−	−
AAH					
Secretory cells	+ + +	−	−	−	+ + +
Basal cells	+ + +	(+) - + +	−	−	−
PIN					
Secretory cells	+ + +	-	−	−	+ +
Basal cells	+ + +	(+) - + +	−	−	−
PC	+ + +	−	−	−	(+) - + + +
SAP					
Scretory cells	+ + +	−	−	−	+ + +
Basal cells/ myoepithelium	+ + +	+ + +	−	−	−

Staining intensity defined in the range − (absent) to + + + (strong).

Key: AAH, atypical adenomatous hyperplasia; BCH, basal cell hyperplasia; BPH, benign prostatic hyperplasia; PC, prostate carcinoma; PIN, prostatic intraepithelial neoplasia; SAP, sclerosing adenosis of the prostate.

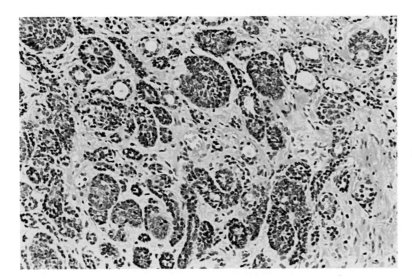

Figure 5–24. Basal cell hyperplasia of the prostate.

epithelial nests and lack of an infiltrative growth pattern. Distinguishing it from the very rare basal cell carcinoma may be difficult. Basal cell carcinoma often produces a desmoplastic stromal response, which is usually absent in benign basal cell hyperplasia and shows perineural invasion.

Postatrophic Hyperplasia

Around the periphery of atrophic parts of prostate glands and mostly in the borderline of dorsoperipheral and anterocentral regions (transition zones), so-called secondary hyperplastic glands can be observed. Atrophic glandular complexes form smaller or larger cysts lined by a single-layer epithelium of flat basal and/or luminal secretory cells (Fig. 5–25). The mitotic and cell kinetics, or immunohistochemical proliferative activity, of atrophic glands is very low. In the case of secondary hyperplasia (so-called postatrophic hyperplasia) in which activated basal cells and secretory cells, often with eosinophilic cytoplasm, occur (Fig. 5–26), proliferative activity increases significantly (see Table 5–3). The surrounding stroma, however, shows no such changes. PSA and PAP can be demonstrated immunohistochemically in the atrophic and postatrophic hyperplastic glands.

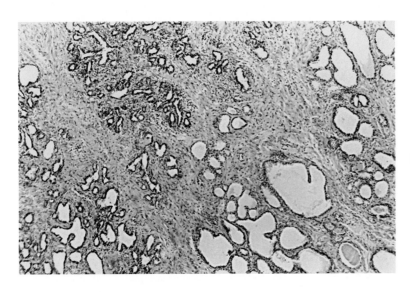

Figure 5–25. Postatrophic hyperplasia of the prostate.

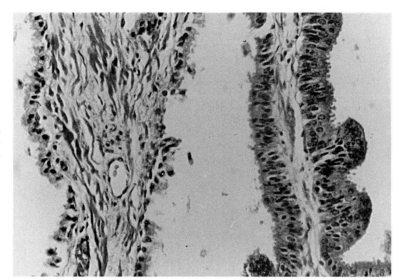

Figure 5–26. Postatrophic hyperplasia of the prostate with activated luminal cells with eosinophilic cytoplasm.

REGRESSIVE CHANGES IN THE HYPERPLASTIC PROSTATE

Infarction

Infarcts of the prostate gland are common and are associated most often with nodular hyperplasia (BPH) (Fig. 5–27). The cause is unknown, but these lesions are thought to be related to vascular compression. Vascular abnormalities have rarely been identified. The infarcts do not exhibit histologic features peculiar to the gland, but the surrounding prostate tissue is frequently the site of squamous or transitional cell metaplasia and can show prostatic glands with high mitotic activity (Fig. 5–28). Patients with prostatic infarcts occasion-

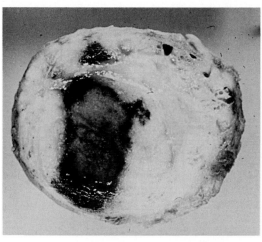

Figure 5–27. Infarction of the prostate.

ally have elevated serum acid phosphatase levels. When this finding is coupled with a highly reactive or metaplastic process, the unwary might be led to misinterpret the findings as carcinoma.

Regressive Changes

Within hyperplastic stromo-glandular regions, regressive changes frequently occur in the prostate. Large and small cystic atrophic glands become lined by a unilayered epithelium with a cuboid pattern. Proliferative activity is very low. Within the periglandular stroma, but also in embryonal-mesenchymal nodules, regressive changes develop very frequently with chronic edema and sclerosis. Alcian blue staining is strongly positive (Fig. 5–29). After long-term anti-inflammatory and antiedema therapy (phytotherapy) this regression may be reversible.[32]

If secondary hyperplasia develops in the atrophic prostate, so-called postatrophic hyperplasia with activated secretory cells showing eosinophilic cytoplasm may be observed (see Figs. 5–25, 5–26). Cellular proliferation and indices continue to increase. While the stroma shows no changes, PSA and PAP expression alter in a manner similar to that in atrophic and postatrophic hyperplastic glands. Immature metaplasia induced by distinct proliferation of basal cells and/or mature squamous metaplasia shows a specific increase of cell proliferation with labeling indices of 4.0% and more. In addition there is an increase of

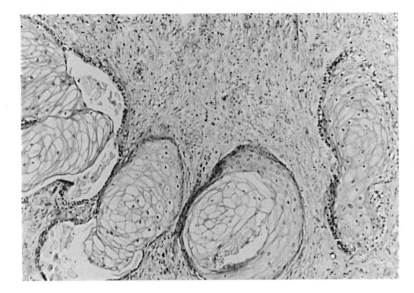

Figure 5–28. Squamous cell metaplasia in neighborhood of infarction of the prostate.

AgNOR in cell nuclei (see Table 5–3). PSA and PAP are not expressed, but the reaction of cytokeratin 34β-E12 is positive. Estrogen receptor staining is positive in squamous metaplasia and in basal cell hyperplasia.

Congestion

Prostatic congestion is a combination of temporary or permanent stasis of secretions together with edematous changes in prostatic tissue. Often this is combined with hyperemia, particularly in the highly vascularized peripheral and subcapsular parts of the prostate. In cases of pure prostate congestion, neither the tissue nor prostatic secretions show evidence of inflammation. This serves as an important diagnostic sign to differentiate from prostatitis, since the clinical pictures of prostatitis and prostatic congestion are often identical. Because of the different therapeutic regimens, however, it is important to distinguish between the two disease entities (e.g., antibiotic treatment in cases of inflammatory prostatitis); (Figs. 5–30, 5–31).

Prostatic congestion is observed mainly in younger patients—between age 20 and 40 years. Because of the typical symptoms it was earlier termed congestive prostatitis or "vegetative adnexitis." It may also be found as congestion associated with other prostatic dis-

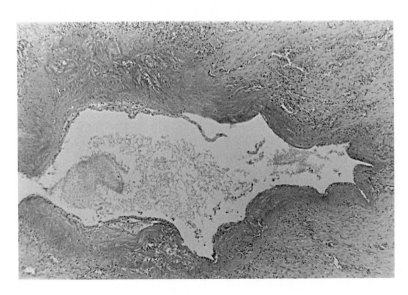

Figure 5–29. Periglandular chronic edema with positive Alcian blue reaction of the stroma.

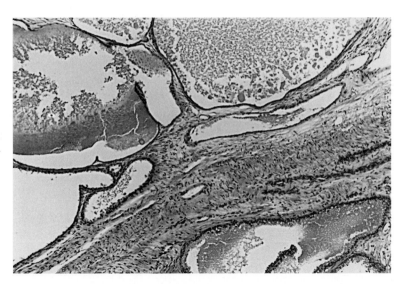

Figure 5–30. Glandular congestion in benign prostatic hyperplasia.

eases, as in cases of acute or chronic prostatitis or in the context of BPH.

The morphologic correlate of prostatic congestion is stasis of secretions in the lumina of glandular acini, which varies in intensity and may lead to the formation of so-called corpora amylacea. These are often found in combination with significant dilatation of lumina and flattening of cylindrical glandular epithelium (Fig. 5–32). Furthermore, edematous changes and myxoid degeneration with Alcian blue–positive reactions are found in the fibromuscular periglandular stroma and within different forms of nodules, as is hyperemia of the peripheral subcapsular venous plexus (Figs. 5–29 and 5–33). Except for small groups of individual (in particular, periglandular) round

cells, no evidence is usually found for acute or chronic inflammatory changes. Both prostatic tissue compartments (glandular and stromal) can be similarly affected by congestive changes. Alternatively, congestive changes may be predominantly glandular or predominantly stromal. In all cases of benign prostatic hyperplasia, predominantly congestive changes are present. These are generally only mild to moderate. Therefore, prostatic congestion is an obligatory phenomenon universally associated with BPH. Congestive changes may be influenced by drug therapy. After phytotherapy, a significant morphologic decrease in congestion can be observed.[32] The cause of prostate congestion might be mechanical compression and blockade of ducts draining the glandular

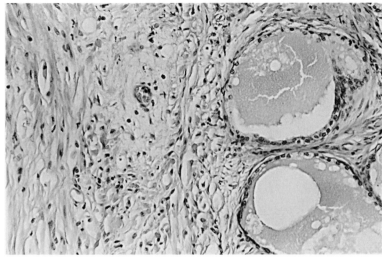

Figure 5–31. Congestive edema in the stroma of benign prostatic hyperplasia.

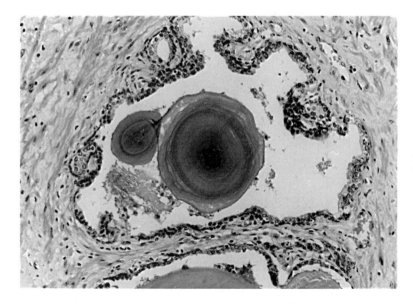

Figure 5–32. Chronic stasis of secretions in the lumina of glands with so-called corpora amylacea.

acini and veins. To what extent other causes such as vegetative functional disturbances, stress, increased sensitivity to cold, nervousness, lack of physical exercise, subvesical obstruction by urethral strictures, blockade of venous drainage in the pelvic area, and spasms of the pelvic floor muscles play a role in prostate congestion is very difficult to determine clinically.[33, 34] Only very little information is available on the morphologic changes after endocrine treatment of BPH. Increased atrophy of secretory cells combined with increased apoptosis (cell loss) may be observed after treatment of BPH with luteinizing hormone–releasing hormone (LHRH) antagonist plus flutamide (see Table 5–3). After hormonal treatment of prostate cancer in a normal or hyperplastic gland increased proliferation of basal cells and squamous metaplasia develop and an atrophy of secretory cells with progressive nuclear pyknosis is observed.[30]

BENIGN PROSTATIC HYPERPLASIA AND INFLAMMATION

In 30% to 50% of hyperplastic prostatic tissue examined histologically, periglandular round cell infiltrates of varying density are found (Fig. 5–34). Occasionally lymph follicles

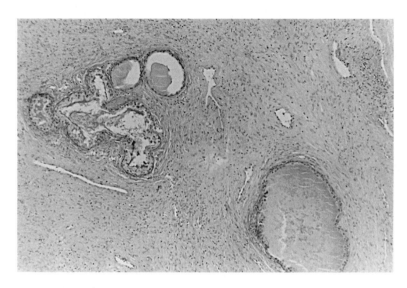

Figure 5–33. Distinct Alcian blue–positive reaction in glandular and stromal prostatic congestion of benign prostatic hyperplasia.

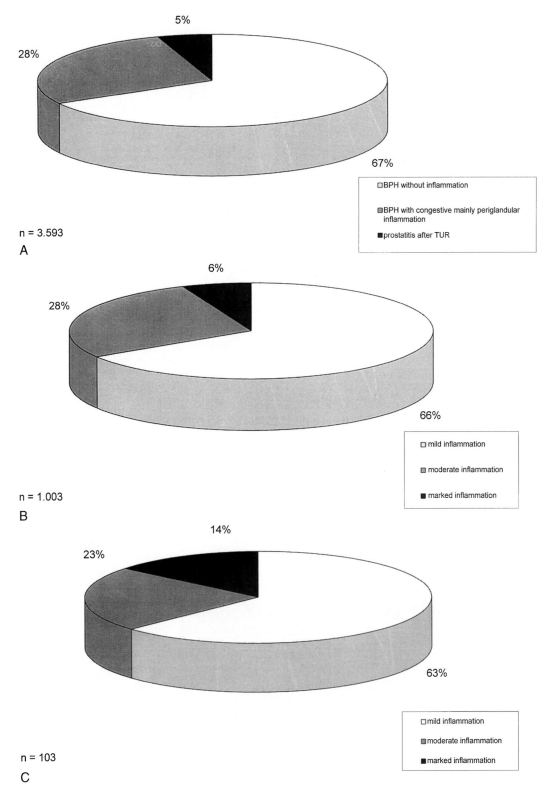

Figure 5–34. *A,* Distribution of benign prostatic hyperplasia with and without prostatitis. *B,* Distribution of mild, moderate, and marked congestive prostatitis. *C,* Distribution of mild, moderate, and marked degrees of inflammation in chronic abacterial prostatitis.

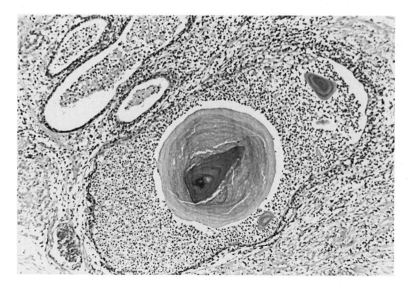

Figure 5–35. Congestive prostatitis in benign prostatic hyperplasia with corpora amylacea.

have formed. In the glandular lumen, macrophages mixed with round cells and polymorphonuclear leukocytes are found. The hyperplastic glandular epithelium is flattened or destroyed. In periglandular areas, round cell infiltrations of varying densities may develop. These loose periglandular round cell infiltrates can, however, be considered an inflammatory concomitant reaction (Figs. 5–35 and 5–36). Stroma and epithelium are activated in the hyperplastic prostate in cases of reactive periglandular round cell infiltration. In cases of nonspecific chronic granulomatous prostatitis with hyperplasia, proliferative indices are found like those seen in cases of chronic prostatitis without hyperplasia (Fig.

5–37). The number of Ki-67–positive proliferative epithelial cells is increased. These are predominantly basal cells that develop a hyperplastic basal cell or squamous epithelial phenotype. The number of AgNORs in BPH with congestive inflammation is increased in glandular epithelial cells and in stromal cells (Figs. 5–38 and 5–39; see Table 5–3).

The inflammatory infiltrate initially comprises a typical mixture of T and B lymphocytes. In advanced stages T lymphocytes predominate (see Table 5–4). Chronic inflammation associated with nodular prostatic hyperplasia is not an independent disease, with the possible exception of acute inflammatory episodes in the context of congestive

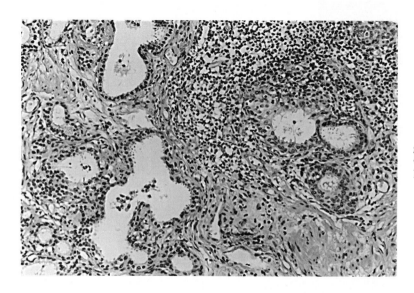

Figure 5–36. Congestive intraglandular and periglandular chronic prostatitis with benign prostatic hyperplasia.

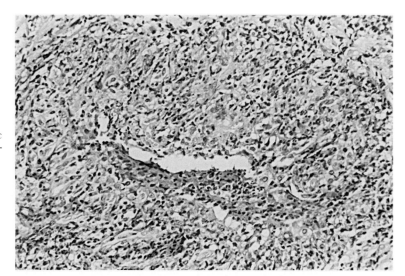

Figure 5–37. Benign prostatic hyperplasia with destructive granulomatous prostatitis.

prostatitis (see Chapter 4). A comparison of the extent of inflammatory infiltrates in BPH prostatitis with chronic recurrent prostatitis without hyperplasia demonstrates that in BPH only minimal periglandular and noncharacteristic cellular infiltrates are seen in 60% to 70% of cases (see Fig. 5–34B, C); therefore the term *prostatitis* does not appear to be justified. BPH prostatitis with moderate or significant cellular infiltrates, the latter already showing glandular destruction, can be characterized as prostatitis; however, this type of BPH prostatitis is seen in 30% of all cases. In cases without evidence of BPH, moderate to severe chronic prostatitis is seen in more than 30% to 40% (Fig. 5–34; see Tables 5–3, 5–4).[35–37]

A longstanding hyperplastic glandular process, and, more importantly, a permanent increase in the proliferation of stromal tissue components, cannot be demonstrated. There is only mild to moderate proliferative activity in cells of the glands and the stroma (Fig. 5–39). The fact that a prerequisite for the development of prostatic hyperplasia is exclusively a chronic destructive prostatitis argues against inflammatory induction of BPH. Prostatectomy specimens of young patients or autopsy specimens without evidence of hyperplasia only very rarely demonstrate inflammatory infiltrates. In this context it is worth mentioning that up to age 40 years, prostatitis is located mainly in the dorsoperipheral gland;

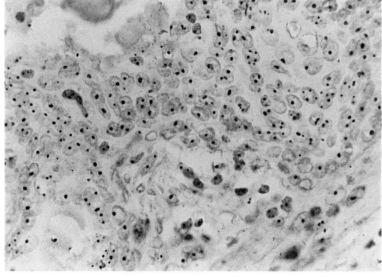

Figure 5–38. Increased number of AgNOR in chronic congestive prostatitis with benign prostatic hyperplasia.

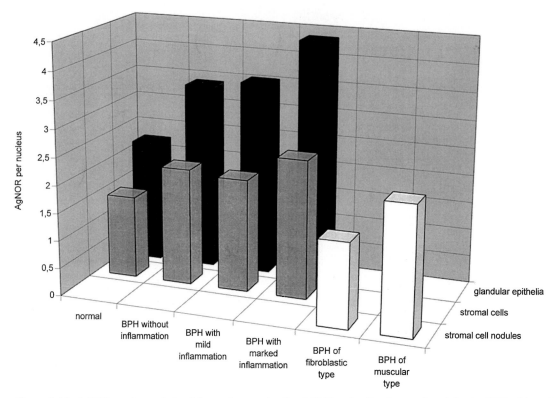

Figure 5–39. AgNOR analyses of glandular and stromal cells of BPH and cells of stromal nodules in BPH, with and without inflammation and diffuse stromal nodules.

only after age 50 is BPH prostatitis found mainly in the central parts (transition zone) of the gland. Moreover, bacteral prostatitis is more often located in atrophic rather than in hyperplastic regions. Finally, the inflammatory infiltrate leads predominantly to destructive, and not to hyperplastic, phenomena. So far, no morphologic evidence has been found to support the theory that stromal or glandular prostatic hyperplasia is induced exclusively by a chronic inflammatory stimulus to the glands. Inflammatory infiltrates in the course of BPH induced by glandular congestion have to be considered a noncharacteristic associated phenomenon; however, this inflammatory reaction may not be confused with T-lymphocyte infiltration of the stromal nodules far from periglandular regions.

TRANSURETHRAL RESECTION PROSTATITIS

Focal prostatitis, which can develop in the residual gland after TURP (Figs. 5–34, 5–40), has a morphologic appearance similar to that of other inflammatory diseases of the prostate.

In addition to necrotic areas with leukocytic infiltrates, which occasionally form abscesses, diffuse or focal lymphocyte or macrophage infiltrates with interspersed polymorphonuclear granulocytes dominate the histologic picture. Much rarer is a predominantly eosinophilic inflammatory infiltrate, as seen in eosinophilic granulomatous or allergic prostatitis.

In common with chronic destructive recurrent and granulomatous prostatitis, T lymphocytes are seen almost exclusively (see Table 5–4). Approximately 7 to 10 days after TURP, and sometimes persisting for several weeks or even months, granulomas rich in macrophages and epithelioid cells with polynuclear giant cells, predominantly of the irregular and occasionally of the regular type, are formed. Frequently these giant cells contain brown pigment that stains positive for iron. These are residual from carbonization of the tissue induced by electrosurgery (Fig. 5–41).

The differential diagnosis during the granulomatous stage with formation of giant cells includes tuberculous prostatitis. This differential diagnosis is particularly difficult if in the post-TURP granuloma small necrotic areas are seen. The exclusive demonstration of Lang-

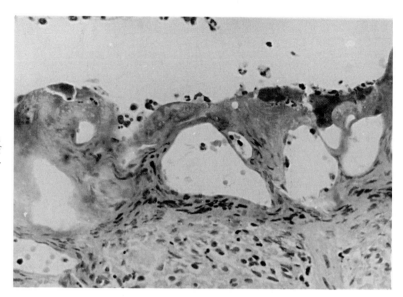

Figure 5–40. Tissue reaction after transurethral resection of the prostate with fresh carbonization.

hans' cells (regular giant cells) and a reaction negative for iron support the diagnosis of tuberculosis. In most cases bacteriologic (and occasionally fluorescence microscopic) demonstration of *Mycobacterium tuberculosis* is possible. Confirmation may now be obtained by PCR technology (see Chapter 4). In both diseases, immunohistochemistry demonstrates T lymphocytes exclusively (Fig. 5–42).[35–38]

BENIGN PROSTATIC HYPERPLASIA AND PROSTATE CARCINOMA

If an advanced, peripherally located glandular prostatic carcinoma grows into the hyperplastic inner parts of the prostate, carcino-matous and hyperplastic glands are seen in close relationship (see Chapter 11). Non-aggressive prostate carcinoma growing peripherally can usually be clearly separated from the hyperplastic glands by the usual histologic staining methods. This differential diagnosis, however, may be difficult in the case of the rare primary anterocentral, very highly differentiated, glandular prostate carcinoma (see Figs. 5–4 and 5–17). The demonstration of a basal cell layer in the hyperplastic glands by the basal cell cytokeratin reaction, and conversely, the lack of these cells from the highly differentiated glandular prostate carcinoma, allow a clear distinction to be made. The expression of estrogen and progesterone in the

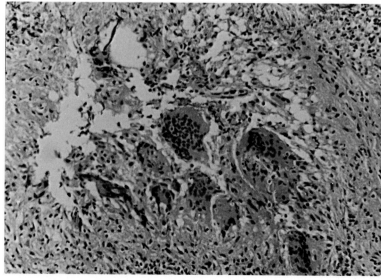

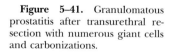

Figure 5–41. Granulomatous prostatitis after transurethral resection with numerous giant cells and carbonizations.

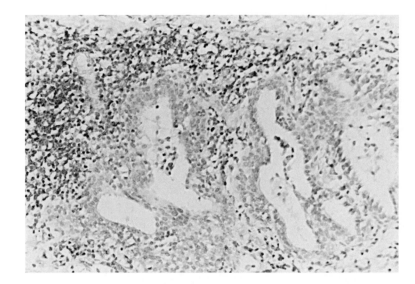

Figure 5–42. Chronic destructive prostatitis with mainly T lymphocytes. (ABC method.)

stroma neighboring the prostate carcinoma is increased.

BENIGN PROSTATIC HYPERPLASIA, ATYPICAL ADENOMATOUS HYPERPLASIA, AND PROSTATIC INTRAEPITHELIAL NEOPLASIA

BPH, AAH, and PIN all represent proliferative processes of the glandular epithelium (see Chapters 6 to 9). Atypical glandular and ductal proliferations of the prostate may be combined with carcinomas but also with BPH without carcinoma. The terms and significances of these atypical lesions, which resemble low- and high-grade carcinoma, are in discussion.[18, 19, 39–42] For the atypical lesion in the anterocentral and/or transition zone of the prostate the terms *atypical adenomatous hyperplasia* (AAH) and in the dorsoperipheral zone of the prostate *prostatic intraepithelial neoplasia* (PIN) are now in use.[43]

AAH is characterized by newly formed microglandular structures with partly incomplete basal cells and secretory cells with different grades of cellular, nuclear, and nucleolar atypias at the border of BPH nodules. The histologic and cytologic patterns are often very similar to those of microglandular carcinoma of low malignancy. One finding is important in differential diagnosis: if the basal cell layer is absent, this lesion corresponds to carcinoma. If the basal cell layer is fragmented, the diagnosis is AAH (Fig. 5–43; see Fig 5–15).[43–45] The morphologic characteristics of, and diagnostic

criteria for, intraepithelial neoplasia are discussed fully in Chapter 6.

CLASSIFICATION AND NOMENCLATURE OF PROSTATIC HYPERPLASIA

Although diagnosis of prostatic hyperplasia may be established, almost conclusively, by clinical tests, morphology may reveal surprises. Atypical formations in the hyperplastic prostate glands and incidental carcinoma are found with a frequency of between 8% and 10%. The importance of proliferative processes has led to a number of different names. The terms *hypertrophy* and *adenoma* are commonly utilized in clinical context. However, since the hyperplastic process is morphologically documented by means of cell kinetics, by DNA cytometry, and immunohistochemically, the terms *hypertrophy* and *adenoma* should no longer be used.

Kastendieck[46] divided primary hyperplasia into several subgroups—namely, *immature, mature, nodular,* and *diffuse* forms—and separated the subgroups from a primary atypical hyperplasia and from the secondary (postatrophic) hyperplasia.[46] Special entities are the dysplasia and the "borderline lesion."

The classification devised by Elbadawi[47] is based on extensive histologic studies. He separated nodular paraurethral stromal-glandular hyperplasia from ductal hyperplasia and distinguished secondary postatrophic hyperplasia from metaplasia. In his staging system, the

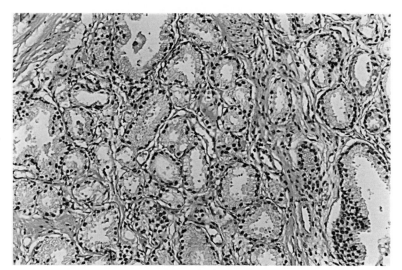

Figure 5–43. Atypical adenomatous hyperplasia of the prostate.

atypia in the stromal and the glandular parts of the gland in juvenile hyperplasia, after prostate infarction, inflammation, and basal cell reaction, are listed separately, as is the atypia in the case of the cribriform median lobe hyperplasia. The World Health Organization (WHO) classification distinguishes nodular hyperplasia and other hyperplasia forms in postatrophic, secondary, and basal cell hyperplasia.[48] In an earlier categorization primary atypical hyperplasia was listed together with primary prostatic glandular and stromal hyperplasia.

Dhom distinguishes among primary hyperplasia, atrophy, and metaplasia. Under the term *primary hyperplasia,* simple hyperplasia, adenomatous small glandular, cribriform, and papillary hyperplasia are summarized.[49] Under *atrophy,* simple atrophy, cystic atrophy, and postatrophic nodular hyperplasia are grouped. For clinicopathologic purposes the following grouping taken from the staging system according to Mostofi (WHO) has been found valuable:[48]

Benign prostatic glandular and stromal hyperplasia (BPH), including the special forms:
BPH and sclerosing adenosis
BPH with basal cell hyperplasia
BPH with secondary hyperplasia/postatrophic hyperplasia/atrophy-associated glandular hyperplasia
BPH and AAH.

REFERENCES

1. Aumüller G, Goebel HW, Bacher M, et al.: Current aspects of prostatic structure and function. Verh Dtsch Ges Pathol 77:1–18, 1993.
2. McNeal JE: Normal histology of prostate. Am J Surg Pathol 12:619–633, 1988.
3. Schmid KW, Helpap B, Tötsch M, et al.: Secretogranin II in normal hyperplastic and neoplastic prostate. Histopathology 24:233–239, 1994.
4. Aumüller G: Benign prostatic hyperplasia: Mechanisms and hypotheses. Urologe A 31:159–165, 1992.
5. Krieg M, Weisser H, Tunn S: Metabolism of androgens and estrogens in the human benign prostatic hyperplasia (BPH). Verh Dtsch Ges Pathol 77:19–24, 1993.
6. Aumüller G: Morphologic and regulatory aspects of prostatic function. Anat Embryol 179:519–531, 1989.
7. Harper ME, Goddard L, Glynne-Jones E, et al.: An immunocytochemical analysis of TGF-α expression in benign and malignant prostatic tumors Prostate 23:9–23, 1993.
8. Yang Y, Chisholm GD, Habib FK: Epidermal growth factor and transforming growth factor alpha concentrations in BPH and cancer of the prostate: Their relationships with tissue androgen levels. Br J Cancer 67:152–155, 1993.
9. Jones EG, Harper ME: Studies on the proliferation, secretory activities, and epidermal growth factor receptor expression in benign prostatic hyperplasia explant cultures. Prostate 20:133–149, 1992.
10. Story MT, Hopp KA, Meier D, et al.: Influence of transforming growth factor beta 1 and other growth factors on basic fibroblast growth factor, level and proliferation of cultured human prostate-derived fibroblasts. Prostate 22:183–197, 1993.
11. Gleason PE, Jones EA, Regan JS, et al.: Platelet derived growth factor (PDGF), androgens and inflammation: possible etiologic factors in the development of prostatic hyperplasia. J Urol 149:1586–1592, 1993.
12. Cunha GR: Epithelio-mesenchymal interactions in primordial gland structures which become responsive to androgenic stimulation. Anat Rec 172:179–196, 1972.
13. Cunha GR, Chung LWK, Shannon JM, et al.: Stromal epithelial interactions in sex differentiation. Biol Reprod 22:19–42, 1980.
14. Cunha GR, Shannon JM, Neubauer BL, et al.: Mesenchymal-epithelial interaction in sex differentiation. Hum Genet 58:68–77, 1981.
15. Cunha GR, Donjacour AA, Sugimura Y: Stromal-epithelial interactions and heterogeneity of proliferative

activity within the prostate. Biochem Cell Biol 64:608–614, 1986.

16. Theyer G, Kramer G, Assmann I, et al.: Phenotypic characterization of infiltrating leucocytes in benign prostatic hyperplasia (BPH). Lab Invest 1:96–106, 1992.

17. Steiner G, Gessl A, Kramer G, et al.: Phenotype and function of peripheral and prostatic lymphocytes in patients with benign prostatic hyperplasia (BPH). J Urol 151:480–484, 1994.

18. Bostwick DG, Amin MB, Dundore P, et al.: Architectural patterns of high-grade prostatic intraepithelial neoplasia. Hum Pathol 24:298–301, 1993.

19. Bostwick DG, Srigley J, Grignon D, et al.: Atypical adenomatous hyperplasia of prostate: Morphologic criteria for its distinction from well-differentiated carcinoma. Hum Pathol 24:819–832, 1993.

20. Rohr HP, Bartsch G: Stereological analysis. An approach to the pathogenesis of benign prostatic hyperplasia. In: Hinman F (ed): Benign Prostatic Hypertrophy. Berlin: Springer Verlag, 1983, pp 112–129.

21. Bartsch G, Rohr H-P: Stereology—a new method to assess normal and pathological growth of the prostate. In: Jacobi E, Hohenfellner R (eds): Prostate Cancer. International Perspectives in Urology, 3. Baltimore: Williams & Wilkins, 1982, pp 433–459.

22. Franks LM: Benign nodular hyperplasia of the prostate: A review. Ann Roy Coll Surg Engl 14:92–106, 1954.

23. Vogel J, Bierhoff E, Pfeifer U, et al.: Modern considerations and investigations in benign prostatic hyperplasia (BPH). In: Vahlensieck W, Rutishauser G (eds): Benign Prostate Diseases. Stuttgart: Thieme, 1992, pp 98–104.

24. Benz M, Giefer T, Bierhoff E, et al.: Morphological classification and comparison of the different types of stromal nodules in benign prostatic hyperplasia. Verh Dtsch Ges Pathol 77:111–116, 1993.

25. Helpap B: Anatomy and physiology of the prostate and pathological anatomy and pathophysiology of the benign prostate hyperplasia (BPH). In: Sökeland J. (ed): Stuttgart: Thieme 1995, pp 3.1–3.27.

26. Hedrick L, Epstein J: Use of keratin 903 as an adjunct in the diagnosis of prostate carcinoma. Am J Surg Pathol 13:389–396, 1989.

27. Wernert N, Gerdes J, Loy V, et al.: Investigations of the estrogen (ER-ICA test) and the progesterone receptor in the prostate and prostatic carcinoma on immunohistochemical basis. Virchows Arch A 412:387–391, 1988.

28. Bonkhoff H, Remberger K: Widespread distribution of nuclear androgen receptors in the basal cell layer of the normal and hyperplastic human prostate. Virchows Arch A 422:35–38, 1993.

29. Bonkhoff H, Remberger K: Differentiation pathways and histogenetic aspects of normal and abnormal prostate growth: a stem cell model. Prostate 28:98–106, 1996.

30. Montironi R, Muzzonigro G, Magi Galluzzi C, et al.: Effect of LHRH agonist and flutamide (combination endocrine therapy) on the frequency and location of proliferating cell nuclear antigen and apoptotic bodies in prostatic hyperplasia. J Urol Pathol 2:161–171, 1994.

31. Sakamoto N, Tsuneyoshi M, Enjoji M: Sclerosing adenosis of the prostate, histopathologic and immunohistochemical analysis. Am J Surg Pathol 15:660–667, 1991.

32. Helpap B, Oehler U, Weisser H, et al.: Morphology of benign prostatic hyperplasia after treatment with the sabal extract IDS 89 (Strogen) or placebo. Results of a prospective, randomized, double-blind trial. J Urol Pathol 3:175–182, 1995.

33. Bierhoff E, Vogel J, Vahlensieck W: Prostatic congestion associated with benign prostatic hyperplasia (BPH) In: Vahlensieck W, Rutishauser G (eds): Benign Prostate Diseases. Stuttgart: Thieme, 1992, pp 105–108.

34. Helpap B: Pathology of benign prostatic hyperplasia (BPH). In: Vahlensieck W, Rutishauser G (eds): Benign Prostate Diseases. Stuttgart: Thieme, 1992, pp 84–97.

35. Helpap B: Pathology of chronic non-specific prostatitis. In: Vahlensieck W, Rutishauser G (eds): Benign Prostate Diseases. Stuttgart: Thieme, 1992, pp 33–48.

36. Helpap B: Histological and immunohistochemical study of chronic prostatic inflammation with and without benign prostatic hyperplasia. J Urol Pathol 2:49–64, 1994.

37. Helpap B, Vogel J: TUR-prostatitis. Histological and immunohistochemical observations on a special type of granulomatous prostatitis. Pathol Res Pract 181:301–307, 1986.

38. McNeal JE, Villers A, Redwine EA, et al.: Microcarcinoma in the prostate. Its association with duct-acinar dysplasia. Hum Pathol 22:644–652, 1991.

39. Brawer MK: Prostatic intraepithelial neoplasia: A premalignant lesion. Hum Pathol 23:242–248, 1982.

40. Amin MB, RO JY, Ayala G: Putative precursor lesions of prostatic adenocarcinoma: Fact or fiction? Mod Pathol 6:476–483, 1993.

41. Weinstein MH, Epstein JI: Significance of high grade prostatic intraepithelial neoplasia on needle biopsy. Hum Pathol 24:624–629, 1993.

42. Helpap B, Bostwick DG, Montironi R: The significance of prostatic intraepithelial neoplasia (PIN) and atypical adenomatous hyperplasia (AAH) for the development of prostate carcinoma. An update. Virchows Arch Pathol 426:425–434, 1995.

43. Epstein JI: Adenosis vs atypical adenomatous hyperplasia of the prostate. Am J Surg Pathol 18:1070–1071, 1994.

44. Gaudin PB, Epstein JI: Adenosis of the prostate. Histologic features in transurethral resection specimens. Am J Surg Pathol 18:863–870, 1994.

45. Bostwick DG: Prostatic intraepithelial neoplasia (PIN). Current concepts. J Cell Biochem 16 H:10–19, 1992.

46. Kastendieck H: Ultrastructural pathology of the human prostatic gland. Prog Pathol 106:1–167, 1977.

47. Elbadawi A: Benign proliferative lesions of the prostate gland. In: Spring-Mills E, Hafez ESE (eds): Male accessory sex glands: Biology and pathology. Amsterdam: Elsevier, 1980, 387–408.

48. Mostofi FK, Sesterhenn J, Sobin LH: Histological Typing of Prostate Tumours. International Histological Classification of Tumours. No 22. Geneva, World Health Organization, 1980.

49. Dhom G: Prostata. In: Doerr W, Seifert G (eds): Pathologie des männlichen Genitale Bd 21 Spezielle pathologische Anatomie. Berlin: Springer, 1991, pp 455–642.

6

PROSTATIC INTRAEPITHELIAL NEOPLASIA

DAVID G. BOSTWICK and WAEL SAKR

The search for the precursor of prostatic adenocarcinoma has in recent years focused on the spectrum of histopathologic changes referred to as *prostatic intraepithelial neoplasia* (PIN).[1] PIN is characterized by cellular proliferation within preexisting ducts and acini with cytologic changes that mimic cancer, including nuclear and nucleolar enlargement. It coexists with cancer in more than 85% of cases but retains an intact or fragmented basal cell layer, unlike cancer, which lacks a basal cell layer.[2-4] The clinical importance of recognizing PIN is based on its strong association with prostate carcinoma. PIN has high predictive value as a marker for adenocarcinoma, and its identification in biopsy specimens of the prostate warrants further search for concurrent invasive carcinoma. Studies to date have not determined whether PIN remains stable, regresses, or progresses, although the implication is that it can progress. In this chapter we describe the diagnostic criteria, differential diagnosis, and clinical significance of PIN, as well as the substantial and growing body of evidence that links PIN and cancer.

DIAGNOSTIC CRITERIA

PIN refers to the putative precancerous (dysplastic) end of the morphologic continuum of cellular proliferations within prostatic ducts, ductules, and acini.[2, 4] The term PIN, introduced in 1987, was endorsed by consensus at a 1989 international conference to replace other appellations used in the literature for the same lesion, including *intraductal dysplasia, large acinar atypical hyperplasia, hyperplasia with malignant change, marked atypia,* and *duct-acinar dysplasia.* This consensus group also proposed that PIN be divided into two grades (low-grade and high-grade) to replace the previous three-grade system (Table 6–1).[2, 5-9] (PIN 1 is considered low-grade and PIN 2 and 3 high-grade lesions.)

In low-grade PIN, the epithelium lining ducts and acini are heaped up, crowded, and irregularly spaced, and marked variation in nuclear size is evident (Fig. 6–1).Elongate hyperchromatic nuclei and small nucleoli are also present but are not prominent. Criteria for the diagnosis of PIN include a combination of cytologic and architectural features, and lesions displaying some but not all features are considered atypical but not neoplastic. Some pathologists prefer not to report low-grade PIN, recognizing the difficulty in separating this lesion from benign epithelium and reactive atypia.

There are four architectural patterns of high-grade PIN: tufting, micropapillary, cribiform, and flat (Figs. 6–2, 6–3).[10] The tufting pattern, the most common, is present in at least 97% of totally embedded radical prostatectomy specimens with PIN and cancer, although most cases have multiple patterns.

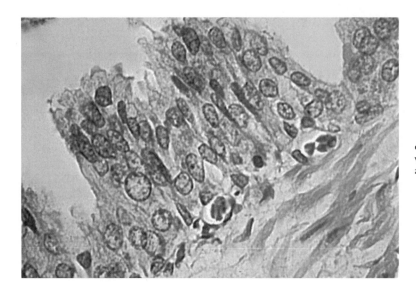

Figure 6–1. Low-grade PIN. The epithelium is proliferative, with variation in nuclear size, shape, and spacing.

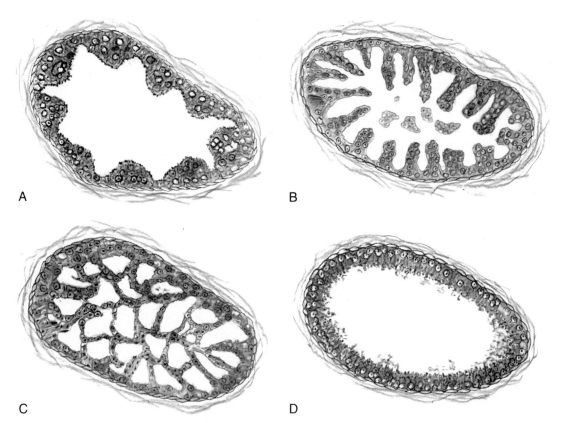

Figure 6–2. Architectural patterns of high-grade PIN. *A,* Tufting pattern; *B,* Micropapillary pattern; *C,* Cribriform pattern; *D,* Flat pattern. (From Bostwick DG, Amin MB, Dundore P, et al.: Architectural patterns of high-grade prostatic intraepithelial neoplasia. Hum Pathol 24:298–310, 1993.)

Table 6–1. Prostatic Intraepithelial Neoplasia (PIN): Diagnostic Criteria

Feature	Low-Grade PIN (Formerly PIN 1)	High-Grade PIN (Formerly PIN 2 and 3)
Architecture	Epithelial cell crowding and stratification, with irregular spacing	Similar to low-grade PIN; more crowding and stratification; four patterns: tufting, micropapillary, cribriform, flat
Cytology		
Nuclei	Enlarged, with marked size variation	Enlarged; some size and shape variation
Chromatin	Normal	Increased density and clumping
Nucleoli	Rarely prominent	Occasionally to frequently large and prominent, similar to invasive carcinoma; sometimes multiple
Basal cell layer	Intact	May show some disruption
Basement membrane	Intact	Intact

From Bostwick DG: High-grade prostatic intraepithelial neoplasia. Cancer 75:1823–1836, 1995.

There are no recognized prognostic differences between the architectural patterns of high-grade PIN, and their recognition appears to have only diagnostic utility. Foci of PIN with solid luminal epithelial proliferation (solid pattern of PIN) and luminal necrosis (comedo pattern of PIN) are very rare in untreated prostates.

At low power, acini with PIN usually appear hyperchromatic owing to proliferation and crowding of the inner layer of cells lining lumina (secretory cell layer). The acini are medium sized or large, with smoothly sculpted, rounded contours similar to those in "benign" glands with which they are usually admixed. Foci of PIN usually involve single glands or small lobular clusters of glands but may be more extensive. The basal cell layer at the periphery is usually inconspicuous and may be difficult to appreciate by routine light

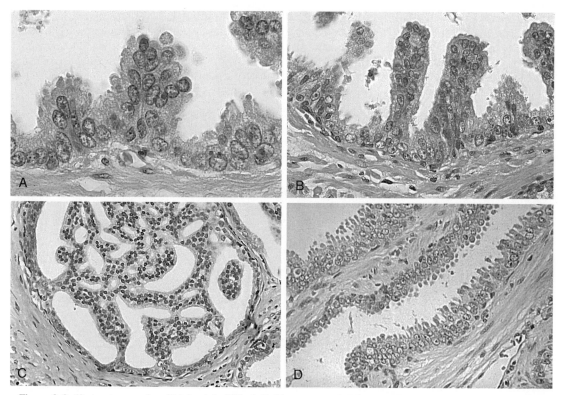

Figure 6–3. Photomicrographs of high-grade PIN. *A,* Tufting pattern; *B,* Micropapillary pattern; *C,* Cribriform pattern; *D,* Flat pattern.

microscopic examination; rarely, it is prominent at low power and partially or completely encircles glands containing PIN.

At medium and high power, crowding and heaping up of the secretory cell layer of PIN is pronounced, in marked contrast with most "benign" acini. The presence of partial acinar involvement is particularly helpful, as this rarely (if ever) occurs with other lesions. Overlapping nuclei are prominent, and cell borders are usually inapparent. Along the luminal surface, the cells often display cytoplasmic blebs reminiscent of apocrine secretion, and this is present regardless of architectural pattern but is not a constant feature and may be subtle. The most striking cytologic findings are nuclear and nucleolar enlargement, diagnostic hallmarks of high-grade PIN. The nuclei are usually uniformly enlarged in the most severe foci of high-grade PIN, although some may be shrunken and hyperchromatic, probably representing degenerative changes; in less severe foci of high-grade PIN (formerly PIN grade 2), greater variability in nuclear size is observed, but some markedly enlarged forms are present. Nucleoli may be single or multiple and are often eccentric or apposed to the chromatinic rim.

PIN spreads in three different patterns, similar to prostate carcinoma.[1, 11] In the first pattern, neoplastic cells replace the normal luminal secretory epithelium, and the basal cell layer and basement membrane are preserved (Fig. 6–4). Foci of high-grade PIN are usually indistinguishable by routine light microscopy from ductal spread of carcinoma. In the second pattern, direct invasion through the ductal or acinar wall is observed, with disruption of the basal cell layer. In the third pattern, neoplastic cells invaginate between the basal cell layer and columnar secretory cell layer ("pagetoid spread"), a very rare finding. Crystalloids are occasionally present in high-grade PIN, but only rarely are prominent. Luminal mucin is sometimes abundant. Unusual findings in PIN include corpora amylacea and mucinous metaplasia.

DIFFERENTIAL DIAGNOSIS

The differential diagnosis includes benign conditions such as lobular atrophy, post-atrophic hyperplasia, atypical basal cell hyperplasia, cribriform hyperplasia, and metaplastic changes associated with radiation, infarction, and prostatitis (Table 6–2). Many of these mimics display architectural and cytologic atypia, including nucleolomegaly, and caution is warranted in interpreting scant specimens, cauterized or distorted specimens, and specimens submitted with incomplete patient history. Malignant mimics include the cribriform pattern of adenocarcinoma, ductal (endometrioid) carcinoma, and urothelial carcinoma involving prostatic ducts and glands.

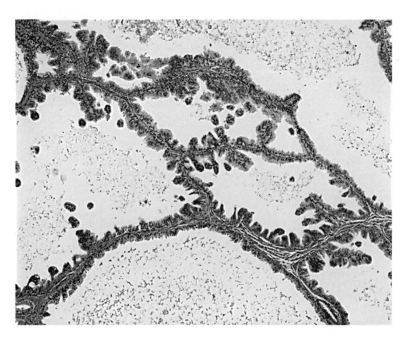

Figure 6–4. High-grade PIN shows extensive involvement of large cystic spaces. This is an unusual pattern of involvement.

Table 6–2. Prostatic Intraepithelial Neoplasia:
Differential Diagnosis

Normal anatomic structures and embryonic rests
    Seminal vesicles and ejaculatory ducts
    Cowper's glands
    Paraganglionic tissue
    Mesonephric remnants
    Ectopic prostatic tissue of the urethra
Hyperplasia
    Benign epithelial hyperplasia
    Cribriform hyperplasia (including clear cell
      hyperplasia)
    Atypical basal cell hyperplasia
    Postatrophic hyperplasia
    Simple lobular atrophy
    Sclerosing adenosis
Metaplasia and reactive changes
    Urothelial metaplasia
    Infarction-induced atypia
    Inflammation-induced atypia
    Radiation-induced atypia
    Nephrogenic metaplasia of the prostatic
      urethra
Carcinoma
    Acinar adenocarcinoma
    Urothelial dysplasia and carcinoma
    Cribriform pattern of prostatic
      adenocarcinoma
    Ductal (endometrioid) prostatic
      adenocarcinoma

From Bostwick DG: High-grade prostatic intraepithelial neoplasia. Cancer 75:1823–1836, 1995.

CLINICAL EVALUATION AND SIGNIFICANCE

The clinical importance of recognizing PIN is based on its strong association with prostate carcinoma. Because PIN has high predictive value as a marker for adenocarcinoma, its identification in biopsy specimens warrants further search for concurrent invasive carcinoma. This is particularly true for high-grade PIN; if this lesion is identified, close surveillance and follow-up biopsy are indicated.

To examine the predictive value of high-grade PIN, Davidson and colleagues conducted a retrospective case-control study of biopsy in 100 patients with high-grade PIN and 112 without PIN matched for clinical stage, age, and serum prostate-specific antigen (PSA). Adenocarcinoma was identified in 36% of subsequent biopsies from cases with PIN, as compared with 13% in the control group (Fig. 6–5). The likelihood of finding cancer was greater in patients with PIN who submitted to more than one follow-up biopsy (44%) than in those with only one biopsy (32%). High-grade PIN, patient age, and serum PSA concentration were jointly highly significant predictors of cancer; PIN was associated with the highest risk ratio (14.93; 95% confidence intervals, 5.6 to 39.8). No other candidate predictor was found to be significant, including patient's race, digital rectal examination findings, transrectal ultrasound results, amount of PIN on biopsy, and architectural pattern of PIN.

Others have reported high predictive value for PIN for cancer (Table 6–3).[13–16] In one study of 37 patients with PIN identified on needle core biopsy, 14 (38%) had carcinoma identified on subsequent biopsy within 8 years.[14] Carcinoma was observed in 39% of 104 follow-up aspiration biopsies of patients with an original diagnosis of high-grade PIN, and an additional 35% had recurrent PIN.[17] Given the clinical suspicion of cancer and negative aspiration biopsy, follow-up aspiration of 48 patients revealed PIN in 15 (31%) and invasive carcinoma in 8 (17%). Another study of PIN diagnosed by fine-needle aspiration revealed that 13 of 32 patients with high-grade PIN developed cancer as compared with 3 of 23 who had low-grade PIN; the patients were followed for 18 months with repeat biopsy.[8] These data underscore the strong association

Table 6–3. Clinical Follow-up of High-Grade Prostatic Intraepithelial Neoplasia

Investigator	Cases (N)	Cancer on Follow-up (No %)	Follow-up* (yr)
Brawer et al.[13]	21	12 (57)†	Immediate 2nd biopsy
Weinstein et al.[16]	19‡	10 (53)	Immediate 2nd biopsy
Davidson et al.[12]	100	33 (33)	≤ 4
Markham[8]	32	13 (41)	≤ 1½
Berner et al.[14]	37	14 (38)	≤ 8

*Interval from diagnosis of PIN to repeat biopsy.
†Includes cases with low-grade *and* high-grade PIN.
‡Of 33 cases presented, 19 had PIN without cancer on first biopsy.
From Bostwick DG: High-grade prostatic intraepithelial neoplasia. Cancer 75:1823–1836, 1995.

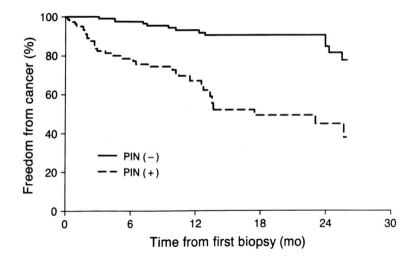

Figure 6–5. Freedom from cancer from time of first biopsy according to the presence or absence of high-grade PIN. (From Davidson D, Bostwick DG, Qian J, et al.: Prostatic intraepithelial neoplasia is a risk factor for adenocarcinoma: Predictive accuracy in needle biopsies. J Urol 154: 1295–1299, 1995.)

of PIN and adenocarcinoma and indicate that vigorous diagnostic follow-up is needed.

High-grade PIN is encountered in as many as 16% of contemporary18-gauge needle biopsies (Fig. 6–6).[18] When PIN is encountered in prostate specimens, all tissue should be embedded and made available for examination; serial sections of suspicious foci may be useful. Antikeratin antibodies such as 34β-E12 (high–molecular weight keratin) may be used to stain tissue sections for the presence of basal cells,

recognizing that PIN retains an intact or fragmented basal cell layer whereas cancer does not (see below). Unfortunately, needle biopsy specimens often fail to show the suspicious focus on deeper concentrations, precluding assessment by immunohistochemistry and compounding the diagnostic dilemma.

Biopsy remains the definitive method for detecting PIN and early invasive cancer, but noninvasive methods are being evaluated. By transrectal ultrasound, PIN may be hypo-

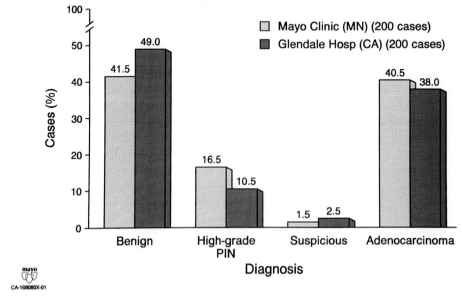

Figure 6–6. Comparative incidence of findings in 200 consecutive needle biopsies from Mayo Clinic (MN) and Glendale Hospital (CA). There is no significant difference in the incidence of benign findings (including low-grade PIN), high-grade PIN, atypical small acinar proliferation suspicious for malignancy, and adenocarcinoma between the two institutions (Data from Bostwick DG, Qian J, Frankel K: The incidence of high grade prostatic intraepithelial neoplasia in needle biopsies. J Urol 154:1791–1794, 1995.)

echoic, indistinguishable from carcinoma, although these findings have been refuted.[19, 20] Transrectal ultrasound-directed biopsy allows localization of the needle and tissue being sampled. If the first attempt is unrevealing some authors suggest repeat biopsy. If all procedures fail to identify carcinoma, close surveillance and follow-up are indicated. Follow-up is suggested at 3-month intervals for 2 years, and thereafter at 12-month intervals for life.[11]

The pathologist must understand the criteria for separating PIN from benign and malignant mimics and should report the presence, severity, and extent of these lesions. Most authors agree that the identification of PIN should not influence or dictate therapeutic decisions. Interobserver agreement on high-grade PIN is "good to excellent," whereas that for low-grade PIN may be too great to justify its diagnostic use.[21, 22] We continue to report low-grade PIN despite this concern, recognizing that this is for research purposes.

PIN also offers promise as an intermediate end point in studies of chemoprevention of prostate carcinoma. Recognizing the slow growth rate of prostate cancer and the considerable amount of time needed in animal and human studies for adequate follow-up, the noninvasive precursor lesion PIN is a suitable intermediate histologic marker to indicate high likelihood of subsequent cancer.[23]

EVIDENCE LINKING PROSTATIC INTRAEPITHELIAL NEOPLASIA AND CANCER

Incidence and Extent of PIN and Cancer Increase with Patient Age

The incidence and extent of PIN appear to increase with age, according to most studies (Fig. 6–7).[6, 19, 24–26] The prevalence of PIN with-cancer in prostates increases with age, predating the onset of carcinoma by more than 5 years.[6] Lee and associates studied 256 ultrasound-guided biopsies of hypoechoic lesions of the prostate and identified 103 cancers and 27 cases of PIN; the mean age of those with PIN (65 years) was significantly lower than that of those with cancer (70 years).[19] The extent (volume) of high-grade PIN increases with patient age, according to a series of 195 radical prostatectomies for cancer.[24]

In a series of recent reports, Sakr and colleagues at Wayne State University described the age distribution of latent prostate cancer and PIN in autopsy prostates obtained in collaboration with the Wayne County Medical Examiner's Office. Intact glands were obtained within 24 hours of death from black and white men over 20 years of age. Following thorough step sectioning and microscopic examination, they showed that carcinoma and

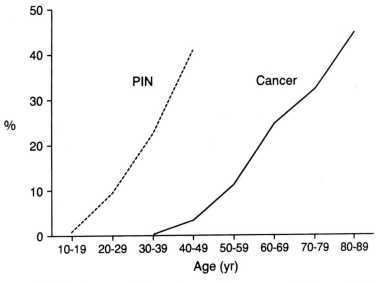

Figure 6–7. Frequency of PIN and cancer with increasing age. There are parallel increases in the frequency of PIN and cancer, according to serially sectioned autopsy prostates, although PIN appears to predate cancer by more than 10 years. (Data on PIN from Sakr WA, Haas GP, Cassin BJ, et al.: The frequency of carcinoma and intraepithelial neoplasia of the prostate in young male patients. J Urol 150:379–385, 1993; data on cancer curve from Bostwick DG, Cooner WH, Denis L, et al.: The association of benign prostatic hyperplasia and cancer of the prostate. Cancer 70:291–301, 1992.)

PIN appeared at an earlier age than had been documented previously and progressively increased in prevalence with age. There was no significant difference between the two races in frequency of cancer, multicentricity of cancer foci, Gleason score, or cancer volume. PIN first appeared in men in their twenties and thirties (9% and 22% prevalence, respectively), and this preceded the onset of carcinoma by more than ten years.[25, 27, 28] In an updated series of the same study, these authors reported their results with 370 consecutive cases—218 black men and 152 whites.[28] High-grade PIN was first identified in the third decade and its prevalence increased steadily with age. It was more prevalent and more extensive in black men: prevalences were 18%, 31%, 69%, 78%, and 86%, respectively, in the fourth, fifth, sixth, seventh, and eighth decades; the corresponding figures for white men were 14%, 21%, 38%, 50%, and 63%, respectively. The prevalence of latent carcinoma increased steadily with age but showed no significant difference between the two races. In black men high-grade PIN appeared to occur about a decade earlier than in Caucasian men. These racial differences have implications in epidemiology, screening, and chemoprevention of prostate cancer and underscore the importance of race as a risk factor.

Increased Frequency, Severity, and Extent of Prostatic Intraepithelial Neoplasia with Cancer

The frequency of PIN in prostates involved with cancer is significantly increased when compared with cancer-free prostates.[2, 6, 24, 29–35] PIN was present in 82% of step-sectioned autopsy prostates with cancer, but in only 43% of benign prostates from patients of similar age.[4] Qian and colleagues found that 86% of a series of 195 whole-mount radical prostatectomy specimens with cancer contained high-grade PIN, usually within 2 mm of the cancer.[24] The severity of PIN in prostates with cancer was also increased over that in prostates without cancer. PIN was more extensive in lower-stage tumors, presumably owing to "overgrowth" or obliteration of PIN by larger high-stage tumors.[9, 32]

Reports about the relationship of volume of PIN and volume of cancer conflict, probably owing to differences in methods of measure-ment or difficulty in identifying PIN in some fields with adenocarcinoma. The positive correlation between PIN and cancer was significant only for PIN within 2 mm of cancer, according to a recent large series[24]; conversely, a negative correlation for PIN and cancer was found by others, and these results were attributed to overgrowth and replacement of PIN by cancer.[29, 32]

The mean volume of PIN in prostates with cancer is 1.2 to 1.32 cc/L.[24, 29] The volume of PIN increases with the pathologic stage, Gleason grade, positive surgical margins, and perineural invasion.[24] These findings underscore the close spatial and biologic relationships between PIN and cancer and may be secondary to the increase in PIN with increasing cancer volume.

Multifocality and Location of Prostatic Intraepithelial Neoplasia and Cancer

PIN and cancer are usually multifocal. One study found that PIN was multifocal in 72% of radical prostatectomies with cancer, including 63% of those involving the nontransition zone and 7% of those involving the transition zone; 2% of cases had concomitant single foci in all zones. These findings agree with those of previous reports.[2, 9, 10, 25, 27, 28, 32]

The peripheral zone of the prostate, the area in which the majority of prostatic carcinomas occur (70%), is also the most common site of PIN.[1, 6, 10, 24, 29, 30] Cancer and PIN are frequently multifocal in the peripheral zone, indicating a "field" effect similar to the multifocality of urothelial carcinoma of the bladder. The majority of foci of high-grade PIN are exclusively in the peripheral zone (in one study, 63% of cases) or simultaneously in the transition and peripheral zones (36%); only rare cases (1%) occur exclusively in the transition zone.[24]

The transition zone and periurethral area, the anatomic areas in which nodular hyperplasia occurs, account for about 20% to 25% of cases of prostate cancer and harbor foci of PIN in 2% to 37% of cases.[6, 9, 24, 25, 26, 28] The highest frequency of involvement of the transition zone (37%) is in radical prostatectomies with cancer[6, 24]; the lowest is in studies of TURP specimens or only small numbers of patients (Table 6–4).[6, 9] These results have important implications for the origin of prostate carcinoma in the transition zone; if PIN is the

Table 6–4. Extent of High-Grade Prostatic Intraepithelial Neoplasia in Serially Sectioned Prostates

Author	Patients (N)	Patient Age (yr)	Specimen Source	Clinical Stage*	Frequency of High Grade PIN†	Method of Measuring	Extent
Prostates without cancer							
McNeal and Bostwick 1986[4]	100	50–90	Autopsy	—	26	Numbers of foci and microscopic fields	39% with ≤ 1 low power field‡ 3% with 1–2 low power fields 1% with > 2 low power fields
Sakr et al., 1993[25]	120	20–50	Autopsy	—	0	Number of foci	NA
Prostates with cancer							
McNeal and Bostwick, 1986[4]	100	50–90	Autopsy	—	72	Numbers of foci and microscopic fields	48% with ≤ 1 low power field‡ 12% with 1–2 low power fields 22% with > 2 low power fields
Troncoso et al., 1989[34]	61	20–90	Cystoprostatectomy	—	77	Numbers of foci	10.68 foci‡
Epstein et al., 1990[22]	32	NA	Radical prostatectomy and TURP	T1	15.6	Semiquantitative (bivariate based on diameter of focus)	43.75% with diameter ≤ 1.8 mm. 56.25% with diameter > 1.8 mm.
Quinn et al., 1990[86]	40	NA	Radical prostatectomy	T2	100	Semiquantitative (bivariate based on diameter of focus)	10% with diameter ≤ 1.8 mm. 90% with diameter > 1.8 mm.
Humphrey et al., 1992[52]	81	NA	Radical prostatectomy	T2	87.7	Estimated percentage of prostate	4.5% of whole prostate
De La Torre, 1993[29]	54	50–80	Radical prostatectomy	T2	85	Volume	About 1.2 cc.‡, §
Qian, Wollan, and Bostwick, 1997[24]	195	40–80	Radical prostatectomy	T1, T2	86	Volume	1.32 cc.

Key: NA, no data given.

*TNM (1992 revision).

†Other studies have evaluated the frequency of PIN in addition to those listed here; this includes only studies that measured extent of PIN.

‡Data include all grades of PIN.

§Data are estimated by analysis of graphs in the paper by De La Torre, 1993.

From Bostwick DG: High-grade prostatic intraepithelial neoplasia. Cancer 75:1823–1836, 1995.

precursor for many cases of prostate cancer, as has been proposed, this level of involvement of the transition zone by PIN is high enough to account for the relative frequency (25%) of cancer at this site. By contrast, atypical adenomatous hyperplasia (AAH), another putative precursor lesion that may be linked with transition zone cancer, is found in as many as 24% of transition zone specimens.[36]

The Basal Cell Layer Is Disrupted in High-Grade Prostatic Intraepithelial Neoplasia

Increasing grades of PIN are associated with progressive disruption of the basal cell layer.[2] Basal cell–specific monoclonal antibodies directed against high–molecular weight keratin (e.g., clone 34β-E12) have been employed immunohistochemically to selectively label the prostatic basal cell layer.[37] Tumor cells consistently fail to display immunoreactivity to this antibody, whereas normal prostate epithelial cells invariably are stained, with a continuous intact circumferential basal cell layer in most instances. Basal cell layer disruption is present in 56% of cases of high-grade PIN and more commonly in glands adjacent to invasive carcinoma than in distant glands (Fig. 6–8). Also, the amount of disruption increases with increasing grades of PIN; more than one third of the basal cell layer is lost in 52% of foci of high-grade PIN.[2]

The basement membrane normally surrounding prostate glands is intact in PIN and in most cases of well-differentiated adenocarcinoma, indicating that this is not a prerequisite of early stromal invasion (Fig. 6–9).[37a, 38] There is also increased expression of type IV collagenase in PIN and cancer as compared with benign epithelium[39]; collagenase is a proteolytic enzyme thought to induce fragmentation of the stroma during invasion.

Early invasive carcinoma occurs at sites of glandular outpouching and basal cell disruption.[1, 2, 4, 9, 24] Although one author has referred to this as *transitive* gland change, we feel that *microinvasion* is the preferred term, as it is applied to other organs and avoids introduction of a new and unnecessary term.[9] A model of prostate carcinogenesis has been proposed based on the morphologic continuum of PIN and the multistep theory of transformation (Fig. 6–10).[2]

Neovascularization Is Greater in Prostatic Intraepithelial Neoplasia and Cancer

Growth and metastasis of prostate cancer require angiogenesis.[40] The number of microvessels in high-grade PIN is greater than that in benign or hyperplastic prostate epithelium but less than that in adenocarcinoma.[40, 41] The microvessels in PIN are shorter than those in benign epithelium, with irregular contours and open lumina, increased number of endothelial cells, and greater distance from the basement membrane.

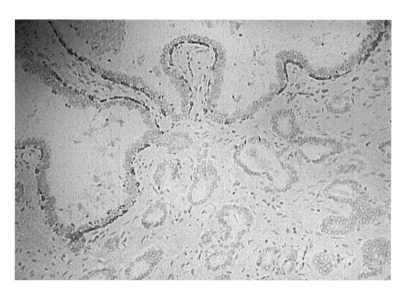

Figure 6–8. The keratin-immunoreactive basal cell layer, identified by the dark brown reaction product within the basal cells, is discontinuous in high-grade PIN *(left and top)* and absent in carcinoma *(bottom and right)*. (Immunoperoxidase stain for keratin 34β-E12.)

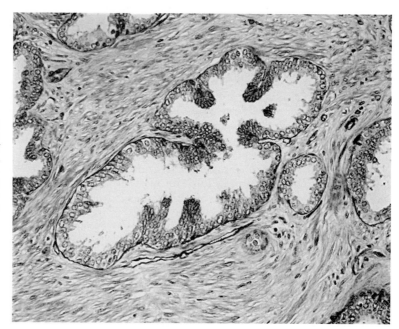

Figure 6–9. The basement membrane is intact in most cases of PIN. Note thin, dark line of immunoreactivity at gland periphery. (Immunoperoxidase stain using a polyclonal antibody directed against heparan sulfate proteoglycan, one of the components of the prostatic extracellular matrix.)

Cell Proliferation and Death (Apoptosis) are Greater with Prostatic Intraepithelial Neoplasia and Cancer

Tumor growth represents a delicate balance between cell proliferation and cell death that is dependent on a variety of influences, including patient age, nutritional and hormone status, and growth factor milieu. This balance is usually altered in malignant transformation, resulting in increased growth secondary to increased cell proliferation, decreased cell death, or a combination of these.

Prostate cancer has a relatively slow doubling time when compared with cancers of other organs—estimated to be between 6 months and 5 years, depending in part on tumor grade. Serial measurements of prostate-specific antigen (PSA) indicate that prostate cancer has a constant log-linear growth rate, with mean doubling times of 2.4 years for lo-

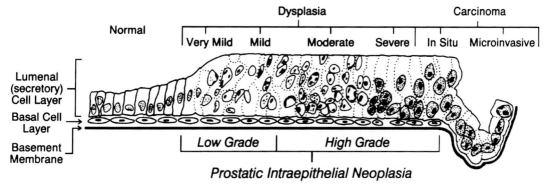

Figure 6–10. Morphologic continuum from normal prostatic epithelium through increasing grades of PIN to early invasive carcinoma, according to the disease-continuum concept. Low-grade PIN (grade 1) corresponds to very mild to mild dysplasia. High-grade PIN (grades 2 and 3) correspond to moderate to severe dysplasia and carcinoma in situ. The precursor state ends when malignant cells invade the stroma; this invasion occurs where the basal cell layer is disrupted. Notice that the dysplastic changes occur in the superficial (luminal) secretory cell layer, perhaps in response to luminal carcinogens. Disruption of the basal cell layer accompanies the architectural and cytologic features of high-grade PIN and appears to be a necessary prerequisite for stromal invasion. The basement membrane is retained with high-grade PIN and early invasive carcinoma. (Modified with permission from Bostwick DG, Brawer MK: Prostatic intraepithelial neoplasia and early invasion in prostate cancer. Cancer 59:788–794, 1987.)

calized cancer and 1.8 years for metastatic cancer.[42, 43] Higher Gleason grades are associated with faster doubling times. The mean growth fraction is 8.7% to 16.3%, according to immunohistochemical studies using antibodies directed against proliferating cell nuclear antigen and Ki-67; the growth rate is fastest at the advancing edge.[44] By comparison, the growth fraction is 0.6% in atrophic prostatic glands, 3.2% to 4.0% in benign prostatic hyperplasia (BPH), 6.0% to 9.5% in low-grade PIN, and 7.9% to 13.8% in high-grade PIN. The intermediate levels of doubling times in PIN, when compared with BPH and cancer, are considered evidence of the role of PIN as a putative premalignant lesion.

Mitotic figures are rare in the epithelium of benign or neoplastic prostate tissue, but there is a progressive increase from BPH through PIN to carcinoma.[45] Mitotic figures are present in BPH only in the basal cell layer, with a mean value of 0.002% (Table 6–5). In PIN the number of mitotic figures was highest in the basal cell layer and decreased progressively through the cell layers to those at the luminal surface. For low-grade PIN the mean value was 0.09% in the basal layer, 0.05% in the intermediate layer, and 0.02% in the superficial layer. For high-grade PIN the mean value was 0.19% in the basal layer, 0.08% in the intermediate layer, and 0.05% in the superficial layer. For low-grade PIN the percentages were slightly lower than for high-grade PIN. The number of mitotic figures in the small acinar pattern of cancer was quite similar to that for low-grade PIN and close to that for the large acinar pattern of cancer: mean values were 0.06% and 0.07%, respectively.

Apoptotic bodies are present throughout the normal prostatic epithelium and in gland lumina in all cases. They are usually seen in intercellular spaces and occasionally within the cytoplasm of epithelial cells, the latter being observed more often in PIN and carcinoma than in benign epithelium.[46] There is a progressive increase in the number of apoptotic bodies from BPH through PIN to adenocarcinoma, and they are invariably most numerous in the basal cell layer (or, in the case of carcinoma, in cells at the periphery of the malignant glands adjacent to the stroma); these trends are virtually identical to those seen with PCNA immunoreactivity (see Table 6–5).[44, 46] The percentage of apoptotic bodies was greater in low-grade PIN, high-grade PIN, and adenocarcinoma than in BPH (0.68%, 0.75%, and 0.92% to 2.10%, versus 0.26%, respectively). There is no apparent association of mitotic figures and apoptotic bodies.

There was greater cytoplasmic expression of the apoptosis-suppressing oncoprotein _bcl_-2 in PIN (100% of epithelial cells) and cancer (62% of cells) than in benign and hyperplastic epithelium (basal cells only).[47] Oncoprotein _bcl_-2 expression might play a role in the progression of PIN and/or low-grade cancer by interfering with apoptosis. Suppression of cell death by _bcl_-2 might result in accumulation of genetic abnormalities, perhaps increasing the clinical aggressiveness of cancer.

Prostatic Intraepithelial Neoplasia and Cancer Are Phenotypically Similar

Virtually all studies of biomarkers have indicated that high-grade PIN is related more

Table 6–5. Cell Proliferation and Cell Death in Benign Prostatic Hyperplasia, Prostatic Intraepithelial Neoplasia, and Cancer

Lesion	PCNA Immunoreactivity (% Positive Cells)	Mitotic Figures Frequency (%)	Apoptotic Bodies (% Positive Cells)
BPH*	3.2	0.002	0.6
PIN, low-grade*	9.5	0.087	0.9
PIN, high-grade*	13.8	0.194	1.0
Adenocarcinoma			
Cribriform pattern	14.4	0.154	1.8
Solid pattern	17.6	0.220	2.2
Small acinar pattern	8.7	0.058	1.0
Large acinar pattern	9.1	0.058	0.9

*Values are means for basal cell layer.
From Bostwick DG: High-grade prostatic intraepithelial neoplasia. Cancer 75:1823–1836, 1995.

closely to carcinoma than to benign epithe-lium.[39, 44, 48–59] There is increased cytoplasmic expression of p160*erb*B-3 and p185*erb*B-2 in PIN and cancer as compared with normal or hyperplastic epithelium,[57] similar to other bio-markers in the prostate, including epidermal growth factor, epidermal growth factor recep-tor,[54] type IV collagenase,[39] Lewis Y antigen, and transforming growth factor-α (TGF-α).[57] Increased cell proliferation is the most likely explanation for this phenotypic similarity of normal basal cells, PIN, and cancer, suggesting that the basal cells are the regenerative or stem cells of the prostate.

Other biomarkers show progressive loss of expression with increasing grades of PIN and cancer, including markers of secretory differ-entiation such as PSA, secretory proteins, cy-toskeletal proteins, glycoproteins, and neuro-endocrine cells. Reduction of cytoplasmic differentiation markers during the preinvasive phase may be followed by abrupt reexpression at the site of microinvasion.[55] There is a pro-gressive decrease in the number of neuroen-docrine cells in normal epithelium, high-grade PIN, and carcinoma.[48] These results indicate progressive impairment of cell differentiation and regulatory control with advancing stages of prostate carcinogenesis. Changes in cy-toskeletal proteins in PIN may affect transport of cell products, accounting for the differences in secretory protein distribution.[58]

MOLECULAR BIOLOGY OF PROSTATIC INTRAEPITHELIAL NEOPLASIA

The continuum that culminates in high-grade PIN and early invasive cancer is charac-terized by progressive basal cell layer disrup-tion, abnormalities in markers of secretory differentiation, increasing nuclear and nucleo-lar alterations, increasing cell proliferation, variation in DNA content, and increasing ge-netic instability. Some biomarkers show up-regulation or gain in the progression from benign prostatic epithelium to high-grade PIN and cancer, whereas others are down-regu-lated or lost (Fig. 6–11; reviewed by Bost-wick[49]). Existing data indicate that more bio-markers are up-regulated, but the relative importance of each is unknown. There is prominent clustering of changes in expression for many biomarkers between benign epithe-lium and high-grade PIN, indicating that this is an important threshold for carcinogenesis in the prostate; PIN shows marked genetic heterogeneity and impairment of cell differen-tiation and regulatory control. A small number of other changes are introduced in the pro-gression from high-grade PIN to localized can-cer, metastatic cancer, and hormone-refractory cancer. This scheme indicates the initial change in expression of a biomarker, but most of these changes become magnified in subse-quent steps.

High-grade PIN shows genetic instability, ac-cording to computer-based static image analy-sis studies of nuclear DNA content in tissue sections and other studies.[14, 29, 49, 60–67] The mean proliferative index and proportion of aneuploid cell nuclei in high-grade PIN are similar to those for cancer, but differ signifi-cantly from those for hyperplastic epithelium and low-grade PIN.[64] Amin and coworkers[60] found an incidence of 32% aneuploidy in high-grade PIN and 55% in carcinoma, some-what lower than the results of Crissman and colleagues[62] (57% and 62%, respectively; Table 6–6). Baretton and colleagues detected aneu-ploidy by image cytometry in 30% of cases of high-grade PIN and found that 70% of aneu-ploid cases were associated with aneuploid in-

Table 6–6. Aneuploidy in Prostatic Intraepithelial Neoplasia

Authors/Year	Patients (N)	Cases of PIN* (N)	Analysis Method	Nondiploid PIN (% Cases)	Nondiploid Cancer (% Cases)
Montironi et al., 1990[63]	20	20	Image	100 (20/20)	80 (16/20)
Weinberg et al., 1993[87]	6	6	Image	20 (1/5)	33 (2/6)
Berner et al., 1993[14]	22	37	Image	73 (26/37)	68 (15/22)
Crissman et al., 1993[62]	52	22	Image	55 (12/22)	62 (21/34)
Amin et al., 1993[60]	51	51	Image	25 (13/51)	41 (21/51)
Takahashi et al., 1994[72]	50	3	FISH	33 (1/3)	48 (24/50)

*High-grade PIN only in studies that separated low-grade and high-grade lesions.
From Bostwick DG: High-grade prostatic intraepithelial neoplasia. Cancer 75:1823–1836, 1995.

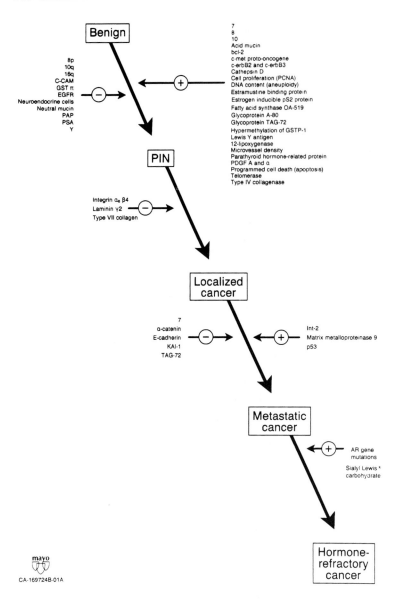

Figure 6–11. Genetic changes and other changes associated with progression of prostate cancer. Some biomarkers show up-regulation, or gain (indicated by + sign), whereas others are down-regulated, or lost (− sign). There is prominent clustering of changes in expression for many biomarkers between benign epithelium and high-grade PIN, indicating that this is an important threshold for carcinogenesis in the prostate. A small number of other changes are introduced in the progression from high-grade PIN to localized cancer, metastatic cancer, and hormone-refractory cancer. The model indicates the initial change in expression of a biomarker; most of these changes become magnified in subsequent steps. This model is based chiefly on studies of human prostate tissue and excludes many biomarkers that have not been evaluated in PIN or different stages of cancer. (From Bostwick DG, et al.: Molecular biology of prostatic intraepithelial neoplasia. Prostate 29: 117–134, 1996.)

vasive carcinoma; conversely, only 29% of cases of aneuploid cancer were associated with aneuploid PIN.[61] Berner and colleagues found that 68% of cases of high-grade PIN were aneuploid.[14]

Allelic loss is common in PIN and prostate cancer. Sakr and colleagues recently identified allelic loss of 8p, 10q, and 16q in as many as 29% of cases of PIN and 42% of primary cancers from 19 cases of stage TxN+ (D1) cancer.[27] Qian and associates used centromere-specific probes directed against chromosomes 7,8,10,12, and Y in a series of 40 whole-mounted prostates and found a similar overall frequency of numeric chromosome anomalies in PIN and carcinoma foci (50% and 51%, respectively), suggesting that these foci share a similar underlying pathogenesis.[65] Carcinoma foci usually contained more anomalies than paired PIN foci, but, within five prostates, one or more PIN foci contained more anomalies than concurrent carcinoma foci. Fluorescence in situ hybridization (FISH) anomalies can be found in one focus of PIN while other multifocal PIN foci may have no apparent FISH anomalies or have other anomalies. Similar intraglandular genetic heterogeneity was observed in multiple foci of carcinoma. Some small, low-grade tumor foci were aneuploid by FISH, whereas concurrent dominant high-grade tumor foci were apparently normal, indicating that small cancers can have significant alterations. In studies that used polymerase chain reaction (PCR), in situ hybridization, and DNA ploidy analysis, similar intraglandular heterogeneity has been reported.[65, 68] Thus, the size of a cancer focus and its degree of histologic dedifferentiation may not fully reflect the extent of its genetic alterations. Gain of chromosome 8 was the most frequent numeric anomaly in PIN and prostate carcinoma. Other studies have also demonstrated gain of the chromosome 8 centromere by FISH and loss of portions of the 8p arm by PCR in specimens of PIN and carcinoma, suggesting that alterations of this chromosome and/or one or more tumor suppressor genes (TSG) on the short arm may be important for the initiation or early progression of prostate cancer.[69]

The role of chromosome 7 in prostate carcinoma is controversial. Positive correlation of trisomy 7 with tumor grade, stage, and prognosis has been reported, and allelic loss studies have also suggested a possible site for a putative tumor suppressor gene.[70–74] However, some authors have reported no association of trisomy 7 with clinical and pathologic parameters.[75, 76] The frequency of trisomy 7 is greater in carcinoma than in PIN, suggesting that gain of chromosome 7 plays a role in the progression of precursor lesions to carcinoma.[72]

Prostatic Intraepithelial Neoplasia and Cancer Are Morphometrically Similar

Virtually all measures of nuclear abnormality by computer-based image analysis reveal the similarity of PIN and cancer, in contrast with normal and hyperplastic epithelium.[51, 63, 64, 77, 78] These changes include nuclear area, DNA content, chromatin content and distribution, nuclear perimeter, nuclear diameter, and nuclear roundness. Also, most measures of nucleolar abnormality reveal the similarities of PIN and cancer, in contrast with normal epithelium. Core and needle biopsies are more reliable than fine-needle aspiration in separating PIN from cancer, this finding based on a morphometric study of 50 "atypical" cases.[78] The cumulative data indicate that the morphologic continuum from PIN to cancer is characterized by progressive morphometric abnormalities of nuclei and nucleoli.

ANDROGEN DEPRIVATION THERAPY DECREASES THE INCIDENCE AND EXTENT OF PROSTATIC INTRAEPITHELIAL NEOPLASIA

After androgen deprivation therapy, the prevalence and extent of high-grade PIN decrease markedly when compared with untreated cases (Fig. 6–12).[79, 80] This decrease is accompanied by epithelial hyperplasia, cytoplasmic clearing, and prominent glandular atrophy, with decreased ratio of glands to stroma. These findings indicate that the dysplastic prostatic epithelium is hormone dependent. In normal prostatic epithelium luminal secretory cells are more sensitive than basal cells to the absence of androgen, and these results show that the cells of high-grade PIN share this androgen sensitivity. The loss of some normal, hyperplastic, and dysplastic epithelial cells with androgen deprivation is probably due to acceleration of programmed single cell death (apoptosis) with subsequent exfoliation into glandular lumina.[81]

EXPRESSION OF PROSTATE-SPECIFIC ANTIGEN

Conflicting findings have been reported about the relationship between PIN and serum PSA concentration. Brawer and coworkers studied 65 men undergoing transurethral or open simple prostatectomy to evaluate the contribution of PIN to serum PSA concentration.[82] Mean serum PSA concentration in patients with PIN alone (5.6 ng/mL), was intermediate between that of benign tissue (2.1 ng/mL) and carcinoma (35.1 ng/mL). Similarly they found that a group of 87 patients with a palpable prostatic abnormality who underwent needle biopsy of peripheral zone hypoechoic lesions and had PIN alone had mean serum PSA concentrations that were intermediate (7.8 ng/mL), between those of benign glands (5.8 ng/mL) and of carcinoma (18.3 ng/mL). Lee and coworkers evaluated 248 consecutive transrectal needle biopsy specimens from prostates with hypoechoic lesions.[19] Mean log serum PSA concentration in patients with high-grade PIN (1.85) were intermediate between those for benign tissue (1.09) and for carcinoma (2.79). These studies suggest that PIN contributes to serum PSA concentration. Conversely, Ronnett and associates studied 65

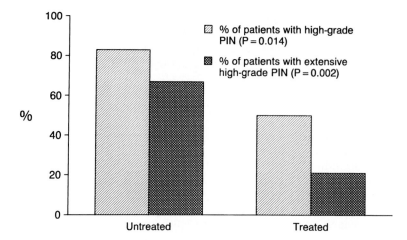

Figure 6–12. Histogram comparing the prevalence and extent of high-grade PIN following androgen deprivation in 24 treated and 24 untreated patients. Dark bars indicate prevalence; crosshatched bars indicate extent in high-power microscopic fields (From Ferguson J, Zincke H, Ellison E, et al.: Decrease of prostatic intraepithelial neoplasia (PIN) following androgen deprivation therapy in patients with stage T3 carcinoma treated by radical prostatectomy. Urology 44:91–95, 1984.)

patients with prostate cancer who underwent radical prostatectomy.[83] Specimens consisted of glands weighing less than 65 g with small-volume cancers (less than 0.5 cm^3); they found that high-grade PIN volume did not correlate with serum PSA concentration or PSA density.

Alexander and associates evaluated the relation of serum PSA and volume of high-grade PIN in a series of 170 radical prostatectomy specimens with high-grade PIN and cancer. PIN volume ranged from 0 to 8.1 ml (mean 1.3 mL), and cancer volume ranged from 0 to 56.9 cc (mean 9.1 mL).[84] In a subset of 93 patients with small cancers (less than 6.0 mL), PIN volume ranged from 0 to 6.1 and did not correlate with serum PSA concentration or PSA density. In the entire study group PIN volume did not correlate with PSA density but did correlate with serum PSA concentration. Multiple regression analysis, which corrected for gland weight and cancer volume, found that PIN volume was not associated with serum PSA concentration or PSA density in small cancers (less than 6.0 mL). They concluded that PIN does not contribute significantly to serum PSA concentration and suggested that patients with high-grade PIN and elevated serum PSA concentration may benefit from early repeat biopsy; patients with high-grade PIN and normal serum PSA also need to be followed clinically, but their risk of cancer may be lower.

Immunohistochemical studies have demonstrated that expression of PSA in PIN is less than that observed in benign epithelium and cancer. PIN is an abnormality within preexisting ducts and acini, and cytoplasmic secretory products such as PSA would be expected

to wash into the lumina and travel downstream rather than escape into the stroma and blood vessels.

SUMMARY

High-grade PIN is the most likely precursor of prostatic adenocarcinoma, according to virtually all available evidence. PIN is associated with progressive abnormalities of phenotype and genotype that are intermediate between normal prostatic epithelium and cancer, indicating impairment of cell differentiation and regulatory control with advancing stages of prostate carcinogenesis. There is progressive loss of some markers of secretory differentiation, including PSA, secretory proteins, cytoskeletal proteins, glycoproteins, and neuroendocrine cells. Other markers show progressive increase, including c-_erb_B-2 oncoproteins, _bcl_-2 oncoprotein, epidermal growth factor, epidermal growth factor receptor, type IV collagenase, Lewis Y antigen, TGF-α, apoptotic bodies, mitotic figures, PCNA expression, aneuploidy and genetic abnormalities, and microvessel density.

The clinical importance of recognizing PIN is based on its strong association with prostate carcinoma. PIN has a high predictive value as a marker for adenocarcinoma, and its identification in biopsy specimens of the prostate warrants further search for concurrent invasive carcinoma. Studies to date have not determined whether PIN remains stable, regresses, or progresses, although the implication is that it can progress. Androgen deprivation therapy decreases the prevalence and extent of high-grade PIN, suggesting a role in chemoprevention. PIN does not appear to elevate serum PSA concentration.

REFERENCES

1. Bostwick DG: High grade prostatic intraepithelial neoplasia: The most likely precursor of prostate cancer. Cancer 75:1823–1836, 1995.
2. Bostwick DG, Brawer MK: Prostatic intra-epithelial neoplasia and early invasion in prostate cancer. Cancer 59:788–794, 1987.
3. Graham SD Jr, Bostwick DG, Hoisaeter A, et al.: Report of the committee on staging and pathology. Cancer 70(Suppl):359–361, 1992.
4. McNeal JE, Bostwick DG: Intraductal dysplasia: A premalignant lesion of the prostate. Hum Pathol 17:64–71, 1986.
5. Drago JR, Mostofi FK, Lee F: Introductory remarks and workshop summary. Urology 34(Suppl):2–3, 1989.
6. Kovi J, Mostofi FK, Heshmat MY, et al.: Large acinar atypical hyperplasia and carcinoma of the prostate. Cancer 61:555–561, 1988.
7. Mostofi FK: Precancerous lesions of the prostate. In: Carter RL (ed). Precancerous States. New York: Oxford University Press, 1984; pp 304–316.
8. Markham CW: Prostatic intraepithelial neoplasia: Detection and correlation with invasive cancer in fine-needle biopsy. Urology 24(Suppl):57–61, 1989.
9. McNeal JE, Villers A, Redwine EA, et al.: Microcarcinoma in the prostate: Its association with duct-acinar dysplasia. Hum Pathol 22:644–652, 1991.
10. Bostwick DG, Amin MB, Dundore P, et al.: Architectural patterns of high grade prostatic intraepithelial neoplasia. Hum Pathol 24:298–310, 1993.
11. Kovi J, Jackson MA, Heshmat MY: Ductal spread in prostatic carcinoma. Cancer 56:1566–1573, 1985.
12. Davidson D, Bostwick DG, Qian J, et al.: Prostatic intraepithelial neoplasia is a risk factor for adenocarcinoma: Predictive accuracy in needle biopsies. J Urol 154:1295–1299, 1995.
13. Brawer MK, Bigler SA, Sohlberg OE, et al.: Significance of prostatic intraepithelial neoplasia on prostate needle biopsy. Urology 38:103–107, 1991.
14. Berner A, Danielsen HE, Pettersen EO, et al.: DNA distribution in the prostate. Normal gland, benign and premalignant lesions, and subsequent adenocarcinomas. Anal Quant Cytol Histol 15:247–252, 1993.
15. Keetch DW, Humphrey P, Stahl D, et al.: Morphometric analysis and clinical follow-up of isolated prostatic intraepithelial neoplasia in needle biopsy of the prostate. J Urol 154:347–351, 1995.
16. Weinstein MH, Epstein JI: Significance of high grade prostatic intraepithelial neoplasia on needle biopsy. Hum Pathol 24:624–629, 1993.
17. Park C, Galang C, Johennig P, et al.: Follow-up aspiration biopsies for dysplasia of the prostate. Lab Invest 60:70A, 1989.
18. Bostwick DG, Qian J, Frankel K: The incidence of high grade prostatic intraepithelial neoplasia in needle biopsies. J Urol 154:1791–1794, 1995.
19. Lee F, Torp-Pedersen ST, Carroll JT, et al.: Use of transrectal ultrasound and prostate-specific antigen in diagnosis of prostatic intraepithelial neoplasia. Urology 24(Suppl):4–8, 1989.
20. Shinohara K, Scardino PT, Carter SSC, et al.: Pathologic basis of the sonographic appearance of the normal and malignant prostate. Urol Clin North Am 16:675–691, 1989.
21. Allam CK, Bostwick DG, Hayes JA, et al.: Interobserver variability in the diagnosis of high grade prostatic intraepithelial neoplasia and adenocarcinoma. Mod Pathol 9:742–751, 1996.
22. Epstein JI, Grignon DJ, Humphrey PA, et al.: Interobserver reproducibility in the diagnosis of prostatic intraepithelial neoplasia. Am J Surg Pathol 19:973–886, 1995.
23. Bostwick DG, Burke HB, Wheeler TM, et al.: The most promising surrogate endpoint biomarkers for screening candidate chemopreventive compounds for prostatic adenocarcinoma in short-term phase II clinical trials. J Cell Biochem Suppl 19:283–289, 1994.
24. Qian J, Wollan P, Bostwick DG: The extent and multicentricity of high grade prostatic intraepithelial neoplasia in clinically localized prostatic adenocarcinoma. Hum Pathol 28:143–148, 1997.
25. Sakr WA, Haas GP, Cassin BJ, et al.: Frequency of carcinoma and intraepithelial neoplasia of the prostate in young male patients. J Urol 150:379–385, 1993.
26. Sakr WA, Haas GP, Grignon DJ, et al.: High grade prostatic intraepithelial neoplasia (HGPIN) and prostatic adenocarcinoma between the ages of 20–69. An autopsy study of 249 cases. In Vivo 8:439–444, 1994.
27. Sakr WA, Macoska JA, Benson P, et al.: Allelic loss in locally metastatic multisampled prostate cancer. Cancer Res 54:3273–3277, 1994.
28. Sakr WA, Grignon DJ, Haas GP, et al.: Epidemiology of high grade prostatic intraepithelial neoplasia. Pathol Res Pract 191:838–941, 1995.
29. De La Torre, Haggman M, Brandstedt S, et al.: Prostatic intraepithelial neoplasia and invasive carcinoma in total prostatectomy specimens: Distribution, volume and DNA ploidy. Br J Urol 72:207–213, 1993.
30. Kastendieck H, Helpap B: Prostatic "dysplasia/atypical hyperplasia." Urology 24(Suppl):28–42, 1989.
31. Melhorn J: Zur diagnostischen Wertigkeit "dysplastischer" Veranderungen der Prostata. [Diagnostic value of "dysplastic" alterations to prostate.] Zentralbl Pathol 137:395–401, 1991.
32. Qian J-Q, Huang S-F: Immunohistochemical and quantitative morphological studies of duct-acinar dysplasia in the prostate. Chin J Pathol 21:198–202, 1992.
33. Sentinelli S, Rondanelli E: La neoplasia intraepiteliale prostatica: Una nuova lesioe displastica della prostata. Pathologica 81:127–137, 1989.
34. Troncoso P, Babaian RJ, Ro JY, et al.: Prostatic intraepithelial neoplasia and invasive prostatic adenocarcinoma in cystoprostatectomy specimens. Urology 24 (Suppl):52–56, 1989.
35. Tsukamoto T, Kumamoto Y, Masumori N, et al.: Studies on incidental carcinoma of the prostate. Nippon Hinyokika Gakkai Zasshi 81:1343–1350, 1990.
36. Bostwick DG, Qian J: Atypical adenomatous hyperplasia of the prostate: Relationship with carcinoma in 217 whole mount radical prostatectomies. Am J Surg Pathol 19:506–518, 1995.
37. Brawer MK, Peehl DM, Stamey TA, et al.: Keratin immunoreactivity in benign and neoplastic human prostate. Cancer Res 45:3665–3669, 1985.
37a. Bostwick DG, Leske DA, Qian J, et al.: Prostatic intraepithelial neoplasia and well differentiated adenocarcinoma retain a basement membrane. Pathol Res Pract 191:850–855, 1995.

38. Schultz DS, Amin MB, Zarbo RJ: Basement membrane type IV collagen immunohistochemical staining in prostatic neoplasia. Appl Immunohistochem 1:123–126, 1993.

39. Boag AH, Young ID: Increased expression of the 72-kd type IV collagenase in prostatic adenocarcinoma. Demonstration by immunohistochemistry and in situ hybridization. Am J Pathol 144:585–591, 1994.

40. Bigler SA, Deering RE, Brawer MK: Comparison of microscopic vascularity in benign and malignant prostate tissue. Hum Pathol 24:220–226, 1993.

41. Montironi R, Magi Galluzzi C, Diamanti L, et al.: Prostatic intra-epithelial neoplasia. Qualitative and quantitative analyses of the blood capillary architecture on thin tissue sections. Pathol Res Pract 189:542–548, 1993.

42. Hanks GE, D'Amico A, Epstein BE, et al.: Prostatic-specific antigen doubling times in patients with prostate cancer: A potentially useful reflection of tumor doubling time. Int J Radiat Oncol Biol Phys 27:125–127, 1993.

43. Schmid HP, McNeal JE, Stamey TA: Observations on the doubling time of prostate cancer. The use of serial prostate-specific antigen in patients with untreated disease as a measure of increasing cancer volume. Cancer 71:2031–2040, 1993.

44. Montironi R, Magi Galluzzi C, Diamanti L, et al.: Prostatic intra-epithelial neoplasia. Expression and location of proliferating cell nuclear antigen (PCNA) in epithelial, endothelial and stromal nuclei. Virchows Arch [A] 422:185–192, 1993.

45. Gainnulis I, Montironi R, Galluzzi CM, et al.: Frequency and location of mitoses in prostatic intraepithelial neoplasia (PIN). Anticancer Res 13:2447–2452, 1993.

46. Montironi R, Magi Galluzzi C, Scarpelli M, et al.: Occurrence of cell death (apoptosis) in prostatic intra-epithelial neoplasia. Virchows Arch [A] Pathol Anat 423:351–357, 1993.

47. Colombel M, Symmans F, Gil S, et al.: Detection of the apoptosis-suppressing oncoprotein bcl-2 in hormone-refractory human prostate cancers. Am J Pathol 143:390–400, 1993.

48. Bostwick DG, Dousa MK, Crawford BG, et al.: Neuroendocrine differentiation in prostatic intraepithelial neoplasia and adenocarcinoma. Am J Surg Pathol 18:1240–1246, 1994.

49. Bostwick DG, Pacelli A, Lopez-Beltran A: Molecular biology of prostatic intraepithelial neoplasia. Prostate 1996 (in press).

50. Algaba F, Trias I, Lopez L, et al.: Neuroendocrine cells in peripheral prostatic zone: Age, prostatic intraepithelial neoplasia and latent cancer-related changes. Eur Urol 27:329–333, 1995.

51. Deschenes J, Weidner N: Nucleolar organizer regions (NOR) in hyperplastic and neoplastic prostate disease. Am J Surg Pathol 14:1148–1155, 1990.

52. Humphrey PA: Mucin in severe dysplasia in the prostate. Surg Pathol 4:137–143, 1991.

53. Ibrahim GK, MacDonald JA, Kerns BJM, et al.: Differential immunoreactivity of her-2/neu oncoprotein in prostatic tissues. Surg Oncol 1:151–155, 1992.

54. Maygarden SJ, Strom S, Ware JL: Localization of epidermal growth factor receptor by immunohistochemical methods in human prostatic carcinoma, prostatic intraepithelial neoplasia, and benign hyperplasia. Arch Pathol Lab Med 116:269–273, 1992.

55. McNeal JE, Alroy J, Leav I, et al.: Immunohistochemical evidence for impaired cell differentiation in the premalignant phase of prostate carcinogenesis. Am J Clin Pathol 90:23–32, 1988.

56. Min KW, Jin J-K, Blank J, et al.: AgNOR in the human prostatic gland. Am J Clin Pathol 95:508, 1990.

57. Myers RB, Srivastava S, Oelschlager DK, et al.: Expression of p160erbB-3 and p185erbB-2 in prostatic intraepithelial neoplasia and prostatic adenocarcinoma. J Natl Cancer Inst 86:1140–1144, 1994.

58. Nagle RB, Brawer MK, Kittelson J, et al.: Phenotypic relationships of prostatic intraepithelial neoplasia to invasive prostatic carcinoma. Am J Pathol 138:119–128, 1991.

59. Perlman EJ, Epstein JI: Blood group antigen expression in dysplasia and adenocarcinoma of the prostate. Am J Surg Pathol 14:810–818, 1990.

60. Amin MB, Schultz DS, Zarbo RJ, et al.: Computerized static DNA ploidy analysis of prostatic intraepithelial neoplasia. Arch Pathol Lab Med 117:794–798, 1993.

61. Baretton GB, Vogt T, Blasenbreu S, et al.: Comparison of DNA ploidy in prostatic intraepithelial neoplasia and invasive carcinoma of the prostate: An image cytometric study. Hum Pathol 25:506–513, 1994.

62. Crissman JD, Sakr WA, Hussein ME, et al.: DNA quantitation of intraepithelial neoplasia and invasive carcinoma of the prostate. Prostate 22:155–162, 1993.

63. Montironi R, Scarpelli M, Sisti S, et al.: Quantitative analysis of prostatic intra-epithelial neoplasia on tissue sections. Anal Quant Cytol Histol 12:366–372, 1990.

64. Petein M, Michel P, Van Velthoven R, et al.: Morphonuclear relationship between prostatic intraepithelial neoplasia and cancers as assessed by digital cell image analysis. Am J Clin Pathol 96:628–634, 1991.

65. Qian J, Bostwick DG, Takahashi S, Borell TJ, Herath JF, Lieber MM, Jenkins RB: Chromosomal anomalies in prostatic intraepithelial neoplasia and carcinoma detected by fluorescence in situ hybridization. Cancer Res 55:5408–5414, 1995.

66. Sakr WA, Haas GP, Drozdowicz SM, et al.: Nuclear DNA content of prostatic carcinoma and intraepithelial neoplasia (PIN) in young males. An image analysis study. Mod Pathol 5:58A, 1992.

67. Weinberg DS, Weidner N: Concordance of DNA content between prostatic intraepithelial neoplasia and concomitant carcinoma. Evidence that prostatic intraepithelial neoplasia is a precursor of invasive prostatic carcinoma. Arch Pathol Lab Med 117:1132–1137, 1993.

68. Cher ML, Ito T, Weidner N, et al.: Mapping of regions of physical deletion on chromosome 16q in prostate cancer cells by fluorescence in situ hybridization (FISH). J Urol 153:249–254, 1995.

69. Emmert-Buck MR, Vocke CD, Pozzatti RO, et al.: Allelic loss on chromosome 8p12-21 in microdissected prostatic intraepithelial neoplasia (PIN). Cancer Res 55:2959–2962, 1995.

70. Alcaraz A, Takahashi S, Brown JA, et al.: Aneuploidy and aneusomy of chromosome 7 detected by fluorescence in situ hybridization are markers of poor prognosis in prostate cancer. Cancer Res 54:3998–4002, 1994.

71. Bandyk MG, Zhao L, Troncoso P, et al.: Trisomy 7: A potential cytogenetic marker of human prostate cancer progression. Genes Chromosom Cancer 9:19–27, 1994.

72. Takahashi S, Qian J, Brown JA, et al.: Potential markers of prostate cancer aggressiveness detected by fluorescence in situ hybridization. Cancer Res 54:3574–3579, 1994.

73. Zenklusen JC, Thompson JC, Troncoso P, et al.: Loss of heterozygosity in human primary prostatic carcinomas: A possible tumor suppressor gene at 7q31.1. Cancer Res 54:6870–6873, 1994.

74. Zitzelsberger H, Szves S, Weier HU, et al.: Numerical abnormalities of chromosome 7 in human prostate cancer detected by fluorescence in situ hybridization (FISH) on paraffin embedded tissue sections with centromere-specific DNA probes. J Pathol 172:325–335, 1994.

75. Alers CA, Krijtenburg PJ, Vissers KJ, et al.: Interphase cytogenetics of prostatic adenocarcinoma and precursor lesions: Analysis of 25 radical prostatectomies and 17 adjacent prostatic intraepithelial neoplasias. Genes Chromosom Cancer 12:241–250, 1995.

76. Brown JA, Alcaraz A, Takahashi S, et al.: Chromosomal aneusomies detected by fluorescence in situ hybridization analysis in clinically localized prostate carcinoma. J Urol 152:1157–1162, 1994.

77. Helpap B: Observations on the number, size and location of nucleoli in hyperplastic and neoplastic prostatic disease. Histopathology 13:203–211, 1988.

78. Layfield LJ, Goldstein NS: Morphometric analysis of borderline atypia in prostatic aspiration biopsy specimen. Anal Quant Cytol Histol 13:288–292, 1991.

79. Ferguson J, Zincke H, Ellison E, et al.: Decrease of prostatic intraepithelial neoplasia (PIN) following androgen deprivation therapy in patients with stage T3 carcinoma treated by radical prostatectomy. Urology 44:91–95, 1994.

80. Montironi R, Magi-Galluzzi C, Muzzonigro G, et al.: Effects of combination endocrine treatment on normal prostate, prostatic intraepithelial neoplasia, and prostatic adenocarcinoma. J Clin Pathol 47:906–913, 1994.

81. Van der Kwast TH, Ruizeveld de Winter JA, Trapman J: Androgen receptor expression in human prostate cancer. J Urol Pathol 3:200–222, 1995.

82. Brawer MK, Lange PH: Prostate-specific antigen and premalignant change: Implications for early detection. CA 39:361–375, 1989.

83. Ronnett BM, Carmichael MJ, Carter HB, et al.: Does high grade prostatic intraepithelial neoplasia result in elevated serum prostate specific antigen levels? J Urol 150:386–389, 1993.

84. Alexander EE, Qian J, Wollan PC, et al.: Prostatic intraepithelial neoplasia does not raise serum prostate specific antigen. Urology 47:693–698, 1996.

85. Sesterhenn IA, Becker RL, Avallone FA, et al.: Image analysis of nucleoli and nucleolar organizer regions in prostatic hyperplasia, intraepithelial neoplasia, and prostatic carcinoma. J Urogen Pathol 1:61–74, 1991.

86. Quinn BD, Cho KR, Epstein JI: Relationship of severe dysplasia to stage B adenocarcinoma of the prostate. Cancer 65:2328–2337, 1990.

87. Weinberg DS, Weidner N: Concordance of DNA content between prostatic intraepithelial neoplasia and concomitant carcinoma. Evidence that prostatic intraepithelial neoplasia is a precursor of invasive prostatic carcinoma. Arch Pathol Lab Med 117:1132–1137, 1993.

7

DIFFERENTIAL DIAGNOSIS OF PROSTATIC INTRAGLANDULAR PROLIFERATIVE LESIONS

Edward C. Jones and Robert H. Young

A number of benign, premalignant, and malignant prostatic lesions may result in an abnormal intraglandular proliferation of cells. A cribriform pattern may be found in each of these categories, and careful assessment of these lesions is necessary for proper interpretation. It is important to recognize prostatic intraepithelial neoplasia (PIN), a lesion that is the most likely precursor of prostate carcinoma,[1, 2] both to avoid misinterpreting it as an infiltrating prostatic adenocarcinoma and to identify patients at increased risk for prostate carcinoma. It is also important to differentiate benign lesions, such as cribriform hyperplasia, basal cell hyperplasia (including atypical forms), and reactive atypia due to inflammation, infarction, and radiation, from neoplastic lesions. Seminal vesicle epithelium can mimic a neoplastic process. Intraductal transitional cell carcinoma may be a diagnostic consideration when examining neoplastic intraglandular epithelium.

PIN is identified on low-power examination by the thickened basophilic epithelium located within a preexisting duct-acinar unit of normal or minimally distorted contour (Fig. 7–1).[1–8] Stratified epithelium several cells thick can usually be appreciated. The initial descriptions of PIN subdivided it into grades 1, 2, and 3—mild, moderate, and severe degrees of intraepithelial dysplasia, respectively.[3, 5, 6] It is now referred to as either high-grade or low-grade PIN with grade 1 lesions designated low-grade.[8, 9] Low-grade PIN, with its mildly crowded, irregularly spaced cells and mild pleomorphism without prominent nucleoli (Fig. 7–2), is a lesion that cannot be reproducibly recognized,[4, 10–12] and the designation correctly identifies its lack of clinical significance. High-grade PIN, a term that encompasses grade 2 and 3 dysplastic lesions and avoids their subjective division, is readily recognized,[12, 13] having many if not all of the cytologic features of a malignant prostatic epithelial cell (Fig. 7–3). In high-grade lesions, the epithelial layer may be arranged in a cribriform, micropapillary, or tufted pattern (Fig. 7–4).[9] Less commonly, it is a flat lesion with only one or two cell layers.[9] The cells are crowded and irregularly spaced with loss of polarity, uniform, oval nucleomegaly, hyperchromaticity, and prominent nucleoli. In fully developed high-grade PIN, these nuclear features are found throughout the atypical epithelium (Figs. 7–1, 7–2, 7–3). PIN may involve the prostate gland diffusely, but it is not an invasive lesion. Often a basal cell layer can be identified (Figs. 7–1, 7–3, 7–5), but it may be discontinuous or even absent in high-grade PIN.[14–16] This cell layer is selectively

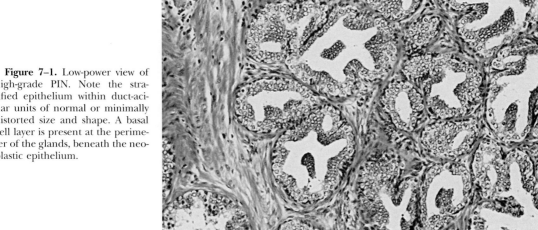

Figure 7–1. Low-power view of high-grade PIN. Note the stratified epithelium within duct-acinar units of normal or minimally distorted size and shape. A basal cell layer is present at the perimeter of the glands, beneath the neoplastic epithelium.

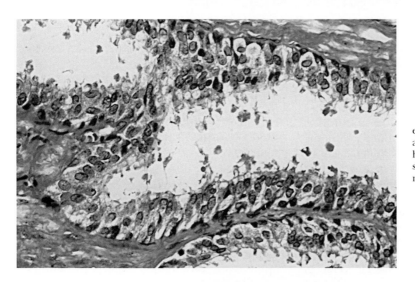

Figure 7–2. Low-grade PIN. The epithelial cells are mildly crowded and irregularly spaced. The nuclei have some variation in size and shape, and they lack prominent nucleoli.

Figure 7–3. High-grade PIN. *A,* The stratified epithelial cells are crowded with uniform nucleomegaly, hyperchromatic nuclei, and prominent nucleoli. *B,* Benign epithelium is present in the upper left. The cytologic features of neoplasia are readily seen in the high-power view.

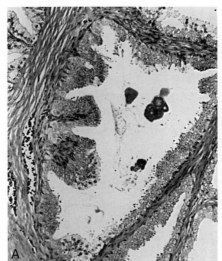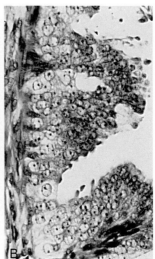

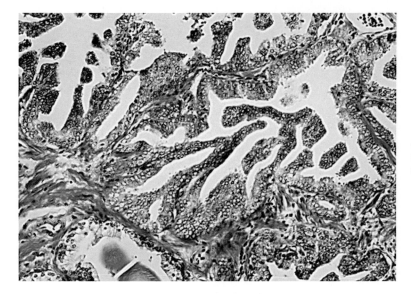

Figure 7–4. High-grade PIN with a range of patterns, including micropapillary, cribriform, tufted, and flat.

stained with a high molecular weight cytokeratin immunostain, and this procedure can be helpful in determining its presence (Fig. 7–5).[14, 15, 17–22]

The key to identifying PIN is recognition of the neoplastic epithelium within noninvasive glands or ducts; that is, the glands with the atypical epithelium are distributed in a manner consistent with preexisting duct-acinar units. When evaluating a small number of acini with malignant cytologic features, it may be difficult to determine whether or not it is an infiltrating prostate carcinoma. In general, PIN is found in larger glands with an orderly arrangement, whereas haphazardly arranged small round acini lined by a single layer of cytologically malignant epithelium are indicative of invasive carcinoma (Fig. 7–6). Topographically, microacinar prostatic carcinoma is often closely associated with PIN,[6, 14, 16, 23–25] and microinvasive foci of carcinoma arising from PIN may be linked to PIN by intermediate-sized "transitive" atypical glands (Fig. 7–7).[23] The presence of a basal cell layer excludes infiltrating carcinoma, but the absence of this layer is less helpful because it can be lost in high-grade PIN lesions.[14, 15] It has been suggested that the presence of luminal acid mucin may be strong evidence for the presence of carcinoma,[26–28] but this finding also occurs in high-grade PIN,[29, 30] and it cannot be relied upon as a differentiating feature. Intraluminal

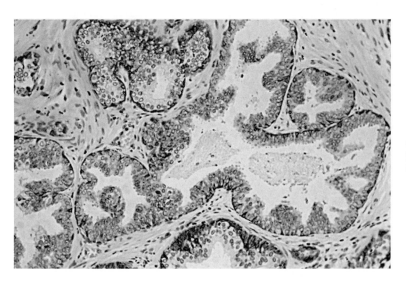

Figure 7–5. Cytokeratin immunostain demonstrates a keratin-positive basal cell layer beneath the high-grade PIN.

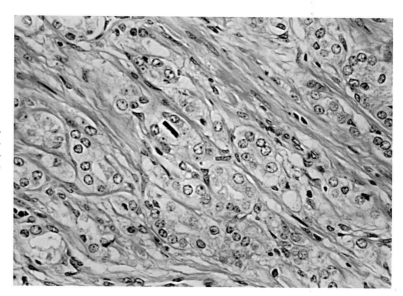

Figure 7–6. Prostatic adenocarcinoma with infiltrating microacini lined by a single layer of malignant epithelial cells. Note the intraluminal crystalloid.

crystalloids, hard-edged, densely eosinophilic needle-shaped or quadrangular structures (see Fig. 7–6), are found much more often in microacinar prostatic adenocarcinoma,[31–35] but they are also found in glands lined by benign epithelium[36] and they have been observed in glands containing PIN.[1] These adjunctive features must be interpreted within the histologic context, and ultimately one must be certain of the presence of infiltrating malignant microacini before rendering a diagnosis of prostatic carcinoma.

Differentiation between cribriform PIN and cribriform carcinoma can be particularly challenging because of the smooth interface between the cribriform masses and the stroma.[5, 19, 37] The distinction obviously has important practical implications, particularly as cribriform prostatic carcinoma is at least a moderately differentiated carcinoma that likely will progress. A florid cribriform or papillary proliferation is suspicious for carcinoma, and the presence of necrosis should raise the index of suspicion. The presence of a basal cell layer at the perimeter of the cribriform proliferation indicates a noninvasive intraglandular lesion,[19, 37] but, as noted above, the absence of this cell layer is less helpful. Prostatic duct or so-called endometrioid carcinoma, a tumor usually found centrally, often with an intraduc-

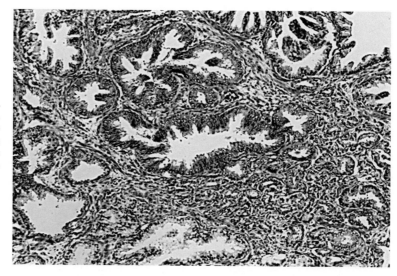

Figure 7–7. A focus of infiltrating microacinar prostatic adenocarcinoma adjacent to larger glands with high-grade PIN. Note the intermediate-sized "transitive glands" budding off from the larger glands.

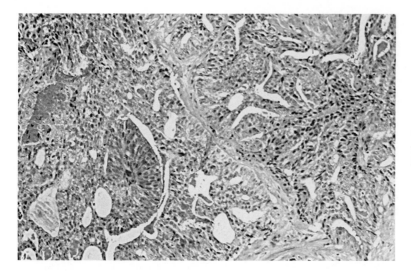

Figure 7–8. Prostatic duct or "endometrioid" adenocarcinoma with a florid papillary-cribriform growth pattern.

tal component, characteristically has a papillary or cribriform pattern that should not be mistaken for PIN (Fig. 7–8).[38-40] If there is confluence of cribriform masses that do not conform to the normal distribution of preexisting duct-acinar units, the diagnosis of cribriform carcinoma is established (Figs. 7–8, 7–9). Cribriform carcinoma is commonly accompanied by a component of infiltrating small acinar carcinoma, and a careful search for this often resolves the differential diagnosis (Fig. 7–10).[1, 20, 21]

Cribriform hyperplasia is a benign lesion that has a prominent and superficially alarming sievelike pattern within duct-acinar units (Fig. 7–11).[1, 11, 41-43] The architectural pattern is similar to that of cribriform PIN. This pattern may also be misinterpreted as prostate carcinoma, and before it was described it was a source of many diagnostic problems.[44] Cribriform hyperplasia lacks the confluence seen in cribriform carcinoma, and the overall contour of the lesional glands often conforms to that of a hyperplastic nodule. Typically, the lining cells have clear cytoplasm, but this feature does not distinguish it from carcinoma, which may also have clear cells. Most importantly, the bland cytologic features of cribriform hyperplasia (Fig. 7–11) contrast with the moderate to severe cytologic atypia in cribriform carcinoma or high-grade PIN. Small foci of basal cell hyperplasia are commonly present at the perimeter of the glands (Fig. 7–11), and a high molecular weight cytokeratin immunoperoxi-

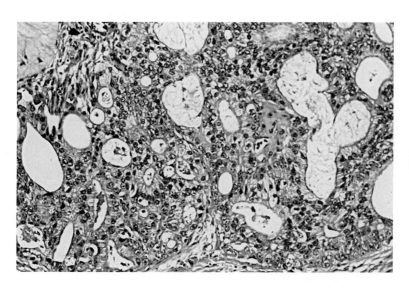

Figure 7–9. Cribriform prostate carcinoma. Confluence of the malignant glands is present.

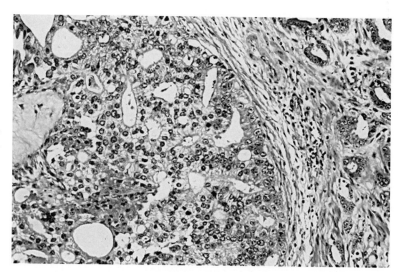

Figure 7–10. Cribriform prostate carcinoma *(left)* with adjacent microacinar carcinoma *(right).*

dase stain consistently highlights the basal cell layer.[42] A flow cytometric study demonstrated diploid DNA content in all 13 cases of cribriform hyperplasia studied, whereas 3 of 4 cribriform carcinomas were aneuploid.[42]

Basal cell hyperplasia is a relatively common finding in prostatic hyperplasia of usual type. It is typically found in nodules of evenly spaced small glands with a noninfiltrative architecture. The expansion of the basal cell compartment may be eccentric or symmetric and there may be small round solid nests of basal cells. When it is prominent, the basal cell hyperplasia may be confused with carcinoma,[43, 45] but usually the oval to elongate, dark-staining basal cells appear bland, without prominent nucleoli. The location of the basal cells be-

tween the columnar secretory cell and the basement membrane can be appreciated, and the multilayered basal cells appear to lift the overlying secretory cells. The long axis of normal basal cells is often oriented parallel to the basement membrane, but in hyperplastic proliferations the basal cells become plump and jumbled (Fig. 7–12). Usually the basal cells have scant cytoplasm, but they may acquire an appreciable amount of pale cytoplasm. Myxoid stroma has been reported in cases of embryonal hyperplasia, a lesion that is probably a variant of basal cell hyperplasia.[46] The basal cells often appear very prominent in the atrophic benign prostate glands of patients who have been treated with antiandrogen hormonal therapy for prostatic carcinoma.[47, 48]

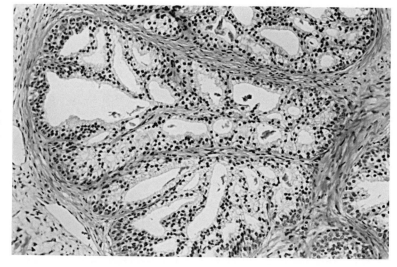

Figure 7–11. Cribriform hyperplasia. The hyperplastic clear cells have bland cytologic features, and a basal cell layer is present at the periphery.

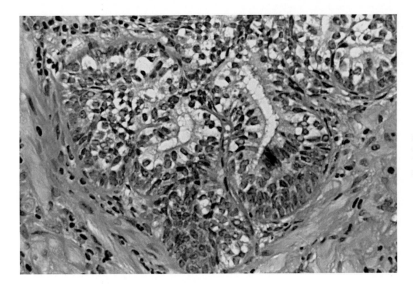

Figure 7–12. Basal cell hyperplasia. There is a proliferation of oval dark-staining basal cells beneath the cuboidal to columnar light-staining secretory cells.

Hyperplastic basal cells may acquire some degree of cytologic atypia, with enlarged nuclei and prominent nucleoli; an appearance that may mimic PIN (Fig. 7–13). The basal cells are usually darker, with less uniformly oval or round nuclei, and smaller, without the fully developed nuclear features of high-grade PIN. However, there may be marked atypia of the basal cells, which has been referred to as atypical basal cell hyperplasia (Fig. 7–13).[49, 50] Careful examination reveals the location of the proliferating basal cell between the luminal secretory cell layer, which may be compressed, and the basement membrane. In contrast to PIN, an abnormality of the secretory cell, the basal cells typically are not immunore-

active for prostate-specific antigen (PSA) or prostatic acid phosphatase (PAP), although some patchy positive reaction for these antigens has been reported in atypical basal cell hyperplasia.[50]

Occasionally, florid basal cell hyperplasia may occur,[51] and the term *basal cell adenoma* has been used to refer to well-circumscribed nodular collections of glands with marked basal cell proliferation (Fig. 7–14).[50, 52] Much less commonly, a cribriform pattern of pseudocysts that resembles adenoid cystic carcinoma of the salivary gland may develop (Fig. 7–15),[43, 53–55] and possibly some of the lesions reported as adenoid cystic carcinoma are examples of a florid cribriform basal cell hyper-

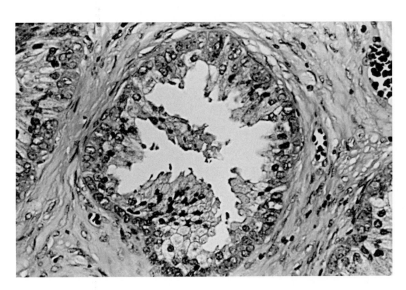

Figure 7–13. Atypical basal cell hyperplasia. Beneath the secretory cell layer there is a proliferation of atypical basal cells with nucleomegaly and prominent nucleoli.

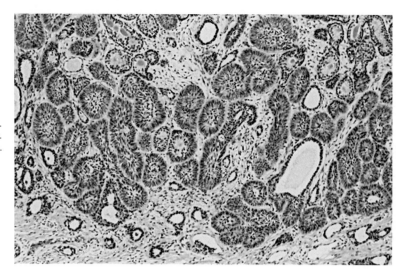

Figure 7–14. A well-circumscribed nodule of basal cell proliferation referred to as *basal cell adenoma.*

plasia.[56–59] Within the spaces of the cribriform basal cell proliferation is a basophilic secretion or hyalinized, eosinophilic material. Cords of basaloid cells may also be found in this lesion, and usually there are glands with nests of hyperplastic basal cells. Squamous metaplasia may be present. This lesion is probably best referred to as an adenoid cystic-like lesion or, alternatively, as an adenoid basal cell tumor,[53, 54] since, although experience is limited, the prognosis appears to be excellent.[55] Rarely, adenoid cystic carcinoma with extensive stromal and perineural invasion has been reported.[53] However, unless there is obvious evidence of infiltration, a diagnosis of adenoid cystic carcinoma is not warranted. Mitotically active, invasive, cytologically malignant basal cell carci-

noma, an extremely rare lesion, has also been reported.[60, 61]

Intraepithelial cytologic atypia with prominent nucleoli may occur in a variety of reactive conditions related to infarction, inflammation, or radiation. Squamous metaplasia is a common response to prostatic glandular injury from a variety of causes, including transurethral prostatectomy, antiandrogen hormonal therapy, radiation therapy, infarction, and inflammation,[47, 48, 62–65] and it may have distinct nucleoli, a finding that might lead to misinterpretation as PIN (Fig. 7–16).[3] It is important to interpret these changes in the clinicopathologic context to avoid overdiagnosis.

Cytologic atypia of benign glands is a common finding in postradiation prostate tissue

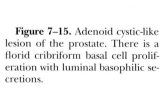

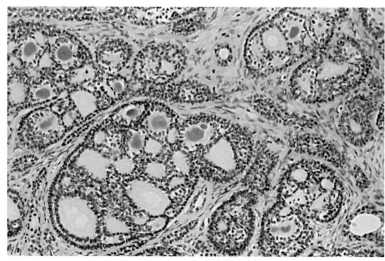

Figure 7–15. Adenoid cystic-like lesion of the prostate. There is a florid cribriform basal cell proliferation with luminal basophilic secretions.

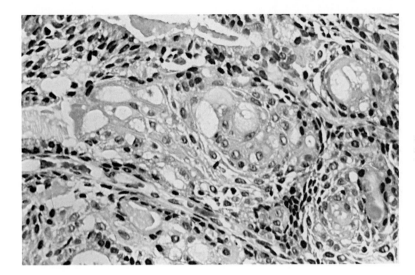

Figure 7–16. Prostate gland squamous metaplasia. An occasional metaplastic cell has a distinct nucleolus.

(Fig. 7–17), and the presence of atypia has been reported in as many as 78% of postradiation prostatic samples.[65] The atypia often varies from cell to cell. When there is a history of radiation, or if there are histologic features to suggest prior radiation, such as a decrease in the gland-to-stroma ratio or stromal fibrosis with glandular atrophy, then the presence of glandular cytologic atypia should be interpreted cautiously. A haphazard infiltrative pattern of the atypical acini is a major clue to the presence of prostatic adenocarcinoma with postradiation effect (Fig. 7–18). In contrast, the distribution of atypical benign glands follows the expected outlines of preexisting duct-acinar units with an atrophic appearance (Fig. 7–17). The transitional cell epithelium lining

the terminal prostatic ducts and prostatic urethra may also develop severe atypia following radiation, and such changes should be interpreted cautiously in this context.

Seminal vesicle tissue may be sampled at the time of prostatic transurethral curettage or needle biopsy, causing concern either because of its crowded glandular pattern or its "atypical" hyperchromatic epithelium (Fig. 7–19).[1, 66] The epithelial changes may be mistaken for PIN.[3] This is more often the case when there is partial sampling of seminal vesicle tissue, making it difficult to recognize its characteristic overall duct-glandular pattern. Correct recognition of this tissue usually is not a problem once one is familiar with the nuclear hyperchromatism and pleomorphism

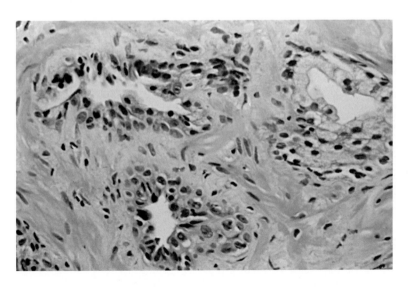

Figure 7–17. Postradiation cytologic atypia of benign glands. The attenuated prostate glands have a noninfiltrative distribution with variable cytologic atypia.

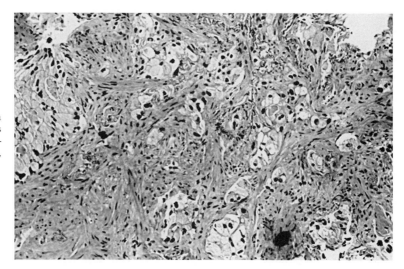

Figure 7–18. Prostate carcinoma with postradiation effect. There is residual carcinoma with an infiltrative pattern, pyknotic nuclei, and cleared cytoplasm.

that can exist in the seminal vesicle (Fig. 7–19).[66] The atypical changes often appear degenerative. As well, the cells vary markedly in nuclear size and shape within the same or immediately adjacent glandular units, an appearance that would be unusual for PIN or prostate adenocarcinoma. The presence of brown lipofuscin pigment within the epithelium is a helpful, but not entirely unique, feature, as it may be seen in benign and neoplastic prostate epithelium as well.[67] Seminal vesicle epithelium is negative for PSA and PAP, and negative immunostains for these markers may be reassuring.

Intraductal transitional cell carcinoma may be confused with PIN, but it usually has malignant cells that are much more pleomorphic, with more angular, hyperchromatic nuclei and darker-staining cytoplasm than those found in high-grade PIN or prostate carcinoma (Fig. 7–20). Transitional cell carcinoma in situ of the prostatic urethra may be present, and a search for this may reveal the true nature of the intraductal disease. A history of bladder carcinoma may be helpful as involvement of the prostate by transitional cell carcinoma is usually associated with primary transitional cell carcinoma of the urinary bladder,[20, 21, 68, 69] although primary transitional cell carcinoma of the prostate uncommonly occurs.[20, 21, 70, 71] Absence of immunoreactivity for PSA and PAP helps to determine the nature of the malignant cells.

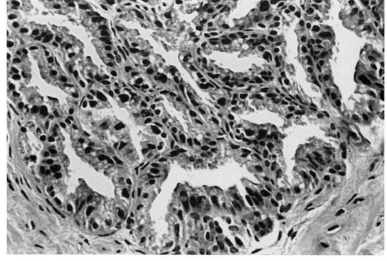

Figure 7–19. Seminal vesicle tissue with characteristic hyperchromatic and pleomorphic epithelium.

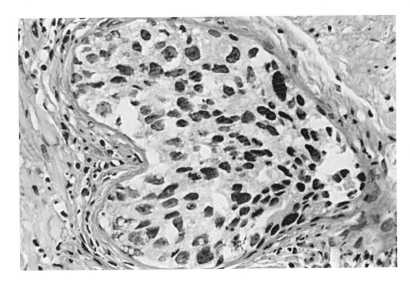

Figure 7–20. Intraductal transitional cell carcinoma. The high-grade malignant cells are pleomorphic with angular and hyperchromatic nuclei.

REFERENCES

1. Jones EC, Young RH: The differential diagnosis of prostatic carcinoma. Its distinction from premalignant and pseudocarcinomatous lesions of the prostate gland. Am J Clin Pathol 101:48–64, 1994.
2. Bostwick DG: High grade prostatic intraepithelial neoplasia: The most likely precursor of prostate cancer. Cancer 75:1823–1836, 1995.
3. Bostwick DG: Premalignant lesions of the prostate. Semin Diagn Pathol 5:240–253, 1988.
4. Mostofi FK, Davis CJ, Sesterhenn IA: Pathology of Carcinoma of the Prostate. Cancer 70 (Suppl):235–253, 1992.
5. McNeal JE, Bostwick DG: Intraductal dysplasia: A premalignant lesion of the prostate. Hum Pathol 17:64–71, 1986.
6. Troncoso P, Babaian RJ, Ro JY, et al.: Prostatic intraepithelial neoplasia and invasive prostatic adenocarcinoma in cystoprostatectomy specimens. Urology 34 (Suppl):52–56, 1989.
7. Kovi J, Mostofi FK, Heshmat MY, Enterline JP: Large acinar atypical hyperplasia and carcinoma of the prostate. Cancer 61:555–561, 1988.
8. Drago JR, Mostofi FK, Lee F, eds: Workshop on prostatic intraepithelial neoplasia: Significance and correlation with prostate-specific antigen and transrectal ultrasound. Urology 34 (Suppl):1–69, 1989.
9. Bostwick DG, Amin MB, Dundore P, et al.: Architectural patterns of high-grade prostatic intraepithelial neoplasia. Hum Pathol 24:298–310, 1993.
10. McNeal JE: Significance of duct-acinar dysplasia in prostatic carcinogenesis. Prostate 13:91–102, 1988.
11. Mostofi FK, Sesterhenn IA, Davis CJ: Prostatic carcinoma: Problems in the interpretation of prostatic biopsies. Hum Pathol 23:223–241, 1992.
12. Epstein JI, Grignon DJ, Humphrey PA, et al.: Interobserver reproducibility in the diagnosis of prostatic intraepithelial neoplasia (PIN). Am J Surg Pathol 19:873–886, 1995.
13. Allam CK, Bostwick DG, Hayes JA, et al.: Interobserver variability in the diagnosis of high grade prostatic intraepithelial neoplasia and adenocarcinoma. Mod Pathol 9:742–751, 1996.
14. Bostwick DG, Brawer MK: Prostatic intraepithelial neoplasia and early invasion in prostate cancer. Cancer 59:788–794, 1987.
15. Shah IA, Schlageter MO, Stinnett P, et al.: Cytokeratin immunohistochemistry as a diagnostic tool for distinguishing malignant from benign epithelial lesions of the prostate. Mod Pathol 4:220–224, 1991.
16. de la Torre M, Haggman M, Brandstedt S, et al.: Prostatic intraepithelial neoplasia and invasive carcinoma in total prostatectomy specimens: distribution, volumes and DNA ploidy. Br J Urol 72:207–213, 1993.
17. Hedrick L, Epstein JI: Use of keratin 903 as an adjunct in the diagnosis of prostate carcinoma. Am J Surg Pathol 13:389–396, 1989.
18. Brawer MK, Peehl DM, Stamey TA, et al.: Keratin immunoreactivity in the benign and neoplastic human prostate. Cancer Res 45:3663–3667, 1985.
19. Amin MB, Schultz DS, Zarbo RJ: Analysis of cribriform morphology in prostatic neoplasia using antibody to high–molecular-weight cytokeratins. Arch Pathol Lab Med 118:260–264, 1994.
20. Bostwick DG, ed: Pathology of the Prostate. New York: Churchill Livingstone, 1990.
21. Epstein JI: Prostate Biopsy Interpretation. New York: Raven Press, 1989.
22. Wojno KJ, Epstein JI: The utility of basal cell–specific anti-cytokeratin antibody (34betaE12) in the diagnosis of prostate cancer: A review of 228 cases. Am J Surg Pathol 19:251–260, 1995.
23. McNeal JE, Villers A, Redwine EA, et al.: Microcarcinoma in the prostate: Its association with duct-acinar dysplasia. Hum Pathol 22:644–652, 1991.
24. Weinstein MH, Epstein JI: Significance of high grade prostatic intraepithelial neoplasia on needle biopsy. Hum Pathol 24:624–629, 1993.
25. Quinn BD, Cho KR, Epstein JI: Relationship of severe dysplasia to stage B adenocarcinoma of the prostate. Cancer 65:2328–2337, 1990.
26. Ro JY, Grignon DJ, Troncoso P, et al.: Mucin in prostatic adenocarcinoma. Semin Diagn Pathol 5:273–283, 1988.
27. Pinder SE, McMahon RFT: Mucins in prostatic carcinoma. Histopathology 16:43–46, 1990.
28. Taylor NS: Histochemistry in the diagnosis of early prostatic carcinoma. Hum Pathol 10:513–520, 1979.

29. Sentinelli S: Mucins in prostatic intra-epithelial neoplasia and prostatic carcinoma. Histopathology 22:271–274, 1993.

30. Humphrey PA: Mucin in severe dysplasia in the prostate. Surg Pathol 4:137–143, 1991.

31. Holmes EJ: Crystalloids of prostatic carcinoma: Relationship to Bence-Jones crystals. Cancer 39:2073–2080, 1977.

32. Jensen PE, Gardner WA, Piserchia PV: Prostatic crystalloids: Association with adenocarcinoma. Prostate 1:25–30, 1980.

33. Furusato M, Kato H, Takahashi H, et al.: Crystalloids in latent prostatic carcinoma. Prostate 15:259–262, 1989.

34. delRosario A, Bui H, Khan M, et al.: Prostatic intraluminal "crystalloids": Significance as an indicator of prostatic malignancy. Mod Pathol 5:52A, 1992.

35. Ro JY, Ayala AG, Ordonez NG, et al.: Intraluminal crystalloids in prostatic adenocarcinoma: Immunohistochemical, electron microscopic and x-ray microanalytic studies. Cancer 57:2397–2407, 1986.

36. Bennett B, Gardner WA: Crystalloids in prostatic hyperplasia. Prostate 1:31–35, 1980.

37. McNeal JE, Reese JH, Redwine EA, et al.: Cribriform adenocarcinoma of the prostate. Cancer 58:1714–1719, 1986.

38. Wernert N, Luchtrath H, Seeliger H, et al.: Papillary carcinoma of the prostate, location, morphology and immunohistochemistry: The histogenesis and entity of so-called endometrioid carcinoma. Prostate 10:123–131, 1987.

39. Bostwick DG, Kindrachuk RW, Rouse RV: Prostatic adenocarcinoma with endometrioid features: Clinical, pathologic, and ultrastructural findings. Am J Surg Pathol 9:595–609, 1985.

40. Kuhajda FP, Gipson T, Mendelsohn G: Papillary adenocarcinomas of the prostate: An immunohistochemical study. Cancer 54:1328–1332, 1984.

41. Ayala AG, Srigley JR, Ro JY, et al.: Clear cell cribriform hyperplasia of prostate. Report of 10 cases. Am J Surg Pathol 10:665–671, 1986.

42. Frauenhoffer EE, Ro JY, El-Naggar AK, et al.: Clear cell cribriform hyperplasia of the prostate. Immunohistochemical and DNA flow cytometric study. Am J Clin Pathol 95:446–453, 1991.

43. Gleason DF: Atypical hyperplasia, benign hyperplasia, and well-differentiated adenocarcinoma of the prostate. Am J Surg Pathol 9 (Suppl):53–67, 1985.

44. Keane PF, Ilesley IC, O'Donoghue EPN, et al.: Pathological classification and follow-up of prostatic lesions initially diagnosed as "suspicious of malignancy." Br J Urol 66:306–311, 1990.

45. Cleary KR, Choi HY, Ayala AG: Basal cell hyperplasia of the prostate. Am J Clin Pathol 80:850–854, 1983.

46. Bennett BD, Gardner WA: Embryonal hyperplasia of the prostate. Prostate 7:411–417, 1985.

47. Tetu B, Srigley JR, Boivin JC, et al.: Effect of combination endocrine therapy (LHRH agonist and Flutamide) on normal prostate and prostatic adenocarcinoma: A histopathologic and immunohistochemical study. Am J Surg Pathol 15:111–120, 1991.

48. Armas OA, Aprikian AG, Melamed J, et al.: Clinical and pathobiological effects of neoadjuvant total androgen ablation therapy on clinically localized prostatic adenocarcinoma. Am J Surg Pathol 18:979–991, 1994.

49. Epstein JI, Armas OA: Atypical basal cell hyperplasia of the prostate. Am J Surg Pathol 16:1205–1214, 1992.

50. Devaraj LT, Bostwick DG: Atypical basal cell hyperplasia of the prostate: Immunophenotypic profile and proposed classification of basal cell proliferations. Am J Surg Pathol 17:645–659, 1993.

51. Van De Voorde W, Baldewijns M, Lauweryns J: Florid basal cell hyperplasia of the prostate. Histopathology 24:341–348, 1994.

52. Lin JI, Cohen EL, Villacin AB, et al.: Basal cell adenoma of prostate. Urology 11:409–410, 1978.

53. Grignon DJ, Ro JY, Ordonez NG, et al.: Basal cell hyperplasia, adenoid basal cell tumor, and adenoid cystic carcinoma of the prostate gland: An immunohistochemical study. Hum Pathol 19:1425–1433, 1988.

54. Reed RJ: Consultation case. Am J Surg Pathol 8:699–704, 1984.

55. Young RH, Frierson HF, Mills SE, et al.: Adenoid cystic-like tumor of the prostate gland: A report of two cases and review of the literature on "adenoid cystic carcinoma" of the prostate. Am J Clin Pathol 89:49–56, 1988.

56. Kuhajda FP, Mann RB: Adenoid cystic carcinoma of the prostate. A case report with immunoperoxidase staining for prostate-specific acid phosphatase and prostate-specific antigen. Am J Clin Pathol 81:257–260, 1984.

57. Shong-San C, Walters MNI: Adenoid cystic carcinoma of prostate. Report of a case. Pathology 16:337–338, 1984.

58. Gilmour AM, Bell TJ: Adenoid cystic carcinoma of the prostate. Br J Urol 58:105–106, 1986.

59. Frankel K, Craig JR: Adenoid cystic carcinoma of the prostate. Report of a case. Am J Clin Pathol 62:639–645, 1974.

60. Sesterhenn I, Mostofi FK, Davis CJ: Basal cell hyperplasia and basal cell carcinoma. Lab Invest 56:71A, 1987.

61. Denholm SW, Webb JN, Howard GCW, et al.: Basaloid carcinoma of the prostate gland: Histogenesis and review of the literature. Histopathology 20:151–155, 1992.

62. Mostofi FK, Morse WH: Epithelial metaplasia in "prostatic infarction." Arch Pathol 51:340–345, 1951.

63. Bainborough AR: Squamous metaplasia of prostate following estrogen therapy. J Urol 68:329–336, 1952.

64. Sutton EB, McDonald JR: Metaplasia of the prostatic epithelium: A lesion sometimes mistaken for carcinoma. Am J Clin Pathol 13;607–615, 1943.

65. Bostwick DG, Egbert BM, Fajardo LF: Radiation injury of the normal and neoplastic prostate. Am J Surg Pathol 6:541–551, 1982.

66. Kuo T, Gomez LG: Monstrous epithelial cells in human epididymis and seminal vesicles: A pseudomalignant change. Am J Surg Pathol 5:483–490, 1981.

67. Brennick JB, O'Connell JX, Dickersin GR, et al.: Lipofuscin pigmentation (so-called "melanosis") of the prostate. Am J Surg Pathol 18:446–454, 1994.

68. Bryan RL, Newman J, Suarez V, et al.: The significance of prostatic urothelial dysplasia. Histopathology 22:501–503, 1993.

69. Wood DP, Montie JE, Pontes JE, et al.: Transitional cell carcinoma of the prostate in cystoprostatectomy specimens removed for bladder cancer. J Urol 141:346–349, 1989.

70. Nicolaisen GS, Williams RD: Primary transitional cell carcinoma of prostate. Urology 24:544–549, 1984.

71. Sawczuk I, Tannenbaum M, Olsson CA, et al.: Primary transitional cell carcinoma of prostatic periurethral ducts. Urology 25:339–343, 1985.

8

SMALL GLANDULAR PATTERNS IN THE PROSTATE: DIFFERENTIAL DIAGNOSIS OF SMALL ACINAR CARCINOMA

JOHN R. SRIGLEY, MARTIN BULLOCK, and MAHUL AMIN

A clear understanding of the differential diagnosis of a small acinar histologic pattern in the prostate gland is important for the accurate interpretation of prostate specimens. A recent review of problem areas in pathology practice cites the increasing frequency of malpractice claims against pathologists in the United States and mentions diagnostic problems with needle biopsy prostate specimens as one area of particular concern.[1] Thus, misdiagnosis has serious repercussions for pathologist and patient alike.

In general, the entities that comprise the differential diagnosis of small acinar adenocarcinoma can be divided into three groups: (1) preexisting normal structures consisting of small glands, such as the seminal vesicles or Cowper's glands; (2) altered native prostate structures, including all forms of atrophy and mucous gland metaplasia; and (3) neoacinar patterns, both benign and malignant (Table 8–1). To arrive at a correct diagnosis, the pathologist must be aware of the normal histologic appearance of the prostate and surrounding structures and must be provided with accurate clinical information, including digital rectal examination and ultrasound findings, serum prostate-specific antigen (PSA) level, history of previous therapy and the sites of the current biopsies.

In evaluating a small glandular lesion it is important to define the type of specimen under consideration. Various small gland lesions have predilections for certain zones of the prostate. For example, transurethral resection of prostate (TURP) samples the transition zone and hence the chief differential diagnostic considerations include lesions that have a proclivity for this zone. Similarly, needle biopsy samples chiefly the peripheral zone, and consideration should first be given to lesions that are more common in this zone. The transition zone normally is not sampled by random needle biopsy but can be targeted with ultrasonographic guidance. Exceptional enlargement of the transition zone by benign prostatic hyperplasia (BPH) can result in "thinning" of the peripheral zone, and in this situation the transition zone may be sampled inadvertently with needle biopsy. The central zone is sampled chiefly by random or sextant needle biopsy but may be included in TURP specimens. Table 8–2 places the small gland proliferations in perspective with respect to zonal anatomy.

The purpose of this review is to provide a comprehensive classification of small acinar patterns in the prostate and an approach to determining the correct diagnosis. In addition, we provide criteria for the diagnosis of small acinar adenocarcinomas and discuss when it

Table 8–1. Small Glandular Patterns in the Prostate in the Differential Diagnosis of Small Acinar Carcinoma

---

Normal histoanatomic structures
    Seminal vesicle
    Ejaculatory duct
    Cowper's gland
    Paraganglion
Alternated native prostatic glands
    Glandular atrophy
        Simple (lobular) atrophy
        Sclerotic atrophy
        Treatment-associated atrophy
            Radiation
            Antiandrogens
    Mucous gland metaplasia
Benign neoacinar proliferations
    Hyperplasia of mesonephric duct remnants
    Nephrogenic metaplasia of prostatic urethra
    Verumontanum mucosal gland hyperplasia
    Prostatic hyperplasia
        Postatrophic hyperplasia
        Benign nodular hyperplasia, small glandular variant
        Basal cell hyperplasia
        Sclerosing adenosis
Atypical adenomatous hyperplasia (adenosis)
Small acinar carcinoma

---

is best to call a lesion "atypical small acinar proliferation of uncertain significance." The clinical relevance of the latter diagnosis is also examined. We can hope that the experience of pathologists in this area will spare patients unnecessary investigations and surgery and protect some physicians from litigation.

In this chapter, we also discuss the staining pattern and the diagnostic utility of basal cell–specific, high–molecular weight cytokeratin (34β-E12). Since complete loss of basal cells is the hallmark of carcinoma, this stain may be used in conjunction with morphology to confirm or rule out the presence of a neoplastic small glandular process.

NORMAL HISTOANATOMIC STRUCTURES WITH A SMALL GLANDULAR PATTERN

Seminal Vesicles and Ejaculatory Ducts

The seminal vesicles are tubular structures generally located posterior and superior to the prostate gland, against the base of the bladder. The excretory ducts of the seminal vesicles join the ampulla of the vas deferens to form the ejaculatory ducts, which enter the prostate and open into the distal prostatic urethra at the verumontanum. The anatomic site of these structures does vary some, and the seminal vesicles may be located farther inferior or can even lie partly within the substance of the gland itself. Misinterpretation of seminal vesicle tissue as adenocarcinoma generally occurs in needle biopsy specimens from the base of the prostate, in which they may be inadvertently sampled.

The tightly-coiled seminal vesicle consists of a single main duct from which emanate secondary and tertiary ducts that ultimately terminate in multiple acini. As patients age, the acini become more complex and develop prominent mucosal folds. Each acinus is lined by two layers of epithelial cells, columnar and basal cells. Especially in older persons, the former may show varying degrees of nucleomegaly, nuclear hyperchromasia, and atypia.[2, 3] Seminal vesicle epithelium frequently contains intranuclear cytoplasmic inclusions. It is precisely the degree of atypia (greater than that in most prostate carcinomas) and the frequent presence of golden-colored lipofuscin pigment in the cytoplasm that distinguish seminal vesicle epithelial cells from those of small acinar adenocarcinoma. That said, however, lipofus-

Table 8–2. Differential Diagnosis of Small Glandular Lesions of Prostate in Relation to Zonal Anatomy of the Prostate

---

Transition zone
    Histoanatomic structures
        Verumontanum
        Mesonephric remnants
        Ejaculatory ducts
    Atrophy (uncommon)
    Neoacinar proliferations
        Nephrogenic adenoma
        Sclerosing adenosis
        Basal cell hyperplasia
        Small gland variant of nodular hyperplasia
        Atypical adenomatous hyperplasia
        Small acinar carcinoma (15–25%)
Peripheral zone
    Histoanatomic structures
        Paraganglia
        Cowper's gland
        Seminal vesicle/ejaculatory duct
    Atrophy
Post-atrophic hyperplasia
    Small acinar carcinoma (70%)
Central zone
    Histoanatomic structures
        Seminal vesicle/ejaculatory duct
        Paraganglia
    Atrophy
    Small acinar carcinoma

---

cin may not be present, especially in a small biopsy specimen, and it is not specific for the seminal vesicles. The pigment of seminal vesicle tends to differ somewhat morphologically from the pigment in prostatic epithelium, although in both it is lipofuscin. The pigment of seminal vesicles is golden yellow and takes the form of large, chunky (granular) deposits that are refractile. The pigment of prostatic epithelium (observed in BPH, preneoplastic (PIN), or cancerous epithelium) is relatively sparse, finely granular, and usually yellow-brown, although it may have a darker gray hue. On occasion, the pigment may appear prominent.[4-6] The acini of seminal vesicles usually maintain a circumscribed, pushing arrangement, although the unwary observer can be fooled by a pseudoinvasive pattern of acini arranged more haphazardly and spread apart (Fig. 8–1). Immunohistochemistry is usually not necessary but can be used to demonstrate absence of staining for PSA if adenocarcinoma of prostate is a diagnostic consideration. A high–molecular weight cytokeratin shows intense staining of the basal cell layer.

Portions of the ejaculatory ducts may be present in TURP or needle biopsy specimens. These paired ducts have a double-layered epithelium, which may contain lipofuscin similar to that of the seminal vesicles. In general, the ejaculatory ducts have wide lumina with mucosal infolding and a prominent fibromuscular band. When the duct is sampled in its entirety, distinguishing it from adenocarcinoma should not be difficult; however, a tangential cut of a portion of the duct can create difficulties. The

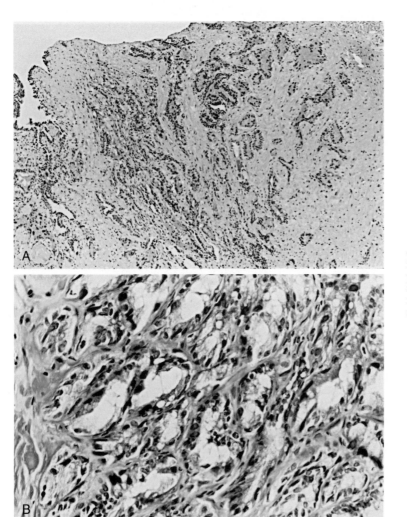

Figure 8–1. *(A)* Seminal vesicle on low-power magnification. Note irregularity and pseudoinvasive pattern (H&E). *(B)* Acini of seminal vesicle display focal enlargement and hyperchromasia of luminal cells (H&E).

presence of pigment similar to that of seminal vesicle, the site of the sample, and the double-layered epithelium should allow the correct diagnosis to be made.

Cowper's Glands

Cowper's glands, paired glands located within the urogenital diaphragm, have ducts that open into the floor of the bulbous urethra.[7] They are mucous glands equivalent to Bartholin's glands in females. Because of their location they may be encountered in needle biopsy specimens from the apex of the prostate. They should not be present in TURP specimens and if noted should be documented, as their presence indicates that the urologist has exceeded the usual limits of TURP, which could cause incontinence.[8, 9] Histologically, they appear as lobules of uniform, closely–packed acini (Fig. 8–2). The Cowper's glands are reminiscent of minor salivary glands because of their mucinous cytoplasm and the presence of an excretory duct. Owing to their location in the urogenital diaphragm, Cowper's glands are frequently bordered by skeletal muscle. The epithelial cells have voluminous, pale, foamy cytoplasm unlike that of small acinar adenocarcinomas. The acini are lined by a single layer of bland cells with uniform, basally located nuclei. Nucleoli are inconspicuous or absent. Mucin stains display intense cytoplasmic positivity. A PSA immunohistochemical stain helps confirm the extraprostatic nature of the tissue.

Paraganglia

Paraganglionic tissue is encountered occasionally in periprostatic connective tissue. These are presumably sympathetic paraganglia, which in the pelvis are associated with urogenital organs, particularly the urinary bladder.[9] Paraganglia encountered in radical prostatectomy specimens should be distinguished from extraprostatic spread of adenocarcinoma, particularly of the hypernephroid type.[10] Paraganglia are most often found along the lateral neurovascular bundle but occasionally are present within the capsule.

Paraganglia consist of organoid collections of polygonal cells with abundant amphophilic or clear and often finely granular cytoplasm and small, ovoid nuclei (Fig. 8–3). They are frequently associated with small nerves and are well-vascularized by small blood vessels. Lumina are not identified. In contrast to the parasympathetic carotid body, nests of neuroendocrine cells forming *Zellballen* are not conspicuous in sympathetic paraganglia. The polygonal chief cells or type 1 cells stain positively for neuron-specific enolase and chromogranin, whereas the network of sustentacular cells is positive for S-100. Paraganglionic tissue is negative for PSA or prostate-specific acid phosphatase (PSAP).

ATROPHY AND RELATED LESIONS

Atrophy is a common finding in the prostate and, according to some experts, is the lesion

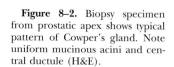

Figure 8–2. Biopsy specimen from prostatic apex shows typical pattern of Cowper's gland. Note uniform mucinous acini and central ductule (H&E).

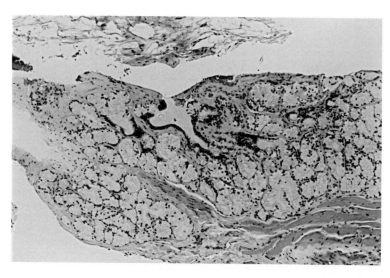

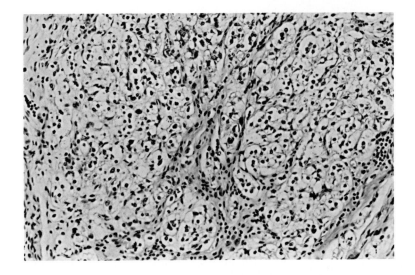

Figure 8–3. Prostatic paraganglia. Note nests of clear cells with uniform central nuclei. A delicate fibrovascular stroma is apparent (H&E).

most frequently confused with carcinoma.[11, 12] In addition to simple (lobular) atrophy, the type with which most of us are familiar, sclerotic and cystic variants also occur. Atrophy may be a morphologic consequence of treatment with radiation or hormone therapy. Postatrophic hyperplasia is discussed later, in conjunction with other forms of hyperplasia.

Simple (Lobular) Atrophy

Lobular atrophy is most often seen in biopsy specimens from the peripheral zone of the gland but can also occur in periurethral tissue and central zone epithelium. It may be seen in adult men of all ages (as young as 20 years) but is most common in the prostates of older

men, where it often coexists with BPH.[13] The causes are multiple—compression due to benign nodular hyperplasia, hormone imbalance, ischemia, inflammation, and perhaps nutritional deficiency.

The atrophic glands appear shrunken and closely packed (Fig. 8–4). The cells lining the glands are inconspicuous, with markedly reduced cytoplasm. The latter leads to an increased nuclear-cytoplasmic ratio. The nuclei usually appear slightly hyperchromatic but are uniform and small, with inconspicuous nucleoli. Basal cells, the hallmark of a benign process, are present but may be difficult to identify by light microscopy; moreover, the shrunken secretory cells resemble basal cells, making distinction between the two difficult. The surrounding stroma also exhibits atrophy

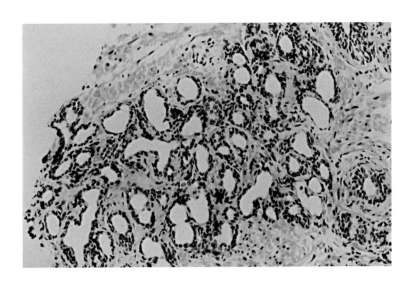

Figure 8–4. Simple atrophy of prostate gland. Note lobular organization and uniformity of glands. Shrunken, hyperchromatic cells are apparent. No atypia is noted (H&E).

of the muscular elements, with fibrous replacement and sometimes thickening of the periacinar collagen.[8, 14] Often, the low-power pattern is the feature most useful in distinguishing atrophy from adenocarcinoma. As the name suggests, lobular atrophy usually maintains its lobular configuration, and smaller glands sometimes arise from or surround a larger, central gland. While this lobular pattern is easy to identify in radical prostatectomy specimens, it can be difficult to appreciate in small biopsy samples. Distinction from adenocarcinoma requires reliance on cytologic features and recognition of basal cells. Cystic atrophy is a variant of simple atrophy that preferentially involves the most peripheral acini, often in a posterolateral site, and that produces a Swiss-cheese appearance on low-power examination. The cysts are lined by atrophic cells, as in simple atrophy; however, the glands are still capable of secretion.[14]

Sclerotic Atrophy

Like simple atrophy, sclerotic atrophy is predominantly a peripheral zone process but is less common. It is characterized by distorted glandular elements separated haphazardly by varying stroma, that can appear desmoplastic (Fig. 8–5). The glands usually show cytologic features similar to those of simple atrophy, but the stromal pattern may be mistaken for tumor-induced desmoplasia.[8] Careful attention to an overall lobular low-power pattern and "benign cytology" should prevent misinterpretation. A characteristic feature is compression, with elongation and sharp angulation of the glands and acini resembling stag horns, which would be unusual in adenocarcinoma (see Fig. 8–5). In the early stages of sclerotic atrophy, a lymphohistiocytic reaction may surround affected acini.[14]

Treatment-Related Atrophy and Other Treatment Effects

Atrophy is the major common pathologic finding in prostates of men treated with external-beam radiation, diethylstilbestrol (DES) or another synthetic estrogen, and luteinizing hormone–releasing hormone (LHRH) agonists or antiandrogens.[15–21] Needle biopsy is routinely used to follow cancer patients treated with radiation therapy, neoadjuvant therapy with LHRH agonists, or antiandrogens before radical prostatectomy.[22] Since hormone therapy is becoming increasingly frequent, pathologists will be faced with evaluating the effects of these therapies and distinguishing treatment-related effects on normal prostate from residual tumor.

In addition to atrophy, external irradiation of nonneoplastic prostate tissue causes squamous metaplasia, accumulation of granular, brown, cytoplasmic pigment,[16] stromal fibrosis, and vascular changes.[15] Both malignant and benign glands exhibit cytologic atypia with marked nuclear enlargement, prominent nucleoli, and cytoplasmic enlargement and vacuolization (Fig. 8–6). The tumor may show

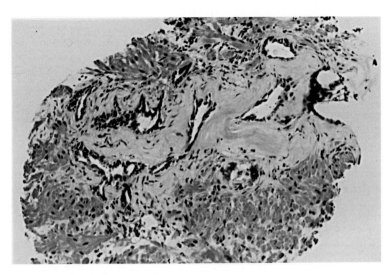

Figure 8–5. Sclerotic atrophy. Note irregular, hyperchromatic acini encircled by dense, hyalinized connective tissue (H&E).

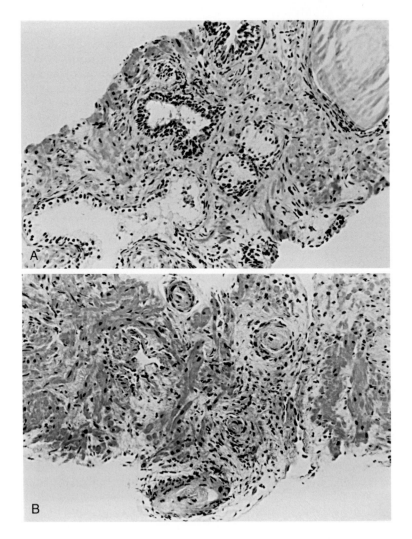

Figure 8–6. *(A)* Radiation effects in a prostatic biopsy specimen. Note glandular atrophy and hyperchromasia with nuclear irregularity of lining cells (H&E). *(B)* Stromal changes of radiation with arteriolar thickening and patchy chronic inflammation (H&E).

loss of gland formation, apparently resembling a higher Gleason grade pattern.[16]

LHRH agonists are commonly combined with an antiandrogen to create total androgen blockade (TAB), and most studies of neoadjuvant therapy have described the effects of TAB. Benign glands show marked atrophy with prominence—and often hyperplasia—of the basal cell layer (Fig. 8–7).[18–21] Squamous and transitional cell metaplasia are seen in some cases, although the former tends to be less frequent than with DES treatment.[17] The secretory cells of non-neoplastic glands exhibit cytoplasmic clearing and vacuolization.[18–21]

Histologic changes in prostate carcinoma cells after TAB include marked clearing, vacuolization, and ultimately loss of cytoplasm with a resultant decrease in the size and density of malignant glands (Fig. 8–8).[20] Less fre-

quently, malignant glands may be dilated and resemble benign atrophic glands.[19] In some cases treated with the antiandrogen cyproterone acetate alone, malignant glands are partially or completely replaced by an accumulation of basophilic mucin. A similar pattern was described by Civantos and coworkers with TAB.[20]

The tumor cells show nuclear pyknosis and small nucleoli.[18–21] Occasionally, the remaining tumor appears simply as branching clefts lined by a few inconspicuous, vacuolized tumor cells, creating the so-called hemangiopericytoma-like pattern described by Têtu and associates.[18] The surrounding stroma may be abundant and hyalinized and a lymphohistiocytic infiltrate is noted in some cases.[19, 20] Diminution of glandular architecture may result in a higher Gleason grade (artifactual upgrading) unless the

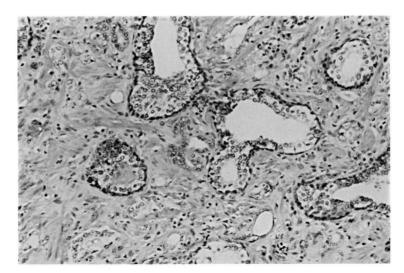

Figure 8–7. Antiandrogen effects in the prostate gland. Note nonneoplastic glands with vacuolization of secretory cells and basal cell prominence. Shrunken and vacuolated neoplastic glands are present in the background (H&E).

scoring system is modified to account for treatment effects.[19–23] The best method of grading these cases has yet to be established. Many studies have included cases in which no residual tumor is identified after treatment[18, 21]; however, we believe that marked hormonal changes can prevent identification of residual tumor in these apparently pT0 cases. In our practice, we have occasionally used a cytokeratin stain to highlight the inconspicuous infiltrating neoplastic cells.

Finally, it is worth noting that, although human data are limited, the 5-α-reductase inhibitor finasteride (Proscar) commonly used to treat BPH has been shown in dog prostates to cause atrophy of both glands and stroma and lymphocytic infiltration of the stroma.[24, 25]

Mucous Gland Metaplasia

Shiraishi and colleagues, in a study of autopsy prostates, described a lesion they termed "mucous gland metaplasia."[26] The pattern is histologically very similar to Cowper's gland epithelium, consisting of lobular collections of small, regular acini lined by a single layer of plump, mucin-containing cells. The nuclei are small and basally located. In contrast to Cowper's glands, the foci may be found in all parts of the gland and are intimately related to normal prostatic epithelium, suggesting a metaplastic process. Mucinous metaplasia may also be found in atrophic foci (Fig. 8–9).[27] Mucinous metaplasia can partially involve acini (incomplete metaplasia) or completely replace

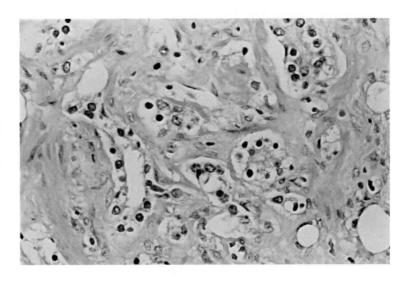

Figure 8–8. Prostate carcinoma shows marked antiandrogen effects. Note vacuolation of cytoplasm and prominent pyknosis (H&E).

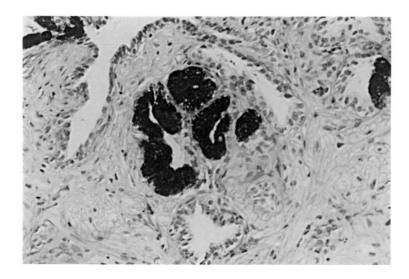

Figure 8–9. Atrophic prostate glands display focal mucinous metaplasia (PAS-diastase).

the secretory epithelium. The foci are usually small, positive for mucicarmine, alcian blue, and high–molecular weight cytokeratin, and negative for PSA.

NEOACINAR PROLIFERATIONS WITH A SMALL GLANDULAR PATTERN

Hyperplasia of Mesonephric Duct Remnants

Florid hyperplasia of mesonephric remnants mimicking prostatic adenocarcinoma was initially reported by Gikas and coworkers in 1993.[28] This process is recognized much more often in the female genitourinary tract, particularly in the uterine cervix.[29] Although rare, hyperplasia of mesonephric duct remnants can be particularly difficult to distinguish from adenocarcinoma, and one of the two cases reported by Gikas and colleagues resulted in radical excision of a prostate that did not contain carcinoma.[28] Mesonephric remnants are usually present in vesicle neck tissues, which may be represented in TURP chips. They may originate in unabsorbed portions of the mesonephric ducts, which give rise to the primordial ejaculatory ducts and ureters in the region of the bladder neck. Hyperplasia of the mesonephric remnants is diagnostically challenging, as it consists of collections of small tubules lined by a single layer of cuboidal or atrophic epithelial cells. The tubules may contain eosinophilic, colloidlike material and thus resemble thyroid follicles (Fig. 8–10). The cells are usually benign-appearing, although the nucleoli

may be conspicuous. In some cases, the tubules are more open, with micropapillary infoldings into the lumen.[28] Particularly troubling is infiltration of these tubules into smooth muscle bundles of the vesicle neck and their frequent association with nerves or ganglion cells.

Several features distinguish mesonephric hyperplasia from adenocarcinoma. First, the tubules often retain a vaguely lobular configuration. The presence of acini that contain colloidlike material, cuboidal cells with scant cytoplasm, or frank atrophy of the epithelial cells and micropapillary infoldings should alert the observer to the possibility of mesonephric hyperplasia. Immunohistochemical analysis has important confirmatory value, as these remnants are negative for PSA and PSAP but positive for high–molecular weight cytokeratin. In some cases of cervical mesonephric hyperplasia the tubules have been described as opening into a central duct; however, to our knowledge this has not been noted in the prostate.

Nephrogenic Adenoma (Metaplasia) of the Prostatic Urethra

Nephrogenic adenoma is most often found in the urinary bladder, but it can involve urothelium in any site.[30] The term is a misnomer, as the lesion neither arises from the kidney (i.e., it is not nephrogenic) nor is a benign neoplasm (not adenoma). It is a metaplastic process that arises as a result of injury to the urothelium, as by a surgical procedure, urinary calculi, infection, or another insult.[31] When this process involves the prostatic urethra it can extend into the prostatic parenchyma and be confused with several other small acinar

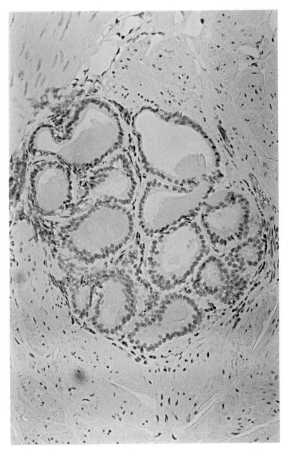

Figure 8–10. Hyperplasia of mesonephric gland remnants. Note lobular arrangement, bland nuclear features, and colloidlike secretion in lumina (H&E).

processes, most importantly carcinoma.[32, 33] The lesion is usually found in the TURP specimens of older men who present with symptoms of urinary obstruction. Patients can also present with hematuria, dysuria, or pyuria, but approximately 20% of such lesions are asymptomatic. Clinical information may be of value, as the lesion often has a shaggy, frondlike, erythematous appearance at cystoscopy.

By light microscopy, nephrogenic adenoma may be seen in association with the urothelium as an exophytic papillary proliferation with tubules extending inward through the underlying lamina propria into prostatic parenchyma. Low-power examination reveals acini that are scattered haphazardly, without lobular organization, and this raises the question of adenocarcinoma (Fig. 8–11). The tubules are small, round to oval, and sometimes cystically dilated. They are lined by a single layer of cuboidal or flattened cells, which sometimes protrude into the lumen in a "hobnail" fashion. The cytoplasm is eosinophilic or clear. On cytologic examination, the cells are bland, with evenly distributed chromatin and usually inconspicuous nucleoli. In some cases, the acini contain colloidlike intraluminal secretions.[33]

Several features distinguish nephrogenic metaplasia from adenocarcinoma. As opposed to the compact stroma that surrounds a malignant process, the stroma of nephrogenic adenoma is usually edematous. Chronic inflammation is noted on occasion.[33] The bland cytologic appearance (especially the absence of prominent nucleoli in most cells and their hobnail appearance), cystic dilatation of some tubules, and the association of the lesion with the urothelium are other useful distinguishing features. Immunohistochemistry reveals no PSA or PAP in the cells of nephrogenic adenoma.

Verumontanum Mucosal Gland Hyperplasia

Verumontanum mucosal gland hyperplasia (VMGH) is an entity that has only recently received formal recognition in the world literature, but its description by Gagucas and colleagues "rings a bell" in the minds of pathologists who examine many radical prostatectomy specimens.[34]

The verumontanum is an elevated ridge on the posterior wall of the prostatic urethra that is easily recognized during cystoscopy and, as such, is used as a landmark during TURP. It is the site where the prostatic ducts, the ejaculatory ducts, and the utricle enter the urethra. The verumontanum is rarely sampled by needle biopsy and is avoided during TURP by urologists who remove hyperplastic tissue proximal to this site but leave the verumontanum intact.

Gagucas' group recognized VMGH in 14% of 341 radical prostatectomy specimens they examined, and Gaudin and coworkers observed it in needle biopsy tissue.[34, 35] The definition of VMGH is rather arbitrary and ill-defined, and no criteria are available to separate it from normal verumontanum glands. Perhaps lesions designated as VGMH are patterned at the extreme end of the histologic spectrum. Nonetheless, those lesions containing 25 acini or more (as defined by Gagucas) may warrant inclusion of VMGH in the differential diagnosis of small acinar proliferations.

The lesion consists of one or more well-

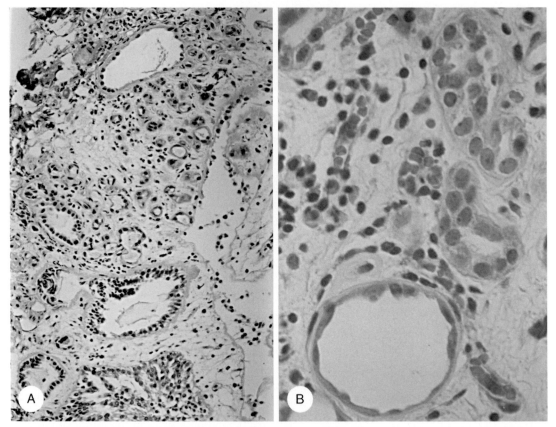

Figure 8–11. *(A)* Nephrogenic adenoma (metaplasia) of the prostatic urethra. Note tiny tubules and cystic spaces, some of which are lined by hobnail-type cells (H&E). *(B)* High-power photomicrograph of nephrogenic adenoma. Note bland, uniform nuclei with tiny chromocenters. These glands stain negatively for PSA (H&E).

circumscribed collections of small acini (i.e., rarely larger than 2 mm in maximum diameter).[34, 35] The acini are arranged back to back and are composed of cuboidal to columnar epithelial cells surrounded by a rim of basal cells (Fig. 8–12). The cuboidal cells are cytologically bland, with small nuclei and inconspicuous nucleoli. Their cytoplasm may contain granular lipofuchsin pigment. A characteristic finding is the presence of corpora amylacea, which are often small and numerous. Fragmented, orange-red luminal concretions, which lack the rounded, concentric morphology of corpora amylacea, are also seen. Crystalloids are not identified, and intraluminal mucin is rare.[35] The foci are well-circumscribed and may consist of fewer than 10 acini or more than 50. The luminal cells are strongly PSA positive, whereas the basal cells stain with high–molecular weight keratin.[34]

Ultimately, precise recognition of VMGH depends on the correct identification of benign-looking acini composed of the two epithelial cell types present in their appropriate location. The presence of urothelium adjacent to the lesion is strong supporting evidence for VMGH. It should rarely be confused with small acinar carcinoma, which, even in its most innocuous form, exhibits nuclear alterations and lacks a basal cell layer (see below).

The histogenesis of VMGH is unclear. Foci are seen to arise from all components of the verumontanum (i.e., the ejaculatory and prostatic ducts, the utricle, and the posterior urethral mucosa). They can arise from more than one of these structures in the same gland.[34] An association with BPH has not been established, and it is unlikely that VMGH is ever symptomatic. For now, the "entity" remains an enigma, but without it the spectrum of small gland proliferations would be incomplete.

Prostatic Hyperplasia

Many forms of hyperplasia occur in the prostate, and most are discussed in earlier chap-

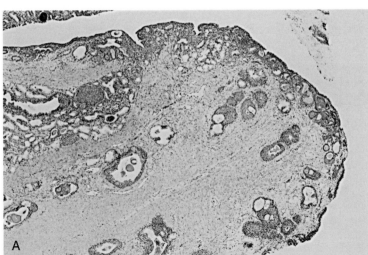

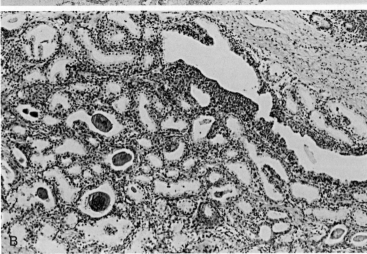

Figure 8–12. *(A)* Normal prostatic verumontanum. Note abundance of ducts lined in part by transitional-type epithelium. A prominent muscular stroma is noted (H&E). *(B)* Hyperplasia of verumontanum mucosal glands. Note tightly packed small acini lined by uniform cells. Corpora amylacea are prominently displayed (H&E).

ters. In this section we concentrate on four types of hyperplasia that have a small acinar pattern: (1) postatrophic hyperplasia (PAH); (2) the small glandular variant of unusual nodular hyperplasia; (3) basal cell hyperplasia; and (4) sclerosing adenosis (which can be confused with adenocarcinoma).

Postatrophic Hyperplasia

In 1954, L.M. Franks documented the first comprehensive description of an atrophy-associated lesion, called postatrophic hyperplasia. He and other workers in this field recognized the potential of this lesion to mimic adenocarcinoma, a problem that persists today.[14, 36, 37]

PAH can be unicentric or multicentric and is principally a peripheral zone lesion. It is generally perceived to be uncommon but in one recent study was identified in 18%

of whole-mount radical prostatectomy specimens.[38] The lesion consists of a lobular collection of small acini, sometimes budding from a central, dilated, atrophic duct (Fig. 8–13). The acini can be round and regular, or irregular, depending on the degree of stromal sclerosis surrounding them. The glands are lined by cuboidal secretory cells that have slightly enlarged, hyperchromatic nuclei.[8, 38] Apical cytoplasmic blebs may be present, with pale eosinophilic secretions in some glands.[36] Rarely, wispy basophilic mucosubstances are noted in the lumina, and these can be highlighted with an acidic mucin stain such as alcian blue. The nuclei are invariably bland and contain fine chromatin and inconspicuous nucleoli. Chronic inflammation may be noted in the stroma.

Franks, who initially divided PAH into two forms, lobular and postsclerotic, proposed that

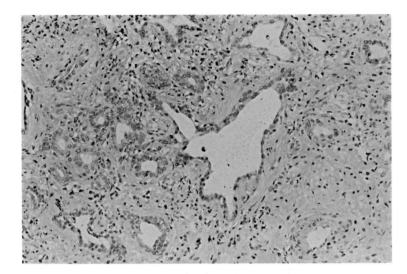

Figure 8–13. Prostatic post-atrophic hyperplasia. Note central, dilated and atrophic gland with adjacent, small acini showing an irregular stromal distribution. Focal chronic inflammation is also evident (H&E).

these entities arose from lobular and sclerotic atrophy, respectively.[36] In postsclerotic PAH, the glands appear irregular and compressed owing to stromal sclerosis resulting in a pseudoinfiltrative pattern as the sclerotic glands become separated from their associated lobules. Further confusion is created as the atrophy of the stroma, which is conspicuous with the lobular form, may be inapparent in the postsclerotic variety. The basal layer is usually less conspicuous in the postsclerotic form, and high–molecular weight keratin stains may be required to accentuate it.

Distinction from prostatic adenocarcinoma is based primarily on low-power observations, including lobular architecture, which usually (but not always) reveals the central atrophic duct, intimate admixture of clearly atrophic acini and hyperplastic ones within a small area, and the association of this lesion with usual atrophy in the surrounding prostate. While the nuclei of PAH are hyperchromatic and slightly enlarged, usually they do not contain prominent nucleoli, or at least not in significant numbers. The cytoplasm is clear, with occasional blebs. Finally, the benign diagnosis is based on the recognition of basal cells.

As both PAH and adenocarcinoma are peripheral zone processes, they are often found together. The proliferative appearance of PAH and its concurrence with carcinoma led Franks and others to propose that PAH is a premalignant lesion.[36, 39] Today, few experts in this field would subscribe to this theory, as there is no convincing evidence to link the two. Nevertheless, little or no phenotypic or genotypic evidence is available that demonstrates that PAH

is not a preneoplastic lesion, and investigators should keep an open mind since some peripheral zone adenocarcinomas are not associated with PIN. At present, we prefer to view PAH as a secondary proliferative response involving atrophic acini, the stimulus for which is unknown. Others have suggested that, in fact, the reverse may be occurring and that PAH is simply a stage in acinar involution.[38]

Small Glandular Variant of Nodular Hyperplasia

The small glandular variant of benign nodular hyperplasia, like the more common glandular and fibromuscular patterns, is principally a transition zone process most often encountered in TURP specimens.[8] It consists of well-circumscribed nests of closely packed, uniform acini that are usually associated with more typical areas of nodular hyperplasia.[40] The acini are composed of two cell types that have bland cytologic features. The secretory cells are often multilayered (a finding consistent with the hyperplastic process) and exhibit clear apical cytoplasm. The glands are separated by variable amounts of cellular (or sometimes fibrotic) mesenchyme, a feature that separates nodular hyperplasia from atypical adenomatous hyperplasia and carcinoma. As the process has been described, it may seem surprising that anyone could mistake it for carcinoma. The problem may arise in small tissue samples such as a prostate chip or sometimes a needle biopsy specimen in which only a small portion of the entire lesion is seen. It may also provide a diagnostic challenge in a TURP specimen artifactually distorted by crush or cautery artifact, or in radical prostatectomy specimens in which nodular hyperplasia, atypical adenomatous hyperplasia (discussed below), and low-grade adenocarcinoma coexist. In the latter case, the pathologist may become exhausted trying to pigeonhole seemingly endless groups of small acini into benign, malignant or possibly premalignant and malignant groups.

Basal Cell Hyperplasia

Basal cell proliferations in the prostate are discussed at length in an earlier chapter. Two forms of basal cell hyperplasia (BCH), specifically the incomplete/acinar type and the atypical type, can be confused with small acinar adenocarcinoma, and relevant aspects will be discussed briefly.[8, 41, 42] Incomplete BCH consists of aggregates of normal-sized and small-caliber glands containing multiple layers of basal cells. There is usually an admixture of solid nests of basal cells along with those that show luminal differentiation (Fig. 8–14). The presence of an inner (luminal) secretory cell layer distinguishes incomplete BCH from the complete form. The basal cells are uniform, with scant, basophilic cytoplasm and round to oval nuclei containing small or inconspicuous nucleoli. Mitotic figures are absent or rare; necrosis is absent; and calcifications may be present. The absence of nuclear grooves in BCH helps distinguish it from transitional metaplasia. The basal cells show gradual maturation to secretory cells, which usually lack nucleoli. The nests of cells commonly maintain a lobular configuration and are evenly spaced by fibromuscular stroma. On rare occasions, BCH may display a pseudoinfiltrative growth pattern. Basal cell hyperplasia is distinguished from carcinoma by several features, including an association or merging with benign fibromuscular and glandular hyperplasia, multilayered nests of basaloid cells, and benign cytologic appearance with central secretory change.

Atypical BCH is a variant in which the architectural features of ordinary BCH are retained but worrisome cytologic abnormalities are seen. Nuclei are enlarged and contain prominent nucleoli, and mitotic figures may be noted within involved glands.[41, 42] As with incomplete BCH, the "multilayering" of basal cells is distinctive from small acinar adenocarcinoma. Atypical BCH is more likely to be confused with PIN or basaloid carcinoma (which are discussed in detail elsewhere).

Finally, it is worth noting that BCH secondary to hormone therapy tends not to form small acini composed of basal cells but appears to result in a proliferation of basal cells within preexisting normal or hyperplastic glands; thus, it is not usually confused with low-grade adenocarcinoma.

Sclerosing Adenosis

Sclerosing adenosis is an uncommon entity that is probably best considered a variant of hyperplasia related to—and possibly derived from—benign nodular hyperplasia. Confusion may occur with prostatic adenocarcinoma if its characteristic morphologic features go unrecognized. The lesion is so named because of its

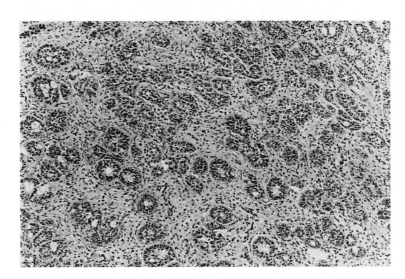

Figure 8–14. Prostatic basal cell hyperplasia. Note mixture of solid nests and ones displaying central lumina (so-called incomplete basal cell hyperplasia).

resemblance to its namesake in the breast[43]; however, before this name was generally accepted, other labels such as adenomatoid prostatic tumor, pseudoadenomatoid tumor, and fibroepithelial nodule has been used to describe it.[8, 44–46] The term "adenomatoid prostatic tumor" was coined by Chen, who published the first case in 1983.[44]

It is unlikely that sclerosing adenosis itself has a characteristic clinical presentation, except for its frequent association with the symptoms of BPH. Most cases are discovered in TURP chips from older men, usually between ages of 60 and 80 years.[47, 48] On histologic examination it appears as well-circumscribed nodules that are several millimeters in diameter but usually not larger than 1 cm. It may be a unifocal or a multifocal process. It is a biphasic lesion composed of proliferating glands (adenosis) distorted by a proliferating stroma

(sclerosing). The lesion is set apart from the surrounding tissue as a coalesced proliferation of small glands within a cellular stroma (Fig. 8–15). The glands may be uniform but most frequently are compressed, distorted, or branched. Compression of the glands can obliterate the lumen, which, along with their haphazard arrangement, may create a pseudoinfiltrative pattern.[47, 48] Many glands exhibit a double cell layer composed of an outer layer of flattened, basal-type cells and an inner columnar or cuboidal layer. The cuboidal cells sometimes have a vacuolated cytoplasm, a feature that led one author to propose the term "pseudoadenomatoid tumor."[45] This feature, however, is inconstant; thus, the term is inappropriate. Most cases exhibit only mild cytologic atypia; however, nuclei are sometimes enlarged with prominent nucleoli. The glands may contain pale, periodic acid-Schiff (PAS)–

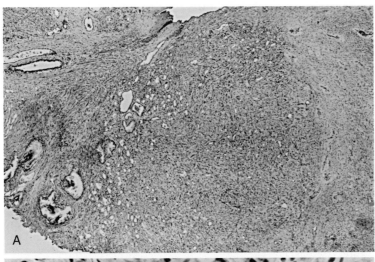

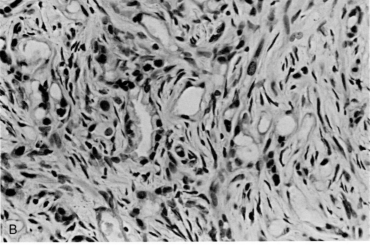

Figure 8–15. *(A)* Low-power view of sclerosing adenosis in prostatic chip. Note irregular pseudoinfiltrative pattern (H&E). *(B)* Tiny irregular glands are embedded in the dense, fibrous matrix (H&E).

or alcian blue–positive secretions. Sakamoto and colleagues emphasized a prominent, eosinophilic basal lamina surrounding the lesional acini, which is highlighted by PAS diastase.[49] Rarely, eosinophilic crystalloids— a feature more common in adenocarcinoma— are noted within the glands.[47, 48]

The other characteristic and integral feature of sclerosing adenosis is the stroma, which contains plump spindle cells of fibroblastic and myofibroblastic origin. Smooth muscle is usually absent. Single epithelial or basal cells, isolated by the sclerotic process from their parent acini, can contribute to the cellularity of the stroma. The collagenous or myxoid matrix has a basophilic appearance on light microscopy. Mild chronic inflammation with lymphocytes and plasma cells may be noted.[47]

The origin of sclerosing adenosis is unclear. Jones and colleagues speculate that the lesion may represent a sclerotic variant of atypical adenomatous hyperplasia.[47] Several studies have documented the observation that basal cells in sclerosing adenosis show evidence of myoepithelial differentiation, determined by the expression of muscle-specific actin and S-100 immunostaining.[47–49] This has been confirmed by electron microscopy.[48, 50] Myoepithelial differentiation is not a feature of normal basal cells in the prostate, and it has been suggested that it may antedate—and possibly initiate—the process of sclerosing adenosis.[47, 48] The fact that myoepithelial differentiation also occurs in some foci of basal cell hyperplasia, with which sclerosing adenosis is sometimes associated, suggests a common origin.[47, 51]

Regardless of the pathogenetic mechanism, there is no evidence that sclerosing adenosis behaves in a malignant fashion or has premalignant potential; thus, it requires no specific treatment or follow-up program. In summary, because of the serious potential for overdiagnosis, it is worth reemphasizing features that distinguish sclerosing adenosis from adenocarcinoma. Both low-grade adenocarcinoma and sclerosing adenosis are well-circumscribed lesions when viewed at low power; however, sclerosing adenosis usually exhibits greater variation in acinar morphology than a low-grade malignancy. The glands are compressed and distorted by a highly cellular stroma, another feature generally not noted in carcinoma; most prostate carcinomas do not elicit a marked desmoplastic response. The acini themselves have two cellular components, the epithelial cells with benign cytologic features and vacuolated cytoplasm and the basal cell layer, which often exhibits myoepithelial differentiation. Although the histomorphologic features are characteristic, immunohistochemistry may be of immense value in difficult cases, particularly if the lesion is encountered in a needle biopsy specimen. Basal cells with myoepithelial features can be demonstrated with high–molecular weight cytokeratin, smooth muscle actin, and S-100 immunoperoxidase stains.

Atypical Adenomatous Hyperplasia

More than 30 years ago, McNeal described what he considered to be two distinct, probably precancerous, patterns of prostate hyperplasia, one associated with small gland formation (postulated to be the product of a budding phenomenon) with architectural atypia resembling carcinoma.[52] The epithelium in this lesion was a "less active involutional epithelium but with continued epithelial activity."[52] The second type of proliferative change described by McNeal arises from an epithelium that shows full persistence of youthful activity in men of an age at which atrophy is usually present. The latter pattern describes what is now referred to as prostatic intraepithelial neoplasia (PIN).[53] The former lesion is generally referred to as atypical adenomatous hyperplasia (AAH), a term that was endorsed in a recent consensus statement.[8, 11, 54–56] Some authors still prefer the term "adenosis."[57, 58] Although the precancerous potential of PIN is convincing, evidence linking AAH to adenocarcinoma is more circumstantial and is not accepted by all workers in the field.[11, 55, 57, 59, 60] (For further discussion of the possible preneoplastic role of AAH, see Transition Zone Carcinoma.)

From a descriptive perspective, we prefer the term "AAH" over "adenosis," for two reasons. First, "adenosis" tends to be used to glorify any exaggerated collection of small glands; second, "AAH" describes a specific atypical proliferation that overlaps with cancer in its architecture, cytology, and ancillary findings such as mucin and crystalloids. AAH is a histologic entity that usually arises in the transition zone and exhibits a spectrum of features, including some that are readily recognizable as benign and ranging to ones that may be indistinguishable from cancer. It is in this specific context that we recommend use of the term "AAH," rather than as a catch-all term for unclassifiable small gland proliferations.

The histologic distinction of AAH from low-grade adenocarcinoma is one of the most difficult problems facing pathologists who evaluate prostate specimens,[8, 11, 12, 54, 59] a fact that has led some respected pathologists to question if these are, indeed, two separate entities.[61] We believe that AAH and small acinar carcinoma can be separated but appreciate that a large "gray zone" exists. The inevitable subjectivity that colors the interpretation of these difficult specimens stimulates healthy skepticism.

AAH is most often found in specimens from the central (periurethral) portion of the prostate, either in TURP chips or in biopsy tissue from the transition zone.[8, 11, 55, 57, 59] Although figures vary considerably, Gaudin and Epstein estimated the incidence of AAH to be less than 1% in needle biopsies and 1.6% in TURP

specimens at the Johns Hopkins Hospital.[57, 58] Bostwick and Qian identified AAH in 23% of radical prostatectomy specimens. It is frequently multifocal.[55] On low-power examination, AAH bears a close resemblance to low-grade acinar adenocarcinoma (Gleason grades 1 and 2). It consists of a nodular, usually well-circumscribed proliferation of closely packed acini (Fig. 8–16). The nodules of AAH usually have a pushing margin; however, occasional single glands appear to infiltrate adjacent stroma, a finding that, by itself, is not necessarily a strong indicator of malignancy. Most acini are small and uniform and vary little in size and shape. A distinctive feature is the presence of larger infolding glands admixed with (and apparently giving rise to) smaller glands. A ductlike structure may be seen as a "feeder" or parent duct in the central portion of the lesion. Individual cells within the acini are cy-

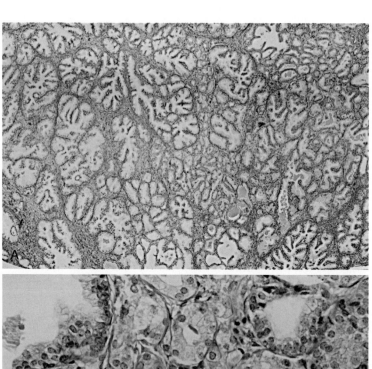

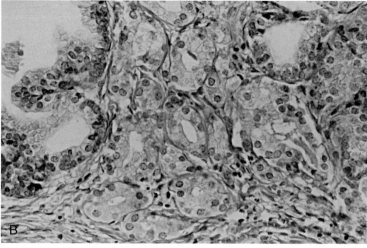

Figure 8–16. Atypical adenomatous hyperplasia. *(A)* Low-power view shows tightly packed, small acini within an otherwise hyperplastic nodule (H&E). *(B)* Tightly packed, small acini are lined by cuboidal cells with bland nuclear features. Nucleoli are inconspicuous (H&E).

tologically benign, with a pale or clear cytoplasm (Fig. 8–16). The nuclei are uniform and round, and nucleoli may be noted, although they are rarely prominent. The bland features of cells in small acini blend with their larger counterparts and with cells in adjacent foci of nodular hyperplasia—a reassuring finding. The basal cell layer lining the small glands is characteristically attenuated and often is difficult to recognize at the light microscopic level. It may be more obvious in the larger glands.

It is important to emphasize further the differentiation between AAH and small acinar adenocarcinoma. Correct diagnosis requires assessment of a range of both architectural and cytologic features, with the realization that there is significant overlap between the entities.[8, 11, 54, 55, 57] On low-power magnification, both low-grade adenocarcinoma and AAH are well-circumscribed lesions. The margins of both are generally of the "pushing" type, often with a minor degree of infiltration into the stroma. While some authors contrast the haphazard dissection of malignant glands with the more subtle wanderings of glands from AAH into the adjacent stroma, we find this to be of little use when Gleason grade 1 carcinoma is a consideration. The admixture of small acini with cytologically similar larger ones is an important feature of AAH but a "soft feature" for differentiation from carcinoma.

AAH and small acinar carcinoma can be compared on the basis of the gland contents. Bostwick and coworkers emphasize that intraluminal crystalloids and basophilic mucin are more frequent findings in adenocarcinoma. They found crystalloids in 75% of cases of low-grade carcinoma but in only 16% of AAH.[54] Gaudin and Epstein, however, located crystalloids in 40% of cases of AAH in TURP specimens and 23% in needle biopsy tissue.[57, 58] Basophilic mucinous secretions (acid mucins) are rarely found in foci of AAH, being present in only 2% to 3% of cases in Gaudin and Epstein's studies.[57, 58] It is our opinion that the coexistence of luminal crystalloids and wispy, basophilic mucosubstances in a small glandular lesion points strongly to a diagnosis of carcinoma.

Ultimately, the distinction often comes down to the time-honored assessment of nucleolar prominence and size and the presence or absence of a basal cell layer.[37, 54] Mean nucleolar diameter, largest nucleolar diameter, and percentage of nucleoli larger than 1 μm in diameter were all found by Bostwick and

colleagues to be significantly greater in low-grade adenocarcinoma than in AAH.[54] Other studies have also shown a higher frequency of prominent nucleoli in adenocarcinoma, using varying definitions of the word "prominent."[62, 63] Kelemen and associates propose that, in suspicious foci the presence of 31% or more of nucleoli larger than 3 μm is very suggestive of carcinoma, whereas Gaudin and Epstein believe that any nucleoli larger than this rule out adenosis (AAH).[62, 63] On light microscopy, of course, this is a judgment call. Gleason considered nucleoli larger than 1 μm to be prominent,[64] and, using this criterion, one would expect to see some prominent nucleoli in foci of AAH. In general, however, increasing nucleolar size and greater numbers of prominent nucleoli increase the likelihood that the lesion is malignant.

Finally, immunohistochemical assessment of the basal cell layer using high–molecular weight cytokeratin plays a very important role in confirming the diagnosis of AAH (Fig. 8–17). Basal cells are perhaps the most reliable indicator of a benign process; however, the basal cell layer is characteristically incomplete in AAH and may be inconspicuous on routine hematoxylin-eosin staining.[11, 54, 65] Pathologists should be careful not to interpret residual benign glands entrapped amidst malignant ones as AAH.

Table 8–3 summarizes the criteria we use to distinguish AAH from low-grade carcinoma. AAH is probably a biologic intermediate between hyperplasia at one end and carcinoma at the other. As such, it is to be expected that the light microscopic features will also form a spectrum, in some cases leaving the physician with the unsatisfying but safe diagnosis of "atypical small acinar proliferation of uncertain significance."

Small Acinar Carcinoma

More than 90% of prostatic adenocarcinomas display acinar histology—predominantly or exclusively. The vast majority of these carcinomas exhibit a small glandular pattern or an admixture of small glands with intermediate-sized ones. Small acinar carcinomas often present a diagnostic challenge that in great part is related to the protean differential diagnosis, as discussed above (see Table 8–4). The problems in the diagnosis of small acinar carcinomas are somewhat different in specimens from TURP and needle biopsy. In TURP specimens

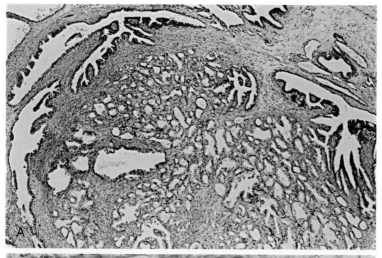

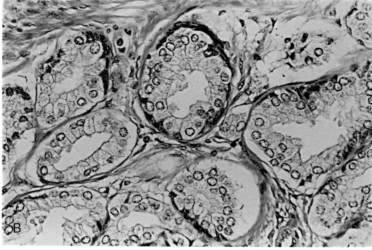

Figure 8–17. Atypical adenomatous hyperplasia. *(A)* Note circumscribed proliferation of small acini within a nodule of glandular and stromal hyperplasia (H&E). *(B)* High-power photomicrograph shows prominent basal cells, which can be highlighted with a high–molecular weight keratin stain (34β-E12) (H&E).

Table 8–3. Atypical Adenomatous Hyperplasia Versus Small Acinar Carcinoma: Comparative Histologic Features

Feature	AAH	SAC
Location	Central	Peripheral and central
Architecture		
Circumscription	Well-circumscribed	Well-circumscribed
Infiltration of stroma	Minimal	Minimal
Glands		
Admixture of small and large	Frequent	Infrequent
Parent duct	Occasional	Absent
Associated PIN	Occasional	Frequent (peripheral zone cases)
		Rare (transitional zone cases)
Luminal crystalloids	Occasional	Frequent
Basophilic mucin (H&E)	Infrequent	Frequent
Corpora amylacea	Occasional	Rare
Basal cells (34β-E12)	Present, discontinuous	Absent
Cytology		
Cytoplasm	Pale or clear	Variable (clear, amphophilic, basophilic)
Nuclei	Slightly enlarged	Slightly enlarged
Nucleoli	Some enlarged (>1 μm)	Many enlarged
Nucleoli >3 μm	Rare	Occasional to frequent

Table 8–4. Summary—Differential Diagnosis of Small Acinar Proliferations of Prostate

Entity	Architecture	Cytology	Other Features
Seminal vesicles/ ejaculatory duct	Well-circumscribed Arise from branching ducts Double-layered epithelium	Nucleomegaly Hyperchromasia Lipofuscin pigment Intranuclear holes	PSA-negative HMCK-positive basal layer
Cowper's gland	Lobular, closely packed acini Single-layered epithelium ± Excretory duct Skeletal muscle at periphery	Voluminous, mucinous cytoplasm Small, basally located bland nuclei	Apical location Mucin-positive
Paraganglion	Organoid Lumina absent	Polygonal cells Oval, dark nuclei Amphophilic finely granular or clear cytoplasm	Associated with small nerves PSA-negative Chromogranin positive
Simple (lobular) atrophy	Lobular configuration Larger, central duct ± Cyst formation Two cell layers	Shrunken, hyperchromatic, uniform, small nuclei	Peripheral zone (usually) ?Treatment related HMCK-positive
Sclerotic atrophy	As for simple (lobular) atrophy ± Stromal sclerosis	As above	Lymphohistiocytic reaction HMCK-positive
Mucous gland metaplasia	Usually peripheral zone Involves pre-existing normal or atrophic glands Double layered	Mucinous cytoplasm Bland nuclei	Mucin-positive HMCK-positive
Hyperplasia of mesonephric duct remnants	Vaguely lobular Single cell layer Micropapillary infolding	Cuboidal cells Bland nuclei	Colloid-like content PSA-negative HMCK-positive May extend beyond prostate or involve nerves
Nephrogenic adenoma	Haphazard arrangement Cystic dilatation of some tubules Suburothelial location	Combination of eosinophilic, cuboidal and hobnail cells Lacks prominent nucleoli	Clinical history Sometimes edema or inflammation PSA-negative
Verumontanum mucosal gland hyperplasia	Well-circumscribed Back-to-back acini Two cell layers	Bland nuclei	Associated transitional epithelial-lined ducts Corpora amylacea Eosinophilic concretions
Postatrophic hyperplasia	Lobular arrangement Central atrophic duct Stromal atrophy or sclerosis	Cytoplasmic blebs Nuclei hyperchromatic Occasional enlarged nucleoli	Inflammation + atrophy nearby HMCK-positive
Small glandular variant of nodular hyperplasia	Well-circumscribed Two cell layers Hyperplastic stroma between glands	Bland nuclei	Associated with ordinary BPH
Basal cell hyperplasia	Multiple layers of basal cells Hyperplastic stroma between nests	Scant, basophilic cytoplasm Central secretory change ± atypia	Occasional calcification Association with ordinary BPH HMCK-positive
Sclerosing adenosis	Well-circumscribed or pseudoinfiltrative Distorted acini Cellular fibrous stroma	Cytoplasmic vacuolation Mild cytologic atypia ± Enlarged nucleoli ± Basal cell noted	S-100, smooth muscle actin and HMCK-positive cells
Atypical adenomatous hyperplasia	Well-circumscribed Variable-sized acini ± Parent duct Two cell layers (discontinuous)	Mild cytologic atypia Occasional enlarged nucleoli	Multifocal TZ lesion HMCK-positive in discontinuous pattern Occasional crystalloids
Small acinar carcinoma	Small, round rigid acini, closely packed, back-to-back	Nucleomegaly Variable cytologic atypia Parachromatic clearing Enlarged nucleoli, some >3 μm	Crystalloids Basophilic mucin Collagenous spherules Perineural/intraneural invasion

BPH = benign prostatic hyperplasia, HMCK = high molecular weight cytokeratin (34β-E12), PSA = prostate specific antigen the chief problem is to differentiate adenocarcinomas of low grade (Gleason patterns 1 and 2) from other small gland proliferations, many of which have a proclivity for the transition zone (see Table 8–2). Crush artifact and thermal injury (cautery injury) can compound the diagnostic dilemma.

In needle biopsy tissue, beside separating adenocarcinoma from its mimics, the greater challenge is to decide whether a small focus of atypical glands shows sufficient abnormality and fulfills the criteria required to render an unequivocal diagnosis of carcinoma. In other words, is there a minimum threshold for the diagnosis of carcinoma? We believe that the diagnostic threshold for a minute focus of carcinoma is not definable but depends on features observed in an individual case. Nonetheless, several features are diagnostically useful and, in combination, help to establish the diagnosis of prostate cancer in most cases.

Before tackling the problem of what criteria constitute a diagnosis of malignancy, it is useful to review the features of Gleason patterns 1 and 2. Gleason pattern 1 carcinomas are well-defined lesions composed of uniform, single, separate, round or ovoid glands. The glands are closely packed but clearly separated by a small amount of stroma. The edge of the lesion is smooth with little evidence of invasion into surrounding prostate. Gleason pattern 2 exhibits slightly greater variability in the size and shape of glands, but the key difference from pattern 1 is more stromal spacing between adjacent glands. On average, they are up to one gland diameter apart. The edge of the lesion shows a greater number of acini infiltrating the surrounding stroma, but at low power the margin is still fairly well-circumscribed.[66]

Minimum criteria for a diagnosis of small acinar carcinoma are easily described on paper; however, the pathologist faced with a difficult needle biopsy sample often considers other factors in addition to the histologic findings. Different pathologists or groups of pathologists have different thresholds for diagnosing cancer, based on their knowledge of current treatment practices in the local urologic community. A pathologist may prefer to be cautious when he or she knows a patient may be indiscriminately treated aggressively. Often, problematic small acinar lesions have some features that support diagnosis of a benign lesion and some that support a diagnosis of cancer. The pathologist must decide if sufficient criteria are met based on the weight of evidence. The importance of carefully examining serial sections from needle biopsy specimens and liberal use of "deepers" cannot be overstated.

To determine whether a small gland pattern represents carcinoma, we recommend a stepwise approach to the diagnosis:

1. Observe architectural features.
2. Analyze cytologic features.
3. Determine presence or absence of ancillary features and other soft criteria for diagnosis of cancer:
   Intraluminal crystalloids
   Intraluminal mucin
   Collagenous micronodules
   Perineural and intraneural invasion
   Tumor within adipose tissue
   Intercurrent high-grade PIN
4. Look for cautionary features:
   Budding from benign glands
   Marked inflammation
   Poor histologic preparation
5. Implement immunohistochemical investigations:
   For a small amount of cancer, high–molecular weight stain to confirm absence of basal cell layer.
   For crushed or cellular epithelioid lesions, PSA/PSAP or cytokeratin to rule out possibilities such as xanthomatous inflammation and malacoplakia.

Architectural Features

Architecturally, acinar carcinoma is composed of small, relatively round glands with rigid contours that are often arranged back to back. At low power they are strikingly distinct from surrounding benign glands (Fig. 8–18). Invasion is characterized by loss of the normal gland-stromal relationship and may be recognized by atypical acini and nests dissecting between the stroma or between morphologically benign glands. Many carcinomas form groups of circumscribed acini, and invasion into these suspect nodules is best assessed at the periphery. If none of these features is helpful, the diagnosis must be established by the major criterion of malignancy—complete absence of the basal cell layer.

Cytologic Features

The nuclear features of prostatic adenocarcinoma are very critical and are characterized by nucleomegaly (nuclei larger than sur-

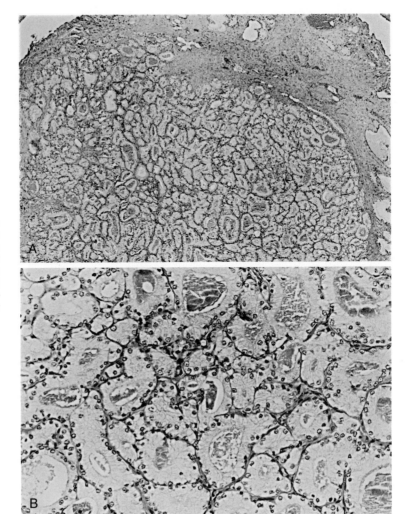

Figure 8–18. Small acinar carcinoma. *(A)* Low-power appearance of Gleason pattern 1 carcinoma: note rounded edge and tightly packed acini with only slight size and shape variations (H&E). *(B)* Tightly packed acini lined by single layer of cells with nucleolar prominence (H&E).

rounding benign glands) and altered nuclear chromatin, which is often clumped, with thickening of the nuclear membrane and zones of parachromatin clearing. The key diagnostic feature is the nucleolus, which in most instances is single, central, eosinophilic, and larger than 1 μm (Fig. 8–19). In spite of atypical nuclear features the nuclei of prostate cancer are, on the whole, relatively monomorphous—and may be deceptively bland. Approximately 20% to 25% of prostate cancers in needle biopsy tissue lack conspicuous nucleoli. In these instances the diagnosis is tenable if an unequivocal infiltrative pattern is observed or absence of the basal cell layer is conclusively demonstrated. Mitoses are uncommon in prostate cancer.

Cytoplasmic features vary from being clear in the clear cell (transition zone) carcinoma pattern or the hypernephroid pattern, to being amphophilic, eosinophilic, or basophilic. The tinctorial quality of the cytoplasm often allows the neoplastic acini to be recognized on low-power magnification, even when they are present in small numbers. Striking eosinophilia of cytoplasm, referred to as "Paneth cell–like change or metaplasia," indicates neuroendocrine differentiation. Finally, the cytoplasm of prostatic carcinoma occasionally contains pigment that is focal, fine, and granular; unlike the coarse, refractile, droplet-like, golden-yellow pigment of seminal vesicle epithelium.

Ancillary Histologic Features
(Soft Criteria for Prostate Carcinoma)

Intraluminal crystalloids are eosinophilic, rhomboid, needle-shaped to prismatic struc-

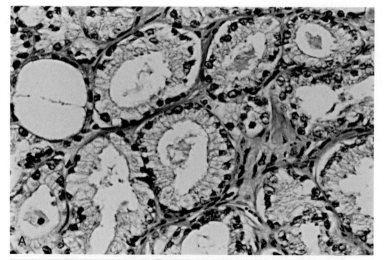

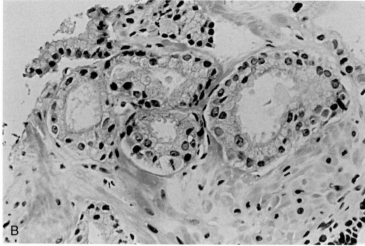

Figure 8–19. Small acinar carcinoma. *(A)* High-power view shows neoplastic acini lined by cells showing mild nuclear pleomorphism and nucleolar prominence (H&E). *(B)* Focus of small acinar carcinoma shows nucleolar prominence and focal mitosis (center) (H&E).

tures that can be seen in neoplastic glands or in uninvolved glands adjacent to cancer foci (Fig. 8–20). Their presence probably reflects a defect in the machinery that normally is responsible for production of corpora amylacea. Crystalloids are not a specific diagnostic feature for cancer. They can also be present in sclerosing adenosis, AAH, and PIN.

Intraluminal, wispy, basophilic mucin that may be observed on routine hematoxylin and eosin–stained sections is of diagnostic value (Fig. 8–21). The normal prostatic acini can produce neutral (PAS-positive) mucin, whereas neoplastic glands produce acidic mucin (alcian blue pH1 and 2.5 positive), which is manifested on routine staining as blue mucin. Acid mucin also is not absolutely specific for carcinoma and may be present within BPH, sclerosing adenosis, AAH, and PIN.

Although perineural invasion, representing spread along the path of least resistance, is a useful clue to the diagnosis of prostate cancer, caution is in order because "benign" glands may be juxtaposed to nerves. Circumferential or nearly circumferential perineural invasion or intraneural invasion is stronger evidence and in the appropriate context can be considered diagnostic of prostate cancer.

Collagenous micronodules are inspissated extracellular mucinous secretions seen in mucin-producing carcinomas and can be a useful clue. The association of collagenous micronodules with benign glands has not been reported to date.

Microvascular invasion or invasion into adipose tissue is an extremely strong indicator of carcinoma. Unfortunately, the former is almost never seen in needle biopsy tissue and the latter is uncommon.

Concurrent high-grade PIN and a suspicious

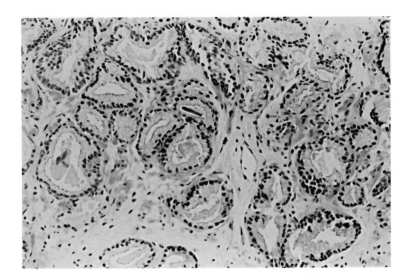

Figure 8–20. Luminal crystalloid in small acinar carcinoma (H&E).

focus of small glands provide supportive evidence of carcinoma. High-grade PIN is seen in 80% to 100% of prostate glands removed for prostate cancer and is a reliable and strong predictor of carcinoma, particularly in the peripheral zone.

Cautionary Features

Small glands emanating from a parent or central benign duct should be viewed with caution as they probably represent not carcinoma but rather a benign process such as atrophy, AAH, PAH, or seminal vesicle or ejaculatory duct epithelium.

Marked inflammation should prompt the examiner to take a step back and reconsider a suspicious small gland lesion. Inflammation can result in atrophic, small-looking glands that may exhibit regenerative nuclear changes and reactive atypia. Carcinoma and prostatitis may, however, coexist within a given focus.

Good histologic sections are a prerequisite for interpreting prostate samples. Prominent nucleoli and the basal cell layer are best recognized on excellent hematoxylin and eosin–stained material. Caution should be exercised with suboptimal histologic preparations (e.g., thick sections, poorly stained or preserved material, crush artifacts, or thermal injury).

Judicious Immunohistochemical Support

Two sets of immunohistochemical stains may be helpful tools for pathologic examination of

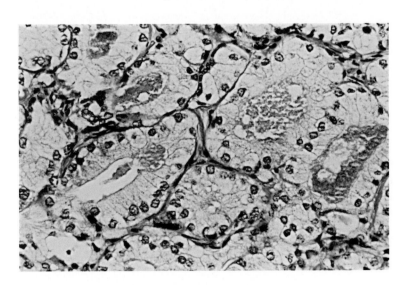

Figure 8–21. Granular luminal mucin secretion in small acinar carcinoma. This material stained positively with the Alcian blue stain (H&E).

prostate tissue: (1) high–molecular weight cytokeratin (clone 34β-E12), which is specific for basal cells, and (2) PSA/PSAP or cytokeratin.

In the appropriate morphologic context, and with strict quality control, high–molecular weight cytokeratin staining may be a very helpful adjunct in the diagnosis of small glandular proliferations (see Table 8–4). All lesions in the extensive differential diagnosis of small acinar carcinoma show varied yet distinctive staining patterns with high–molecular weight cytokeratin. Small acinar adenocarcinoma, by definition, is totally negative with this antibody. A common problem is loss of the focus in question on deeper sections. An intermediate-level section can be saved on gelatin-coated slides for possible future hematoxylin-eosin or immunohistochemical staining. If the focus in question is present on the two adjacent slides, the intermediate-level slide is probably suitable for immunohistochemistry. Decolorized, hematoxylin-eosin–stained slides can also be used where intermediate levels are unavailable. These cases must be handled meticulously, as the sections may become detached from the slides. Since the diagnosis of carcinoma is based on negative immunoreactivity strict attention to quality control is imperative, and we cannot overstate the importance of proper staining of adjacent or admixed morphologically benign glands and external tissue controls (Fig. 8–22). The entire focus under study

must be completely negative on 34β-E12 immunohistochemical staining, excluding obviously benign glands between which the neoplasm may be infiltrating. The critical step is to correlate the immunostaining findings with the morphologic ones. The indications for high–molecular weight cytokeratin immunostaining of prostate biopsy or TURP specimens include (1) confirming cancer in an extremely small focus, (2) ruling out other lesions in the differential diagnosis, (3) confirming cancer in patients receiving radiation or hormone therapy, (4) establishing a diagnosis of high-grade PIN when a back-to-back glandular arrangement raises the question of ductal carcinoma (see Chapter 6).

PSA/PSAP or cytokeratin can be used if the "epithelial" nature of the lesion is in question. Possible indications include (1) a small cell lesion with a differential diagnosis of lymphoma, rhabdomyosarcoma, florid inflammation, or carcinoma, (2) clear cell lesions, (e.g., prostatic xanthomas versus carcinoma), (3) epithelioid lesions (e.g., malacoplakia versus granulomatous prostatitis versus carcinoma), and (4) in a crushed cellular infiltrate, where immunostaining may help accentuate an infiltrative pattern and confirm the epithelial nature of the infiltrate.

We suggest the following algorithm be used for the diagnosis of malignancy in a small acinar process:

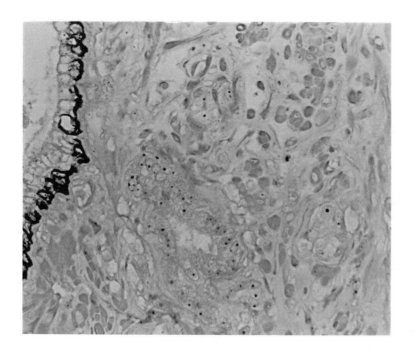

Figure 8–22. Small acinar carcinoma shows negativity for high–molecular weight keratin (34β-E12). A normal gland that displays intense positivity of the basal cell layer is visible at the left of the field (immunoperoxidase-34β-E12).

1. Identify a small acinar process on low-power examination.

2. Confirm the absence of a normal basal cell layer by intermediate-power microscopy.

3. Confirm the presence of significant nuclear abnormalities, especially enlarged nucleoli, on high-power examination.

4. Look for other evidence (e.g., crystalloids, cytoplasmic features, collagenous micronodules, perineural invasion) to support the diagnostic impression and, finally, if necessary to judiciously apply immunohistochemistry with careful morphologic control. In our opinion, the gold standard for diagnosis of prostatic carcinoma is still the hematoxylin and eosin slide.

Transition Zone Carcinoma

Approximately 70% to 80% of prostatic acinar carcinomas arise in the peripheral zone, 15% to 25% in the transition zone, and 8% to 10% in the central zone.[67] Most of these acinar carcinomas exhibit the histologic features described above, but about 60% of transition zone cancers have a distinctive morphology of tall columnar cells with basally situated nuclei (this is also referred to as the "tall columnar cell variant of prostatic adenocarcinoma.")[68]

On low-power examination, this pattern of well-differentiated adenocarcinoma is extremely deceptive, as it merges with and is closely related to nodules of BPH. The difficulty in diagnosis is further compounded by the architecture of this pattern of cancer, which tends to exhibit considerable variability in gland size, including some rather large and sometimes cystically dilated glands (Fig. 8–23). The gland contours may be regular, with occasional papillary infoldings. The tall, columnar cells contain abundant clear cytoplasm. In contrast to BPH, in which the nuclei may be found at various levels, the nuclei of transition zone cancer are aligned basally, consistently enlarged and hyperchromatic, with prominent nucleoli. The glands may contain granular eosinophilic secretions, but crystalloids and corpora amylacea are generally absent.

The clear cell pattern of acinar carcinoma is not peculiar to transition zone cancer: it can be found in peripheral zone cancers in radical prostatectomy specimens. Since most clear cell adenocarcinomas occur in the transition zone they are most often seen in TURP specimens, though we have personally seen this pattern in needle biopsy tissue, where the large gland diameter and marked variations in size and contour may lead to an incorrect diagnosis of a benign process. All cases of clear cell acinar carcinoma of the transition zone are Gleason pattern 1, 2, or 3, in contrast to the "other" clear cell (hypernephroid) pattern of prostatic adenocarcinoma, which is a Gleason pattern 4 and usually occurs in the peripheral zone.[13]

McNeal, in 1965 and 1969, proposed that AAH is a precursor lesion of prostate carcinoma.[52, 69] AAH and clear cell acinar carcinoma are predominantly transition zone lesions associated with BPH. Both lesions are characterized by variable gland diameter and contours, and McNeal has documented cases which appear transitional between AAH and carcinoma.[52, 68] In routine diagnostic practice, it is perhaps similar cases that provide the greatest challenge in distinguishing AAH from transition zone carcinoma. The principal difference between the two entities remains the complete absence of the basal cell layer which points to a diagnosis of carcinoma. Based on the aggregate evidence in the literature, transition zone cancers may have a favorable outcome and indolent course as compared with peripheral zone cancers.[70]

The morphologic overlap of AAH and transition zone carcinoma, and the histologic transition from one to the other provide the strongest available arguments that AAH is a precursor lesion to adenocarcinoma of the prostate. In AAH, the basal cell layer is variably attenuated and focally lost, suggesting that it is a stage along a morphologic continuum with carcinoma in which this layer is absent. Other data supporting the precursor potential include increased incidence in association with cancer (at autopsy, 15% in 100 cancer-free prostates and 31% in 100 cancerous glands); its spatial relationship with cancer; increased silver nucleolar–organizing region count; increased nuclear diameter and area; and a proliferative cell index similar to that for carcinoma.[54, 55, 57, 59] In spite of these findings, the precursor potential of AAH remains unestablished. Very few studies have addressed the biology of this lesion, and to date direct evidence linking AAH with carcinoma is not documented. In the only available study that documents clinical follow-up and outcome of AAH, Brawn reported that 6.5% of AAH cases developed into carcinoma during 5 to 15 years follow-up.[60] Unfortunately, Brawn's criteria are all-encompassing, and one might argue that

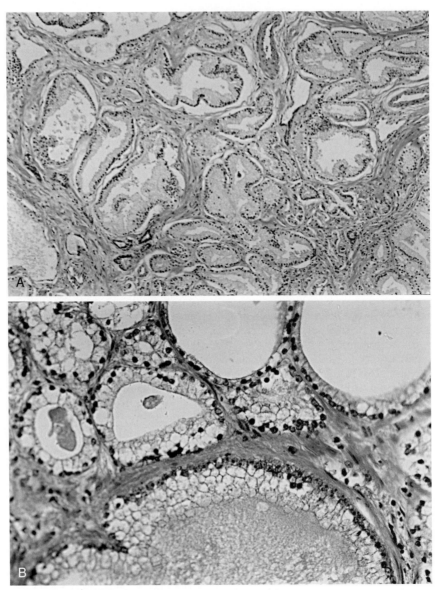

Figure 8–23. Low-grade transition zone carcinoma. *(A)* Note irregular proliferation of variably sized glands, some of which appear dilated. Many glands are lined by tall columnar cells with clear cytoplasm (H&E). *(B)* The glands are lined by a single layer of cells containing basally located enlarged nuclei and nucleolar prominence (H&E).

examples of "severe adenosis" are actually well-differentiated adenocarcinoma. Information of DNA index, ploidy status, and genetic and molecular studies of AAH may enhance our understanding of this lesion.

Atypical Small Acinar Proliferation of Uncertain Significance

In some truly borderline cases, accurate categorization as a benign or malignant lesion is not possible. This is especially problematic when the suspect focus consists of only a few glands, sometimes along the edge or at the tip of a core (Fig. 8–24). It is best not to be dogmatic but rather to diagnose such lesions as atypical small acinar proliferations of uncertain significance (ASAPUS). Sometimes lesions that lack an infiltrative pattern and contain nucleoli of intermediate size between those of benign and of malignant cells create the greatest problem.[53, 54] From a practical standpoint, it is important to ensure that all available tissue

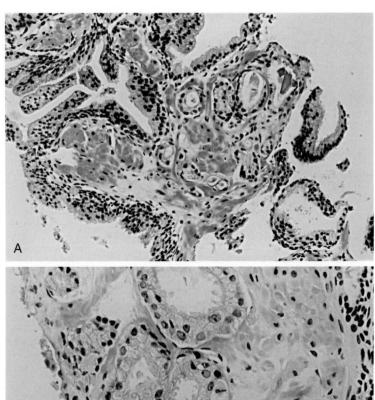

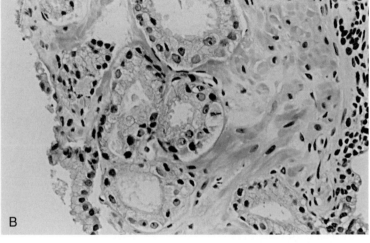

Figure 8–24. Atypical small acinar proliferation of uncertain significance. *(A)* A small fragment of a prostatic core biopsy displays a tiny collection of irregular, small acini adjacent to nonneoplastic glands (H&E). *(B)* Collection of atypical small acini along edge of prostatic biopsy. While suspicious, findings are insufficient to make an unequivocal diagnosis of carcinoma (H&E).

has been examined and to provide the clinician with as much information as possible on which to base a clinical decision. In many instances, the patient is treated conservatively and followed closely with repeat serum PSA measurements, digital rectal examinations, and transrectal ultrasonography. Repeat biopsies should be obtained when there is strong morphologic or clinical suspicion of carcinoma. In our experience, a diagnosis of ASAPUS is made in 1% to 2% of biopsy specimens. It is of utmost importance that the meaning of this term is conveyed to the referring urologists and that appropriate follow-up is generated.

REFERENCES

1. Troxel DB, Sabella JD: Problem areas in pathology practice uncovered by a review of malpractice claims. Am J Surg Pathol 18:821–831, 1994.

2. Kuo T, Gomez LG: Monstrous epithelial cells in human epididymis and seminal vesicles: A pseudomalignant change. Am J Surg Pathol 5:483–490, 1981.
3. Trainer TD: Testis and excretory duct system. In Sternberg SS (ed): Histology for Pathologists. New York: Raven, 1992, pp 731–748.
4. Brennick JB, O'Connell JX, Dickersin GR, et al.: Lipofuschin pigmentation (so-called "melanosis") of the prostate. Am J Surg Pathol 18:446–454, 1994.
5. Leung CS, Srigley JR: Distribution of lipochrome pigment in the prostate gland: Biological and diagnostic implications. Hum Pathol 26:1302–1307, 1995.
6. Amin MB, Bostwick DG: Pigment in prostatic epithelium and adenocarcinoma: A potential source of diagnostic confusion with seminal vesicular epithelium. Mod Pathol 9:791–795, 1996.
7. Bourne CW, Kilcoyne RF, Kraenzlar EJ: Prominent lateral mucosal folds in the bulbous urethra. J Urol 126:326–330, 1981.
8. Srigley JR: Small acinar patterns in the prostate gland with emphasis on atypical adenomatous hyperplasia and small-acinar carcinoma. Semin Diagn Pathol 5:254–272, 1988.
9. Melcher MP: Bulbourethral glands of Cowper (letter). Arch Pathol Lab Med 110:991, 1986.

10. Ostrowski ML, Wheeler TM: Paraganglia of the prostate. Location, frequency, and differentiation from prostatic adenocarcinoma. Am J Surg Pathol 18:412–420, 1994.

11. Jones EC, Young RH: The differential diagnosis of prostatic carcinoma. Its distinction from premalignant and pseudocarcinomatous lesions of the prostate gland. Am J Clin Pathol 101:48–64, 1994.

12. Epstein JI: Diagnostic criteria of the prostate on needle biopsy. Hum Pathol 26:223–229, 1995.

13. Gardner WA Jr, Culberson DE: Atrophy and proliferation in the young adult prostate. J Urol 137:55–56, 1987.

14. Franks LM: Atrophy and hyperplasia in the prostate proper. J Pathol Bacteriol 68:617–621, 1954.

15. Bostwick DG, Egbert BM, Fajardo LF: Radiation injury of the normal and neoplastic prostate. Am J Surg Pathol 6:541–551, 1982.

16. Siders DB, Lee F: Histologic changes of irradiated prostatic carcinoma diagnosed by transrectal ultrasound. Hum Pathol 23:344–351, 1992.

17. Grignon D, Troster M: Changes in immunohistochemical staining in prostatic adenocarcinoma following diethylstilbestrol therapy. Prostate 7:195–202, 1985.

18. Têtu B, Srigley JR, Bovin JC, et al.: Effect of combination endocrine therapy (LHRH agonist and flutamide) on normal prostate adenocarcinoma. Am J Surg Pathol 15:111–120, 1991.

19. Armas OA, Aprikian AG, Melamed J, et al.: Clinical and pathobiologic effects of neoadjuvant total androgen ablation therapy on clinically localized prostatic adenocarcinoma. Am J Surg Pathol 18:979–991, 1994.

20. Civantos F, Marcial MA, Banks ER, et al.: Pathology of androgen deprivation therapy in prostate carcinoma. Cancer 75:1634–1641, 1995.

21. Vaillancourt L, Têtu B, Fradet Y, et al.: Effect of neoadjuvant endocrine therapy (combined androgen blockade) on normal prostate and prostatic carcinoma: A randomized study. Am J Surg Pathol 20:86–93, 1996.

22. Witjes WP, Horenblas S, Oosterhof GO, et al.: Neoadjuvant therapy in prostate cancer—is it of any use? Eur Urol 4:433–437, 1993.

23. Goldenberg SL, Klotz LH, Srigley JR, et al.: Randomized, prospective, controlled study comparing radical prostatectomy alone and neoadjuvant androgen withdrawal in the treatment of localized prostate cancer. J Urol 156:873–877, 1996.

24. Laroque PA, Prahalada S, Grodon LR, et al.: Effects of chronic oral administration of a selective 5-alpha-reductase inhibitor, finasteride, on the dog prostate. Prostate 24:93–100, 1994.

25. Civantos F, Soloway M: Prostatic pathology after androgen blockade: Effects on prostatic carcinoma and on nontumor prostate. Adv Anat Pathol 3:259–265, 1996.

26. Shiraishi T, Kusano I, Wantanabe M, et al.: Mucous gland metaplasia of the prostate. Am J Surg Pathol 17:618–622, 1993.

27. Grignon DJ, O'Malley FP: Mucinous metaplasia in prostate gland. Am J Surg Pathol 16:1205–1214, 1992.

28. Gikas PW, Del Buono EA, Epstein JI: Florid hyperplasia of mesonephric remnants involving prostate and periprostatic tissue. Possible confusion with adenocarcinoma. Am J Surg Pathol 17:454–460, 1993.

29. Ferry JA, Scully RE: Mesonephric remnants, hyperplasia and neoplasia in the uterine cervix. A study of 49 cases. Am J Surg Pathol 14:1100–1111, 1990.

30. Ford TF, Watson GM, Cameron KM: Adenomatous metaplasia (nephrogenic adenoma) of urothelium: An analysis of 70 cases. Br J Urol 57:427–433, 1985.

31. Oliva E, Young RH: Nephrogenic adenoma of the urinary tract: A review of the microscopic appearance of the 80 cases with emphasis on unusual features. Mod Pathol 8:722–730, 1995.

32. Young RH: Nephrogenic adenomas of the urethra involving the prostate gland: A report of two cases of a lesion that may be confused with prostatic adenocarcinoma. Mod Pathol 5:617–620, 1992.

33. Malpica A, Ro JY, Troncosco P, et al.: Nephrogenic adenoma of the prostatic urethra involving the prostate gland: A clinicopathologic and immunohistochemical study of eight cases. Hum Pathol 25:390–395, 1994.

34. Gagucas RJ, Brown RW, Wheeler TM: Verumontanum mucosal gland hyperplasia. Am J Surg Pathol 19:30–36, 1995.

35. Gaudin PB, Wheeler TM, Epstein JI: Verumontanum mucosal gland hyperplasia in prostatic needle biopsy specimens. A mimic of low grade prostatic adenocarcinoma. Am J Clin Pathol 104:620–626, 1995.

36. Franks LM: Benign nodular hyperplasia of the prostate: A review. Ann R Coll Surg 68:617–642, 1954.

37. Totten RS, Heineman MW, Hudson PB, et al.: Microscopic differential diagnosis of latent carcinoma of the prostate. AMA Arch Pathol 55:131–141, 1953.

38. Cheville JC, Bostwick DG: Postatrophic hyperplasia of the prostate. A histologic mimic of prostatic adenocarcinoma. Am J Surg Pathol 19:1068–1076, 1995.

39. Liavag I: Atrophy and regeneration in the pathogenesis of prostatic carcinoma. Acta Pathol Microbiol Scand 73:338–350, 1968.

40. Kovi J: Microscopic differential diagnosis of small acinar adenocarcinoma of prostate. Pathol Annu 20:157–196, 1985.

41. Epstein JI, Armas OA: Atypical basal cell hyperplasia of the prostate. Am J Surg Pathol 16:1205–1214, 1992.

42. Devaraj LT, Bostwick DG: Atypical basal cell hyperplasia of the prostate. Immunophenotypic profile and proposed classification of basal cell proliferations. Am J Surg Pathol 17:645–659, 1993.

43. Young RH, Clement PB: Sclerosing adenosis of the prostate: Report of a case. Arch Pathol Lab Med 111:363–366, 1987.

44. Chen KT, Schiff JJ: Adenomatoid prostatic tumor. Urology 21:88–89, 1983.

45. Hulman G: "Pseudoadenomatoid" tumor of prostate. Histopathology 14:317–323, 1989.

46. Sesterhenn IA, Mostofi FK, Davis CJ: Fibroepithelial nodules of the prostate simulating carcinoma. Lab Invest 68:83A, 1988.

47. Jones EC, Celment PB, Young RH: Sclerosing adenosis of the prostate gland. A clinicopathological and immunohistochemical study of 11 cases. Am J Surg Pathol 15:1171–1180, 1991.

48. Grignon DJ, Ro JY, Srigley JR, et al.: Sclerosing adenosis of the prostate gland. A lesion showing myoepithelial differentiation. Am J Surg Pathol 16:383–391, 1992.

49. Sakamoto N, Tsuneyoshi M, Enjoji M: Sclerosing adenosis of the prostate. Histopathologic and immunohistochemical analysis. Am J Surg Pathol 15:660–667, 1991.

50. Collina G, Botticelli AR, Martinelli AM, et al.: Sclerosing adenosis of the prostate. Report of three cases with electron microscopy and immunohistochemical study. Histopathology 20:505–510, 1992.

51. Ronnett BM, Epstein JI: A case showing sclerosing adenosis and an unusual form of basal cell hyperplasia of the prostate. Am J Surg Pathol 13:866–872, 1989.

52. McNeal JE: Morphogenesis of prostate carcinoma. Cancer 18:1659–1666, 1965.

53. Bostwick DG, Brawer MK: Prostatic intra-epithelial neoplasia and early invasion in prostatic cancer. Cancer 59:788–794, 1987.

54. Bostwick DG, Srigley J, Grignon D, et al.: Atypical adenomatous hyperplasia of the prostate: Morphologic criteria for its distinction from well-differentiated carcinoma. Hum Pathol 24:819–832, 1993.

55. Bostwick DG, Junqi Q: Atypical adenomatous hyperplasia of the prostate. Relationship with carcinoma in 217 whole-mount radical prostatectomies. Am J Surg Pathol 19:506–518, 1995.

56. Bostwick DG, Algaba F, Amin MB, et al.: Consensus statement on terminology: Recommendation to use atypical adenomatous hyperplasia in the place of adenosis of the prostate. Am J Surg Pathol 18:1069–1072, 1994.

57. Gaudin PB, Epstein JI: Adenosis of the prostate. Histologic features in transurethral resection specimens. Am J Surg Pathol 18:863–870, 1994.

58. Gaudin PB, Epstein JI: Adenosis of the prostate. Histologic features in needle biopsy specimens. Am J Surg Pathol 19:737–747, 1995.

59. Amin MB, Ro JY, Ayala AG: Putative precursor lesions of prostatic adenocarcinoma: Fact or fiction? Mod Pathol 6:476–483, 1993.

60. Brawn PN: Adenosis of prostate. A dysplastic lesion that can be confused with prostate adenocarcinoma. Cancer 49:826–833, 1982.

61. Koss LG, Suhrland MJ: Atypical hyperplasia and other abnormalities of prostatic epithelium. Hum Pathol 24:817–818, 1993.

62. Kelemen PR, Buschmann RJ, Weisz-Carrington P: Nucleolar prominence as a diagnostic variable in prostatic carcinoma. Cancer 65:1017–1020, 1990.

63. Kramer CE, Epstein JI: Nucleoli in low-grade prostate adenocarcinoma and adenosis. Hum Pathol 24:618–623, 1993.

64. Gleason DF: Atypical hyperplasia, benign hyperplasia, and well-differentiated adenocarcinoma of the prostate. Am J Surg Pathol 9(Suppl):53–67, 1985.

65. Wojno KJ, Epstein JI: The utility of basal cell–specific anti-cytokeratin antibody (34BE12) in the diagnosis of prostate cancer. A review of 228 cases. Am J Surg Pathol 19:251–260, 1995.

66. Gleason DF: Histologic grading and clinical staging of prostatic carcinoma. In Tannenbaum M (ed): Urologic Pathology: The Prostate. Philadelphia: Lea & Febiger, 1977, pp 171–197.

67. McNeal JE, Redwine EA, Freiha FS, et al.: Zonal distribution of prostatic adenocarcinoma: Correlation with histologic pattern and direction of spread. Am J Surg Pathol 12:897–906, 1988.

68. McNeal JE, Price HM, Redwine EA, et al.: Stage A versus stage B adenocarcinoma of the prostate: Morphological comparison and biological significance. J Urol 139:61–65, 1988.

69. McNeal JE: Origin and development of carcinoma of the prostate. Cancer 23:24–34, 1969.

70. Bostwick DG, Cooner WH, Denis L, et al.: The association of benign prostatic hyperplasia and cancer of the prostate. Cancer 70:291–301, 1992.

9

BASAL CELL PROLIFERATIONS AND TUMORS OF THE PROSTATE

DAVID G. BOSTWICK **and** LEENA T. DEVARAJ

Basal cell proliferations in the prostate exhibit a morphologic continuum ranging from focal basal cell hyperplasia in the setting of nodular hyperplasia to florid adenoid cystic/basal cell carcinoma. These uncommon lesions are present in 5.8% and 8.9% of biopsies and transurethral resection specimens, respectively.[1, 2] Basal cell proliferations have been called a variety of names, including *fetalization of the prostate*,[3] *embryonal hyperplasia*,[4] *basal cell atypia*,[5] *basal cell hyperplasia*,[5–8] *basal cell tumor*,[7] *basal cell adenoma*,[9] *basaloid carcinoma*,[10] *adenoid basal cell tumor*,[11, 12] *prostatic adenoma of ductal origin*,[13] *adenoid cysticlike tumor*,[14] *basal cell carcinoma*, and *adenoid cystic carcinoma*.[11, 15]

Light microscopic findings are usually sufficient to separate basal cell proliferations from other lesions. Immunohistochemical staining with antibodies directed against high–molecular weight keratin such as clone 34β-E12 is useful in confirming the presence of basal cells in equivocal cases, but it is used infrequently in our laboratory and others.[3, 16–25] Some basal cell proliferations may be mistaken for high-grade prostatic intraepithelial neoplasia (PIN) or carcinoma due to the presence of significant cytologic abnormalities, including nuclear and nucleolar enlargement.[26, 27] These cases are often a source of diagnostic confusion, particularly in small samples such as needle biopsy specimens.

This chapter reviews the diagnostic criteria for basal cell proliferations, including basal cell hyperplasia, atypical basal cell hyperplasia, basal cell adenoma, and adenoid cystic/basal cell carcinoma; cribriform hyperplasia is also included because it is probably within the spectrum of basal cell proliferations. Recognition of basal cells in suspicious lesions is a useful diagnostic feature that effectively excludes adenocarcinoma from consideration.

NORMAL BASAL CELLS

In benign prostatic acini, basal cells form an inconspicuous and almost continuous circumferential layer at the periphery of prostatic ducts, ductules, and acini (Fig. 9–1). These elongate cells have scant cytoplasm, and are surmounted by a cuboidal to columnar secretory luminal cell layer.[26, 28, 29] The long axis of the basal cells is usually parallel to the underlying basement membrane and perpendicular to the secretory cell layer. Nuclei are small, thin, and tapering, with delicate uniform chromatin. Nucleoli are usually single and inconspicuous, measuring less than 0.3 μm. The cytoplasm is difficult to identify by light microscopy and often appears as a dark narrow rim with inconspicuous cell margins. Many basal cells display fine dendritic extensions that partially encircle acini. These cytoplasmic extensions frequently abut one another, forming a continuous—but thin and inconspicuous—layer. The normal prostatic epithelium fre-

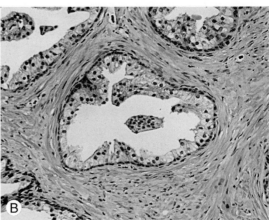

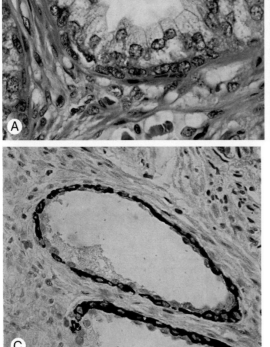

Figure 9–1. Normal prostatic acinus with prominent basal cell layer. *A* and *B*, The basal cells are cigar shaped, with the long axis parallel to the basement membrane, in contrast to the overlying secretory cell layer. *C*, Immunohistochemical staining for high–molecular weight keratin 34β-E12 reveals selective intense cytoplasmic immunoreactivity in the basal cells.

quently contains foci of basal cell proliferation that are not considered sufficient to warrant the diagnosis of basal cell hyperplasia.

Basal Cell Development

At puberty, the immature prostatic epithelium differentiates into basal cells and secretory cells under the influence of androgens.[30] The fetal and prepubertal prostatic epithelium expresses a broad spectrum of keratins, including high–molecular weight keratin, with a progressive dichotomy with age of keratin immunoreactivity of the basal cell and secretory cell layers.

Basal Cells Are the Most Likely Stem Cells of the Prostate

Basal cells are the most likely "reserve," or stem, cells, capable of dividing and replenishing the prostatic epithelium, and of dif-ferentiating into other cell types such as secretory cells,[28, 30–34] but this is not invariably accepted.[35–37] A recent consensus group determined that a small subset of the basal cell layer houses the stem cell population.[38] Although both basal cells and secretory cells retain the ability to divide,[35] the usual proliferative compartment is the basal cell layer.[34] Transition forms have been identified between basal cells and secretory luminal and neuroendocrine cells, although rarely and usually in tissue culture.[32, 34] Prostate-specific antigen (PSA) and prostatic acid phosphatase (PAP) immunoreactivity is present in a subset of basal cells, suggesting that basal cells can acquire the immunophenotype of secretory cells.[2, 15] Basal cells also retain the ability to undergo metaplasia, including squamous differentiation in the setting of prostatic infarction[34] and myoepithelial differentiation in the setting of sclerosing adenosis.[39–41]

Other evidence supporting the stem cell origin of basal cells includes the identification of the apoptosis-suppressing *bcl*-2 oncoprotein exclusively in basal cells[42] and the androgen independence but androgen responsiveness of basal cells as documented by the presence of 5-alpha-reductase-2 and the nuclear androgen receptor.[43]

BENIGN BASAL CELL PROLIFERATIONS

There are three patterns of benign basal cell hyperplasia: typical basal cell hyperplasia, atypical basal cell hyperplasia, and basal cell adenoma.[2, 15] A fourth histologic pattern, cribriform hyperplasia, is often considered a form of basal cell proliferation.[44, 45] Adenoid cystic/basal cell carcinoma is considered the malignant counterpart of basal cell hyperplasia.

Basal Cell Hyperplasia

Basal cell hyperplasia consists of a thickness of two or more cells at the periphery of prostatic acini (Figs. 9–2, 9–3). A minimum thickness of two basal cells is required for diagnosis, although this criterion is arbitrary.[2] Basal cell hyperplasia sometimes appears as small nests of cells surrounded by a few concentric layers of compressed stroma, often associated with chronic inflammation. The nests may be solid or cystically dilated, and occasionally are punctuated by irregular round luminal spaces, creating a cribriform pattern. Basal cell hyperplasia frequently involves only part of an acinus and sometimes protrudes into the lumen, retaining the overlying secretory cell layer; less often symmetric duplication of the basal cell layer is observed at the periphery of the acinus.

The cells in basal cell hyperplasia are enlarged, ovoid, or round and plump, with large, pale ovoid nuclei, finely reticular chromatin, and a moderate amount of cytoplasm. Nucleoli are usually inconspicuous, (smaller than 1 μm diameter), although they are enlarged in atypical basal cell hyperplasia (see below). Basal cell hyperplasia is rarely associated with atypical adenomatous hyperplasia.[2, 46]

Basal cell hyperplasia with sclerosis refers to the presence of delicate, lacelike fibrosis or dense irregular sclerotic fibrosis and hyperplastic smooth muscle surrounding and distorting hyperplastic basal cell aggregates.

Clear cell change is common in basal cell hyperplasia and other forms of basal cell proliferation, often with a cribriform pattern.

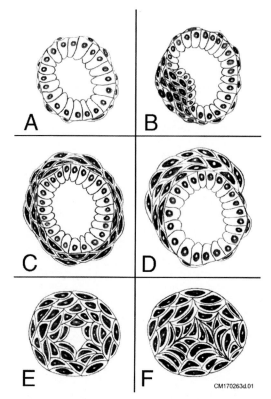

Figure 9–2. Schematic illustration of basal cell hyperplasia in the prostate. *A*, Normal prostate gland with thin peripheral layer of basal cells and cuboidal to low columnar secretory luminal cell layer. *B*, Focal basal cell proliferation with mild distortion of the glandular luminal contour. *C*, Symmetric circumferential proliferation of basal cells, at least two cells in thickness. *D*, Eccentric focus of atypical basal cell hyperplasia with prominent nucleoli, eccentric pattern. *E*, Basal cell hyperplasia with loss of secretory cell layer (note retention of glandular lumen); compare with *F*. *F*, "Solid" pattern of basal cell hyperplasia, with absence of lumen. (From Devaraj LT, Bostwick DG: Atypical basal cell hyperplasia of the prostate. Immunophenotypic profile and proposed classification of basal cell proliferations. Am J Surg Pathol 17:645–659, 1993.)

Squamous metaplasia is found infrequently, usually in association with infarction. Chronic inflammation is common but not specific. Nuclear grooves are infrequent. Nuclear "bubble" artifact, appearing as intranuclear vacuoles, is commonly observed in formalin-fixed specimens but not in frozen sections, and appears more prominent in basal cells than in secretory luminal cells. Focal calcification is evident in some lesions and may be present within the basal cell nests. Basal cell hyperplasia associated with orchiectomy or diethylstilbesterol usually shows prominent squamous metaplasia (Fig. 9–4).

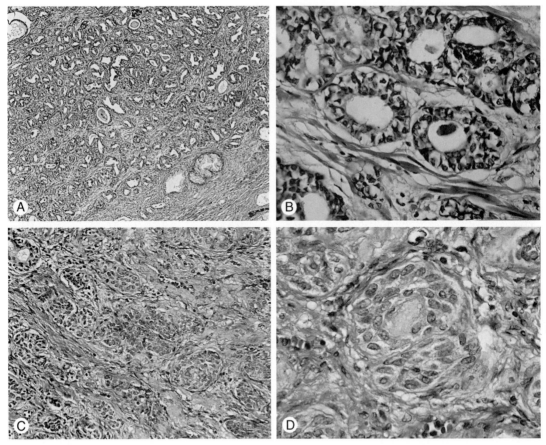

Figure 9–3. Basal cell hyperplasia architecturally mimicking adenocarcinoma. *A* and *B,* This proliferation consists of prostatic acini with prominent basal cells with abundant clear cytoplasm and hyperchromatic, wizened nuclei. *C* and *D,* Another case shows solid nests of proliferating basal cells, occasionally punctuated by small lumens with scant mucin *(D)*.

Atypical Basal Cell Hyperplasia

Atypical basal cell hyperplasia is identical to basal cell hyperplasia except for the presence of large, prominent nucleoli (Fig. 9–5); the mean diameter is 1.96 μm (maximum, 4.8 μm).[2, 47] The nucleoli are round to oval and lightly eosinophilic. There is chronic inflammation in the majority of cases, suggesting that the characteristic nucleolomegaly is reactive.

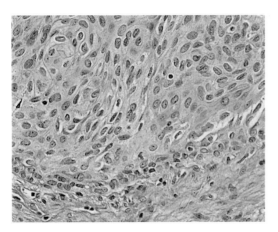

Figure 9–4. Basal cell hyperplasia with prominent squamous metaplasia. Note that some of the nuclei contain central linear grooves. The patient had a history of bilateral orchiectomy and diethylstilbesterol treatment for prostatic adenocarcinoma.

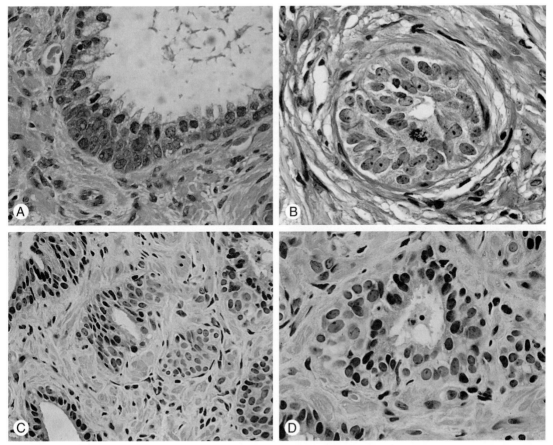

Figure 9–5. Atypical basal cell hyperplasia. *A,* The basal cells are enlarged and round, with central enlarged nucleoli. *B,* In another case, atypical basal cells have replaced the acinus; there is a single mitotic figure. *C* and *D,* In a third case, the basal cell nuclei are hyperchromatic or display dark chromatin with prominent nucleoli.

A morphologic spectrum of nucleolar size is observed in basal cell proliferations; they are considered atypical only when more than 10% of cells exhibit prominent nucleoli. There is no apparent clinical significance to atypical basal cell hyperplasia, but it is a pitfall of a histopathologic diagnosis.

Basal Cell Adenoma

Basal cell adenoma consists of a large, round, usually solitary, circumscribed nodule of acini with hyperplastic basal cells in the setting of nodular hyperplasia (Fig. 9–6). The nodule contains aggregates of basal cells that form small solid nests or cystically dilated acini. Condensed stroma is seen at the periphery of the nodule. In addition, stromal connective tissue traverses the adenomatous nodule, creating incomplete lobulation in some cases.

The stroma may be basophilic, sometimes with myxoid change adjacent to cell nests.

The cells in basal cell adenoma are plump, with large nuclei, scant cytoplasm, and inconspicuous nucleoli, although large, prominent nucleoli are rarely observed. Many cells are cuboidal or epithelioid, particularly centrally in the cell nests, and some contain clear cytoplasm. Prominent calcific debris is often present within acinar lumina. Multiple basal cell adenomas (basal cell adenomatosis) invariably arise in association with nodular hyperplasia and appear to be a variant of basal cell hyperplasia.

Cribriform Hyperplasia

Cribriform hyperplasia, including clear cell cribriform hyperplasia, consists of acini with a distinctive cribriform pattern, sometimes form-

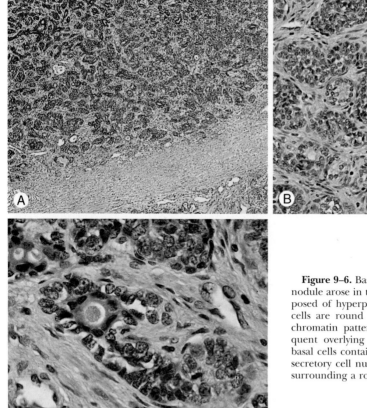

Figure 9–6. Basal cell adenoma. *A,* This circumscribed nodule arose in the setting of nodular hyperplasia, composed of hyperplastic acini of basal cells. *B,* The basal cells are round to oval, with uniform finely punctate chromatin pattern, inconspicuous nucleoli, and infrequent overlying secretory cell layer. *C,* Some of the basal cells contain small punctate nucleoli; the residual secretory cell nuclei are smudged and hyperchromatic, surrounding a round lumen with mucin.

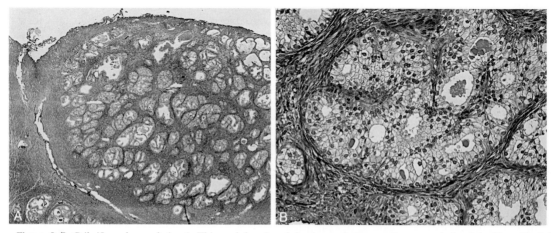

Figure 9–7. Cribriform hyperplasia. *A,* This nodule of nodular hyperplasia contains expanded acini with epithelial proliferation with irregular fenestrations. *B,* The epithelial cells are uniform, without nuclear or nucleolar enlargement, and there is abundant clear or pale, finely vacuolated cytoplasm.

ing a nodule (Fig. 9–7). The cells from such acini usually have pale to clear cytoplasm and small, uniform nuclei with inconspicuous nucleoli.[44, 45] This lesion is benign.

ADENOID CYSTIC/BASAL CELL CARCINOMA (ADENOID BASAL CELL TUMOR; ADENOID CYSTICLIKE TUMOR)

The rarest neoplastic basal cell proliferation in the prostate is adenoid cystic/basal cell carcinoma. Fewer than 50 cases are documented, and most have little or no clinical follow-up.[2, 10, 14, 15, 48–53] The age, presenting symptoms, and clinical findings are similar to those of typical acinar adenocarcinoma. Almost all reported cases were confined to the prostate at presentation, and follow-up has not extended

beyond 6 years after diagnosis. Serum PSA and PAP concentrations are not elevated.

Adenoid cystic/basal cell carcinoma of the prostate is histologically similar to adenoid cystic carcinoma or basal cell carcinoma at other sites (Figs. 9–8, 9–9). The criteria for distinguishing these lesions were recently refined (Table 9–1), and the malignant nature of cases previously reported as adenoid cystic carcinoma has been questioned.[2, 14, 15] Young and colleagues reclassified four previously reported cases of adenoid cystic carcinoma as adenoid cystic-like tumor following review of the histologic slides, and added two cases from their files.[14] Published cases illustrated in the 1973 Armed Forces Institute of Pathology (AFIP) fasicle[54] have been reclassified as variants of adenoid basal cell tumor.[14] Young and coworkers stated that virtually all cases of adenoid cystic carcinoma of the prostate in the litera-

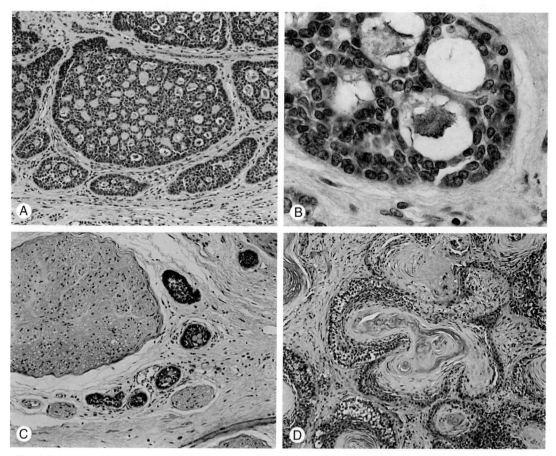

Figure 9–8. Adenoid cystic/basal cell carcinoma. *A, B,* and *C,* This florid proliferation displayed a prominent adenoid cystic pattern, with large, dilated spaces filled with flocculent mucinous material. Perineural invasion *(C)* and extraprostatic extension were prominent. *D,* Another case, with central keratinous debris within the basal cell nests. In other fields, the basal cells have variable amounts of optically clear cytoplasm, with a distinctive clear cell appearance.

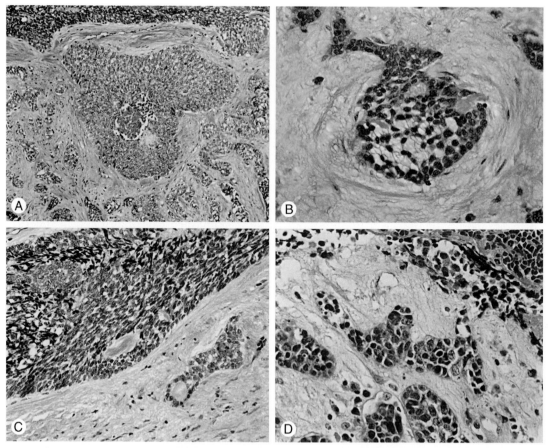

Figure 9–9. Adenoid cystic/basal cell carcinoma with liver metastases in an 87-year-old man. *A, B,* and *C,* The tumor in the prostate was extensive and infiltrating, composed chiefly of basal cell pattern, sometimes with luminal necrosis. *D,* Fine-needle aspiration biopsy of the liver revealed basal cell carcinoma identical to the primary prostate lesion.

ture resemble basal cell hyperplasia and should not be considered malignant.[14] Metastases have never been documented from these tumors, although we recently encountered a case with liver metastases in an elderly man (see Fig. 9–9).

Adenoid cystic/basal cell carcinoma is histologically similar to basal cell hyperplasia and

Table 9–1. Basal Cell Proliferations of the Prostate: Diagnostic Criteria

	Normal Basal Cell Layer	Basal Cell Hyperplasia (BCH)	Atypical Basal Cell Hyperplasia	Basal Cell Adenoma	Adenoid Cystic / Basal Cell Carcinoma
Architecture	Nearly continuous, single cell layer	Small cell nests (solid or cystic), usually in nodular hyperplasia, two-cell layer minimum	Same as BCH	Round circumscribed nodule of BCH	Infiltrating adenoid cystic pattern or basaloid pattern, myxoid stroma
Cytologic findings	Small elongated cells, ovoid nuclei, scant cytoplasm	Large, ovoid nuclei, indistinct nucleoli, scant cytoplasm (may be clear)	Same as BCH but with nucleolomegaly	Same as BCH, may have nucleolomegaly	Basaloid cells with large nuclei

basal cell adenoma, but the tumor involves large areas of the prostate with no circumscription.[14] It shows varying proportions of two distinct architectural patterns, occasionally consisting exclusively of one: adenoid cystic carcinoma or basal cell carcinoma.[2, 10, 11, 14] The adenoid cystic pattern consists of irregular clusters of crowded basaloid cells punctuated by round fenestrations, many of which contain mucinous material; the findings are virtually identical to those of salivary gland adenoid cystic carcinoma, including a propensity for perineural invasion. The basaloid pattern consists of variably sized round basaloid cell nests with prominent peripheral palisading. These patterns are usually intimately admixed.[14]

The basal cell nests of adenoid cystic/basal cell carcinoma are large and irregular in outline and separated by benign myxoid stroma, and the tumor cells are predominantly elongated, with narrow, tapering nuclei and peripheral palisading. Cell crowding is prominent, and the basal cell masses frequently display multiple lumens, some of which are sharply circumscribed and round, with a punched-out appearance. Nucleoli are inconspicuous, similar to those of basal cell hyperplasia. In limited samples such as needle biopsy specimens, it may be difficult to separate basal cell adenoma and adenoid cystic/basal cell carcinoma. Squamous differentiation with keratin production is frequent in the prostate, unlike adenoid cystic carcinoma arising at other sites. Grignon and associates described an adenoid cystic/basal cell carcinoma with extensive perineural invasion; however, the tumor lacked significant cytologic atypia, and no extraprostatic extension or follow-up was reported.[15]

In some areas, tumor nests are punctuated by small cystic spaces, imparting a prominent adenoid pattern. These spaces are filled with hyaline material, mucin, or eosinophilic deposits. Two cell types are present: (1) basaloid cells with delicate stippled chromatin and scant cytoplasm, and (2) cuboidal to columnar duct cells with moderate amounts of pale, eosinophilic cytoplasm. Rarely, mitotic figures and mild cytologic atypia are present. In some areas, prominent keratinization of the secretory luminal cells is observed; foci of benign basal cell hyperplasia are often present in adjacent acini. These tumors are expansive, extending into the stroma of the prostate and often accompanied by a myxoid matrix. Adenocarcinoma may be adjacent, but it has not

been reported in direct contact with the adenoid cystic/basal cell carcinoma.

Ultrastructurally, the basaloid cells in adenoid cystic/basal cell carcinoma form cohesive nests surrounded by prominent basal laminae. Well-formed desmosomes are present, and intercellular spaces occasionally are lined by microvilli or, rarely, cilia. In nests with true lumina, the cells exhibit superficial microvilli and have nuclei with conspicuous heterochromatin. The lumina are filled with abundant vesicles, granular material, and cellular debris. In solid nests, the tumor cells have round nuclei with uniform chromatinic rims and prominent euchromatin. There is no evidence of myoepithelial differentiation.

HISTOCHEMICAL AND IMMUNOHISTOCHEMICAL FINDINGS

Normal Basal Cells

Keratin 34β-E12 (Keratin 903; High–Molecular Weight Keratin)

Basal cell–specific anti–keratin 34β-E12 stains virtually all of the normal basal cells of the prostate, with continuous intact circumferential staining in most instances (Table 9–2; see Fig. 9–1C); there is no staining in the secretory and stromal cells. Increasing grades of prostatic intraepithelial neoplasia (PIN) are associated with progressive disruption of the basal cell layer. Basal cell layer disruption is present in 56% of cases of high-grade PIN and is more frequent in acini adjacent to invasive carcinoma than in distant acini. The amount of disruption increases with increasing grades of PIN. Early invasive carcinoma occurs at sites of glandular outpouching and basal cell discontinuity.[26] Cancer cells consistently fail to react with this antibody. Basal cell layer disruption also occurs in inflamed acini, atypical adenomatous hyperplasia, and postatrophic hyperplasia.[16, 17, 21–24, 26, 27, 55]

Other Markers of Basal Cells

Basal cells display immunoreactivity, at least focally, for keratins 5, 10, 11, 13, 14, 16, and 19; of these, only keratin 19 is also found in secretory cells.[17–28, 30] Keratins found exclusively in the secretory cells include 7, 8, and 18.

Basal cells usually do not display immunore-

Table 9–2. Basal Cell Proliferations of the Prostate: Immunohistochemical Findings

	Staining Rate (%)			
	Basal Cell Hyperplasia	Atypical Basal Cell Hyperplasia	Basal Cell Adenoma	Adenoid Cystic / Basal Cell Carcinoma
Basal cell–specific keratin 34β-E12	100	100	83	100
PSA	71	75	83	50
PAP	71	75	66	50
Chromogranin	57	50	33	25
S-100 protein	14	33	16	0
Neuron-specific enolase	43	0	0	0

Data from Devaraj LT, Bostwick DG: Atypical basal cell hyperplasia of the prostate. Immunophenotypic profile and proposed classification of basal cell proliferation. Am J Surg Pathol 17:645–659, 1993.

activity for PSA, PAP, and S-100 protein, and only rare single cells stain with chromogranin and neuron-specific enolase. Conversely, the normal secretory luminal cells invariably stain with PSA and PAP. Prostatic basal cells do not usually display myoepithelial differentiation,[12, 24] in contrast with basal cells in the breast, salivary glands, pancreas, and other sites.[51]

Numerous immunohistochemical markers have recently been identified in the prostate, and many of them are preferentially found in the basal cell layer of the epithelium (Table 9–3). These markers include proliferation markers, differentiation markers, and genetic markers. The preferential localization of many of these markers in basal cells but not in secretory cells suggests that they play a role in growth regulation.

Basal Cell Hyperplasia and Basal Cell Adenoma

Basal cell hyperplasia and adenoma display intense cytoplasmic immunoreactivity in virtually all cells with keratin 34β-E12 (see Table 9–2).[2] PSA and PAP immunoreactivity is scant or absent. Rare basal cells stain with chromogranin, S-100 protein, and neuron-specific enolase.

Adenoid Cystic/Basal Cell Carcinoma

The watery basophilic material in the cystic spaces of adenoid cystic carcinoma stains with Alcian blue at pH 2.5 but is eliminated by hyaluronidase digestion. PAS stain after diastase digestion is positive, as is mucicarmine. The myxoid stroma that often surrounds the tumor nests stains strongly with Alcian blue at pH 2.5, weakly with PAS, and does not stain with mucicarmine.

Adenoid cystic/basal cell carcinoma shows variable immunoreactivity with anti–keratin 34β-E12 (see Table 9–2).[2, 56] Also, rare scattered cells near the lumen show PSA and PAP immunoreactivity, and rare cells display chromogranin staining. S-100 protein and neuron-specific enolase stains are negative.

TREATMENT AND PROGNOSIS

Treatment is the same for basal cell hyperplasia, basal cell adenoma, and cribriform hyperplasia as for benign prostatic hyperplasia, and is based largely on the severity of symptoms. Options include expectant management, medical management, (alpha blockers, androgen deprivation therapy, among others), and surgery (transurethral resection, laser ablation, transurethral hyperthermia, and others).

Most patients with adenoid cystic/basal cell carcinoma are treated by transurethral resection, although other forms of therapy have been employed, including radical prostatectomy and radiation therapy. At present, adenoid cystic/basal cell carcinoma is probably best considered as a tumor of low malignant potential pending long-term follow-up study of other cases.

DIFFERENTIAL DIAGNOSIS

Basal cell proliferations may be mistaken for a wide variety of benign, hyperplastic (Table 9–4) and malignant lesions. Atypical adenomatous hyperplasia is a benign, small, glandular

Table 9–3. Immunophenotypic Profile of Prostatic Basal Cells: Recent Selected Findings

Biomarker	Function	Findings	Selected References
PCNA*	Cell proliferation marker	≤79% of labeled cells are basal cells	Montironi et al.,[62] Bonkhoff et al.[62a]
MIB 1	Cell proliferation marker	≤77% of labeled cells are basal cells	Bonkhoff et al.[62a]
Ki-67	Cell proliferation marker	≤81% of labeled cells are basal cells	Bonkhoff et al.[62a]
Androgen receptors	Nuclear receptors which are necessary for prostatic epithelial growth	Strong immunoreactivity; also present in cancer cells	Bonkhoff et al.,[62a] van der Kwast et al.[63]
PSA	Enzyme which liquefies the seminal coagulum	Present in rare basal cells; mainly in secretory luminal cells	Bonkhoff et al.[34]
Keratin 8.12	Keratins 13, 16	Strong immunoreactivity	Srigley et al.[24]
Keratin 4.62	Keratin 19	Moderate immunoreactivity	Srigley et al.[24]
Keratin PKK1	Keratins 7, 8, 17, 18	Moderate immunoreactivity	Srigley et al.[24]
Keratin 312C8-1	Keratin 14	Strong immunoreactivity	Srigley et al.,[24]
Keratin 34β-E12	Keratins 5, 10, 11	Strong immunoreactivity; most commonly used for diagnostic purposes	Brawer et al.,[16] Bostwick and Brawer,[26] Grignon et al.[15]
Epidermal growth factor receptor (EGF)	Membrane-bound 170-kd glycoprotein that mediates EGF activity	Strong immunoreactivity; rare in cancer	Maygarden et al.,[64] Ibrahim et al.,[65] Robertson et al.,[66] Turkeri et al.,[67] Myers et al.,[68] Visakorpi et al.[69]
CuZn-superoxide dismutase	Enzyme that catalyzes superoxide anion radicals	Strong immunoreactivity	Nonogaki et al.[70]
Type IV collagenase	Enzyme involved in extracellular matrix degradation	Strong immunoreactivity; decreased in cancer	Boag and Young,[71] Stearns and Stearns,[72] Hamdy et al.[73]
Type VII collagen	Part of the hemidesmosomal complex	Strong immunoreactivity; lost in cancer	Knox et al.[74]
Integrins alpha 1,2,4,6, and v; beta 1 and 4	Extracellular matrix adhesion molecules	Strong immunoreactivity; decreased in most with cancer, although alpha 6 and beta 1 are retained	Nagle et al.[75, 76]
Estrogen receptors	Hormone receptor	Moderate immunoreactivity	Wernert et al.[77]
bcl-2	Oncoprotein that suppresses apoptosis	Strong immunoreactivity; also found in most cancers	Columbel et al.[42]
c-erb B2	Oncogene protein in the EGF family	Strong immunoreactivity; also found in most cancers	Visakorpi et al.,[69] Ibrahim et al.,[78] Giri et al.,[79] McCann et al.,[80] Ware,[81] Grizzle et al.,[82] Zhau et al.,[83] Lee et al.[84]
Glutathione S transferase gene (GSTP1)	Enzyme that inactivates electrophilic carcinogens	Strong immunoreactivity; rare in cancer	Lee et al.,[84] Kuhn et al.,[88] Mellon et al.,[89] Myers et al.[90]
C-CAM	Epithelial cell adehsion molecule	Strong immunoreactivity; absent in cancer	Kleinerman et al.[85]
TGF-B	Growth factor that regulates cell proliferation and differentiation	Strong immunoreactivity; absent in cancer	Myers et al.,[68] Eklov et al.[86]
Cathepsin B	Enzyme that degrades basement membranes; may be involved in tumor invasion and metastases	Present in many basal cells and rarely in luminal secretory cells; also found in cancer cells	Sinha et al.[87]
Progesterone receptors	Hormone receptor	Moderate immunoreactivity	Wernert et al.[77]

*PCNA: Proliferating cell nuclear antigen.

Table 9–4. Histopathologic Variants of Benign Prostatic Hyperplasia (BPH)

Variant	Microscopic Features	Usual Location
Basal cell hyperplasia	Proliferation of basal cells two or more cells thick; may have prominent nucleoli (atypical basal cell hyperplasia) or form a nodule (basal cell adenoma)	Transition zone
Stromal hyperplasia with atypical giant cells	Stromal nodules in the setting of BPH with increased cellularity and nuclear atypia	Transition zone
Postatrophic hyperplasia	Atrophic acini with epithelial proliferative changes; easily mistaken for adenocarcinoma owing to architectural distortion	All zones
Cribriform hyperplasia	Acini with distinctive cribriform pattern, often with clear cytoplasm; easily mistaken for proliferative acini of the central zone	Transition zone
Atypical adenomatous hyperplasia	Localized proliferation of small acini in association with BPH nodule, which architecturally mimics adenocarcinoma but lacks cytologic features of malignancy	Transition zone
Sclerosing adenosis	Circumscribed proliferation of small acini in dense spindle cell stroma without significant cytologic atypia; usually solitary and microscopic	Transition zone
Verumontanum mucosal gland hyperplasia	Small benign acinar proliferation involving the verumontanum	Verumontanum
Hyperplasia of mesonephric remnants	Rare benign lobular proliferation of small acini with colloid-like material in lumina; may mimic nephrogenic metaplasia focally. Acini apparently do not express PSA or PAP	All zones (very rare)

From Bostwick DG: The pathology of benign prostatic hyperplasia. In: Kirby R, McConnell J, Fitzpatrick J, Roehrborn P, Boyle P (eds): Textbook of Benign Prostatic Hyperplasia. Oxford: ISIS Medical Media Ltd., 1996.

proliferation that usually arises in the setting of nodular hyperplasia and may be confused with basal cell hyperplasia, although atypical adenomatous hyperplasia displays a discontinuous keratin 34β-E12–immunoreactive basal cell layer that is not thickened.[57, 58]

Sclerosing adenosis may be confused with basal cell hyperplasia with sclerosis, and these lesions may coexist; however sclerosing adenosis displays myoepithelial differentiation and lacks smooth muscle in the sclerotic stroma (intense cytoplasmic immunoreactivity with keratin 34β-E12, S-100 protein, and muscle-specific actin, as well as ultrastructural evidence of cytoplasmic myofilaments).[39–41]

Seminal vesicle and ejaculatory duct epithelium may mimic basal cell hyperplasia and adenoma, particularly in small specimens such as those from needle biopsy and, rarely, from transurethral resection. The proliferation and stratification of lining cells with cytologic atypia may resemble small foci of solid basal cell hyperplasia. Seminal vesicular epithelium is distinguished by the presence of secretory luminal cells with significant cytologic atypia (particularly in senile seminal vesicles) and distinctive abundant yellow to golden brown lipochrome pigment; however, pigment is oc-

casionally present in prostate epithelium.[59–61] Immunohistochemical stains for PSA and PAP are negative in seminal vesicular epithelium and in most basal cell proliferations.

The normal urothelium of the prostatic urethra and periurethral ducts resembles basal cell hyperplasia, histologically and immunohistochemically.[16] Also, urothelial metaplasia may occur in the small and medium-sized ducts in the prostate, sometimes in association with inflammation and reactive atypia with mild nucleolomegaly.

Urethral polyp, although uncommon, may be confused with basal cell hyperplasia and adenoma, particularly in small cystoscopic and needle biopsy specimens. The spectrum of polyps includes proliferative papillary urethritis, ectopic prostate tissue, nephrogenic metaplasia, and inverted papilloma.

High-grade PIN may be mistaken for atypical basal cell hyperplasia.[27] It is distinguished by the presence of cytologic abnormalities in secretory luminal cells of medium-sized to large acini, intense cytoplasmic PSA and PAP immunoreactivity in the abnormal cells, and an intact or fragmented keratin 34β-E12–immunoreactive basal cell layer.

Well-differentiated adenocarcinoma is distinguished from basal cell hyperplasia by the presence of PSA and PAP-immunoreactive luminal secretory cells with nucleolomegaly, frequent luminal crystalloids, and absence of a keratin 34β-E12–immunoreactive basal cell layer. Similar criteria are used to separate the cribriform variant of adenocarcinoma, adenoid cystic/basal cell carcinoma, basal cell hyperplasia with or without clear cell change, and clear cell cribriform hyperplasia.[44]

SUMMARY

Prostatic basal cells contain a subset of reserve or stem cells that are capable of dividing and replenishing the prostatic epithelium and of differentiating into other cell types such as secretory cells. They have a distinctive immunophenotype, including expression of high–molecular weight keratin and markers of cell proliferation.

Recognition of the presence of basal cells in suspicious lesions is a useful diagnostic feature that effectively excludes adenocarcinoma from consideration. In difficult cases, antibodies directed against high–molecular weight keratin and other basal cell–specific markers may be of value. The most important basal cell proliferation to recognize is adenoid cystic/basal cell carcinoma, a tumor of low-grade malignancy.

REFERENCES

1. Mittal BV, Amin MB, Kinare SG: Spectrum of histological lesions in 185 consecutive prostatic specimens. J Postgrad Med 35:157–161, 1989.
2. Devaraj LT, Bostwick DG: Atypical basal cell hyperplasia of the prostate. Immunophenotypic profile and proposed classification of basal cell proliferations. Am J Surg Pathol 17:645–659, 1993.
3. Schlegel R, Banks-Schlegel S, McLeod JA, et al.: Immunoperoxidase location of keratin in human neoplasms. Am J Pathol 101:41–50, 1980.
4. Bennett BD, Gardner WA: Embryonal hyperplasia of the prostate. Prostate 7:411–417, 1985.
5. Elbadawi A: Benign proliferative lesions of the prostate gland. Male Accessory Sex Glands: Biology and Pathology. In Spring-Mills E, Hafez ESE (eds): New York, Elsevier, 1980, pp 387–408.
6. Kasman LP, Gold J: Metaplastic changes in the prostate gland. J Lab Clin Med 301–308, 1933.
7. Krompecher E: Uber Basalzellenhyperplasien und Basalzellenkrebse der Prostata. Eingegangen 284–293, 1925.
8. McNeal JE: Normal histology of the prostate. Am J Surg Pathol 12:619–633, 1988.
9. Lin JI, Cohen EL, Villacin AB, et al.: Basal cell adenoma of prostate. Urology 11:409–410, 1978.
10. Denholm SW, Webb JN, Howard GCW, et al.: Basaloid carcinoma of the prostate gland: histogenesis and review of the literature. Histopathology 20:151–155, 1992.
11. Reed RJ: Consultation case. Am J Surg Pathol 8:699–704, 1984.
12. Howat AJ, Mills PM, Lyons TJ, et al.: Absence of S-100 protein in prostatic glands. Histopathology 13:468–470, 1988.
13. Min KW, Gyorkey F: Prostatic adenoma of ductal origin. Urology 16:95–96, 1980.
14. Young RH, Frierson HF, Mills SE, et al.: Adenoid cystic-like tumor of the prostate gland. A report of two cases and review of the literature on "adenoid cystic carcinoma" of the prostate. Am J Clin Pathol 89:49–56, 1988.
15. Grignon DJ, Ro JY, Ordonez NG, et al.: Basal cell hyperplasia, adenoid basal cell tumor, and adenoid cystic carcinoma of the prostate gland: an immunohistochemical study. Hum Pathol 19:1425–1433, 1988.
16. Brawer MK, Peehl DM, Stamey TA, et al.: Keratin immunoreactivity in the benign and neoplastic human prostate. Cancer Res 45:3663–3667, 1985.
17. Kitajima K, Tokes ZA: Immunohistochemical localization of keratin in human prostate. Prostate 9:183–190, 1986.
18. Nagle RB, Ahmann FR, McDaniel KM, et al.: Cytokeratin characterization of human prostatic carcinoma and its derived cell lines. Cancer Res 47:281–286, 1987.
19. Purnell DM, Heatfield Anthony RL, Trump BF: Immunohistochemistry of the cytoskeleton of human prostatic epithelium. Evidence for disturbed organization in neoplasia. Am J Pathol 126:384–395, 1987.
20. Guinan P, Shaw M, Targonski P, et al.: Evaluation of cytokeratin markers to differentiate between benign and malignant prostatic tissue. J Surg Oncol 42:175–180, 1989.
21. Hedrick L, Epstein JI: Use of keratin 903 as adjunct in the diagnosis of prostate carcinoma. Am J Surg Pathol 13:389–396, 1989.
22. O'Malley FP, Grignon DJ, Shum DT: Usefulness of immunoperoxidase staining with high-molecular-weight cytokeratin in the differential diagnosis of small-acinar lesions of the prostate gland. Virchows Archiv [A] Pathol Anat 417:191–196, 1990.
23. Shah IA, Schlageter MO, Stinnett P, et al.: Cytokeratin immunohistochemistry as a diagnostic tool for distinguishing malignant from benign epithelial lesions of the prostate. Mod Pathol 4:220–224, 1991.
24. Srigley JR, Dardick I, Hartwick RWJ, et al.: Basal epithelial cells of human prostate gland are not myoepithelial cells. A comparative immunohistochemical and ultrastructural study with the human salivary gland. Am J Pathol 136:957–966, 1990.
25. Okada H, Tsubura A, Okamura A, et al.: Keratin profiles in normal/hyperplastic prostates and prostate carcinoma. Virchows Arch [A] Pathol Anat 421:157–161, 1992.
26. Bostwick DG, Brawer MK: Prostatic intra-epithelial neoplasia and early invasion in prostatic cancer. Cancer 59:788–794, 1987.
27. Bostwick DG: High grade prostatic intraepithelial neoplasia: The most likely precursor of prostate cancer. Cancer 75:1823–1836, 1995.
28. Dermer GB: Basal cell proliferation in benign prostatic hyperplasia. Cancer 41:1857–1862, 1978.

29. Bostwick DG, Qian J: Atypical adenomatous hyperplasia of the prostate. Relationship with carcinoma in 217 whole-mount radical prostatectomies. Am J Surg Pathol 19:506–518, 1995.

30. Wernert N, Seitz G: Immunohistochemical investigation of different cytokeratins and vimentin in the prostate from the fetal period up to adulthood and in prostate carcinoma. Pathol Res Pract 182:617–626, 1987.

31. Cleary KR, Choi HY, Ayala AG: Basal cell hyperplasia of the prostate. Am J Clin Path 80:850–854, 1983.

32. Heatfield BM, Sanefuji H, Trump BF: Long-term explant culture of normal human prostate. Methods Cell Biol 21:171–194, 1980.

33. Merchant DJ, Clarke SM, Ives K, et al.: Primary explant culture: an in vitro model of the human prostate. Prostate 4:523–542, 1983.

34. Bonkhoff H, Stein U, Remberger K: The proliferative function of basal cells in the normal and hyperplastic human prostate. Prostate 24:114–118, 1994.

35. Evans GS, Chandler JA: Cell proliferation studies in the rat prostate: The effects of castration and androgen-induced regeneration upon basal and secretory cell proliferation. Prostate 11:339–351, 1987.

36. Aumüller G: Morphologic and endocrine aspects of prostatic function. Prostate 4:195–196, 1983.

37. English HF, Santen RJ, Isaacs JT: Response of glandular versus basal rat ventral prostatic epithelial cells to androgen withdrawal and replacement. Prostate 11:229–242, 1987.

38. Montironi R, Bostwick DG, Bonkhoff H, et al.: Workshop #1: Origins of Prostate Cancer. Cancer 78:362–365, 1996.

39. Jones EC, Clement PB, Young RH: Sclerosing adenosis of the prostate gland. Am J Surg Pathol 15:1171–1180, 1991.

40. Sakamoto N, Tsuneyoshi M, Enjoji M: Sclerosing adenosis of the prostate. Am J Surg Pathol 5:660–667, 1991.

41. Young RH, Clement PB: Sclerosing adenosis of the prostate. Arch Pathol Lab Med 11:363–366, 1987.

42. Columbel M, Symmans F, Gil S, et al.: Detection of the apoptosis-suppressing oncoprotein bcl-2 in hormone-refractory human prostate cancer. Am J Pathol 143:390–400, 1993.

43. Bonkhoff H, Stein U, Aumüller G, et al.: Differential expression of 5 alpha-reductase isoenzymes in the human prostate and prostatic carcinomas. Prostate 29:261–267, 1996.

44. Ayala AG, Srigley JR, Ro JY, et al.: Clear cell cribriform hyperplasia of prostate. Am J Surg Pathol 10:665–672, 1986.

45. Frauenhoffer EE, Ro JY, El-Naggar AK, et al.: Clear cell cribriform hyperplasia of the prostate: Immunohistochemical and flow cytometric study. Am J Clin Pathol 95:446–453, 1991.

46. Bonkhoff H, Remberger K: Widespread distribution of nuclear androgen receptors in the basal cell layer of the normal and hyperplastic prostate. Virchows Arch [A] Pathol Anat 422:35–38, 1993.

47. Epstein JI, Armas O: A. Atypical basal cell hyperplasia of the prostate. Am J Surg Pathol 16:1205–1214, 1992.

48. Frankel KC Jr: Adenoid cystic carcinoma of the prostate. Report of a case. Am J Clin Pathol 62:639–645, 1974.

49. Tannenbaum M: Adenoid cystic or "salivary gland" carcinomas of prostate. Urology 6:2338, 1975.

50. Kramer SA, Bredael JJ, Krueger RP: Adenoid cystic carcinoma of the prostate: Report of a case. J Urol 120:383–384, 1978.

51. Lawrence JB, Mazur MT: Adenoid cystic carcinoma: A comparative pathologic study of tumors in salivary gland, breast, lung, and cervix. Hum Pathol 13:916–924, 1982.

52. Shond-San C, Walters MNI: Adenoid cystic carcinoma of prostate. Report of a case. Pathology 16:337–338, 1984.

53. Gilmour AM, Bell TJ: Adenoid cystic carcinoma of the prostate. Br J Urol 58:105–106, 1986.

54. Mostofi FK, Price EB Jr: Tumors of the Male Genital System. Fascicle 8, second series, Atlas of Tumor Pathology. Washington, DC: Armed Forces Institute of Pathology, 1973, pp 244–245.

55. Cheville J, Bostwick DG: Post-atrophic hyperplasia of the prostate. A histologic mimick of prostatic adenocarcinoma. Am J Surg Pathol 19:1068–1076, 1995.

56. Kuhajda FP, Mann RG: Adenoid cystic carcinoma of the prostate. A case report with immunoperoxidase staining for prostate-specific acid phosphatase and prostate-specific antigen. Am J Clin Pathol 81:257–260, 1984.

57. Srigley JR: Small-acinar patterns in the prostate gland with emphasis on atypical adenomatous hyperplasia and small-acinar carcinoma. Semin Diagn Pathol 5:254–27, 1988.

58. Bostwick DG, Srigley J, Grignon D, et al.: Atypical adenomatous hyperplasia of the prostate: Morphologic criteria for its distinction from well-differentiated carcinoma. Hum Pathol 24:819–832, 1993.

59. Brennick JB, O'Connell JX, Dickersin GR, et al.: Lipofuscin pigmentation (so-called "melanosis") of the prostate. Am J Surg Pathol 18:446–454, 1994.

60. Leung CS, Srigley JR: Distribution of lipochrome pigment in the prostate gland: Biological and diagnostic implications. Hum Pathol 26:1302–1307, 1995.

61. Amin MB, Bostwick DG: Pigment in prostatic epithelium and adenocarcinoma: A potential source of diagnostic confusion with seminal vesicular epithelium. Mod Pathol 9:791–795, 1996.

62. Montironi R, Magi Galluzzi C, Diamanti L, et al.: Prostatic intra-epithelial neoplasia: Expression and location of proliferating cell nuclear antigen in epithelial, endothelial and stromal nuclei. Virchows Arch [A] Pathol Anat 422:185–192, 1993.

62a. Bonkhoff H, Stein V, Remberger K: Multidirectional differentiation in the normal, hyperplastic, and neoplastic human prostate: Simultaneous demonstration of cell-specific epithelial markers. Hum Pathol 25:42–46, 1994.

63. Van der Kwast TH, Ruizeveld de Winter JA, Trapman J: Androgen receptor expression in human prostate cancer. J Urol Pathol 3:200–222, 1995.

64. Maygarden S, Strom S, Ware JL: Localization of epidermal growth factor receptor by immunohistochemical methods in human prostatic carcinoma, prostatic intraepithelial neoplasia, and benign hyperplasia. Arch Pathol Lab Med 116:269–273, 1992.

65. Ibrahim GK, Kerns BM, MacDonald JA, et al.: Differential immunoreactivity of epidermal growth factor receptor in benign, dysplastic and malignant prostatic tissues. J Urol 149:170–173, 1993.

66. Robertson CN, Robertson KM, Herzberg AJ, et al.: Differential immunoreactivity of transforming growth factor alpha in benign, dysplastic, and malignant prostatic tissues. Surg Oncol 3:237–242, 1994.

67. Turkeri LN, Sakr WA, Wykes SM, et al.: Comparative

analysis of epidermal growth factor receptor gene expression and protein product in benign, premalignant, and malignant prostate tissue. Prostate 25:199–205, 1994.

68. Myers RB, Kudlow JE, Grizzle WE: Expression of transforming growth factor-alpha, epidermal growth factor and the epidermal growth factor receptor in adenocarcinoma of the prostate and benign prostatic hyperplasia. Mod Pathol 6:733–737, 1993.

69. Visakorpi T, Kallioniemi O-P, Koivula T, et al.: Expression of epidermal growth factor receptor and ERBB2 (Her-2/Neu) oncoprotein in prostatic carcinomas. Mod Pathol 5:643–648, 1992.

70. Nonogaki T, Noda Y, Narimoto K, et al: Localization of CuZn-superoxide dismutase in the human male genital organs. Hum Reprod 7:81–85, 1992.

71. Boag AH, Young ID: Immunohistochemical analysis of type IV collagenase expression in prostatic hyperplasia and adenocarcinoma. Mod Pathol 6:65–68, 1993.

72. Stearns ME, Stearns M: Autocrine factors, type IV collagenase secretion and prostatic cancer cell invasion. Cancer Metas Rev 12:39–52, 1993.

73. Hamdy FC, Fadlon EJ, Cottam D, et al.: Matrix metalloproteinase 9 expression in primary human prostatic adenocarcinoma and benign prostatic hyperplasia. Br J Cancer 69:177–182, 1994.

74. Knox JD, Cress AE, Clark V, et al.: Differential expression of extracellular matrix molecules and the alpha-6 integrins in the normal and neoplastic prostate. Am J Pathol 145:167–174, 1994.

75. Nagle RB, Brawer MK, Kittelson J, et al.: Phenotypic relationships of prostatic intraepithelial neoplasia to invasive prostatic carcinoma. Am J Pathol 1138:119–128, 1991.

76. Nagle RB, Hao J, Knox JD, et al.: Expression hemidesmosomal and extracellular matrix proteins by normal and malignant human prostate tissue. Am J Pathol 146:1498–1507, 1995.

77. Wernert N, Gerdes J, Loy V, et al: Investigations of the estrogen (ER-ICA-test) and the progesterone receptor in the prostate and prostatic carcinoma on immunohistochemical basis. Virchows Arch [A] 412:387–391, 1988.

78. Ibrahim GK, MacDonald JA, Kerns BJM, et al.: Differential immunoreactivity of her-2/neu oncoprotein in prostatic tissues. Surg Oncol 1:151–155, 1992.

79. Giri DK, Wadhwa SN, Upadhaya SN, et al.: Expression of neu/her-2 oncoprotein (p185neu) in prostate tumors: An immunohistochemical study. Prostate 23:329–336, 1993.

80. McCann A, Dervan PA, Johnston PA, et al.: c-erbB-2 oncoprotein expression in primary human tumors. Cancer 65:88–94, 1990.

81. Ware JL, Maygarden SJ, Koontz WW Jr, et al.: Immunohistochemical detection of c-erbB-2 protein in human benign and neoplastic prostate. Hum Pathol 22:254–259, 1991.

82. Grizzle WE, Myers RB, Arnold MM, et al.: Evaluation of biomarkers in breast and prostate cancer. J Cell Biochem Suppl 19:259–266, 1994.

83. Zhau HE, Wan DS, Zhou J, et al.: Expression of c-erbB-2/neu proto-oncogene in human prostatic cancer tissues and cell lines. Mol Carcinog 5:320–327, 1992.

84. Lee WH, Morton RA, Epstein JI, et al.: Cytidine methylation of regulatory sequences near the Pi-class glutathione S-transferase gene accompanies human prostatic carcinogenesis. Proc Natl Acad Sci USA 91:11733–11737, 1994.

85. Kleinerman DI, Troncoso P, Lin S-H, et al.: Consistent expression of an epithelial cell adhesion molecule (C-CAM) during human prostate development and loss of expression in prostate cancer: Implication as a tumor suppressor. Cancer Res 55:1215–1220, 1995.

86. Eklov S, Funa K, Nordgren H, et al.: Lack of the latent transforming growth factor beta binding protein in malignant, but not benign, prostatic tissue. Cancer Res 53:3193–3197, 1993.

87. Sinha AA, Gleason DF, Deleon OF, et al.: Localization of a biotinylated cathepsin B oligonucleotide probe in human prostate including invasive cells and invasive edges by in situ hybridization. Anat Rec 235:233–240, 1993.

88. Kuhn EJ, Kurnot RA, Sesterhenn IA, et al.: Expression of the c-erbB-2 (HER2/neu) oncoprotein in human prostatic carcinoma. J Urol 150:1427–1433, 1993.

89. Mellon K, Thompson S, Charlton RG, et al.: p53, c-erbB-2 and the epidermal growth factor receptor in the benign and malignant and malignant prostate. J Urol 147:496–499, 1992.

90. Myers RB, Srivastava S, Oelschlager DK, et al.: Expression of p160erbB-3 and p185erbB-2 in prostatic intraepithelial neoplasia and prostatic adenocarcinoma. J Natl Cancer Inst 86:1140–1145, 1994.

10

EXAMINATION OF RADICAL PROSTATECTOMY SPECIMENS: THERAPEUTIC AND PROGNOSTIC SIGNIFICANCE

DAVID G. BOSTWICK **and** CHRISTOPHER S. FOSTER

Accurate examination of radical prostatectomy specimens by the pathologist is crucial for predicting patient outcome. However, many diagnostic histopathology laboratories, particularly outside the United States, receive radical prostatectomy specimens only infrequently. For pathologists handling such tissues, routine protocol-based tissue sampling ensures consistent and thorough examination by trainees and consultants. This issue has been addressed recently by the College of American Pathologists (CAP),[1] the Association of Directors of Anatomic and Surgical Pathology (ADASP),[2] and a recent consensus conference sponsored by the American Cancer Society, World Health Organization, and Mayo Clinic.[3] In this report, we incorporate the conclusions of each of these contemporary statements to create a standardized approach to examination of radical prostatectomy specimens. Also included is a brief evaluation of pathologic staging and the "vanishing cancer phenomenon." We begin with a comparison of partial and complete tissue sampling (Figs. 10–1, 10–2).

METHODS OF SAMPLING RADICAL PROSTATECTOMY SPECIMENS

Numerous methods for partial and complete sampling of prostatectomy specimens

have been described, and the completeness of sampling affects the determination of pathologic stage.[1, 4–7] Haggman and colleagues compared the results of partial sampling (sections of palpable tumor and two random sections of apex and base) with those of complete sampling and found a significant increase in positive surgical margins (12% and 59%, respectively) and pathologic stage with complete sectioning.[6] Others have shown that the presence and extent of extraprostatic extension in clinical stage T2 adenocarcinoma (and thus clinical staging error) was directly related to the number of tissue blocks submitted.[5] Donahue and Miller noted that 40% of patients had extraprostatic extension of cancer determined by standard study, as compared with 60% determined by whole-mount evaluation.[8] Cohen and colleagues found that partial sampling with alternate sections missed 15% of cases with extraprostatic extension, which were identified by complete sampling.[9] Partial sampling methods are reportedly equivalent to whole-mount sections for determining cancer volume,[5] but we question this finding.

Current guidelines for the evaluation of radical prostatectomy specimens emphasize information that should be included in the pathology report but leave the decision on partial or complete sampling to the individual patholo-

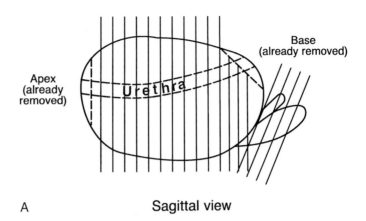

Apex
(already
removed)

Urethra

Base
(already removed)

A

Sagittal view

Figure 10–1. Slicing protocol for radical prostatectomy specimens. *A,* Parallel transverse cuts are made after amputating the apex and base (see text). *B,* The apex may be submitted as a conization specimen by quadrants.

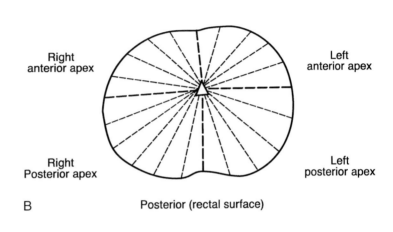

Right
anterior apex

Left
anterior apex

Right
Posterior apex

Left
posterior apex

B

Posterior (rectal surface)

gist.[1] Sampling methods for harvesting tissue for research purposes often vary from routine methods and are discussed elsewhere.[10–12] Regardless of which sampling method is employed, the initial handling of the specimen is similar or identical.

In the Department of Anatomic Pathology at Liverpool University, radical prostatectomy specimens are received fresh and unfixed, immediately after removal from the patient. The specimen is weighed, measured, and described before being photographed in monochrome using Polaroid to provide a working illustration and color transparencies for demonstration purposes. Thereafter, the outer surfaces are coated with orienting colors. Suspensions of artists' pigments cadmium red or cobalt blue (50% w/v in acetone) provide useful markers of left- and right-hand resection margins. Since they contain heavy metals, these pigments have the additional advantage of being radiopaque; however, this feature is also

potentially hazardous if the cut surfaces of the dissected prostate become contaminated by these pigments, giving the spurious appearance of microcalcification. Alternative media for marking resection margins include acrylic paints (green, yellow, etc.), which dry rapidly and resist processing. After the macroscopic description is completed, the prostate is sliced transversely at 2- to 3-mm intervals and the slices laid out, in a standard anatomic sequence, onto a clear acetate sheet. The entire sliced specimen is then photocopied to provide a working visual reference sheet, and is also x-rayed within the dissection laboratory using a Microfocus 50 Imaging System (at 20 kV for 18 to 25 seconds using Kodak MIN-R MREI mammography film) to identify regions of contrasting radiopacity, including microcalcification. Thereafter, the slices of prostate are sampled. The amputated upper (bladder) and lower (penile) resection slices are conized, either radially or transversely. The shape and

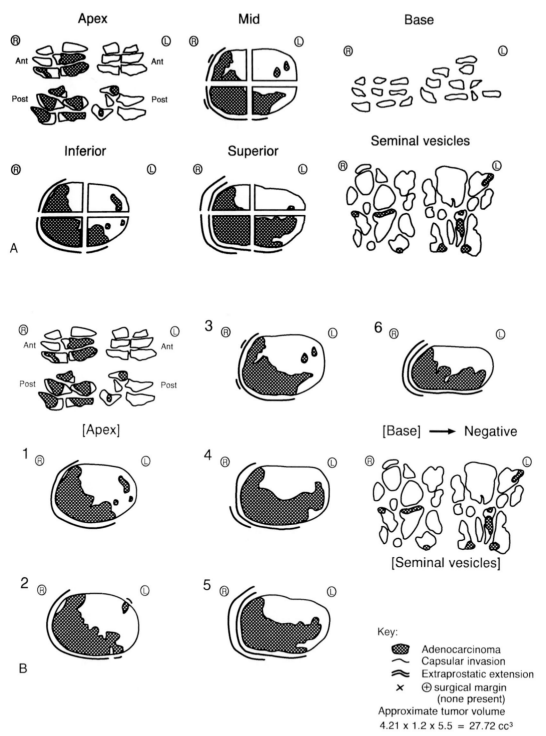

Figure 10–2. Sample prostate cancer maps used at the Mayo Clinic for radical prostatectomy specimens. *A,* Partial sampling. *B,* Complete sampling with whole-mount sections. (From Bostwick DG, Eble JE: Urologic Surgical Pathology. St. Louis: Mosby–Year Book, 1997.)

location of individual blocks taken are recorded directly onto the xerogram. Brief notes accompanying each site sampled, such as appearance, questions about imaging, and invasion or resection margins are written onto the xerogram and used when performing microscopy. It is our experience that unfixed radical prostatectomy tissue is sufficiently resilient that fixation is not necessary before completing the dissection and block sampling, including the removal of tissue for culture, biochemistry, or molecular analyses.

Initial Handling of the Prostatectomy

All methods begin with weighing the fresh specimen and measuring it in three dimensions. Weight may be more reproducible than linear dimensions because the resected prostate is an irregular structure.[15] For ultrasonographic measurements, radiologists often describe the shape of the prostate as a prolate ellipsoid (length × height × width × 0.532),[13] but this is only a rough estimate that shows considerable variability. Separate measurements are made of the attached seminal vesicles.

Subsequent handling of the specimen can be performed when it is fresh or fixed. For fixation, the prostatectomy specimen should be submerged in 5 to 10 volumes of 10% neutral buffered formalin. Care should be taken to avoid touching the sides of the container to avoid tissue compression and distortion. Some investigators cannulate the prostatic urethra with a tube attached to an aquarium pump to create a constant gentle bathing stream of formalin during fixation,[5] but we find that simple immersion is sufficient. The fresh (or fixed) prostate is inked by brief immersion in a small container of India ink or by painting the surface with different colors of ink to allow unequivocal identification of left and right sides. Subsequently, the wet specimen is immersed briefly in acetone or Bouin's fixative and air dried or blotted dry. Some pathologists use different colors of ink for the anterior and posterior prostate, apex, and base to ensure proper orientation.

Disruption of the attached periprostatic soft tissues by the surgeon or pathologist may cause ink to seep into tissue crevices. This creates the potential for misinterpretation of an inked surface as a true surgical margin (i.e., false-positive diagnosis of involved surgical margin).

Consequently, it is important to note whether the attached tissue was disrupted and at which sites.

The apex and base are amputated at a thickness of 4 to 5 mm, and these margins are submitted as 3- to 4-mm thick conization slices in the vertical parasagittal plane[14]; alternatively, some pathologists prefer 1- to 2-mm thick shave margins. For conization, the apex usually requires quadrant sectioning, and we routinely use abbreviations for the right anterior apex (RAX), left anterior apex (LAX), right posterior apex (RPX), and left posterior apex (LPX). Similarly, the base is sampled, usually into left and right halves as left bladder base (LBB) and right bladder base (RBB), respectively. Although some protocols include circular ("doughnut") sections of the urethral stump at the apex and base, we do not routinely submit these; unlike some cancers, prostate cancer rarely demonstrates pagetoid spread or submucosal spread without involving large areas of adjacent tissue.

The remaining specimen is serially sectioned at 3- to 5-mm thickness by knife to create transverse sections perpendicular to the long axis of the prostate from its apex to the tip of the seminal vesicles. Some investigators employ commercial meat slicers[14] or unique prostate-slicing devices,[5] but these are not widely used. Partial and complete sampling differ by the amount of prostate tissue submitted after this point. According to a 1994 survey, 88% of pathologists prefer partial sampling, probably owing to time and cost considerations (Table 10–1).[15]

Macroscopic Identification of Cancer

Macroscopic identification of prostatic adenocarcinoma may be difficult or in some cases impossible, and definitive diagnosis requires microscopic examination. Grossly apparent tumor foci are usually at least 5 mm in greatest dimension and appear yellow-white with a firm consistency due to stromal desmoplasia. Some cancers appear as yellow, granular masses that contrast sharply with the normal spongy prostatic parenchyma. Gross mimics of cancer include tuberculosis, granulomatous prostatitis, and acute and chronic prostatitis. One study noted that 92% of cases of clinically organ-confined biopsy-proven cancer were grossly identifiable in prostatectomy specimens,[16] but

Table 10–1. Examination of Radical Prostatectomy Specimens: Practice Survey by the American Society of Clinical Pathologists, 1994 (True, 1994)

Practice Characteristic	"Yes" Responses (%)
Processing and sampling	
Record weight	95
Record measurements	97
Cut specimen before fixing	40
Fix specimen overnight	53
Ink margins	86
Use different colors of ink	29
Section prostate coronally	82
Label each section by site	88
Describe size of lesions	97
Complete sectioning	12
Embed 1–4 blocks	5
Embed 5–8 blocks	19
Embed 9–12 blocks	29
Embed > 12 blocks	34
Embed entire apex	64
Embed entire bladder base	62
Submit all lymph nodes	99
Reporting	
Assign Gleason score	73
Use other grading system	35
Assign nuclear grade	21
Report involvement of apex	83
Report involvement of seminal vesicles	99
Report extraprostatic extension	100
Report prostatic intraepithelial neoplasia	50
Report distance of cancer from surgical margin of resection	61
Report vascular invasion	89
Report perineural invasion	90
Report multifocal cancer	90
Report nonneoplastic changes	81

From True LD: Surgical pathology examination of the prostate gland. Practice survey by American Society of Clinical Pathologists. Am J Clin Path 10:572–579, 1994.

most investigators, including us, find a much lower incidence.

Partial (Limited) Sampling

Partial sampling results in histopathologic submission of a fraction of the prostate, usually less than half, including all grossly apparent cancer. Given the limitations of macroscopic identification of cancer, partial sampling protocols sometimes require submission of additional tissue to identify cancer (see Vanishing Cancer Phenomenon, below). The partial sampling protocol used at the Mayo Clinic since 1968 is equivalent to that recently endorsed by consensus at the American Cancer Society meeting[3] and fulfills all of the requirements of the CAP[1] and the ADASP.[2]

Complete (Unlimited or Totally Embedded) Sampling

Complete sampling results in the entire prostate being submitted for histopathologic examination; however, this method is subject to sampling error since generation of a single 5-μm thick section from each 3-mm tissue block still results in microscopic review of only 0.17% of all embedded tissue. Theoretically, 15,600 slides per case would be required to review the entire specimen.[17] Two alternative methods exist for complete sampling: routine sections and whole-mount sections.

(1) *Complete sampling with routine sections:* This method refers to submitting the entire prostate after cutting tissue samples sufficiently small to fit into routine cassettes, obviating the special handling required for whole-mount sections. Sections are obtained by slicing each transverse section into four quadrants; larger prostates often generate six, or even eight, sections per transverse slice, whereas smaller prostates may generate only two sections per slice. This method of complete sampling yields, on average, 26 routine slides per case.[5] In rare cases of a very small prostate (fewer than one in 300 cases in our experience), intact transverse sections can fit into a cassette, thus allowing routine sections of whole mounts.

(2) *Complete sampling with whole mount sections:* In this method the entire prostate is submitted as intact transverse serial slices without subdivision (Fig. 10–3). This method is preferred by some investigators, but it requires special handling of tissue samples that are larger than routine sections. It may be the optimal method for teaching and research purposes but is infrequently used in routine practice.

REPORTING OF PATHOLOGIC FINDINGS FROM RADICAL PROSTATECTOMY SPECIMENS

Examination of radical prostatectomy specimens should include the information in Table 10–2.

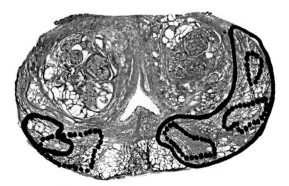

Figure 10–3. Organ-confined prostate cancer. Note extensive bilateral cancer in the peripheral zone (*outlined with solid lines*) accompanied by high-grade prostatic intraepithelial neoplasia (*outlined with dotted lines*). The cancer was confined to the prostate (stage T2c) but was close to the lateral surgical margins.

Histopathologic Type

More than 95% of cases of prostate carcinoma are acinar adenocarcinoma; in recent years, a number of new and unusual histopathologic variants have been identified. The biologic behavior of many of these variants may differ from that of typical adenocarcinoma, and proper clinical management depends on accurate diagnosis and separation from tumors arising in other sites. Unusual tumors arising in the prostate also raise questions of histogenesis. The diagnostic features of variants of carcinoma are described elsewhere in this volume.

Histologic Grade

Grade is one of the strongest and most useful predictors of pathologic stage and other

Table 10–2. Examination of Radical Prostatectomy Specimens: Information to Be Included in the Surgical Pathology Report

Histopathologic type of carcinoma
Histologic grade (Gleason score)
Location and size of cancer(s)
Extraprostatic extension: amount and location
Seminal vesicle involvement
Surgical margin status
Apex
Base
Neurovascular bundles
Posterior prostate
Anterior prostate
Lymph nodes
Sites, number, and status
pTNM

clinical and pathologic features according to numerous univariate and multivariate studies. This predictive weight applies to virtually every measure of pathologic stage, including extraprostatic extension, seminal vesicle invasion, lymph node metastases, and bone metastases. Some investigators claim that a Gleason score of 8 or higher is strongly predictive of lymph node metastases, and they suggest dispensing with staging lymph node dissections in these cases. Despite the optimism about grading as a predictor of stage, the predictive value is not great enough to permit its application to individual patients, particularly in cases of moderately differentiated adenocarcinoma. Grade is discussed elsewhere in this volume.

Site of Cancer

The site of origin of cancer appears to be a significant prognostic factor. When cancer arises in the transition zone, it is apparently less aggressive than typical acinar adenocarcinoma arising in the peripheral zone (Table 10–3). The majority of transition zone cancers arise next to nodules of hyperplasia, and a third actually originate within nodules. These adenocarcinomas are better differentiated than those in the peripheral zone, accounting for the majority of Gleason primary grade 1 and 2 tumors. The volume of low grade tumors tends to be smaller than that of those arising in the peripheral zone, although frequent exceptions are seen. The confinement of transition zone adenocarcinoma to its anatomic site of origin may account in part for the favorable prognosis of clinical stage T1 tumors. The transition zone boundary may act as a relative barrier to tumor extension, as malignant acini appear frequently to fan out along this boundary before invading the peripheral and central zones.

Cancer Volume

Cancer volume has been proposed as an adjunct to digital rectal examination–based staging of prostatic adenocarcinoma because of its powerful prognostic capability.[18–20] This approach may be feasible in the future, with improvements in imaging techniques such as transrectal ultrasonography (TRUS). A cancer volume–based prognostic index has been proposed as an adjunct for staging, based on evi-

Table 10–3. Prostatic Carcinoma: Comparison Based on Anatomic Site of Origin*

	Transition Zone	Peripheral Zone
Prevalence (%)		
Stage T1a	75	——
Stage T1b	79	——
All stage T1a and T1b	78	——
All stages	24	70
Origin		
In or near BPH?	Yes	No
Near apex?	Yes	Yes
Detection rate by TURP (%)	78	——
Pathologic features		
Tumor volume	Usually small	Small to large
Tumor (Gleason) grade	Usually 1 or 2	Usually 2, 3, or 4
Clear cell pattern	Most cases	Rare
Stromal fibrosis	Uncommon	Common
Associated putative premalignant changes	AAH or PIN	PIN
Aneuploidy (%)	6	31
Clinical behavior		
Extraprostatic extension (%)	11	44
Site of extracapsular extension	Anterolateral and apical	Lateral
Average tumor size with extracapsular extension	4.98 cc	3.86 cc
Risk of seminal vesicle invasion (%)	0	19
Risk of lymph node metastases	Low	High

*Central zone cancers (5–10% of total) were excluded.

Key: BPH, benign prostatic hyperplasia; TURP, transurethral resection of the prostate; AAH, atypical adenomatous hyperplasia; PIN, prostatic intraepithelial neoplasia.

From Bostwick DG et al.: The association of benign prostatic hyperplasia and cancer of the prostate. Cancer 70:291–301, 1992.

dence linking adenocarcinoma volume with patterns of progression (extraprostatic extension, seminal vesicle invasion, and lymph node metastases).[19] For organ-confined cancer, three main categories were recognized: V1, cancer lesions smaller than 1 cm³; V2a, cancer 1 to 5 cm³; and V2b, tumor larger than 5 cm³. The goal of the prognostic index is to achieve greater precision in predicting outcome for individual patients.[20]

Several studies have shown a positive correlation between cancer volume and serum prostate-specific antigen (PSA) concentration, suggesting that PSA can serve as a surrogate of volume.[21–23] The additive and confounding effect of nodular hyperplasia, however, limits the usefulness of PSA in estimating preoperative cancer size and extent.[22] As adenocarcinoma enlarges, it usually becomes less differentiated and may lose some of its capacity for PSA production. PSA concentration increases with increasing Gleason grade, but, when tumor volume is held constant, PSA decreases (PSA concentration declines as Gleason grade increases).[22] This finding results from production of less PSA per cell in poorly differentiated tumors as compared with well- and moderately differentiated tumors.[23] No ac-

cepted standard exists for reporting cancer volume in prostatectomy specimens. The easiest and most practical approach is to estimate the percentage of cancer in the entire specimen. After accounting for pathologic stage, tumor volume may not provide significant additional prognostic information, but this observation has not been confirmed.[24]

Extraprostatic Extension

The term "extraprostatic extension" (EPE) was accepted at a recent consensus conference to replace other terms, including "capsular invasion," "capsular penetration," and "capsular perforation."[3] To define EPE, it is first necessary to understand the anatomy of the capsule of the prostate.

Anatomy of the Prostatic Capsule

The capsule is an extension of the prostatic parenchyma that consists of variable amounts of transverse fibers of compressed smooth muscle and collagen (Fig. 10–4, see Color Plate 1 following p. 190). The mean thickness of the capsule varies from 0.5 to 2 mm, and the mean percentage of smooth muscle fibers is 31%, a figure similar to that within the prostate.[25] At the outer edge of the apex and bladder base, the acinar elements are often sparse, and the capsule is thin and ill-defined, precluding reliable evaluation. Anteriorly, the smooth muscle and fibrous stroma of the prostate interdigitate with the smooth muscle and skeletal muscle of the pelvic wall; although this constitutes a useful surgical plane of dissection, it does not provide the sharp microscopic line of demarcation usually expected from a capsule. As a result, the prostatic capsule is not regarded as a well-defined anatomic structure with constant features.[14, 25] We use the term "capsule" to refer to the surface or edge of the fibromuscular stroma of the prostate, recognizing that this is the only stable and reproducible anatomic landmark. We consider the capsule as an extension of the parenchymal stroma, which is compressed.

The capsule at the apex and bladder base is difficult or impossible to identify (see Fig. 10–4, Color Plate 1 following p. 190). Consequently, it is not possible to determine, reliably and consistently, the presence of extraprostatic extension of cancer at these sites, and we limit our evaluation there to surgical margin status.

Definition of Extraprostatic Extension

Extension of cancer beyond the edge or capsule of the prostate is diagnostic of EPE. There are three criteria for EPE, depending on the site and composition of the extraprostatic tissue: (1) cancer in adipose tissue; (2) cancer in perineural spaces of the neurovascular bundles; and (3) cancer in anterior muscle (Fig. 10–5, see Color Plate 2 following p. 190).

Cancer in Adipose Tissue. EPE is easily diagnosed when malignant acini are in contact with adipose tissue. There is no adipose tissue in the prostate, so this finding constitutes unequivocal EPE; it is useful in biopsy specimens and in poorly oriented sections from a prostatectomy. Adipose tissue is usually present adjacent to the lateral, posterolateral, and posterior surfaces of the prostate.

Difficulty is occasionally encountered when cancer has provoked a dense desmoplastic response in the extraprostatic tissue, particularly in cases treated by androgen deprivation therapy. We resolve this uncommon problem by scanning the smooth, rounded external contour of the prostate to determine if the focus of concern has breached this contour and is enmeshed within an extraprostatic nodule of fibrous tissue.

Cancer in Perineural Spaces of the Neurovascular Bundles. The neurovascular bundles are a path of least resistance by which cancer can escape from the prostate. These bundles are clustered in the posterolateral corners of the prostate (at about 5:00 o'clock and 7:00 o'clock in transverse sections) and are best appreciated at scanning magnification in whole-mount sections of non–nerve sparing radical prostatectomy specimens. Although cancer may not be in contact with adipose tissue, involvement of perineural spaces of the neurovascular bundles represents EPE.

Perineural invasion alone does not constitute EPE, and there are often large nerve twigs within the prostate that can be mistaken for neurovascular bundles. Accordingly, it is best to diagnose cancer in the neurovascular bundles (and, thus, EPE) only when the malignant acini are present beyond the reasonable contour (edge) of the prostate.

Cancer in Anterior Muscle. The anterior muscle is a very uncommon site of EPE and is observed only with large, bulky cancers within the transition zone. The anterior fibromuscular stroma of the prostate interdigitates with external smooth muscle and skeletal muscle adjacent to the pubic bone, and there is usually insufficient adipose tissue in this area to define the extraprostatic tissue. Consequently, it may be difficult to identify EPE. We diagnose EPE at this site only when there is unequivocal evidence of cancer extending beyond the reasonable confines of the prostate's edge into skeletal muscle and beyond the rounded interface between the fibromuscular stroma and skeletal muscle.

Frequency of Extraprostatic Extension

In patients treated by radical prostatectomy for clinically localized cancer, the frequency of EPE (stage pT3 cancer) has variously been reported as 23%,[26] 41%,[27] 43%,[28] 45%,[29] or 52%.[30] There is a strong association between tumor volume and extraprostatic extension and seminal vesicle invasion.[7] An autopsy study showed EPE in 2% of cancers smaller than 0.46 cc in volume, as compared with 52% of larger cancers.[18]

Clinical Significance of Extraprostatic Extension

Patients with EPE have a worse prognosis than those with organ-confined cancer.[29, 31] Cancer-specific survival 10 years after radical prostatectomy in patients with pT3 cancer is 54%,[32] 62%,[33] 70%,[34] or 80%[35]; at 15 years, it is 69%.[35] Cancer-specific survival 10 years after definitive radiation therapy for clinical stage T3 lesions is 44%[36] or 59%[37]; at 15 years, survival is 36%,[36] 33%,[38] or 39%.[37] Cancer-specific survival after expectant management (watchful waiting or observation) of patients with clinical stage T3 cancer is 70%.[39] Direct comparison of surgical and nonsurgical series may be inaccurate owing to significant differences in methods of patient selection, evaluation, and staging. Furthermore, no prospective comparative study has been performed to settle the debate about optimal treatment.

Most patients with EPE also have positive surgical margins with a frequency of 57% to 81%[30] (57%[24] to 81%[30]). The combination of EPE and positive margins carries a worse prognosis than EPE alone.[24, 34]

Recent studies have questioned the value of substaging T3 adenocarcinoma in patients treated by radiation therapy. In two studies, there were no differences in relapse rates for those with clinical stage T3a and T3c adenocarcinoma.[40, 41] Substaging is useful, however, for predicting outcome in patients treated by radical prostatectomy.[24] Consequently, substaging based on digital rectal examination alone (used in radiation therapy studies) does not distinguish among meaningful prognostic substages in patients with T3 cancer.[41]

Surgical Margins

Definition of Positive Surgical Margin

"Positive surgical margin" is defined as cancer cells touching the inked surface of the prostate (Fig. 10–6, see Color Plate 3 following p. 190). Care must be taken to avoid interpreting ink within tissue crevices created by postoperative handling of the specimen as positive margins. Careful handling of the specimen and awareness of this potential problem are usually sufficient.

Surgical margins are not included in pathologic staging; however, many studies have erroneously equated positive margins with extraprostatic extension, particularly when the surgeon has cut into the prostate and intraprostatic cancer. The recent Mayo Clinic consensus conference emphasized this distinction and called on investigators to carefully describe surgical margin status separately from extraprostatic extension.[3]

Confusion may persist in interpretation of prostatectomy specimens in which there is focally no extraprostatic tissue for examination. At such sites, the surgical resection margin corresponds exactly with the outer surface of the prostate or cuts into the prostatic capsule or parenchyma. If the surgical margin at this site contains cancer, does this represent extraprostatic extension? Participants at the recent Mayo Clinic consensus conference agreed that these foci should be considered T2+ rather than T3 (the plus sign is a "telescopic ramification" of the TNM staging system that is added to emphasize that the available evidence indicates T2 cancer but there may be cancer outside of the prostate that cannot be evaluated in the specimen submitted (see Fig. 10–6, Color Plate 3 following p. 190).[3]

Frequency of Positive Surgical Margins

The prevalence of positive surgical margins has steadily declined in the past decade, probably owing to refinements in surgical technique and earlier detection of cancer of smaller volumes (Table 10–4). Ohori and colleagues found positive surgical margins in 24% of whole-mount radical prostatectomy specimens obtained at their hospital before 1987,

Table 10–4. Incidence of Positive Surgical Margins in Totally Embedded Radical Prostatectomy Specimens According to Pathologic Stage

Investigator/Stage	Specimens with Positive Margins/Proportion (%)
Epstein et al., 1993[24]	
Less than pT3c (stages not provided)	100/185 (54)
Ravery et al., 1994[74]	
pT3a + b	17/26 (65)
pT3c	14/19 (74)
All pT3	31/45 (69)
Ohori et al., 1995[28]	
pT1 and pT2	23/247 (9)
pT3a + b	33/150 (22)

From Bostwick DG, Montironi R: Evaluating radical prostatectomy specimens: therapeutic and prognostic importance. Virch Archiv 430:1–19, 1997.

Table 10–5. Frequency of Positive Surgical Margins by Location in Radical Prostatectomy Specimens*

Location	Stamey et al., 1990[42]†	Ackerman et al., 1993[46]
Apex	21%	23%
Superior pedicle	4%	
Lateral surface	4%	
Rectal surface	7%	
"Mid-portion"		22%
Bladder neck	7%	6%
Anterior fibromuscular stroma	1%	
All cases with positive surgical margins/All cases	63/189 (33%)	37/101 (37%)

*Frequencies are percentages of positive surgical margins by location among all cases; consequently, the cumulative frequencies do not add up to 100% because more than one margin is often involved.

†Used totally embedded specimens.

From Bostwick DG, Montironi R: Evaluating radical prostatectomy specimens: Therapeutic and prognostic importance. Virch Arch 430:1–19, 1997.

usually in the posterolateral region near the neurovascular bundles. By modifying surgery to approach the neurovascular bundles laterally and to widely dissect the apex of the prostate, they observed a positive surgical margin rate of only 8% by 1993,[28] despite similar volumes, grades, and pathologic stages of cancer. Earlier reports noted frequencies of positive surgical margins of 33%,[42] 46%,[43] and 57%,[44] with no difference in specimens from nerve-sparing and non–nerve-sparing operations.[43] Positive surgical margins are strongly correlated with cancer volume[27, 28, 34, 42, 45] and number of needle biopsies containing cancer.[46, 47] Most positive surgical margins in prostates with cancer smaller than 4 cc are caused by surgical incision.[45]

Positive margins are variously located at the apex (48%), rectal and lateral surfaces (24%), bladder neck (16%), and superior pedicles (10%)[42] (Table 10–5).

Clinical Significance of Positive Surgical Margins

The significance of positive surgical margins in patients treated by prostatectomy is unclear (Table 10–6). Paulson and colleagues noted that patients with organ-confined cancer and positive surgical margins have a 60% chance of dying from cancer, a risk significantly greater than the 30% possibility for patients without positive surgical margins.[34] Another study found that surgical margin status was the only predictor of cancer progression other than Gleason score in patients without seminal vesicle invasion or lymph node metastases.[24, 48] Conversely, Ohori and colleagues found that positive surgical margins had no effect on prognosis.[28] Currently, there is no consensus on the utility of postoperative adjuvant therapy in patients with positive surgical margins, probably owing to uncertainty about the clinical significance of this finding.[49]

Lymph Nodes

Staging pelvic lymph node biopsy is usually performed before prostatectomy, and most

Table 10–6. Correlation of Positive Surgical Margins and Progression in Totally Embedded Radical Prostatectomy Specimens

Investigator/Stage	Months of Follow-up Mean (Range)	Progression/ Proportion (%)
Epstein et al., 1993[24]		
Less than pT3c	Minimum 60	
(Stages not provided)	(Range not provided)	40/85 (47)
Ravery et al., 1994[77]		
pT1c and T2	24 (6–48)	6/7 (86)
pT3a+b	24 (6–48)	14/26 (54)
pT3c	24 (6–48)	18/19 (95)
All pT3	24 (6–48)	32/45 (71)
Ohori et al., 1995[28]		
pT1 and pT2	39 (1–126)	0/23 (0)
pT3a+b	39 (1–126)	14/33 (42)

From Bostwick DG, Montironi R: Evaluating radical prostatectomy specimens: Therapeutic and prognostic importance. Virch Arch 430:1–19, 1997.

urologists discontinue surgery if metastases are identified. Lymph node dissection is performed by an open or laparoscopic procedure. Radical perineal prostatectomy and lymph node dissection are performed as separate procedures because the surgical approaches are different, whereas radical retropubic prostatectomy and lymphadenectomy are often performed as a single procedure. The pathologist should carefully evaluate the fibroadipose tissue obtained by lymphadenectomy and submit all lymph nodes for pathologic examination. It may not be necessary to submit obvious adipose tissue, although it is our policy to do so. Sampling error by frozen section accounts for a false-negative rate of lymph node metastases of 3% in our experience (D.G. Bostwick, unpublished observations). Surgeons at Wayne State University and at some other centers do not undertake frozen section evaluation of pelvic lymph nodes that are not palpably enlarged because of the potential for histopathologic sampling error (D. Grignon, personal communication). The surgical pathology report should include the number and sites of all lymph nodes submitted, as well as sites of involvement and the size of cancer foci.

The incidence of micrometastatic, occult prostate carcinoma in pelvic lymph nodes that cannot be detected by routine hematoxylin and eosin staining is low (Table 10–7).[50] Using immunohistochemical studies directed against cytokeratin, Moul and colleagues found lymph node micrometastases in 3% of patients with clinically localized prostatic adenocarcinoma[50]; their results are similar to those of Gomella and coworkers.[51]

Stage

Current clinical and pathologic staging of early prostatic adenocarcinoma separates patients into two groups: those with palpable tumors and those with impalpable tumors.[7, 52, 53] This reliance on palpability of the tumor as determined by digital rectal examination is unique among organ-staging systems and is

Table 10–7. Micrometastases in Patients with Prostate Cancer

Site	Investigator/Year	Patients (no.)	Method of Detection	Results
Lymph nodes	Deguchi et al., 1993[78]	22	RTPCR and immunohistochemistry (anti-PSA)	Micrometastases by RT in six patients (27.3%), including four with both histologic and immunohistochemical confirmation
	Gomella et al., 1993[51]	32	Immunohistochemistry (anti-PSA, PAP, and cytokeratin)	Micrometastases in one of 32 patients (3%)
	Moul et al., 1994[50]	32	Immunohistochemistry (anti-PSA and cytokeratin)	Micrometastases in 1 of 32 patients (3%)
Bone marrow	Mansi et al., 1988[79]	40	Immunohistochemistry (anti-PSA)	Mirometastases in 73% of patients with clinically metastatic cancer and 13% with clinically organ-confined cancer
	Wood et al., 1994[80]	55	RTPCR and immunohistochemistry (anti-PSA)	Micrometastases in 65% of patients with extraprostatic cancer; immunohistochemistry confirmed micrometastases in 79% of those with positive RTPCR
Serum	Hamdy et al., 1992[81]	40	Flow cytometry and immunohistochemistry (anti-PSA)	PSA-positive cells in 47% of patients with stage M − cancer and 100% with stage M + cancer
	Moreno et al., 1992[82]	12	RTPCR (PSA)	PSA-positive cells in 4 patients with stage N + cancer (33%)
	Katz et al., 1994[83]	83	RTPCR (PSA)	PSA-positive cells in 78% of patients with stage N + cancer, and 38.5% with clinically organ-confined cancer

Key: RTPCR, reverse-transcriptase PCR for PSA mRNA sequence; PSA, prostate-specific antigen; PAP, prostatic acid phosphatase.
Modified from Bostwick DG, Dundore PD: Biopsy Interpretation of the Prostate. New York, Chapman and Hall, 1997.

hampered by the low sensitivity, low specificity, and low positive predictive value of digital rectal examination.[54] Recent refinements in staging have led to the introduction of a new stage of nonpalpable adenocarcinoma, detected by elevated serum PSA level and referred to as "stage T1c"; however, this new stage was introduced without supportive clinical evidence, and recent studies show that it does not identify a distinct group of patients.[55–58] The question remains whether patients who will benefit from early detection and intervention can be separated from those who will not.

The 1992 revision of the tumor-node-metastasis (TNM) system is the international standard for prostatic adenocarcinoma staging.[7, 52, 53, 59] (Fig. 10–7). The Commission on Cancer of the American College of Surgeons has required it for accreditation since 1995.[60] Efforts directed toward standardization of staging, including guidelines for pathologic evaluation

of specimens, are useful in allowing comparison of results from different centers.[1]

The two principal clinical staging systems currently in widespread use are the TNM system and American system (modified Whitmore-Jewett) (Table 10–8).[7] These two systems are similar, although the TNM system contains a greater number of subdivisions for most stages. Also, the TNM system includes stage groupings, which consist of combined clinical stage and tumor grade.

TNM Staging System

The TNM classification for prostatic adenocarcinoma was first published by the American Joint Committee on Cancer (AJCC) and the Union Internationale Contre le Cancer (UICC) in 1978, but their definitions at that time contained significant differences.[53] By 1987, these differences were resolved, but the

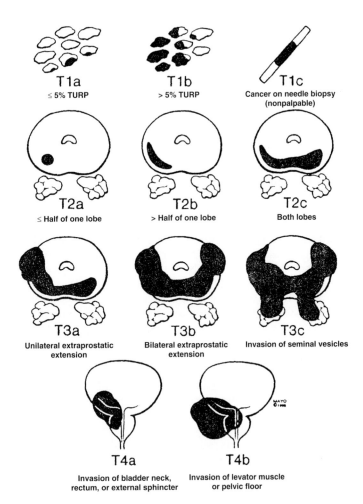

Figure 10–7. Prostate cancer staging using the TNM system, 1992 revision, for the T (tumor) category. Black indicates extent of cancer. (From Bostwick DG, Eble JE: Urologic Surgical Pathology. St. Louis: Mosby–Year Book, 1997.)

Table 10–8. Staging of Prostatic Adenocarcinoma

Clinical Findings	American	TNM*†
Nonpalpable cancer		
≤ 5% of TURP tissue‡	A1	T1a
> 5% of TURP tissue‡	A2	T1b
Cancer detected by biopsy (e.g., elevated PSA)	B0	T1c
Palpable or visible cancer clinically confined within the capsule		
≤ Half of one lobe	B1	T2a
> Half of one lobe, but not both lobes	B1	T2b
Both lobes	B2	T2c
Cancer with local extraprostatic extension		
Unilateral	C1	T3a
Bilateral	C1	T3b
Seminal vesicle invasion	C2	T3c
Invasion of bladder neck, rectum, or external sphincter	C2	T4a
Invasion of levator muscle or pelvic wall	C2	T4b
Metastatic cancer		
Single regional lymph node, ≤ 2 cm in greatest dimension	D1	N1§
Single regional lymph node, 2–5 cm, or multiple regional lymph nodes ≤ 5 cm	D1	N2
Single regional lymph node, > 5 cm	D1	N3
Distant metastasis	D2	M1
Nonregional lymph node(s)	D2	M1a
Bone(s)	D2	M1b
Other sites	D2	M1c

*N0 or Nx M0 for T1-T4.

†Stage groupings for TNM staging system (G = grade on 1–4 scale):

Stage 0	T1a	N0	M0	G1	Stage II	T2	N0	M0	Any G
Stage I	T1a	N0	M0	G2, 3, 4	Stage III	T3	N0	M0	Any G
	T1b	N0	M0	Any G	Stage IV	T4	N0	M0	Any G
	T1c	N0	M0	Any G		Any T	N1, 2, 3	M0	Any G
	T1	N0	M0	Any G		Any T	Any M	M1	Any G

‡Different definitions exist for substaging A1 and A2 cancers.

§Nx: Regional lymph nodes are not assessable. Mx: distant metastasis is not assessable.

resulting classification was criticized by the European Organization for Research on Treatment of Cancer (EORTC) Genitourinary Group and others, particularly for the T (primary tumor) category and the proposed stage groupings. A consensus conference held to resolve discrepancies included representatives from the AJCC, UICC, EORTC Genitourinary Group, and the American Urological Association; as a result of this meeting, a revised and uniform TNM classification was published in 1992.[53]

The 1992 revision of the TNM system included four significant changes from the 1987 version.[53] First, a new category (T1c) was introduced to recognize nonpalpable, invisible adenocarcinomas identified by random biopsy following detection of elevated serum PSA level. Second, palpable adenocarcinoma confined to the prostate (T2) was subdivided into three groups, rather than two, based on the relative involvement of the prostate (involvement of half a lobe or less, more than half a lobe

but not both lobes, or both lobes) instead of absolute tumor size as determined by digital rectal examination. Third, adenocarcinoma with local extraprostatic extension (T3) was subdivided into three groups rather than two, based on laterality and seminal vesicle invasion (unilateral, bilateral, and seminal vesicle invasion) (Fig. 10–8, see Color Plate 4 following p. 190). Finally, the concept of "telescopic ramification" was introduced, to allow introduction of additional prognostic factors without altering existing categories.

American (Modified Whitmore-Jewett) Staging System

The American staging system, introduced by Whitmore in 1956, consists of letters A though D to denote stages. It was modified by Jewett to allow substaging of stage B. He and others noted that patients with a palpably discrete nodule (B1 nodule, "Jewett nodule") had longer cancer-free survival time. Recently, the

American system was modified to accommodate PSA-detected adenocarcinoma.[53] The current stage divisions are similar to those of the TNM system (see Table 10–8), but do not include tumor grade except to separate stages A1 and A2.

Limitations of Current Staging Systems

Current staging systems are limited by a number of factors: (1) clinical understaging with transurethral resection; (2) clinical understaging with digital rectal examination; (3) limited ability of imaging studies to evaluate the presence and extent of prostatic adenocarcinoma; (4) heterogeneity of stage T1c adenocarcinoma; (5) variability in pathologic staging of stage T1 adenocarcinoma; and (6) variability in examination of radical prostatectomy specimens.

Clinical Understaging with Digital Rectal Examination

Current staging of palpable organ-confined adenocarcinoma relies on digital rectal examination to separate unilateral tumors from bilateral ones or small tumors from large ones (less than half of one lobe, between one half and one lobe, and more than one lobe). There is, however, a high level of inaccuracy and interobserver variability in determining tumor size and pathologic stage by digital rectal examination. Prostatic adenocarcinoma staging is unique among organ-staging systems because it relies on the presence or absence of palpability and substage T2 adenocarcinoma based on the proportion of prostatic induration identified.

Bostwick identified clinical understaging in 59% of cases and clinical overstaging in 5% in a series of 311 serially sectioned radical retropubic prostatectomies removed for clinically localized prostatic adenocarcinoma (excluding stages T1a, T1b, and T1c. Note that there is no equivalent pathologic stage for clinical stage T1c, so this group will always be restaged pathologically).[27] These results were similar to those reported by others who have also undertaken careful pathologic sectioning of prostatectomy specimens. This substantial error rate must be accounted for when evaluating recurrence and survival rates, especially when comparing studies of clinically staged patients followed with active surveillance (watchful waiting) and surgically (pathologically) staged patients. There was considerable overlap in the volume of adenocarcinoma in clinical stages T2a + b and T2c, with tumors measuring up to 41 and 43 cc, respectively. These data indicate that digital rectal examination is inaccurate for preoperative assessment of tumor volume.

Limitations of Imaging Studies

Imaging studies to assess tumor volume and extent would be invaluable in clinical staging; however, the current accuracy of such methods is not sufficient to be useful for all patients. The accuracy of correctly identifying extraprostatic extension is 63% with TRUS,[61] 71% with body coil magnetic resonance imaging (MRI),[60] and 83% with endorectal and surface coil MRI.[62]

Pathology of PSA-Detected Adenocarcinoma (Clinical Stage T1c)

Before clinical use of PSA became widespread, most organ-confined adenocarcinoma was discovered by digital rectal examination (clinical stage T2) or at the time of transurethral resection (clinical stage T1). Routine use of serum PSA increased the detection rate of prostatic adenocarcinoma and uncovered some adenocarcinomas that would not have been detected by digital rectal examination.[63–67] There was a sevenfold increase in PSA-detected adenocarcinomas at the Mayo Clinic in the 3-year period from 1988 to 1991 (14 versus 118 cases, respectively).[55]

There is no pathologic stage equivalent for clinical stage T1c, and such tumors are invariably "upstaged" at surgery, usually to pathologic stage T2 or T3 (see Table 10–8). Oesterling and colleagues found that clinical stage T1c adenocarcinoma and clinical stage T2a + b adenocarcinoma had similar maximum tumor diameters, frequencies of multifocality, tumor grades, DNA content results, pathologic stages, and tumor locations. Interestingly, they had different serum PSA values, tumor volumes, rates of positive surgical margins, and prostate gland sizes, the T1c tumors having higher values for each feature.[55] These findings indicate that PSA detects adenocarcinoma, which is clinically important and potentially curable. Also, PSA-detected tumors that are visible on TRUS have pathologic features similar to those of lesions that are not visible.[58] Further long-term follow-up of PSA-detected prostatic adenocarcinoma is necessary to establish the prognosis of these tumors and determine whether a separate staging category is warranted for them.

Problems with TNM Staging (1992 Revision) of Radical Prostatectomy Specimens

Three practical problems have been described for pathologic staging using the TNM system for radical prostatectomy specimens. First, separation of substages T2a (less than half of one lobe) and T2b (more than half of one lobe) is difficult, particularly in specimens that are partially sampled rather than whole mounted. This problem is resolved by reporting such cases as T2a+b, an approach that necessarily compresses data. Second, the pathologist rarely (if ever) has access to clinical information pertaining to distant metastases at the time of histologic evaluation of the prostatectomy specimen and thus cannot accurately report the *M* of TNM. This problem is resolved by reporting all cases as "Mx," with a brief qualification that refers to the clinical record. The third problem is pathologic "upstaging" of adenocarcinoma, which usually occurs with prostatectomy following transurethral resection; as noted above, transurethral resection–detected adenocarcinomas are T1a and T1b, yet additional adenocarcinoma identified on prostatectomy frequently results in upstaging to T2 and T3. This problem is resolved by reporting both TNM stages (transurethral resection and prostatectomy) with a brief note describing this issue. Alternatively, it may be better to exclude the T1 category from pathologic staging of radical prostatectomy specimens.

Perineural Invasion

Perineural invasion is common in adenocarcinoma and may be the only evidence of malignancy in a biopsy specimen. This finding is strong presumptive evidence of malignancy but is not pathognomonic because it occurs rarely with benign acini.[68–70] Complete circumferential growth, intraneural invasion, and ganglionic invasion are found only with cancer.

Perineural invasion indicates tumor spread along the path of least resistance and does not represent lymphatic invasion. When present in needle biopsy specimens, perineural invasion indicates the possibility of extraprostatic extension[70]; however, it does not appear to have independent prognostic value after other factors are evaluated.[71]

Vascular/Lymphatic Invasion

Microvascular invasion is a strong indicator of malignancy, and its presence correlates with histologic grade, although it is sometimes difficult to distinguish from fixation-associated retraction artifact of acini.[72, 73] Microvascular invasion may also be an important predictor of outcome, and it carries a fourfold greater risk of tumor progression and death.[72] The CAP[1] recommends reporting microvascular invasion for all prostate specimens, presumably using routine light microscopic examination. Despite this recommendation, most laboratories including ours do not evaluate microvascular invasion in prostate specimens unless it is obvious and extensive. Immunohistochemical stains directed against endothelial cells, such as Factor VIII–related antigen or *Ulex europaeus*, may increase the detection rate.[73]

Microvascular invasion is defined as the unequivocal presence of tumor cells in endothelium-lined spaces. We do not require the presence of a cellular reaction in the adjacent stroma with hemosiderin and fibrin deposition to diagnose microvascular invasion. Also, we do not differentiate vascular and lymphatic channels because of the difficulty and lack of reproducibility among different observers on routine light microscopic examination.[73]

Microvascular invasion is most often confused with perineural invasion and cell clusters in empty spaces owing to retraction artifact. Equivocal foci and spaces without an identifiable endothelial lining are not considered evidence of perineural invasion. Microvascular invasion is present in 38% of radical prostatectomy specimens and is commonly associated with extraprostatic extension and lymph node metastases (62% and 67% of cases, respectively).[72, 73] It is not, however, an independent predictor of progression when stage and grade are included in the multivariate analysis.[71]

VANISHING CANCER PHENOMENON

Some thoroughly studied radical prostatectomy specimens contain little or no residual cancer. This "vanishing cancer phenomenon" is probably increasing in incidence as more low-stage cancers are being treated by radical prostatectomy.[74] The inability to identify cancer in a prostate removed for needle biopsy–proven carcinoma does not necessarily indicate technical failure, although it is important to exclude the possibility of improper patient identification. DNA "fingerprinting" has been used as a research tool to compare formalin-fixed, paraffin-embedded biopsy and prostatectomy tissues.[74]

Substantial resources may be needed to identify minimal residual cancer, and even exhaustive sectioning may fail. How many sections is it reasonable to obtain in such cases? When can one stop in such cases sectioning if no cancer is found? We believe that it is appropriate for the pathologist to submit for histologic evaluation routine sections of the entire prostate; however, after submission and examination of the entire prostate, further levels and block flipping probably are not necessary, as at that point any residual cancer is likely to be extremely small and of no clinical significance.

CONCLUSION

Significant progress has been made in recent years in standardizing the handling of radical prostatectomy specimens. Most practitioners utilize selected partial sampling rather than whole-mount sectioning. Practice protocols published by multiple authoritative groups contain similar suggestions about which information should be included in pathology reports. Definitions of extraprostatic extension and positive surgical margins are also standardized, although methods of quantitating EPE and the clinical significance of positive margins remain uncertain. The 1992 revision of the TNM system is now the international standard for staging, but future refinements may increase its predictive accuracy for individual patients.

REFERENCES

1. Henson DE, Hutter RVP, Farrow GM: Practice protocol for the examination of specimens removed from patients with carcinoma of the prostate gland. A publication of the Cancer Committee, College of American Pathologists. Arch Pathol Lab Med 118:779–783, 1994.
2. Association of Directors of Anatomic and Surgical Pathology: Recommendations for the reporting of resected prostate carcinomas. Hum Pathol 27:321–323, 1996.
3. Sakr W, Wheeler T, Blute M, et al: Staging and reporting of prostate cancer. Sampling of the radical prostatectomy specimen. Cancer 78:366–368, 1996.
4. Hall GS, Kramer CE, Epstein JI: Evaluation of radical prostatectomy specimens: A comparative analysis of sampling methods. Am J Surg Pathol 16:315–324, 1992.
5. Schmid H-P, McNeal JE: An abbreviated standard procedure for accurate tumor volume estimation in prostate cancer. Am J Surg Pathol 16:184–191, 1992.
6. Haggman M, Norberg M, de la Torre M, et al.: Characterization of localized prostatic cancer: Distribution, grading and pT-staging in radical prostatectomy specimens. Scand J Urol Nephrol 27:7–13, 1993.
7. Bostwick DG, Myers RP, Oesterling JE: Staging of prostate cancer. Semin Surg Oncol 10:60–73, 1994.
8. Donahue RE, Miller GJ: Adenocarcinoma of the prostate: Biopsy to whole mount. Denver VA experience. Urol Clin North Am 18:449–452, 1991.
9. Cohen MB, Soloway MS, Murphy WM: Sampling of radical prostatectomy specimens. How much is adequate? Am J Clin Pathol 101:250–252, 1994.
10. Sakr WA, Grignon DJ, Visscher DW, et al.: Evaluating the radical prostatectomy specimen, Part I. A protocol for establishing prognostic parameters and harvesting fresh tissue samples. J Urol Pathol 3:355–364, 1995.
11. Bova GS, Fox WM, Epstein JI: Methods of radical prostatectomy specimen processing: A novel technique for harvesting fresh prostate cancer tissue and review of processing techniques. Mod Pathol 6:201–207, 1993.
12. Wheeler TM, Lebovitz RM: Fresh tissue harvest for research from prostatectomy specimens. Prostate 25:274–279, 1994.
13. Littrup PJ, William CR, Egglin TK, et al.: Determination of prostate volume with transrectal US for cancer screening. Part II. Accuracy of in vitro and in vivo techniques. Radiology 179:49–53, 1991.
14. Ayala AG, Ro JY, Babaian R, et al.: The prostatic capsule: Does it exist? Its importance in the staging and treatment of prostatic carcinoma. Am J Surg Pathol 13:21–27, 1989.
15. True LD: Surgical pathology examination of the prostate gland. Practice survey by American Society of Clinical Pathologists. Am J Clin Pathol 10:572–579, 1994.
16. Hall GS, Kramer CE, Epstein JI: Evaluation of radical prostatectomy specimens: A comparative analysis of sampling methods. Am J Surg Pathol 16:315–324, 1992.
17. Humphrey PA: Complete histologic serial sectioning of a prostate gland with adenocarcinoma. Am J Surg Pathol 17:468–472, 1993.
18. McNeal JE, Bostwick DG, Kindrachuk RA, et al.: Patterns of progression in prostate cancer. Lancet 1:60–63, 1986.
19. Graham SD Jr, Bostwick DG, Hoisaeter A, et al.: Report of the committee on staging and pathology. Cancer 70(Suppl):359–361, 1992.

20. Bostwick DG, Graham SD Jr, Napalkov P, et al.: Staging of early prostate cancer: A proposed tumor volume-based prognostic index. Urology 41:403–411, 1993.

21. Stamey TA, Yang N, Hay AR, et al.: Prostate-specific antigen as a serum marker for adenocarcinoma of the prostate. N Engl J Med 317:909–916, 1987.

22. Partin AW, Carter HB, Chan DW, et al.: Prostate specific antigen in the staging of localized prostate cancer: Influence of tumor differentiation, tumor volume, and benign hyperplasia. J Urol 143:747–752, 1990.

23. Blackwell KL, Bostwick DG, Zincke H, et al.: Combining prostate specific antigen with cancer and gland volume to predict more reliably pathologic stage: The influence of prostate specific antigen cancer density. J Urol 151:1565–1570, 1994.

24. Epstein JI, Carmichael M, Partin AW, et al.: Is tumor volume an independent predictor of progression following radical prostatectomy? A multivariate analysis of 185 clinical stage B adenocarcinomas of the prostate with 5 years of followup. J Urol 149:1478–1485, 1993.

25. Sattar AA, Noel J-C, Vanderhaeghen J-J, et al.: Prostate capsule: Computerized morphometric analysis of its components. Urology 46:178–181, 1995.

26. Theiss M, Wirth MP, Manseck A, et al.: Prognostic signficance of capsular invasion and capsular penetration in patients with clinically localized prostate cancer undergoing radical prostatectomy. Prostate 27:13–17, 1995.

27. Bostwick DG: Significance of tumor volume in prostate cancer. Urol Annu 8:1–22, 1994.

28. Ohori M, Wheeler TM, Kattan MW, et al.: Prognostic significance of positive surgical margins in radical prostatectomy specimens. J Urol 154:1818–1824, 1995.

29. McNeal JE, Villers AA, Redwine EA, et al.: Capsular penetration in prostate cancer: Significance for natural history and treatment. Am J Surg Pathol 14:240–247, 1990.

30. Zeitman AL, Edelstein RA, Coen JJ, et al.: Radical prostatectomy for adenocarcinoma of the prostate: The influence of preoperative and pathologic findings on biochemical disease-free outcome. Urology 43:828–833, 1994.

31. Epstein JI, Partin AW, Suavageot J, et al.: Prediction of progression following radical prostatectomy. A multivariate analysis of 721 men with long-term follow-up. Am J Surg Pathol 20:286–292, 1996.

32. Schellhammer PF: Radical prostatectomy. Patterns of local failure and survival in 67 patients. Urology 31:191–197, 1988.

33. Stein A, deKernion JB, Smith RB, et al.: Prostate specific antigen levels after radical prostatectomy in patients with organ confined and locally extensive prostate cancer. J Urol 147:942–947, 1992.

34. Paulson DF, Moul JW, Walther PJ: Radical prostatectomy for clinical stage T1-2N0M0 prostatic adenocarcinoma: Long-term results. J Urol 144:1180–1185, 1990.

35. Lerner SE, Blute ML, Zincke H: Primary surgery for clinical stage T3 adenocarcinoma of the prostate. In Vogelzang NJ, Scardino PT, Shipley WU (eds): Comprehensive Textbook of Genitourinary Oncology. Baltimore: Williams & Wilkins, 1996, pp 803–811.

36. Scardino PT: Is radiotherapy effective for locally advanced (stage C or T3) prostate cancer? Prog Clin Biol Res 303:223–239, 1989.

37. Scardino PT, Frankel JM, Wheeler TM, et al.: The prognostic significance of post-irradiation biopsy results in patients with prostatic cancer. J Urol 135:510–516, 1986.

38. Bagshaw MA, Cox RS, Ray GR: Status of radiation treatment of prostate cancer at Stanford University. Natl Cancer Inst Monogr 7:47–60, 1988.

39. Adolfsson J: Deferred treatment of low grade, stage T3 prostate cancer without distant metastases. J Urol 149:326–329, 1993.

40. Zagars GK, Geara FB, Pollack A, et al.: The T classification of clinically localized prostate cancer. An appraisal based on disease outcome after radiation therapy. Cancer 73:1904–1912, 1994.

41. Corn BW, Hanks GE, Lee WR, et al.: Do the current subclassifications of stage T3 adenocarcinoma of the prostate have clinical relevance? Urology 45:484–490, 1995.

42. Stamey TA, Villers AA, McNeal JE, et al.: Positive surgical margins at radical prostatectomy: Importance of the apical dissection. J Urol 143:1166–1173, 1990.

43. Jones EC: Resection margin status in radical retropubic prostatectomy specimens: Relationship to type of operation, tumor grade, and local extension. J Urol 144:89–93, 1990.

44. Catalona WJ, Dresner SM: Nerve-sparing radical prostatectomy: Extraprostatic tumor extension and preservation of erectile function. J Urol 134:1149–1151, 1985.

45. Voges G, McNeal JE, Redwine EA, et al.: Morphologic analysis of surgical margins with positive findings in prostatectomy for adenocarcinoma of the prostate. Cancer 69:520–526, 1992.

46. Ackerman DA, Barry JM, Wicklund RA, et al.: Analysis of risk factors associated with prostate cancer extension to the surgical margin and pelvic node metastasis at radical prostatectomy. J Urol 150:1845–1850, 1993.

47. Schmid HP, Ravery V, Billebaud T, et al.: Early detection of prostate cancer in men with prostatism and intermediate prostate-specific antigen levels. Urology 47:699–703, 1996.

48. Epstein JI: Pathology of prostatic intraepithelial neoplasia and adenocarcinoma of the prostate: Prognostic influences of stage, tumor volume, grade, and margins of resection. Semin Oncol 21:527–541, 1994.

49. Montie JE: Significance and treatment of positive margins or seminal vesicle invasion after radical prostatectomy. Urol Clin North Am 17:803–811, 1990.

50. Moul JW, Kahn DG, Lewis DJ, et al.: Immunohistologic detection of prostate cancer pelvic lymph node micrometastases: Correlation to preoperative serum prostate-specific antigen. Urology 43:68–73, 1994.

51. Gomella LG, White JL, McCue PA, et al.: Screening for occult nodal metastases in localized carcinoma of the prostate. J Urol 149:776–778, 1993.

52. Montie JE: Staging of prostate cancer. Current TNM classification and future prospects for prognostic factors. Cancer 75:1814–1818, 1995.

53. Shroder FH, Hermanek P, Denis L, et al.: The TNM classification of prostate carcinoma. Prostate 4(Suppl):129–138, 1992.

54. Friedman GD, Hiatt RA, Quesenberry CP, et al.: Case-control study of screening for prostate cancer by digital rectal examinations. Lancet 337:1526–1529, 1991.

55. Oesterling JE, Suman VJ, Zincke H, et al.: PSA-detected (Clinical stage T1c or B0) prostate cancer: Pathologically significant tumors. Urol Clin North Am 20:687–693, 1993.

56. Epstein JI, Walsh PC, Carmichael M, et al.: Pathologic

and clinical findings to predict tumor extent of non-palpable (stage T1c) prostate cancer. JAMA 271:368–374, 1994.

57. Scaletscky R, Koch MO, Eckstein CW, et al.: Tumor volume and stage in carcinoma of the prostate detected by elevations in prostate specific antigen. J Urol 152:129–131, 1994.

58. Ferguson JK, Bostwick DG, Suman V, et al.: Prostate-specific antigen detected prostate cancer. Pathological characteristics of ultrasound visible versus ultrasound invisible tumors. Eur Urol 27:8–12, 1995.

59. British Association of Urological Surgeons TNM Subcommittee, 1995: The TNM classification of prostate cancer: A discussion of the 1992 classification. Br J Urol 76:279–285, 1995.

60. Donaldson ES, Glen JF: The 1995 staging requirement for approved cancer programs. Urology 47:455–456, 1996.

61. Rifkin MD, Zerhouni EA, Garsonis CA, et al.: Comparison of magnetic resonance imaging and ultrasonography in staging early prostate cancer: Results of a multi-institutional cooperative trial. N Engl J Med 323:621–627, 1990.

62. Ramchandani P, Schnall MD: Magnetic resonance imaging of the prostate. Semin Roentgenol 28:74–82, 1993.

63. Cooner WH, Mosley BR, Rutherford CL Jr, et al.: Prostate cancer detection in a clinical urological practice by ultrasonography, digital rectal examination and prostate-specific antigen. J Urol 143:1146–1151, 1990.

64. Catalona WJ, Smith DS, Ratliff TL, et al.: Measurement of prostate-specific antigen in serum as a screening test for prostate cancer. N Engl J Med 324:1156–1161, 1991.

65. Mettlin C, Lee F, Drago J, et al.: Findings on the detection of early prostate cancer in 2425 men. Cancer 67:2949–2957, 1991.

66. Brawer MK, Chetner MP, Beatie J, et al.: Screening for prostatic carcinoma with prostate-specific antigen. J Urol 147:841–844, 1992.

67. Labrie F, Dupont A, Suburu R, et al.: Serum prostate-specific antigen as pre-sceening test for prostate cancer. J Urol 147:846–850, 1992.

68. Hasson MO, Maksem J: The prostatic perineural space and its relation to tumor spread. An ultrastructural study. Am J Surg Pathol 4:143–148, 1980.

69. McIntire TL, Franzina DA: The presence of benign prostate glands in perineural spaces. J Urol 135:507–509, 1986.

70. Bastacky SI, Walsh PC, Epstein JI: Relationship between perineural tumor invasion on needle biopsy

71. Egan AJM, Bostwick DG: Prediction of extraprostatic extension of prostate cancer based on needle biopsy findings: Perineural invasion lacks significance on multivariate analysis. Am J Surg Pathol 1997 (in press).

72. Bahnson RR, Dresner SM, Gooding W, Becich MJ: Incidence and prognostic significance of lymphatic and vascular invasion in radical prostatectomy specimens. Prostate 15:149–155, 1989.

73. Salamao DR, Graham SD, Bostwick DG: Microvascular invasion in prostate cancer correlates with pathologic stage. Arch Pathol Lab Med 119:1050–1054, 1995.

74. Goldstein NS, Begin LR, Grody WW, et al.: Minimal or no cancer in radical prostatetomy specimens. Report of 13 cases of the "vanishing cancer phenomenon. Am J Surg Pathol 19:1002–1009, 1995.

75. Bostwick DG, Cooner WH, Denis L, et al.: The association of benign prostatic hyperplasia and cancer of the prostate. Cancer 70:291–301, 1992.

76. Bostwick DG, Montironi R: Evaluating radical prostatectomy specimens: Therapeutic and prognostic importance. Virch Archiv 430:1–19, 1997.

77. Ravery V, Delmas V, Boccon-Gibod LA, et al.: Systematic biopsies accurately predict extracapsular extension of prostate cancer and persistent/recurrent detectable PSA after radical prostatectomy. Urology 44:371–377, 1994.

78. Deguchi T, Doi T, Ehara H, et al.: Detection of micrometastatic prostate cancer cells in lymph nodes by reverse transcriptase-polymerase chain reaction. Cancer Res 53:5350–5355, 1993.

79. Mansi JL, Berger U, Wilson P, et al.: Detection of tumor cells in bone marrow of patients with prostatic carcinoma by immunocytochemical techniques. J Urol 139:545–548, 1988.

80. Wood D Jr, Banks E, Humphreys S, et al.: Identification of bone marrow micrometastases in patients with prostate cancer. Cancer 74:2533–2538, 1994.

81. Hamdy FC, Lawry J, Anderson JB, et al.: Circulating prostate specific antigen-positive cells correlate with metastatic prostate cancer. Br J Urol 69:392–396, 1992.

82. Moreno JG, Croce CM, Fischer R, et al.: Detection of hematogenous micrometastasis in patients with prostate cancer. Cancer Res 52:6110–6112, 1992.

83. Katz A, Olsson C, Raffo A, et al.: Molecular staging of prostate cancer with the use of an enhanced reverse transcriptase polymerase chain reaction assay. Urology 43:765–772, 1994.

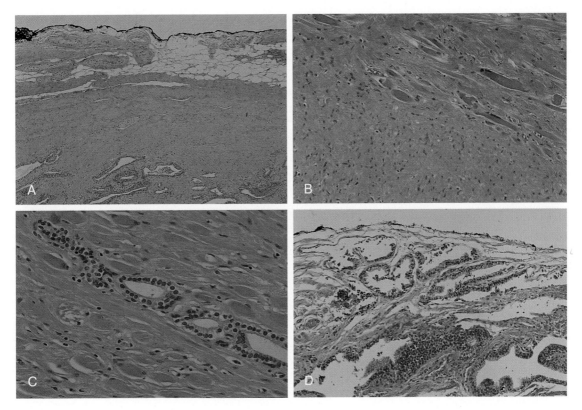

Figure 10–4. The edge of the prostate at different sites. *A,* Lateral prostate with abundant fibromuscular stroma of the capsule at the periphery. *B,* Anterior prostate, with interdigitation of smooth muscle and skeletal muscle. *C,* Anterior prostate skeletal muscle with benign prostatic acini. *D,* External edge of the apex following conization; the benign acini extend to the edge of the sections with no apparent fibromuscular stroma, precluding assessment of the capsule at this site.

Plate 1

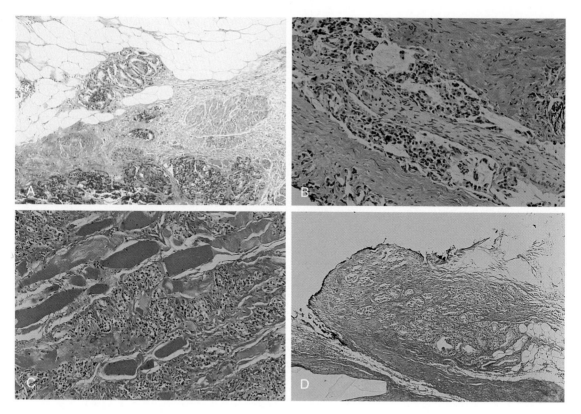

Figure 10–5. Extraprostatic extension. *A*, Cancer in adipose tissue. *B*, Cancer in perineural spaces of the neurovascular bundles. *C*, Cancer in the anterior muscle above the urethra. *D*, Positive surgical margins with extraprostatic extension. Note the presence of cancer in the extraprostatic soft tissue with extension to the inked surface (stage T3 cancer with positive surgical margins).

Plate 2

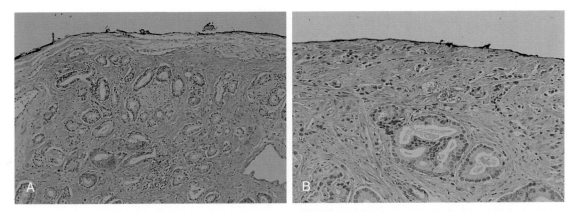

Figure 10–6. Surgical incision of the prostate. *A,* Cancer is close to the margin, but not in contact with the inked surface. *B,* Compare with this view from the same patient, showing positive surgical margins elsewhere with surgical incision into the prostatic parenchyma (stage T2+).

Plate 3

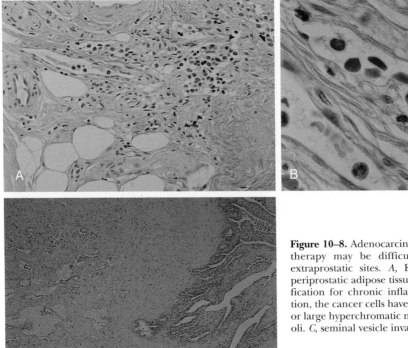

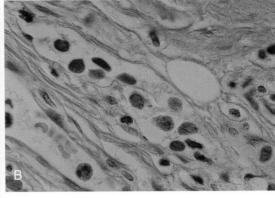

Figure 10–8. Adenocarcinoma after androgen deprivation therapy may be difficult to identify, particularly in extraprostatic sites. *A,* Extraprostatic extension in the periprostatic adipose tissue may be mistaken at low magnification for chronic inflammation. *B,* At high magnification, the cancer cells have abundant clear cytoplasm, small or large hyperchromatic nuclei, and often indistinct nucleoli. *C,* seminal vesicle invasion.

Plate 4

11

GRADING PROSTATE CANCER

Nayneeta Deshmukh and Christopher S. Foster

Identification of cellular features that accurately predict the behavior of an individual patient's tumor is a major challenge facing contemporary pathologists. Despite the rising prevalence of prostate cancer, little progress has yet been made in identifying parameters that accurately determine the biologic activities of specific prostate cancers.[1] Anatomically localized prostate cancer is not a benign disease and although progression might be slow, it is inexorable. However, it is paradoxical that not all primary prostate carcinomas discovered incidentally exhibit similar lethal potential. Unfortunately, current conventional therapy is of little value in controlling the phenotypically malignant primary prostate tumors. Thus, the dilemma of this disease is that clinically unimportant cancers do not require urgent or aggressive treatment (from which patients should be spared to lessen overall morbidity) while it is not yet possible to recognize clinically important cancers while they remain curable.[2]

Traditionally, diagnostic histopathologists have attempted to forecast the behavior of individual carcinomas by comparing specific morphologic features of the neoplastic tissues with their nonneoplastic tissues of origin. Although this approach has identified some features that are common to prostate cancers as a group, it has been of limited value in predicting the future behavior of individual tumors. During recent years, unassisted morphologic criteria have been supported by the concomitant use of now routine analytic methods, which include immunohistochemistry, flow cytometry, and a range of in situ and other nucleic acid hybridization techniques. This multiparametric approach to classifying and grading prostate cancer is presently receiving detailed evaluation in many laboratories worldwide. Some of these approaches are discussed in appropriate chapters elsewhere. Within the past decade, accelerating development and application of molecular biologic methods has reinforced the notion that ''molecular profiling'' of malignant diseases, including prostate cancer, is likely to supplant morphology as the preferred technique for predicting biologic behavior. However, until the gene sequences that determine behavior are identified, appropriate oligonucleotide probes synthesized, and the necessary diagnostic techniques developed and evaluated, accurate morphologic grading will remain the gold standard by which prostate cancers are assessed.

PRINCIPLES OF GRADING

The majority of prostate malignancies are adenocarcinomas derived from tubuloalveolar glands situated in the outer zone of the prostate gland (see Chapters 1 and 2). Unusual morphologic variants of prostate cancer account for fewer than 10% of all cases (see Chapter 21). The wide spectrum of biologic malignancy encountered in prostate cancer is strongly correlated with its extensive and diverse morphologic appearances. Although staging is important in determining the treatment of patients with prostate adenocarcinomas, it does not necessarily predict the biologic behavior of the tumor. Grading has been advocated as a method of improving the pathologist's ability to accurately predict a particular tumor's biologic behavior. Methods of grading prostate cancer apply only to the adenocarcinomas; uncommon tumors are assessed by independent criteria.

Many systems have been proposed to assess morphologic features of prostate adenocarcinomas and hence to derive a histologic grade that is indicative of the degree of malignancy (Table 11–1). Such attempts have employed the classical approach, first advocated by Broders, by making comparison between specific cytoarchitectural features of normal and malignant tissues.[3]

Normal Histology

The normal prostate is composed of complex tubular alveolar glands within a fibromuscular stroma. The glandular epithelium is either of low cuboidal or tall columnar secretory type, which is frequently arranged into papillary folds. Acini drain by individual intralobular ducts, which unite into interlobular ducts. Ducts may be lined by cuboidal or by columnar epithelium. Surrounding the acinar and ductular epithelium is an incomplete layer of basal "reserve" cells, the prostatic homolog of human breast myoepithelial cells. Anatomically, human prostate is comprised of two main groups of glands: central and peripheral. Although controversy remains about their precise microanatomic distribution,[25, 26] it is now accepted that benign enlargement of the prostate arises from the central group whereas prostate cancer generally arises from peripheral glands.[27] Owing to the structural arrangement of the glands, biopsy confirmation of early prostate cancer is frequently difficult to obtain since preurethral biopsy is unlikely to provide neoplastic tissue until the tumor is extensive. While significant tumor enlargement usually occurs before involvement of adjacent structures produces symptoms, invasion of the prostatic capsule is an early phenomenon that frequently results in periprostatic lymphatic and vascular invasion before the development of local symptoms caused by an enlarging tumor.

Atypical Hyperplasia

Alterations to normal morphology suggestive of malignancy are frequently encountered in prostate biopsy specimens. Such changes have been variously described as "atypical prostatic hyperplasia," "dysplasia," and "adenosis."[28, 29] The most important features to differentiate foci of morphologic abnormality are the cytologic changes that accompany structural acinar change, including formation of cribriform, papillary, or microacinar patterns.

Table 11–1. Morphological Methods of Grading Prostate Cancer

Authors	System Criteria
Broders, 1926[3]	Histologic patterns of tumor differentiation
Young & Davis, 1926[4]	Histologic patterns of tumor growth
Muir, 1934[5]	Tubule formation, cytomorphology, and mitoses
Kahler, 1938[6]	Distinction of squamous and adenocarcinoma
Evans et al., 1942[7]	Gland morphology, cell shape, fibrosis, and inflammation
Edwards et al., 1953[8]	Morphologic differentiation of neoplastic glands
Shelley et al., 1958[9]	Cytomorphology, tubule formation, and nuclear morphology
Vickery & Kerr, 1963[10]	Two morphologic categories: well- and poorly differentiated
Gleason, 1966[11]	Glandular architecture and stromal involvement
Jewett et al., 1968[12]	Morphologic, grades 1–3
Mobley & Frank, 1968[13]	Acinar architecture and nuclear morphology
Utz & Farrow, 1969[14] (Mayo Clinic System)	Seven morphologic and cytologic criteria
Corriere et al., 1970[15]	Modified Gleason's classification
Mostofi (AFIP), 1975[16]	Nuclear anaplasia and glandular differentiation
Müller et al., 1980[17]	Glandular differentiation and nuclear anaplasia
Gaeta, 1981[18]	Combination of glandular pattern and nuclear morphology
Brawn et al., 1982[19]	Percentage of tumor containing glandular and solid components
Böcking & Sinagowitz, 1982[20]	Combined glandular pattern and nuclear morphology
Schröder et al., 1984[21–23]	Combined tumor architecture, nuclear anaplasia, and mitosis

From Foster CS: Pathological grading systems for prostatic cancer. In Waxman J, Williams G (eds): Prostatic Cancer: A Consensus. London, Edward Arnold, 1991.

In such areas, acini are lined by cuboidal or columnar cells with increased nuclear-cytoplasmic ratio and prominent nucleoli. The basal or "reserve" layer of cells is maintained. The biologic significance of such structural changes remains controversial.[30] Most frequently observed in operative specimens removed for carcinoma, the suggestion has been made that they are premalignant and represent early generalized "field change" within the gland.[31] When encountered, differentiation of benign from well-differentiated adenocarcinoma rests with cytologic criteria. Detailed appraisals of these appearances, and a practical consideration of the criteria employed in the differentiation of benign hyperplastic conditions from prostatic cancer, are presented in Chapters 5 through 9.

Unfortunately, few systems advocated for grading prostate cancer are reproducible when performed by diagnostic pathologists who are insufficiently trained in the particular method and, thus, neither rigorous nor consistent in their approach to different specimens. Of the many problems associated with the principle of grading, a fundamental consideration is to determine the precise histologic features of the tumor that are important in assigning a grade. A major limitation of most systems is that the procedure is subjective. Systems based on sophisticated morphometric techniques might be highly reproducible but require expensive equipment, extensive operator training, and much time, all of which restrict their routine application. In diagnostic surgical pathology laboratories, the systems most frequently adopted are those devised by Gleason and Mostofi-World Health Organization (WHO). Each of these two systems is clinically useful for relating patterns of tumor progression with parameters that include tumor volume, serum prostate-specific antigen (PSA) levels, the probability of pelvic lymph node metastasis, and tumor recurrence after surgical or radiation therapy; however, conceptually and in practice, Gleason's system has found greatest application worldwide.

GLEASON GRADING SYSTEM

Gleason's unique approach to grading prostate cancer was developed following a detailed, prospective, case-controlled, and fully randomized clinical study performed by the Veterans Administration Co-operative Urological Research Group (VACURG), which analyzed the histomorphologic appearances of more than 4000 specimens in 20 Veterans Administration hospitals between 1960 and 1975.[32] Histologic patterns were categorized at low magnification according to the extent of glandular differentiation and the pattern of growth of the tumors within the prostatic stroma. Identified glandular patterns varied from "well-differentiated" (grade 1) to "anaplastic" (grade 5). Characteristic morphologic appearances of the different patterns encountered in Gleason's grading system for human prostate carcinoma are summarized in Table 11–2. A schematic drawing emphasizing the salient architectural features of each pattern is presented in Figure 11–1.

Most prostate cancers contain more than one histologically recognizable pattern. To account for this variability, Gleason assigned a primary grade to the "dominant" pattern and a secondary grade to the next most frequent or "subdominant" pattern. Both grades are scored as integers, which are then summed over a range of 1 through 5 to give the histologic score.[34] Early reports also described the

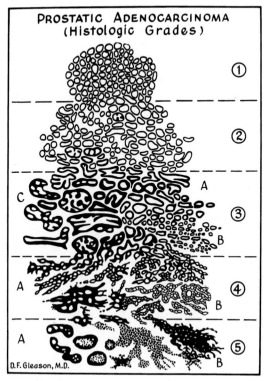

Figure 11–1. Histologic patterns of prostatic adenocarcinoma. Standardized drawing for Gleason grading system. (From Gleason DF: Classification of prostatic carcinoma. Cancer Chemother Rev 50:125–128, 1966.)

Table 11–2. Gleason Grading System for Prostatic Adenocarcinoma: Histologic Pattern

Pattern	Peripheral Borders of Tumor	Stromal Invasion	Appearance of Glands	Size of Glands	Architecture of Glands	Cytoplasm
1	Circumscribed, pushing, expansile	Minimal	Simple, round, monotonously replicated	Medium, regular	Closely packed, rounded masses	Similar to benign epithelium
2	Less circumscribed, early infiltration	Mild, with definite separation of glands by stroma	Simple, round, some variability in shape	Medium, less regular	Loosely packed, rounded masses	Similar to benign epithelium
3A	Infiltration	Marked	Angular, with variation in shape	Medium to large	Variably packed, irregular masses	More basophilic than patterns 1 and 2
3B	Infiltration	Marked	Angular, with variation in shape	Small	Variably packed, irregular masses	More basophilic than patterns 1 and 2
3C	Smooth, rounded	Marked	Papillary and cribriform	Irregular	Round to elongate masses	More basophilic than patterns 1 and 2
4A	Ragged infiltration	Marked	Microacinar, papillary, and cribriform	Irregular	Fused, with chains and cords	Dark
4B	Ragged infiltration	Marked	Microacinar, papillary, and cribriform	Irregular	Fused, with chains and cords	Clear (hypernephroid)
5A	Smooth, rounded	Marked	Comedocarcinoma	Irregular	Round to elongate masses	Variable
5B	Ragged infiltration	Marked	Difficult to identify gland lumina	Sheets of glands	Fused sheets and masses	Variable

From Bostwick DG: Grading prostate cancer. Am J Clin Pathol 102(Suppl 1):S38, 1994.

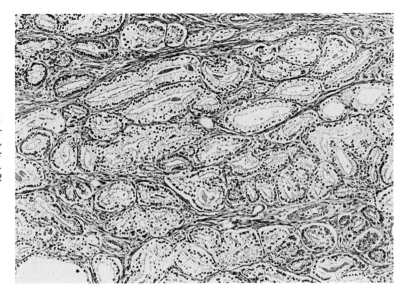

Figure 11–2. Gleason grade 1 carcinoma comprising, throughout all regions of the tumor, closely packed, uniform, separate glands, each with rounded edge. This field also contains grade 2 and 3 lesions. (×50.)

addition of clinical stage (on a scale of 1 to 4) to create the Gleason "sum," but this has not achieved widespread acceptance.

Morphologic Criteria

Grade 1 (Very Well-Differentiated)

The architecture of the prostate gland and of contained tumors is little distorted. The neoplastic glands are closely packed, round, single, separate, uniform in shape and diameter, and sharply delineated from surrounding, scant fibrovascular stroma (Fig. 11–2). Since some forms of benign or atypical hyperplasia also fulfill these criteria, the final requirement for grade 1 tumors is the presence of at least a few cells, frequently as few as 1%, or many cells containing very definitely enlarged nucleoli, each >1 μm in diameter (Fig. 11–3). Within Gleason grade 1 carcinomas, patterns 1 and 2 both appear as very pale tumors following hematoxylin and eosin staining, given that they contain abundant eosinophilic cytoplasm. Furthermore, in grades 1 and 2, glands tend to be larger than intermediate-grade carcinomas.

Grade 2 (Well-Differentiated)

The characteristic features of Gleason grade 2 tumors are: (1) mild but definite separation

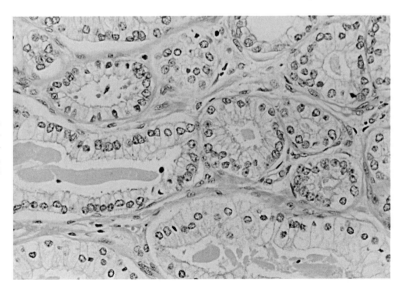

Figure 11–3. Higher magnification (×400) of specimen in Figure 11–2 shows glands with abundant pale eosinophilic cytoplasm. A few glands include tumor cells containing prominent nucleoli.

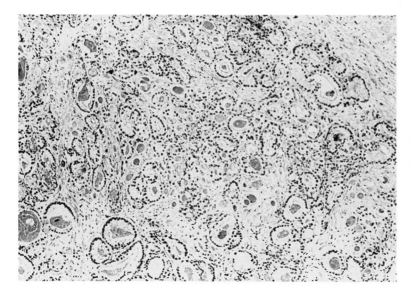

Figure 11–4. Gleason grade 2 tumors, showing increased variation in gland size with some separation of malignant glands by stroma. (×50.)

of the tumor glands by stroma and (2) more variation in the size and shape of the glands (Fig. 11–4) than are observed in grade 1 tumors, although not as much as in grade 3. The tumor remains circumscribed, although separation of the neoplastic glands is apparent at the periphery of the tumor (Fig. 11–5) and suggests some restricted ability to spread into the surrounding stroma. Separation of tumor glands is usually less than one average gland diameter, although some random variation occurs. While not an infrequent finding in radical prostatectomy specimens, occurrence of Gleason (1 + 2) or (2 + 2) tumors on needle biopsy is unusual since most peripherally lo-

cated prostate carcinomas sampled by needle biopsy are of intermediate or higher grade.

Grade 3 (Glands with Variable and Distorted Architecture)

Three distinct histologic forms of grade 3 prostate carcinomas (3A, 3B, and 3C) are identified according to architectural dispersion of the neoplastic glands (Fig. 11–6). Grades 3A and 3B exhibit more extreme variation in the shape, size, and separation of individual glands than in grade 2. The glands are usually spaced more than one average gland diameter apart. There is irregular extension of glands into

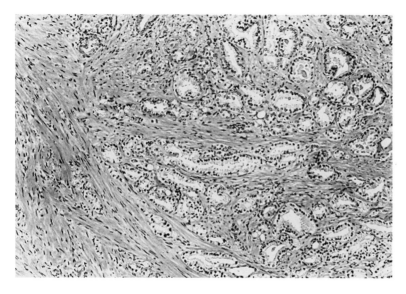

Figure 11–5. Separation of the neoplastic glands at the periphery of a grade 2 tumor. The margin is less distinct or regular than that of grade 1 tumors. (×100.)

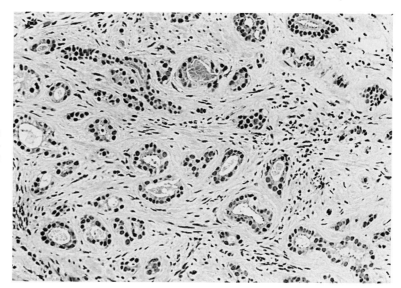

Figure 11–6. Gleason grade 3 tumor shows single, separate, irregularly spaced, very variable glands. (×100.)

the surrounding prostatic stroma (Fig. 11–7), giving the edges of the tumors a "ragged" appearance. Tumor cell cytoplasm tends to be more basophilic than that of grade 1 and 2 carcinomas. Nuclei are variable in appearance but are larger than those found in grades 1 and 2. Typically, they are vesicular in appearance with an open and irregularly distributed chromatin pattern. Nucleoli are almost always present.

Grade 3A and 3B carcinomas differ only in the average size of the tumor glands. The convention is that grade 3A glands are moderate to large, whereas 3B glands are small,

sometimes only tiny clusters of a very few cells (Fig. 11–8). Of these some contain only tiny lumina, or even no lumina. The crucial feature is complete absence of any form of linking between these small clusters into cords or chains, a criterion characteristic of grade 4 carcinomas. Grade 3C carcinomas consist of masses and cords of papillary and/or cribriform tumors (Fig. 11–9); however, the tumor masses have smooth, rounded peripheries with no hint of ragged invasive edges. Since grades 3A, 3B, and 3C exhibit similar prognostic features and are often found together, they are grouped together.

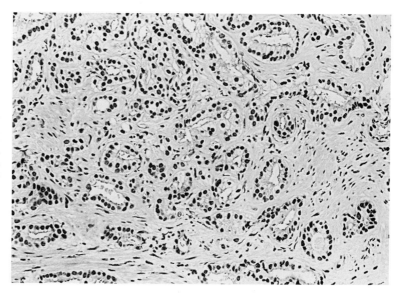

Figure 11–7. Gleason grade 3 tumor with an infiltrative pattern in which there is variation in size and shape of neoplastic glands together with extension of the neoplastic glands into surrounding prostatic stroma. (×100.)

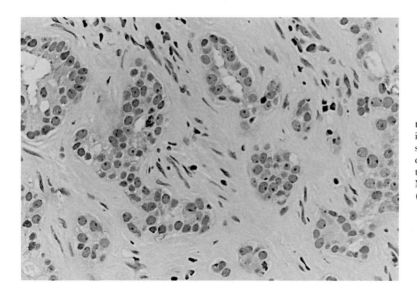

Figure 11–8. Higher-power illustration of Gleason grade 3 tumor in which variation in size and shape of glands range from small clusters of only a few cells with tiny lumina to larger, open glands. Note the prominent nucleoli. (×400.)

Grade 4 (Poorly Differentiated)

Grade 4 prostate cancers may be solid, cribriform, microacinar, or papillary. The cribriform pattern is characterized by large tumor cells arranged in solid masses that are punctuated by sievelike spaces. According to Gleason criteria, these tumors should be a histologically distinct form of Grade 3 intraductal prostate adenocarcinoma[35] and, in contrast to cribriform prostatic intraepithelial neoplasia (PIN), should not have an identifiable basal layer at the periphery of the malignant glands (Fig. 11–10). However, following examination of 46 cases, McNeal and colleagues suggested

that the "cribriform" variant represents a particular type of intraductal carcinoma that, most probably, develops by evolution from the premalignant lesion, PIN.[36] In contrast to Gleason's opinion, they concluded that the majority of, if not all, examples of cribriform carcinoma are equivalent to grade 4 carcinoma growing within pre-existing gland lumina. As an exception to Foulds' hypothesis that full biologic malignant potential is not present in early cancers but evolves with the progress of time,[37] they made the further suggestion that grade 4 (cribriform) cancer evolves within a duct by direct, single-step progression from dysplasia, thus giving rise to the

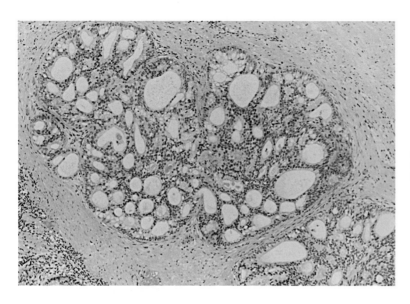

Figure 11–9. Gleason grade 3 carcinoma comprising a well-circumscribed cribriform tumor mass. (×100.)

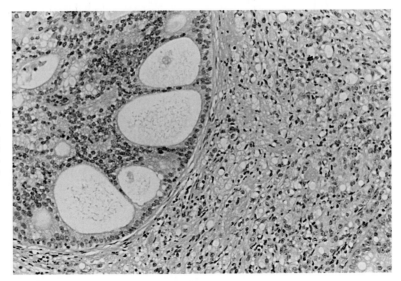

Figure 11–10. Higher magnification of grade 3 cribriform pattern carcinoma shows round, smooth edge with no identifiable basal layer. There is also adjacent infiltrative microacinar carcinoma. (×100.)

coincidental finding of high-grade cancer surrounded by immunohistochemically identifiable (using monoclonal antibody 34β-E12) basal cells and superimposed on a pre-existing grade 3 carcinoma. The biologic behavior of all variants of cribriform carcinoma is the same as other forms of grade 4 prostate cancer and is simultaneously associated with large-volume tumors. Based upon the cumulative available data, we suggest that the term "cribriform" be used only descriptively, if it is used at all. It should not be used to define a specific entity and should refer only to this one particular histogenetic category of prostate cancer.

The distinctive feature of all grade 4 tumors is their ragged and invading edges, in contrast to the smooth, "pushing" edges characteristic of grade 3C cancers. Illustrated examples include microacinar (Figs. 11–11, 11–12), cribriform (Figs. 11–13, 11–14), or papillary (Figs. 11–15, 11–16) tumors. The more common form (grade 4A) is marked by dark-staining tumor cells. The "hypernephroid clear cell form" (grade 4B) resembles renal cell carcinoma (Figs. 11–17, 11–18). Both of these forms of prostate cancer are often found together.

Grade 5

Grade 5 prostate cancers show no glandular differentiation. The tumors may be composed

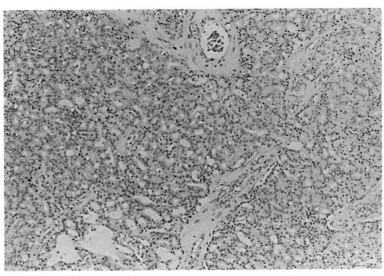

Figure 11–11. Gleason grade 4 carcinoma in which there is loss of glandular differentiation with fusion of glands. Microacinar pattern. (×10.)

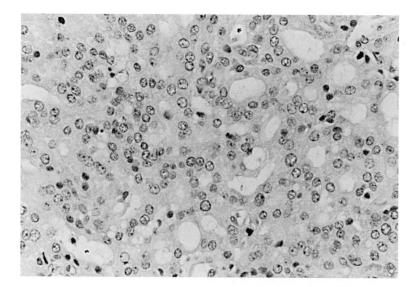

Figure 11–12. Higher magnification of specimen in Figure 11–11 reveals microacinar pattern with some luminal differentiation. (×400.)

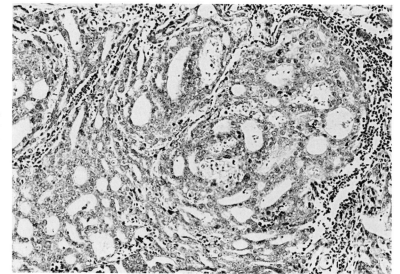

Figure 11–13. Infiltrative masses of cribriform carcinoma surrounded by stroma containing a dense, chronic inflammatory cell infiltrate. Gleason grade 4 tumor. (×100.)

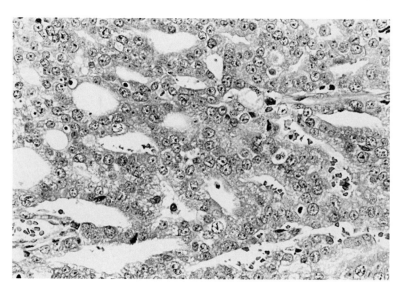

Figure 11–14. Higher magnification of specimen in Figure 11–13. Nuclei are enlarged and contain prominent nucleoli. (×400.)

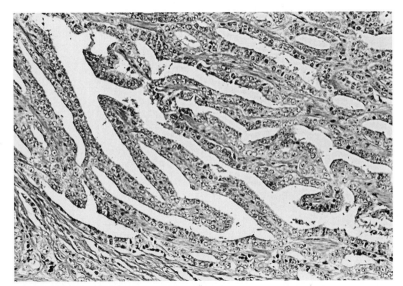

Figure 11–15. Papillary pattern prostatic carcinoma. Gleason grade 4 tumor. (×50.)

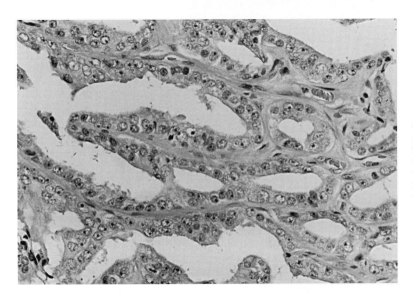

Figure 11–16. Higher magnification of Figure 11–15 reveals papillary architecture comprising tumor cells containing large nuclei with prominent nucleoli. The tumor cells are supported on a fine fibrovascular stromal framework. (×400.)

Figure 11–17. "Hypernephroid clear cell form" carcinoma. Gleason grade 4. (×200.)

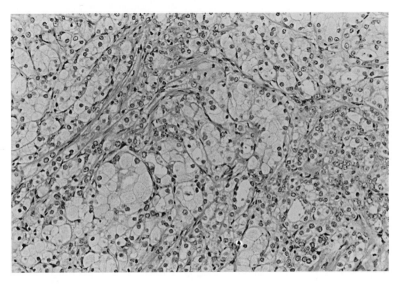

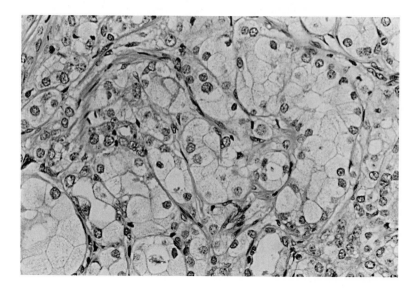

Figure 11–18. Higher magnification of specimen from Figure 11–17. Tumor cells are large and contain relatively small nuclei with indistinct nucleoli. (×400.)

of solid masses of cells, trabeculae, or cords of tumor, or they may appear as single cells infiltrating prostate stroma. Grade 5A carcinomas may superficially resemble grade 3C tumors since they consist of smooth, rounded, packed, papillary or cribriform cylinders with variable foci of central necrosis (comedocarcinoma; Fig. 11–19). The category of grade 5 carcinomas also includes anaplastic tumors growing in infiltrating trabecular or nonglandular solid tumor masses (grade 5B). The appearance of these tumors may be identical to small cell carcinomas (Figs. 11–20 to 11–23),or to undifferentiated anaplastic carcinomas of nonprostatic origin (Fig. 11–24). Differentia-

tion of this latter group is considered in detail in Chapter 13.

APPLICATION OF THE GLEASON GRADING SYSTEM IN PRACTICE

Specimens to Grade

Three types of specimen are now received routinely by most diagnostic histopathology laboratories: (1) radical prostatectomy tissue, (2) transurethral resection (TURP) chippings, and (3) needle biopsy tissue. Morphologic assessment of aspiration cytology specimens in-

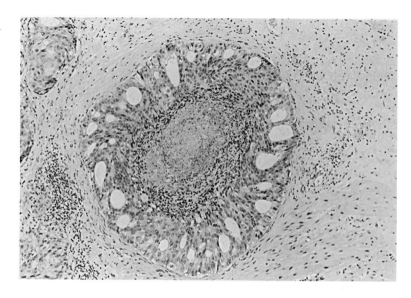

Figure 11–19. Masses of cribriform tumor with central necrosis—comedocarcinoma. This entity is always Gleason grade 5. (×100.)

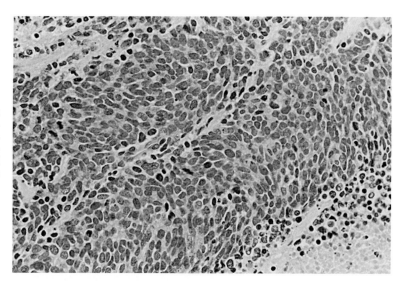

Figure 11–20. Infiltrating small malignant cells with scant cytoplasm, hyperchromatic ovoid nuclei, and a high nuclear-cytoplasmic ratio, resembling "small cell carcinoma" of lung. Gleason grade 5. (×200.)

volves different techniques and criteria from those applied to solid tissues and is considered in Chapter 3. We consider it an important practice to assign a Gleason grade to all histologic specimens of prostate cancer—however small—although special considerations apply to needle biopsy specimens.

Lumping of Grades

Many authors have simplified the Gleason grading system by compressing the scores into groups ("grade lumping" or "grade compression") thus creating only three groups: (2-3-4) well-differentiated, (5-6-7) moderately differentiated, and (8-9-10) poorly differentiated. Unfortunately, lumping significantly weakens the inherent and very particular clinical value of the Gleason grading system by reducing the correlation between histologic and biologic malignancy. Lumping scores 5, 6, and 7 does recognize a subset of intermediate malignancy; however, grade 4 carcinoma (poorly differentiated) generally emerges in score 7 (e.g., 4 + 3 = 7), which is a mixture of low- and high-grade tumors. Since scores 6 and 7 are the most common scores of clinically diagnosed tumors, it would be preferable to maintain a strict demarcation between scores 6 and 7, thus establishing only two groups (2-3-4-5-6) and (7-8-9-10), if the goal is to make

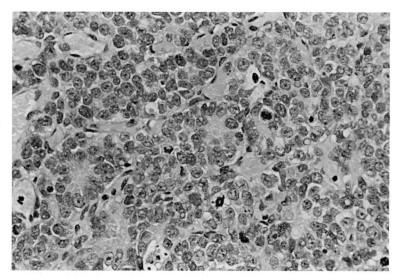

Figure 11–21. Infiltrating carcinoma in which there is morphologic neuroendocrine differentiation. Tumor mitoses are prominent. The rosettes of malignant tumor cells are supported on a delicate and characteristically interlacing fibrovascular stromal network. Gleason grade 5. (×400.)

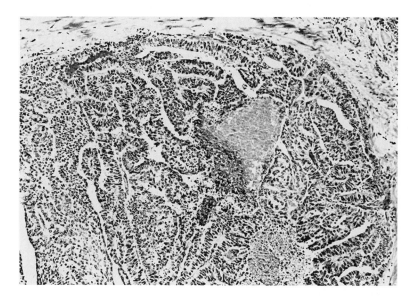

Figure 11–22. Masses of papillary tumor with areas of necrosis. Gleason grade 5. (×25.)

some comparison between "good" and "bad" tumors. Unfortunately, the most common basis for grade lumping appears to be failure to apply the Gleason grading system with sufficient diligence and rigor necessary to achieve clinical and biological validity. The importance of strictly applying the grading system is emphasized by the knowledge that the probability of lymph node metastases is substantially greater in patients with score 7 than in those with score 6.

Grading After Radiation Therapy

After local irradiation for cancer, biopsy of the prostate is unlikely to be of any diagnostic or therapeutic value until about 12 months after completion of therapy because of the delayed effect of ionizing radiation on tumor cell death. However, after this time needle biopsy appears to provide a useful objective assessment of local tumor control, with a low level of sampling error being minimized by the taking of several serial specimens. A detailed consideration of the histologic appearances of postirradiated prostate carcinoma specimens may be found in Chapter 17.

Grading of specimens after radiation therapy has yielded conflicting results. Some observers note no difference from the pretherapy grade, whereas others have reported a substantial increase in grade. Bostwick and colleagues

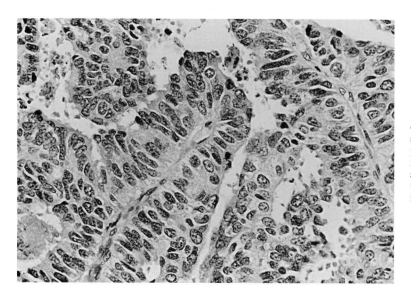

Figure 11–23. Higher magnification of papillary carcinoma shown in Figure 11–22 reveals pseudostratified columnar arrangement of cells supported on a fine fibrovascular stroma. Some tumor cells contain only small and indistinct nucleoli. (×400.)

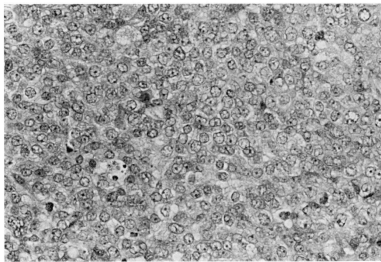

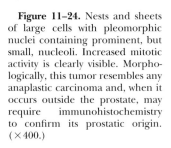

Figure 11–24. Nests and sheets of large cells with pleomorphic nuclei containing prominent, but small, nucleoli. Increased mitotic activity is clearly visible. Morphologically, this tumor resembles any anaplastic carcinoma and, when it occurs outside the prostate, may require immunohistochemistry to confirm its prostatic origin. (×400.)

found no apparent difference in grade before and after external-beam therapy in a series of 40 patients.[38] Conversely, Wheeler's group found a substantial increase in tumor grade after treatment, and which they attributed to time-dependent tumor progression.[39] Similarly, when Siders and Lee evaluated matched tissue specimens from 58 men before radiation therapy and more than 18 months after therapy, they found a substantial increase in Gleason score. There were 24% more poorly differentiated cancers (scores 8 to 10) with an associated shift toward aneuploid DNA content in 31% of pretreatment diploid tumors, indicating increasing histologic and biologic tumor aggressiveness.[40]

No definitive method exists to assess tumor viability after irradiation. Musselman and colleagues obtained monolayer epithelial growth from explants of prostate carcinoma 2 years or more after therapeutic irradiation[41]; however, Mollenkamp and associates could not culture any of 19 irradiated tumors examined and concluded that radiation suppressed mitotic activity and growth potential.[42] Unfortunately, these data are unreliable, since growth in tissue culture is not a valid assay of carcinoma cell viability. Markers of proliferation, such as Ki-67, were not available when this study was performed. Some reports have claimed that if prostate cancer is not histologically ablated by radiotherapy after 12 months, it probably remains biologically active. Specific systems for grading prostate cancer following therapy-induced tumor regression have been proposed, chiefly by German investigators; how-

ever, they have not been universally accepted or adopted.

Grading After Androgen-Deprivation Therapy

Distinctive changes to prostate cancer morphology, following androgen deprivation therapy, were first noted more than 50 years ago. Schenken and colleagues reported that estrogen therapy for prostate cancer reduced nuclear size by 56% as compared with untreated controls.[43] In addition, loss of recognizable nucleoli, condensation of chromatin, nuclear pyknosis, and cytoplasmic vacuolation were all identified as features characteristic of androgen deprivation (Fig. 11–25). It is essential that pathologists are aware of these changes, because of the reliance on nuclear and nucleolar size as a reliable criterion when identifying prostate cancer, particularly in small biopsy specimens and lymph node metastases.

Ellison and Murphy and their colleagues have found a substantial increase in the Gleason grade for cases treated by androgen deprivation therapy.[44, 45] Their independent observations raise the question, Does the high grade reflect aggressive androgen-insensitive clones or merely the collapse cancer of low viability? Murphy suggested that the apparent increase in grade can have two possible explanations: (1) The apparent change in grade could be the result of incomplete sampling (by core needle biopsy) of a widely distributed tumor having foci of different grades; or (2) the

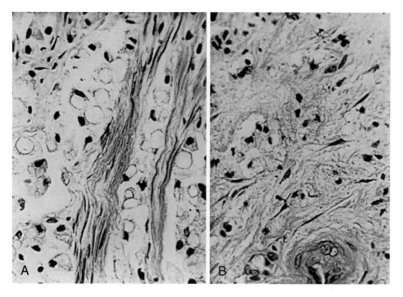

Figure 11–25. *(A)* Autopsy specimen of prostatic carcinoma treated with estrogens for 30 months before death and showing marked intracytoplasmic vacuolation and nuclear pyknosis. (×915.) *(B)* Cytoplasmic vacuolation, nuclear pyknosis, dissolution of epithelial-stromal margins, and marked stromal changes. (×870.) (From Fergusson JD, Franks LM: Response of prostatic carcinoma to estrogen treatment. Br J Surg 40:422–428, 1953.)

changes could relate to gland shrinkage with apparent loss of lumina and increased periglandular connective tissue due to leuprolide (Fig. 11–26). In this latter situation, pathologists might be prompted by the absence of gland lumina to consider the neoplasms poorly differentiated when they were actually responding favorably to the treatment. Measurements of gland density, together with a decrease in serum PSA or prostatic acid phosphatase (PAP) levels after treatment, tend to support this hypothesis. DNA ploidy analysis by Ellison and coworkers revealed no difference between treated and untreated cases.[44] They showed that treated prostate cancer retains its immunophenotype although the clinical importance of high grade remains uncertain.

TURP Chippings and Radical Prostatectomies

Gleason noted that more than 50% of cancers in his series contained two or more patterns, but he limited his reports to two grades since he could never acquire sufficient three-grade tumors to evaluate their behavior. If a particular tumor contains three or more patterns, the approach is as follows:

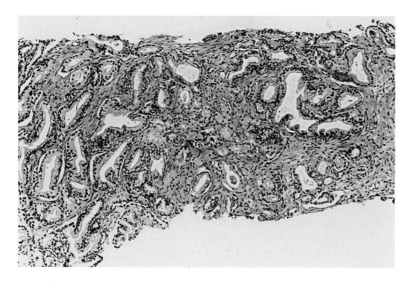

Figure 11–26. Prostatic needle biopsy specimen contains a small amount of gland-forming tumor *(center)*, which is infiltrating between normal/benign glands. The neoplastic glands are smaller than the surrounding normal ones. (×200.)

1. The individual patterns are identified and assigned a grade, and their appropriate quantitative contribution is assessed as the relative proportions of the entire tumor occupied by each grade.

2. The lowest grade is omitted if it comprises less than 5% of the tumor.

3. If the highest and lowest grades each constitute at least 5% of the tumor, they are recorded and the middle grade is omitted.

4. If the highest grade is less than 5% of the tumor and the volume of the other two grades is very extensive, the highest grade is omitted.

5. If the highest grade is more than 5% of the tumor and one of the other grades is very extensive, that predominant grade is recorded as the *primary grade* and the highest grade as the *secondary grade.*

Frequently, discordant grading is due to overlap of two consecutive grades. Under such circumstances, grading is liable to become highly subjective. Errors and problems commonly occur with low-grade carcinomas (i.e., Gleason score 2 through 5), particularly with patterns that give Gleason scores of between 2 and 3 and between scores 3 and 4. Figure 11–27 shows a moderately circumscribed tumor composed of large and small cells with pale eosinophilic cytoplasm. Glands are closely packed, but separate, and are of uniform size. While there is some separation of glands at the periphery, this tumor should be classified as grade 2 and not *underdiagnosed* as grade 1.

Grade 3 carcinoma should be diagnosed, instead of grade 2, wherever well-formed glands are small in size and composed of cells containing amphophilic cytoplasm, or where neoplastic glands vary in size and are to be seen infiltrating between adjacent nonneoplastic prostate glands (Fig. 11–28). Grade 4 should be recognized wherever there is fusion of neoplastic glands, even though the glandular structure might be uniform and composed of cells with bland cytology (Fig. 11–29).

Conventional (14-Gauge) Needle Biopsies or Small Samples

When assigning Gleason grades to needle biopsies or to small tissue samples, the convention is that the two highest grades are recorded, to avoid sampling errors. If only one small focus is present, then one grade only is recorded. Undergrading of needle biopsy specimens is the most common problem and tends to occur in low-grade cancers. An accepted approach to grading a needle biopsy is as follows:

1. If the specimen contains well-formed malignant glands showing a variation in size, then this is regarded as being an element of Gleason grade 3. If that is the only pattern in the sample, the grade is given as "3 + 3" (Fig. 11–30).

2. When glands start to fuse, in addition to appearing discrete and well-formed, such tumors are defined as Gleason grade "3 + 4" or "4 + 3," depending on the relative amounts of each pattern (Fig. 11–31).

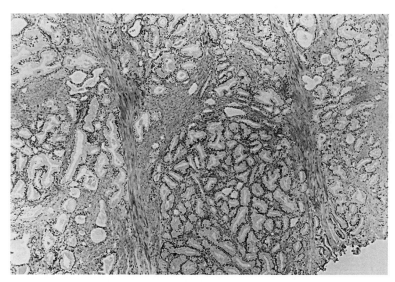

Figure 11–27. A well-circumscribed tumor comprising closely packed glands (grade 1), although there is also some separation of the glands at the periphery (grade 2) (i.e., combined Gleason grade 1 + 2). (×100.)

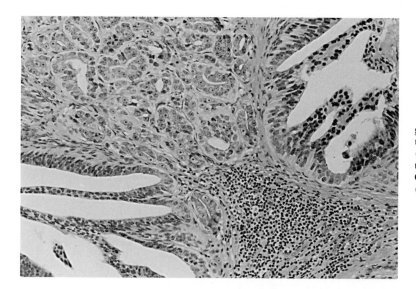

Figure 11–28. When neoplastic glands vary in size and are infiltrating between adjacent glands (which, in this example, also contain PIN), the tumor is considered Gleason grade 3 instead of 2. (×200.)

Figure 11–29. Prostate carcinoma composed of cytologically low-grade tumor cells arranged into well-formed glands (right field, grade 3) and fused glands (left field, grade 4). Gleason grade 3 + 4. (×100.)

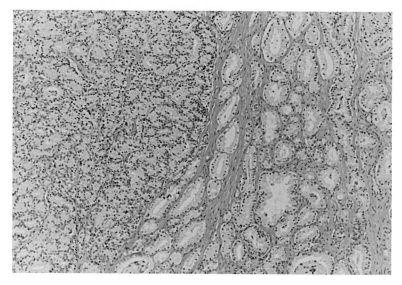

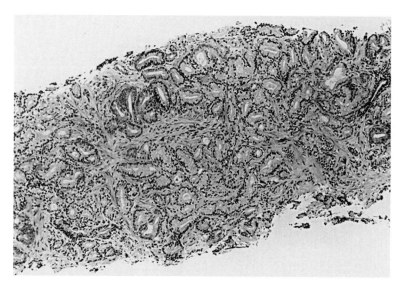

Figure 11–30. Needle biopsy contains well-formed malignant glands that vary in size. Gleason grade 3 tumor. (×100.)

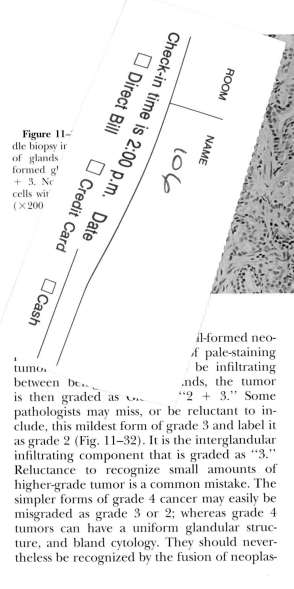

Figure 11-
dle biopsy in
of glands
formed g
+ 3. No
cells wit
(×200

l-formed neo-
f pale-staining
tumo be infiltrating
between ben nds, the tumor
is then graded as t. "2 + 3." Some
pathologists may miss, or be reluctant to include, this mildest form of grade 3 and label it
as grade 2 (Fig. 11–32). It is the interglandular
infiltrating component that is graded as "3."
Reluctance to recognize small amounts of
higher-grade tumor is a common mistake. The
simpler forms of grade 4 cancer may easily be
misgraded as grade 3 or 2; whereas grade 4
tumors can have a uniform glandular structure, and bland cytology. They should nevertheless be recognized by the fusion of neoplas-

tic tubules (Fig. 11–33). On needle biopsy, two
overlapping grades are frequently recognizable; however, occasionally, two discrete foci
comprising two different grades may be identified, in which case both grades should be recorded.

Contemporary (18-Gauge) Needle Biopsies

Throughout the past decade, the amount of
previously standard core biopsy prostate tissue
available for pathologic examination has
decreased—for two reasons:

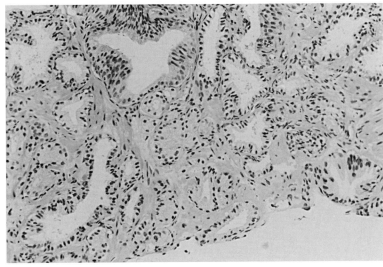

Figure 11–32. Needle biopsy
containing mildest form of Gleason grade 3 tumor. Well-formed
neoplastic glands are composed of
pale-staining tumor cells which
are infiltrating between benign
prostate glands. (×400.)

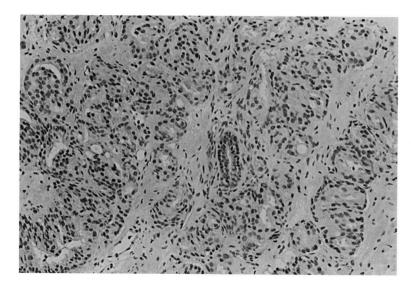

Figure 11–33. Needle biopsy of prostatic carcinoma in which there is fusion of the neoplastic glands. The tumor, composed of cytologically bland cells without prominent nucleoli, is infiltrating through, and is effacing, normal prostatic glands *(center)*. Gleason grade 4. (×200.)

1. The traditional 14-gauge biopsy needle has been replaced by that of 18-gauge.

2. More biopsies contain smaller amounts of tumor than were formerly identified because of the dramatic success of efforts made during recent years to detect smaller tumors at an earlier stage.

Since underdiagnosis of carcinoma in biopsies containing only small amounts of tumor is a relatively frequent occurrence, the first important step is to confirm the presence of tumor in needle biopsy material. If such small amounts of tumor are missed on needle biopsy, the chance is greater than 20% that a repeat biopsy also will be negative. Recogni-

tion of prostate cancer in fine-needle biopsy specimens rests on identification of architectural and cytologic abnormalities.[46]

It is important to survey the entire needle biopsy specimen at low power, in order to appreciate the distribution of the nonneoplastic prostate glands and to identify glands that do not correspond with the appearance of normal glands. The following criteria are used to diagnose *limited amounts of gland-forming carcinoma* on needle biopsy:

Abnormal Architecture. First is identification of glands that are smaller than normal and that may be found infiltrating and occupying the stroma between the benign glands (Fig. 11–34). After recognizing, on low power, that

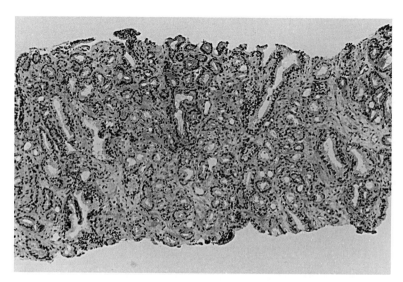

Figure 11–34. Needle biopsy in which neoplastic glands are smaller than normal glands and are infiltrating the stroma between benign glands. Gleason grade 3. (×100.)

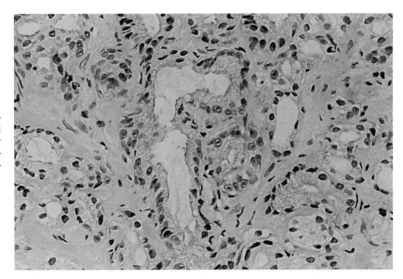

Figure 11–35. Higher magnification of Figure 11–34 shows small neoplastic glands with single layer of epithelium. Some nuclei contain small but prominent nucleoli. (×400.)

some glands are suspicious, evaluation of cytologic details can be made at higher magnification (Fig. 11–35).

Cytoplasm. The gland-forming carcinomas found on needle biopsy are usually of intermediate grade and have a more granular amphophilic cytoplasm than the surrounding benign glands (Fig. 11–36). Against a background of very atrophic nonneoplastic glands, however, infiltrating prostate carcinoma may stand out as glands with distinctly pale cytoplasm. The observation that such cells contain enlarged nuclei with prominent nucleoli is common in prostate carcinomas of intermediate grade.

Nuclear Details. Intermediate gland forming tumors also contain some atypical nuclear features. One seen on needle biopsy most frequently is enlarged nuclei, often with small nucleoli. These nuclear features are, however, also a frequent finding in benign glands with an associated intense inflammation. The appropriate abnormal architectural pattern must be present before assigning the diagnosis of carcinoma through recognition of such cytologic features as prominent nucleoli.

Basal Cell Layer. An unequivocal lack of a basal cell layer is the prerequisite for the diagnosis of carcinoma. Use of monoclonal antibody 34β-E12, which recognizes 49-, 57-, 59-, and 66-kd cytokeratin proteins, makes it possible to selectively stain basal cells of normal and hyperplastic prostate.[47, 48] While negative

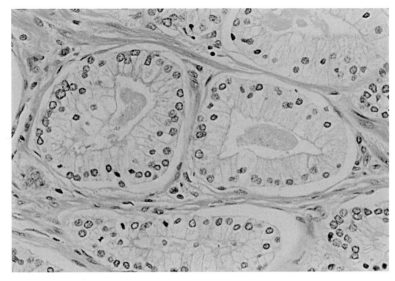

Figure 11–36. Detail to show well-formed glands composed of cells containing amphophilic cytoplasm. Nuclei are "open," when compared to those of the surrounding benign glands (not shown), but nucleoli are not prominent. (×400.)

immunohistochemical staining for basal cells should not be used as the sole criterion for malignancy, strategic use of this feature in conjunction with other morphologic aspects may add significant weight to the diagnosis of prostate cancer.

Other Features. Two morphologic features formerly considered of assistance in distinguishing benign from malignant prostate tissue are (1) perineural invasion with malignant glands encircling nerve and (2) the presence of apparently specific microcrystalline structures within malignant acini and/or in adjacent benign glands. The former is a difficult criterion to apply, particularly in small samples, since perineural infiltration by epithelium has been identified in benign prostatic disease in a manner analogous to that of mammary epithelium occurring in benign fibroadenomatous disease of the human breast.[49] Nevertheless, when applied judiciously, the observation of perineural invasion may be helpful in confirming the diagnosis of prostate cancer. The glands in question should completely encircle the nerve (Fig. 11–37), thus distinguishing the appearance from that of the perineural infiltration that has been reported in benign disease.[50, 51] The second feature, microcrystalline structures can be a useful adjunctive indicator of the presence of malignancy (Fig. 11–38); however, it is not reliable as a firm diagnostic feature, nor is the presence of crystals of any value in either grading or in making statements about the prognosis of confirmed prostate cancer.[52, 53] Nevertheless, the presence of intraluminal

crystalloids should significantly heighten a suspicion of associated malignancy, just as in the breast,[54] and this possibility must be investigated by a detailed evaluation of all adjacent tissues.[55, 56]

Undergrading the Original Biopsy

As many as 45% to 50% of original biopsy specimens have been reported to be undergraded by a number of investigators when the grades of prostate carcinoma in whole resected specimens were compared with those of the initial biopsy material. A proportion of "undergrading" is simply the result of errors incurred in sampling through the use of small needle biopsies; however, some pathologists actually seem reluctant to recognize a higher-grade tumor if the total amount of tumor tissue in a biopsy is very small. Other pathologists do not identify the mildest form of grade 3—presumably through failure to appreciate the fine cytoarchitectural details required to make the diagnosis—and label it as grade 2 (see Fig. 11–28). When compared with matched prostatectomy specimens, contemporary 14-gauge needle biopsy samples underestimate tumor grades in some 33% to 45% of cases and overestimate tumor grade in 4% to 32%. The findings are somewhat similar with 18-gauge needle biopsy specimens (Table 11–3). Grading errors are common in biopsy specimens with small amounts of tumor, particularly low-grade tumors. Most often, these are due to errors in tissue sampling, tumor hetero-

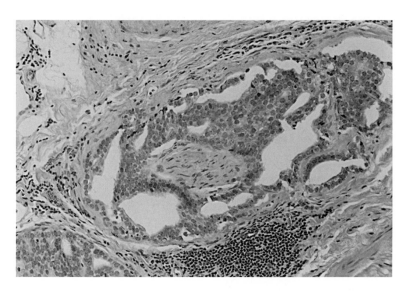

Figure 11–37. Perineural invasion in which malignant glands are present within the perineurium and encircling the nerve bundle. (×400.)

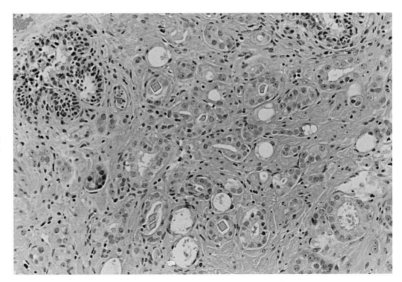

Figure 11–38. Microcrystalline structures within malignant acini. (×200.)

geneity, and observer error in undergrading needle biopsy samples.

So-called undergrading is not a failure of histologic grading itself; rather, it is a situation that will always prevail during investigation of any bivariate distribution in which there is less than perfect correlation between the x and y values (i.e., all biologic bivariate distributions).[63] Gleason has examined the apparent discrepancy between low grades reported on needle biopsy and higher grades found subsequently in the resected specimen and has provided a mathematical explanation of the apparent paradox (defined as, "A situation in which relationships appear to be inconsistent or false but, in fact, are constant and true") that confirms the inevitability of the relationship. The false notion of "undergrading" is further accentuated by the reporting of low biopsy grades leading to prostatic resections, whereas high grades (8, 9, or 10) deter further radical surgery. However, there is an identical probability that *lower* grades would be discovered in these latter specimens if radical prostatectomy were performed. Such "overgrading" of these biopsy specimens has gone unnoticed because few high-grade tumors are resected. Unfortunately, such disappointing discrepancies are inherent in the model and cannot be eliminated simply by more detailed examination of the initial biopsy specimens.

The histologic score and other details of the tumor in a prostatectomy specimen provide a superior level of predictive information (surgical and pathologic staging) that is important to the study of cancer biology, as well as desir-

able for formulating follow-up treatment. However, such new information is not available until the initial biopsy *proves* that cancer is present within a particular prostate and, together with other clinical information, determines whether or not that prostate should be resected. It is probable that the histologic score in the radically resected specimen is better correlated with the biologic malignancy of the tumor than the score in the smaller biopsy; however, to prove such a simple hypothesis will require a large and prolonged study. At such a time, it will be of relatively minor clinical value since the major decision (whether to perform prostatectomy or not) will already have been made, but with the biopsy score having played a pivotal role in formulating that decision.

Presently, no correlation has been established between the amount of tumor on needle biopsy and the total amount of tumor within the prostate gland. This question has been addressed by Kubota and colleagues, who reviewed 284 needle biopsy specimens of prostate cancer from patients who underwent subsequent androgen deprivation endocrine therapy.[64] They measured the area occupied by poorly differentiated tumor (defined according to Mostofi-WHO criteria) and compared it to the total area of adenocarcinoma in each specimen. The survival of each patient after endocrine therapy was then related to the percentage of the area occupied by these different components. The data revealed that patients whose biopsy specimens were diagnosed as prostatic adenocarcinoma containing

Table 11–3. Correlation of Biopsy Grade and Prostatectomy Grade: Review of the Literature

Author/Year	Patients (n)	Biopsy Specimens (n)	Grading System	Correlation of Biopsy and Prostatectomy Grades (Gleason Score) (%)				Other
				Exact	± 1 Unit	Needle Higher	Needle Lower	
14-Gauge Biopsies								
Kastendieck, 1980[57]	120	Needle biopsies: 120	Glandular differentiation Well, moderately, poorly	63	—	—	—	No correlation of grading error and clinical understaging
Catalona et al., 1982[58]	66	Needle biopsies: 66	Glandular differentiation Well, moderately, poorly	59	—	8	33	No correlation of grading error and clinical understaging
Lange & Narayan, 1983[59]	72	Needle biopsies: 66 TURP: 6	Gleason score	74	—	14	39	Grading error greatest with low-grade tumors
Garnett et al., 1984[60]	115	Needle biopsies: 111 TURP: 4	Gleason score	30	72	32	38	Grading error greatest with low-grade tumors
Mills & Fowler, 1986[61]	53	Needle biopsies: 38 TURP: 15	Gleason score	51	74	4	45	Grading error greatest with low-grade tumors and small amounts of tumor No correlation of grading error and clinical understaging
18-Gauge Biopsies								
Spires et al., 1994[62]	67	Needle biopsies: 67	Gleason score	58	94	15	27	No correlation of grading error and clinical understaging
Bostwick, 1994[38]	316	Needle biopsies: 316	Gleason score	35	74	25	40	Grading error greatest with low-grade tumors and small amounts of tumor No correlation of grading error and clinical understaging

From Bostwick DG: Grading prostate cancer. Am J Clin Pathol 102(Suppl 1):S38, 1994.

no solid or trabecular element showed an extremely good prognosis, regardless of their clinical stage. Conversely, even in small needle biopsy specimens there was a strong tendency for higher percentages of occupation of solid/trabecular elements to correlate with worse survival. When all patients were divided into three groups according to occupancy of solid/trabecular elements (0%, 0% to 20%, and more than 20% occupancy), clear statistical differences were revealed between survival times within the three groups. Again, this was independent of the stage of the particular prostate cancer. Thus, accurate identification of the presence of prostate cancer and detailed evaluation of its degree of differentiation can provide important information to the clinician with respect to the likely biologic behavior of the particular tumor in individual patients.

While needle biopsies may be associated with apparent errors in tumor grading, these grading errors do not affect the capacity of needle biopsies to predict lymph node involvement. Careful and rigorous assessment of such tissues permits accurate selection of those patients who are at least risk, or at greatest risk, of local nodal disease. Based on these findings, many pathologists have recommended that a carefully applied Gleason score may be assigned to all needle biopsy specimens, even those with small amounts of tumor, and similar to the original recommendations of Gleason.

Grading on Fine-Needle Aspiration Cytology

Fine-needle aspiration cytology has proved to be an extremely valuable modality when making the diagnosis of many different malignant diseases. A detailed evaluation of cytologic appearances in prostate carcinoma may be found in Chapter 3. In establishing the primary diagnosis of prostate cancer, the diagnostic accuracy of fine-needle aspiration was initially considered to be superior to that of core biopsy when performed by trained and dedicated cytologists experienced in this work. Except in relatively undifferentiated cancers, however, fine-needle aspiration is a poor predictor of final pathologic grade or likely tumor behavior. Recently, the technique has been compared with core biopsy for diagnosis and monitoring of prostate cancer.[65] In an unselected series of 121 patients undergoing both core biopsy and fine-needle aspiration before transurethral resection or radical prostatec-

tomy, diagnostic accuracy was greater for fine-needle aspiration than for core biopsy (82% versus 74%). Except in poorly differentiated cancers, fine-needle aspiration was a poor predictor of final pathologic grade. Fine-needle aspiration was not useful in detecting stage A_1 prostate cancer. Another controlled study of benign and malignant prostate disease revealed significant discordance between cytologic evaluation of disease and that found on examination of conventionally processed tissue blocks from the same prostates.[66] The results of these two studies, performed by experienced diagnostic cytopathologists, cast doubt upon the value of fine-needle aspiration as a routine technique for diagnosing and grading prostate cancer. It appears probable that those cancers most likely to be missed by this technique are the stage A_1, well-differentiated (grade 1 or 2) tumors. Unfortunately, it is precisely this group of prostate carcinomas that requires early diagnosis.

OTHER MORPHOLOGIC GRADING SYSTEMS

Several other grading systems based upon a variety of different morphologic features have been devised; however, none has gained the widespread clinical acceptance of Gleason's system because they all failed to take account of the regional pattern heterogeneity intrinsic to prostate cancers and have not been shown to be as reproducible or prognostically reliable.

Mostofi-WHO

The system devised by Mostofi (1975) has been adopted by the WHO and the International Union Against Cancer (UICC).[16] However, it does not have the clinical significance established by Gleason. The Mostofi-WHO grading system is based on degree of glandular differentiation and cytologic anaplasia. Tumors that form glands are regarded as differentiated neoplasms, whereas those that do not form glands are regarded as undifferentiated. The glands formed by differentiated tumors may be large, intermediate, or small; they may be fused, have a cribriform gland-in-gland pattern, or a papillary configuration.

Grade 1: Well-differentiated glands with nuclei that show slight nuclear anaplasia.

Grade 2: Gland formation but nuclei that show moderate nuclear anaplasia.

Grade 3: Glands with marked nuclear anaplasia or tumors that are undifferentiated (do not form glands).

Schröder-Mostofi later recommended a revised scoring system for grading prostate carcinoma. This system considers the three independent parameters of tumor architecture, nuclear anaplasia, and the presence or absence of mitoses. Five significantly different prognostic groups were distinguished using these criteria.[23] By this process, the large "group in the middle" that is usually seen in other grading system disappeared and a more equal distribution of patients over the five prognostic groups was achieved.

M.D. Anderson Hospital

This system of grading prostate cancer was proposed by Brawn and colleagues and is based on the percentage of a tumor containing differentiated (gland-forming) or undifferentiated (solid) components.[19] The system extended in four equal steps from Grade 1 tumors, in which gland formation occurred in between 75% and 100% of the biopsy specimens, to Grade 4 tumors, in which fewer than 25% of the specimen showed gland formation.

Gaeta

This now unused grading system devised by Gaeta's group was established to include a separate evaluation of the architectural arrangement of glandular structures or lack of them, as well as a separate scale system of assessment of nuclear characteristics of individual tumor cells.[67] This is a four-grade system based on a combination of glandular and nuclear cytologic features of the tumor (Table 11–4). The system has been demonstrated to be straightforward, objective, and reproducible. Through incorporation of cytologic parameters it was designed to be more sensitive than the Gleason system. Retrospective studies demonstrated good correlation between tumor grade and death from prostate cancer. This system has since undergone modification from its earlier description by the National Prostatic Cancer Treatment Group (NPCTG), in order to obtain a score that is the sum of the glandular and nuclear grades of the tumor. However, analysis relating progression-free survival to Gleason and Gaeta grading systems has indicated the Gleason score to predict, more successfully than that of Gaeta, the probable biologic behavior of a primary prostatic malignancy.

Other Morphologic Systems

A combined assessment of glandular differentiation and nuclear anaplasia was devised by Müller and colleagues.[17] Tumors were graded histologically as highly or poorly differentiated, cribriform, and solid. These were scored as 0, 1, 2, and 3, respectively. Nuclear anaplasia was graded as mild, moderate or pronounced and scored 0, 1, and 2. The sum of the scores assigned to glandular differentiation and to nuclear anaplasia was then used to determine the degree of malignancy: grade 1 (score 0 or 1), grade 2 (score 2 or 3), and grade 3 (score 4 or 5). Böcking devised a scoring system intended to indicate the probable prognosis of a tumor. Scores of 1 to 3 were assigned to a variety of nuclear and nucleolar characteristics, which included area, regularity, and size, together with the extent of dissociation of tumor cells.[20]

Table 11–4. Histologic Grades of Prostate Cancer: Gaeta System

Grade	Glands	Cells
I	Well-defined and separated by scant stroma	Uniform and normal size; nucleoli not conspicuous; chromatin dark and dense
II	Medium and small, scattered and infiltrating prostatic stroma	Slightly pleomorphic; nucleoli conspicuous and small
III	Small, irregular or poorly formed acini combined with areas devoid of organization	Significant pleomorphism; nuclei vesicular and show large, often acidophilic nucleoli
IV	Round and solid masses of cells or diffuse infiltration of small cells with no glands	Small or large, uniform or pleomorphic with significant mitotic activity ($\geq$3 per high-power field)

From Gaeta JF: Glandular profiles and cellular patterns in prostatic cancer grading: National prostatic cancer project system. J Urol 17(Suppl 1)33–37, 1981.

RELATIVE VALUE OF MORPHOLOGIC CRITERIA

In many of the reported studies, a fundamental assumption is that morphologic grade (e.g., Gleason score) remains unaltered throughout the life span of a particular tumor. This assumption is not supported by data derived from examination of the natural history of individual prostate cancers, particularly from metastatic sites where the grade may be significantly different than that of the primary tumor.[68] The likelihood that morphologic variants within cribriform/epidermoid group of prostate carcinomas provide important exceptions to Foulds' hypothesis[37] that there is a systematic and sequential progression in the malignant behavior of all carcinomas has already been discussed. The prognostic effects of particular architectural features, considered either singly or combined, have been analyzed by Schröder and associates.[21, 22] In tumors that exhibit only one pattern, tumor gland architecture and nuclear pleomorphism appeared to influence overall survival. Amounts of tumor, cellular pleomorphism, and mitoses were of secondary significance. In tumors containing multiple architectural patterns, prognosis did not reflect the "worst" part of the tumor; this emphasizes Gleason's original observation, and the rationale upon which his two-pattern scoring system is based. Although survival was poor in carcinomas comprising exclusively grade 3 formations, morphologically similar tumors containing areas of well-differentiated neoplastic glands exhibited significantly better survival. Thus, the anticipated effect of poorly differentiated carcinoma appeared to be modulated by adjacent better-differentiated regions.[22] These and similar analyses support the original concept underlying Gleason's grading system by confirming tumor architecture to be the most important morphologic indicator of probable behavior, only then followed by nuclear anaplasia and the presence or absence of mitoses.

Grading Variants of Prostate Carcinoma

A number of distinctive histologic variants of prostatic adenocarcinoma are recognizable and have been characterized. Awareness and recognition of these variants are important, especially because some of them have a clinical course significantly different from that of conventional prostatic adenocarcinoma. These variants may occur either in pure form or in association with the acinar component. Table 11–5 lists the Gleason pattern with each pathologic variant.

QUANTITATIVE METHODS OF GRADING

Three distinct hypotheses underlie recent efforts to quantify structural features of prostate cancer and to relate those features to the prognosis of individual prostate cancers. First is the concept of tumor progression as defined by Foulds, in which he stated that cancers do not express their full range of malignant biologic attributes from the outset but rather progress toward increasing malignancy with time.[37, 69] Support for this thesis has come from the recognition of tumor cell heterogeneity,[70, 71] and the spontaneous emergence of new biologic phenotypes such as metastatic ability and drug resistance.[72] However, Foulds appeared not to appreciate the relationship between tumor morphology, tumor biology, and time. McNeal and coworkers subsequently devised the second hypothesis that biologic progression of prostate cancer correlates directly with tumor volume and hence identified this parameter to be central to predicting biologic behavior.[73] The third thesis is that morphometric information, if sufficiently detailed and suitably analyzed, might accurately predict future behavior of prostate adenocarcinoma.

Table 11–5. Variants of Prostate Adenocarcinoma: Gleason Patterns and Clinical and Pathologic Features

Histologic Variants	Gleason Pattern
1. Ductal (endometrioid) adenocarcinoma	Without necrosis, 3 With necrosis, 5
2. Small cell undifferentiated (high-grade neuroendocrine) carcinoma	5
3. Mucinous (colloid) cancer	4
4. Signet ring cell cancer	5
5. Sarcomatoid cancer	5
6. Carcinosarcoma	5
7. Adenoid basal cell tumor(adenoid cystic cancer or basal cell cancer)	3–5
8. Lymphoepithelioma-like cancer	5
9. Squamous carcinoma	N/A
10. Transitional cell carcinoma	N/A

From Bostwick D. G.: Grading prostate cancer. Am J Clin Pathol 102(Suppl 1):S38, 1994.

During recent years, advent of image analysis techniques, coupled with powerful data-processing computer software, have stimulated renewed interest in obtaining morphologic grading of human prostate cancer based upon accurately quantified tumor volumes. While automated image analysis is an invaluable technique for obtaining large amounts of accurate data that would not be available from manual techniques alone, if the basic parameters being determined are biologically irrelevant to prostate tumor behavior, then they will be useless as prognostic indices, however precisely they may be measured.

Volumetric Parameters

Detailed examination of small prostatic tumors found incidentally and large cancers presenting with symptoms indicated a strong correlation between Gleason grade and tumor volume.[74] A further correlation was demonstrated between prevalence of large prostatic neoplasms found at autopsy and clinical incidence and mortality rates for disseminated prostatic cancer. According to McNeal and coworkers, approximately 20% of "latent" cancers found incidentally at autopsy are sufficiently large to be potentially life-threatening.[73] Although small tumors of grades 1 or 2 are common incidental findings, large prostate cancers invariably contain a mixture of different morphologic appearances and are always at least grade 3. Thus, McNeal concluded that the uniquely broad range of histologic differentiation seen in prostate cancer is a morphologic reflection of biologic progression. Unfortunately, these are comparative data obtained from different persons with morphologically similar tumors but for which functional and behavioral characteristics are unknown.

Although volumetric parameters are important indices of malignant potential in assessing prostate cancer, the majority of studies report findings from radical prostatectomies[75] or from autopsy studies. Humphrey and Vollmer originally showed that, in patients undergoing transurethral prostatic resection, the ratio of prostatic chippings containing cancer to the total number of chippings removed may be considered a relatively accurate approximation of tumor stage and volume.[76] Foucar and colleagues extended this approach by employing a computerized interactive morpho-metric technique to determine relative areas of cancer in transurethrally resected prostatic chippings.[77] The two morphometrically determined parameters of actual area of cancer and percentage area of cancer were compared with the total number of chippings and the percentage of chippings involved by cancer. Although they identified no statistical value for the total number of chippings involved by cancer, the percentage of chippings involved by malignancy, the two morphometrically determined parameters, and the Gleason score were all found to be significant predictors of survival. Although these are valuable observations, the data were collected from a retrospective series of 79 prostatic cancers for which survival information was already available. In keeping with many different morphologic parameters in other malignancies, despite excellent correlation being demonstrated between groups of patients and trends in the alteration of certain parameters, this study confirmed that morphology and morphometry, alone, are not reliable predictors of behavior for any individual prostate tumor.

Nuclear Morphology

Recent techniques of quantitation and computer-based image analysis have been variously employed as methods of obtaining more detailed and reliable data with which to predict biologic behavior of specific tumors. Diamond and coworkers attempted to relate nuclear roundness to the probability of metastatic potential of human prostate cancer.[78] This same group compared their morphometric data with Gleason grade for the same cohort of 27 patients followed for up to 15 years after radical prostatectomy for stage B_1 and stage B_2 carcinomas.[79] Computerized image analysis of relative or absolute nuclear roundness in these prostatic tumors could accurately separate the stage B lesions into two distinct groups, one with high lethal metastatic potential and one with a benign clinical course. The Gleason grading system could not separate these metastatic and nonmetastatic groups without significant overlap.

Nucleolar Morphology

The value of nucleolar surface area measurements as objective parameters for predicting the biologic behavior of prostatic carcinomas has been reported.[80] Scanning electron microscopy data from at least 100 nucleoli in each specimen were examined from the primary and subsequent prostatic biopsies of 40 stage B and 12 stage D patients. Comparison was made between these obtained data and Gleason grading of the same tumors. Nucleolar surface area measurements appeared to correlate with biologic behavior of individual tumors. Cancers from stage B patients with no evidence of disseminated disease for 3 years or more contained small nucleoli with values from 0.82 to 3.4 μm^2. For patients who died of prostate cancer or developed metastases following radical prostatectomy, values from 4.1 to 5.6 μm^2 were obtained. Nucleolar surface area values for patients with stage D disease ranged up to 10 μm^2 (mean of 5.36 μm^2). In this cohort of patients, correlation between Gleason's histologic grading and disease progression was significantly less accurate. Myers and colleagues examined and graded prostate cancer nucleoli according to size, and classified from large and prominent to difficult to identify, following assignment of primary and secondary Gleason patterns.[81] Regardless of Gleason grade, the mean interval from diagnosis to disease progression was shorter in patients whose tumor nucleoli were designated as prominent or intermediate than in those whose nucleoli graded as nonprominent.

Examination of prostate cancer nucleolar organizer region–associated proteins (AgNORs) has been attempted in several laboratories. Colloidal silver-staining techniques for AgNORs are thought to identify proteins involved in regulating DNA-RNA transcriptional activity, and thus their presence might be regarded as a measure of cell proliferative activity. Hitherto, unlike many other malignancies of both epithelial and mesenchymal origin, this technique has not been shown to be of either diagnostic or prognostic value in assessing human prostate cancer.

PROBLEMS OF GRADING

The fundamental concept of tumor grading is that, within any tumor, specific morphologic features relate to the biology of the disease. Any grading system should fulfill the following criteria:

1. It should be simple, reliable, accurate, and easily mastered.

2. It should be applied without needing techniques beyond those used for routine diagnoses and capable of being self-taught from brief, simple instructional materials.

3. It should be reproducible.

4. It should predict biologic behavior.

Prostate cancer is a slowly growing tumor. Microscopic examination reveals a wide range of histologic appearances and behavior of any individual tumor is unpredictable. Mostofi has suggested that the basic problem in grading carcinoma of the prostate lies in confusion over the criteria for *anaplasia* and for *differentiation*. Anaplasia refers to variation from normal size, shape, staining, and chromatin distribution of nuclei whereas differentiation refers to formation of glands. The five grade levels of the Gleason system have effectively satisfied the diversity of architectural patterns into a prognostically valuable scale.

Reproducibility

Inter- and intraobserver variability have been reported with Gleason and other grading systems. Gleason noted exact reproducibility of score in 50% of needle biopsies and within ±1 histologic score in 86% of cases, similar to the findings of Bain and associates.[82] Some investigators have expressed concerns about Gleason grading because of the significant incidence of observer variability in their studies. Di Loreto and colleagues found a high level of disagreement in grading among three pathologists evaluating 41 cases of Gleason grade 2 and 3 (well- to moderately differentiated) adenocarcinomas.[83]

De Las Morenas and coworkers graded 100 cases of prostate adenocarcinomas according to the Gleason, Mostofi, Böcking, and M.D. Anderson (MDAH) systems. The MDAH system was the most reproducible but had a clear tendency to undergrade prostate tumors.[84] The Gleason system was least reproducible, although it provided better correlation with the clinical stage than the MDAH system. The Böcking and the Mostofi systems were second and third in reproducibility and provided the best correlation between grade and stage; however, Gleason has doubted grading in these studies, with a systematic bias toward low histologic scores. The feasibility of applying Gleason's grading method depends on whether practicing pathologists can grade prostate cancers with acceptable accuracy and precision. Intraobserver variation of three grading systems—Mostofi, Gleason, and Böcking—was examined in 139 cases of prostatic carcinomas, by Cintra and Billis (1991).[85] No significant difference between the histologic grades was found in two examinations by any of the three methods employed. Neither the type of surgical procedure nor the number of slices containing tumor influenced the reproducibility of histologic grading within each system studied. The highest level of disagreement between observers using the Gleason system would not have resulted in a change of therapy; however, the same level of disagreement would have altered management in 2% of tumors graded according to the Mostofi system. Despite questions over exact reproducibility, the collective experience of practicing pathologists and urologists supports the clinical utility of grading prostate cancer. Furthermore, for this purpose, the Gleason system is widely accepted because of its relative simplicity and prognostic accuracy.

OBJECTIVE MARKERS OF DIFFERENTIATION

Biologic Implications from Histologic Grading

In any malignancy, two principal effects contribute to the behavior of the particular disease: (1) expression (or absence) of intrinsic properties of the tumor cells and (2) the local host interaction with that specific tumor. A variety of such features related to the cell biology of individual prostate carcinomas may be demonstrated in both histologic and cytologic preparations.

Correlation of Grade with Recurrence and Survival

Every measure of recurrence and survival is strongly correlated with cancer grade, including crude survival, tumor-free survival after treatment (or watchful waiting), metastasis-free survival, and cause-specific survival (Table 11–6). Schröder and colleagues quantitated the effect on cancer-specific survival of 12 histopathologic characteristics used to grade prostate cancer.[21] In their analysis of 346 patients treated by perineal radical prostatectomy, they recommended only three independent parameters of significance for grading prostate cancer: tumor architecture, nuclear anaplasia, and the presence or absence of mitoses. PSA level is an important marker for adenocarcinoma of prostate and is of clinical utility in assessment of residual carcinoma after radical prostatectomy. Humphrey and associates found that Gleason score was a significant, but less reliable, predictor of elevated initial postoperative PSA levels.[110]

Correlation of Grade and Tumor Volume

The strong correlation between Gleason grade and cancer volume has been shown in both transurethral and radical prostatectomy specimens. The volume of high-grade cancer appears to be an important prognostic factor; as the tumor volume increases, the frequency and volume of high-grade tumor increases. McNeal and associates found a strong correlation between cancer volume, percentage of poorly differentiated cancer, and nodal metastasis.[111] Of 38 patients with more than 3.2 cm^3 of prostatic cancer comprising histologic Grades 4 and 5, 22 had tumor-positive nodes, in comparison with only one of 171 patients with less than 3.2 cm^3 of grade 4 or 5 cancer. Gleason grade 1 and 2 cancers are almost always small, usually measuring less than 1 cm^3, and are indolent, localized, and frequently located in the transition zone. Bostwick also found similar results with 405 completely embedded radical prostatectomy samples.[112] Egawa and associates and Gaffney's group independently confirmed the volume of poorly differentiated cancer to be the strongest predictor of tumor progression.[104, 113] The studies from the Johns Hopkins University and Duke University found that grade and tumor volume were the two strongest predictors of tumor progression; when tumor volume was held constant, the predictive value of histologic grade decreased markedly, indicating that these two prognostic factors are closely linked.

Correlation of Grade and PSA

Cancer associated with an elevated serum PSA value is more likely to be of higher grade, larger volume, and more advanced pathologic stage than cancer with normal PSA levels. Blackwell and coworkers found a significant positive correlation between serum PSA, primary Gleason grade, percentage of Gleason grades 4 and 5, nuclear grade, and DNA con-

Table 11–6. Prostate Cancer Grade: Contemporary Correlation with Clinical Measures

Outcome Measure	First Author and Year	Positive Predictive Factors (Univariate)	Positive Predictive Factors (Multivariate)
Crude survival	Neilsen, 1993[86]	Grade/ploidy/nuclear volume	Grade/ploidy
Tumor-free survival after prostatectomy	Humphrey, 1991[87]	Grade/stage/% tumor/ploidy	% Tumor
	Anscher, 1991[88]	Grade/surgical margins/prostatic acid phosphatase/seminal vesicle invasion	Grade/surgical margins
	Wirth, 1993[89]	Grade/stage/ploidy	Grade/stage/ploidy
	Voges, 1993[90]	% Grade 4,5/ploidy/volume	% Grade 4,5/ploidy/volume
	Epstein, 1993[91]	Grade/stage/volume/surgical margins	Grade/surgical margins
	Cheng, 1993[92]	Grade/volume	Grade/volume
Tumor-free survival after radiation	Pisansky, 1993[93]	Grade/PSA	Grade/PSA
	Zagars, 1993[94]	Grade/clinical stage	Grade/clinical stage
AgNOR-free survival (watchful waiting vs. hormonal therapy)	Van den Ouden, 1993[95]	No correlation with grade	
Metastasis-free survival after prostatectomy	Irinopoulou, 1993[96]	Grade/chromatin texture	
Metastasis-free survival after radiation	Zagars, 1993[94]	Grade/TURP/age/PAP	All
Metastasis-free survival (watchful waiting)	Chodak, 1994[97]	Grade/age/place of residence	Grade
Cause-specific survival (all treatments)	Brawn, 1990[98]	Grade in metastases	
	Forsslund, 1992[99]	Grade/stage/ploidy	Grade/stage/ploidy
	Visakorpi, 1992[100]	Grade/stage/S phase/PCNA	Grade/stage/S phase
	Ritter, 1992[101]	Grade/PSA/PAP/stage	Grade/PAP/stage
	Partin, 1992[102]	Grade/clinical stage/age/nuclei	Grade/clinical stage/age/nuclei
	Cheng, 1993[92]	Grade/volume	Grade/volume
	Zagars, 1993[94]	Grade/TURP	Grade/TURP
	Bagshaw, 1993[103]	Grade/stage (both inverse)	Grade/stage (both inverse)
	Egawa, 1993[104]	Grade/clinical stage	Grade
	Tribukait, 1993[105]	Grade/age/clinical stage/ploidy/metastases	Grade/age/clinical stage/ploidy/metastases
	Cadeddu, 1993[106]	Grade/nuclear roundness	
Cause-specific survival (watchful waiting)	Chodak, 1994[97]	Grade/age/place of residence	Grade
	Egawa, 1993[104]	Grade/clinical stage	Grade
Time to recurrence after prostatectomy	Humphrey, 1991[87]	Grade/stage/% tumor/ploidy	Grade/ploidy
PS doubling time	Schmid, 1993[107, 108]	Grade/clinical stage	
	Hands, 1993[109]	Grade/stage	

From Bostwick DG: Grading prostate cancer. Am J Clin Pathol 102(Suppl 1):S38, 1994.

tent in a large series of completely embedded prostatectomy specimens.[114] Cancer specimens with Gleason scores greater than 7 had a significantly higher median serum PSA value and median cancer volume than cancer with Gleason scores less than 7; also, cancer consisting of more than 30% of Gleason patterns 4 and 5 had a significantly higher median serum PSA and cancer volume than cancer specimens with less than 30% Gleason patterns 4 and 5. Partin and colleagues evaluated the usefulness of serum PSA in the staging of prostate cancer in 350 men with clinically localized disease, and they found negative correlation between PSA and Gleason score, which they attributed to the decrease in production of PSA by higher-grade lesions as tumor volume increases.[115] However, this finding is not supported by others'. Although the cells in poorly differentiated cancer produce less PSA than do cells in well- to moderately differentiated cancer, they are usually present in large numbers (greater tumor volume) and replace more of the prostate, resulting in higher serum PSA level. A detailed appraisal of the relative status of morphology and PSA as predictive modalities in prostate cancer is given in Chapter 14.

Correlation of Grade and PSA Doubling Time

Serial measurement of PSA indicates that prostate cancer has a constant log-linear growth rate, with mean doubling time of 2.4 years for localized cancer and 1.8 years for metastatic cancer. Higher Gleason grades are associated with faster doubling times. See Chapter 14 for the most comprehensive survey of the relationship between grade and PSA as combined predictive modalities in the progression of prostate carcinoma.

Correlation of Grade and Pathologic Stage

Grade is one of the strongest and most useful predictors of pathologic stage and other clinical and pathologic features, according to many univariate and multivariate studies. This predictive ability applies to every measure of pathologic stage, including capsular perforation, seminal vesicle invasion, lymph node metastases, and bone metastases. Some investigators claim that a Gleason score of 8 or higher on biopsy is strongly predictive of lymph node metastases, and lymph node dissections can be omitted for these patients. Despite the optimism for grading to determine clinical stage, the predictive value is not high enough to permit its application for individual patients, particularly those with moderately differentiated cancer.

Correlation of Grade and Tumor Location

Grade may be related to the site of origin of cancer within the prostate. Cancer arising in the transition zone of the prostate appears to be lower grade and less aggressive clinically than the more common cancer arising in the peripheral zone. Most transition zone cancers arise in foci adjacent to nodular hyperplasia, and one third actually originate within nodules. In general, these cancers are better differentiated than those in the peripheral zone and account for most Gleason pattern 1 and 2 tumors.

Correlation of Grade and Growth Receptors

Interaction between neoplastic cells and either humoral or structural components of the surrounding environment is a powerful modulator of tumor biology. Differential expression of specific hormone receptors by particular malignancies is recognized to be associated with disease progression. Evidence of the complexity of the relationship between hormone receptors, tumor morphology, and behavioral phenotype is provided by the observation that both androgen and antiandrogen therapy enhance proliferation rate of some prostate cancer cell-lines through differential modulation of epidermal growth factor receptor (EGFr) expression.[116] At the same time, ploidy levels, often considered to be an independent predictor of prostate cancer behavior, appear to be independent of androgen, EGF, and other growth factors.[117] With respect to the metastatic behavior of prostate cancer cells, treatment with EGF or retinoic acid causes increased expression of urinary plasminogen activator (uPA) with a secondary rise in invasive capacity.[118] This is a somewhat surprising observation since retinoic acid is also able to enhance expression of major histocompatibility complex (MHC) Class I and Class II antigens by prostate cancer cells, thus reversing the loss of these determinants that accompanies progression from normal prostate tissue through dysplasia to frankly malignant, and ultimately metastatic, carcinoma.[119] Current evidence indicates that elevated levels of EGF or EGFr, either individually or together, appear able to potentiate prostate tumor cell invasion.[120] With respect to intact human tissues, expression of a series of growth factors and their receptors has been examined in prostatic hyperplasia and neoplasia.[121] Concentrations of EGF receptor in hyperplastic tissues were significantly higher than those in prostate carcinomas. Furthermore, within the cancers, expression of EGF receptors appeared to be a function of Gleason histologic grade. Thus, EGF receptor status might be employed as an adjunct marker of prostate cancer differentiation; however, if the data from the prostate cell lines are reliable and can be extrapolated to the intact tissues, then enhanced EGF or EGFr expression signify more aggressive tumor behavior. Unfortunately, little information is available on the structure of these molecules in prostate cancer. Current data suggest that a mutational event may be one explanation for their apparently autocrine behavior in this disease.[122]

Androgen receptor–binding activity has been investigated as a possible predictor of response to endocrine therapy by primary and metastatic prostate carcinomas, and thus as a marker of tissue differentiation. Tissues removed by conventional transurethral resection were assessed for androgen-binding activity and the data were correlated with time to disease progression, clinical stage, and histologic (Gleason) grade. No association was demonstrated between time to progression and clinical stage; however, correlation was demonstrated between time to progression and histologic grade. When grade 4 carcinomas were excluded from analysis, androgen-binding activity became predictive of disease progression, independently of histologic grade and clinical stage.[123]

Whereas cytoplasmic androgen receptors are labile molecules, prostate membrane prolactin-binding sites are relatively stable. Expression of prolactin receptors has been examined in a range of hyperplastic and neoplastic prostate tissues removed by transurethral resection.[124] Using a histologic grading system of G1-G3, free prolactin receptors were found in none of the poorly differentiated (G1) carcinomas. While only 62.5% of G2 carcinomas were positive, all G1 tumors and benign hyperplastic tissues contained measurable levels of free prolactin membrane–binding components. When treated with combined chemotherapy and hormone manipulation, subsequent tumor biopsy specimens revealed increased expression of prolactin receptors in the tumors that responded.

These many different, and apparently frequently conflicting, observations emphasize the multifactorial nature of prostate cancer in which morphologic grade remains the strongest predictor of tumor behavior, morphologic or otherwise, although it is influenced by a wide range of functional constraints.

Grading and the Multiple Prognostic Index

A prognostic index that combines multiple variables (multiple prognostic index) should be more precise at predicting patient outcome than current methods of clinical staging, which rely on only a few variables. Such an index for prostate cancer would, almost certainly, include Gleason grade and percentage of Gleason patterns 4 and 5, as well as tumor volume, serum PSA level, tumor origin, anddDNA content. Preliminary efforts to create a multiple prognostic index for prostate cancer have focused on serum PSA and ultrasound findings. Wolfe and colleagues combined serum PSA and ultrasound findings and enhanced the accuracy of preoperative tumor staging by considering tumor grade as a third variable.[125] They calculated the "expected" PSA level for each patient as "K" × volume of ultrasonographic hypoechoic area + 0.07 ng/mL × ultrasonographic gland volume; where "K" was 2.1 ng/mL if the Gleason score was 7 or more, and 4.2 if the score was less than 7. Inclusion of the level of PSA into this formula allowed preoperative prediction of clinical stage in 48 men undergoing radical prostatectomy with 84% sensitivity, 82% specificity, 94% positive predictive value, and 83% diagnostic accuracy. According to Pisansky and colleagues, the combination of pretherapy grade and serum PSA accurately identified a cohort of patients at high risk for tumor recurrence following radiation therapy.[93]

FUTURE PROSPECTS

Histologic grading is a strong prognostic factor in prostate cancer and appears to be reasonably reproducible, even with contemporary thin-needle biopsy specimens. Its success is limited by several factors, including small sample size, tumor heterogeneity, "undergrading" of biopsy samples, and changes following irradiation and androgen deprivation therapy. Despite a low but significant level of interobserver and intraobserver variability, grading is important in predicting patient outcome in univariate and multivariate analysis.[126] Future refinements that combine grade with other prognostic factors should allow more precise stratification of patients for particular types of therapy. Advent of modern molecular biologic techniques, particularly those based on polymerase chain reaction (PCR), are likely to allow identification of distinct behavioral phenotypes through analysis of important genotypic markers at a time when relatively small populations of cancer cells that express those markers have emerged. Already, the finding of genetically distinct (for example, with respect to different mutations of the p53 gene) but histologically indistinguishable prostate cancers occurring simultaneously within a single specimen is emphasizing the fundamental weakness of strictly morphologic approaches and the urgent requirement for new functional methods to identify biologically and behaviorally relevant phenotypes at the time prostate cancer is first diagnosed.[127]

REFERENCES

1. Foster CS, McLoughlin J, Bashir I, Abel PD: Markers of the metastatic phenotype in prostate cancer. Hum Pathol 23:381–394, 1992.
2. Foster CS, Abel PD: Clinical and molecular techniques for diagnosis and monitoring of prostate cancer. Hum Pathol 23:395–401, 1992.
3. Broders AC: Carcinoma grading and practical application. Arch Pathol Lab Med 2:376–381, 1926.
4. Young HH, Davis DM: Young's Practice of Urology. Philadelphia: WB Saunders, 1926.
5. Muir EG: Carcinoma of the prostate. Lancet i:667–672, 1934.
6. Kahler JE: Carcinoma of the prostate gland. Mayo Clin Proc 13:589–592, 1938.
7. Evans N, Barnes RW, Brown AF: Carcinoma of the prostate. Correlation between the histologic observations and the clinical course. Arch Pathol 34:473–483, 1942.
8. Edwards CN, Steinthorsson E, Nicholson D: An autopsy study of latent prostatic cancer. Cancer 6:531–554, 1953.
9. Shelley HS, Auerbach SH, Classen KL, et al.: Carcinoma of the prostate. A new system of classification. Arch Surg 77:751–756, 1958.
10. Vickery AL, Kerr WS: Carcinoma of the prostate treated by radical prostatectomy. Cancer 16:1598–1608, 1963.
11. Gleason DF: Classification of prostatic carcinoma. Cancer Chemother Rep 50:125–128, 1966.
12. Jewett HJ, Bridges RW, Gray GF, et al.: The palpable nodule of prostatic cancer. Results 15 years after radical excision. JAMA 203:403–406, 1968.
13. Mobley TL, Frank IN: Influence of tumor grade on survival and on serum acid phosphatase levels in metastatic cancer of prostate. J Urol 99:321–323, 1968.
14. Utz DC, Farrow GM: Pathological differentiation and prognosis of prostatic carcinoma. JAMA 209:1701–1703, 1969.
15. Corriere JN, Cornog JL, Murphy JJ: Prognosis in patients with carcinoma of the prostate. Cancer 25:911–918, 1970.
16. Mostofi FK: Grading of prostatic carcinoma. Cancer Chemother Rep 59:111–117, 1975.
17. Müller H-A, Ackermann R, Frohmüller HGW, et al.: The value of perineal punch biopsy in estimating histological grade of carcinoma of the prostate. Prostate 1:303–309, 1980.
18. Gaeta JF: Glandular profiles and cellular patterns in prostatic cancer grading: National prostatic cancer project system. J Urol 17(Suppl 1):33–37, 1981.
19. Brawn PN, Ayala AG, Von Eschenbach AC, et al.: Histologic grading study of prostatic adenocarcinoma: The development of a new system and comparison with other methods—a preliminary study. Cancer 49:525–532, 1982.
20. Böcking A, Sinagowitz E: Histologic grading of prostatic carcinoma. Pathol Res Pract 168:115–125, 1980.
21. Schröder FH, Blom JHM, Hop WCJ, et al.: Grading of prostatic cancer: I. An analysis of the prognostic significance of single characteristics. Prostate 6:81–100, 1985.
22. Schröder FH, Blom JHM, Hop WCJ, et al.: Grading of prostatic cancer: II. The prognostic significance of the presence of multiple architectural patterns. Prostate 6:403–415, 1985.
23. Schröder FH, Hop WCJ, Blom JHM, et al.: Grading of prostate cancer. III. Multivariate analysis of prognostic parameters. Prostate 7:13–20, 1985.
24. Foster CS: Pathological grading systems for prostatic cancer. In Waxman J, Williams G (eds): Prostatic Cancer: A Consensus. London: Edward Arnold, 1991.
25. Franks LM: Benign nodular hyperplasia of the prostate: A review. Ann R Coll Surg Eng 14:92–106, 1954.
26. McNeal JE, Redwine EA, Freiha FS, et al.: Zonal distribution of prostatic adenocarcinoma. Correlation with histologic pattern and direction of spread. Am J Surg Pathol 12:897–906, 1988.
27. Price H, McNeal JE, Stamey TA: Evolving patterns of tissue composition in benign prostatic hyperplasia as a function of specimen size. Hum Pathol 21:578–585, 1990.
28. Tannenbaum M: Atypical epithelial hyperplasia or carcinoma of the prostate gland: The surgical pathologist at an impasse? Urology 4:758–760, 1974.
29. Kastendieck H: Correlations between atypical hyperplasia and carcinoma of the prostate. Pathol Res Pract 169:366–378, 1980.
30. Helpap B: The biological significance of atypical hyperplasia of the prostate. Virch Arch Path Anat 387:307–317, 1980.
31. McNeal JE: Origin and development of carcinoma in the prostate. Cancer 23:24–34, 1969.
32. Gleason DF: Classification of prostatic carcinoma. Cancer Chemother Rev 50:125–128, 1966.
33. Bostwick DG: Grading prostate cancer. Am J Clin Pathol 102(Suppl 1):S38–56, 1994.
34. Gleason DF: Histologic grading of prostate cancer: A perspective. Hum Pathol 23:273–279, 1992.
35. Gleason DF: Veterans Administration Cooperative Urological Research Group: Histological grading and clinical staging of prostatic carcinoma. In Tannenbaum M (ed): Urologic Pathology: The Prostate. Philadelphia: Lea & Febiger, 1977.
36. McNeal J, Reese JH, Redwine EA, et al.: Cribriform adenocarcinoma of the prostate. Cancer 58:1714–1719, 1986.
37. Foulds L: The experimental study of tumor progression: A review. Cancer Res 14:327–329, 1954.
38. Bostwick DG: Gleason grading of prostatic needle biopsies: Correlation with grade in 316 matched prostatectomies. Am J Surg Pathol 18:796–803, 1994.
39. Wheeler JA, Zagars GK, Ayala AG: Dedifferentiation of locally recurrent prostate cancer after radiation therapy. Cancer 71:3783–3787, 1993.
40. Siders DB, Lee F: Histologic changes of irradiated prostatic carcinoma diagnosed by transrectal ultrasound. Hum Pathol 23:344–351, 1992.
41. Musselman PW, Tubbs R, Connelly RW, et al.: Biological significance of prostatic carcinoma after definitive radiation therapy [Abstract]. J Urol 137:114A, 1987.
42. Mollenkamp JS, Cooper JF, Kagan AR: Clinical experience with supervoltage radiotherapy in carcinoma of the prostate: A preliminary report. J Urol 113:374–377, 1975.
43. Schenken JR, Burns EL, Kahle PJ: The effect of diethylstilbestrol dipropionate on carcinoma of the prostate gland II. Cytologic changes following treatment. J Urol 48:99–112, 1942.
44. Ellison E, Ferguson J, Zincke H, et al.: "Nucleolus-poor" clear cell adenocarcinoma of the prostate. A distinctive histologic variant in patients receiving total androgen blockade [Abstract]. Lab Invest 68:59A, 1993.

45. Murphy WM, Soloway MS, Barrows GH: Pathologic changes associated with androgen deprivation therapy for prostate cancer. Cancer 68:821–828, 1991.

46. Eble JN, Angermeier PA: The roles of fine needle aspiration and needle core biopsies in the diagnosis of primary prostatic cancer. Hum Pathol 23:249–257, 1992.

47. Brawer MK, Peehl DM, Stamey TA, et al.: Keratin immunoreactivity in the benign and neoplastic human prostate. Cancer Res 45:3663–3667, 1985.

48. Grignon DJ, Ro JY, Ordóñez NG, et al.: Basal cell hyperplasia, adenoid basal cell tumor, and adenoid cystic carcinoma of the prostate gland: An immunohistochemical study. Hum Pathol 19:1425–1433, 1988.

49. Taylor HB, Norris HJ: Well-differentiated carcinoma of the breast. Cancer 25:687–692, 1970.

50. Carstens PHB: Perineural glands in normal and hyperplastic prostates. J Urol 123:686–688, 1980.

51. McIntyre TL, Franzini DA: The presence of benign prostatic glands in perineural spaces. J Urol 135:507–509, 1986.

52. Bennett BD, Gardner WA: Crystalloids in prostatic hyperplasia. Prostate 1:31–35, 1980.

53. Jensen PE, Gardner WA, Piserchia PV: Prostatic crystalloids: Associations with adenocarcinoma. Prostate 1:25–30, 1980.

54. Foster CS, Neville AM: The histopathology of breast cancer. In Coombes RC, Powles TJ, Ford HT, et al. (eds): Breast Cancer Management. London: Academic Press, 1981.

55. Holmes EJ: Crystalloids of prostatic carcinoma: Relationship to Bence Jones crystals. Cancer 39:2073–2080, 1977.

56. Ro JY, Ayala AG, Ordóñez NG, et al.: Intraluminal-crystalloids in prostatic adenocarcinoma. Cancer 57:2397–2407, 1986.

57. Kastendieck H: Morphologie des Prostatacarcinoms in Stanzbiopsien und totalen Prostatektomein. Untersuchungen zur Frage der Relevanz bioptischer Befundaussagen. Pathologe 2:31–43, 1980.

58. Catalona WJ, Stein AJ, Fair WR: Grading errors in prostatic needle biopsies: Relation to the accuracy of tumor grade in predicting pelvic lymph node metastases. J Urol 127:919–922, 1982.

59. Lange PH, Narayan P: Understaging and undergrading of prostate cancer. Urology 21:113–118, 1983.

60. Garnett JE, Oyasu R, Grayhack JT: The accuracy of diagnostic biopsy specimens in predicting tumour grades by Gleason's classification of radical prostatectomy specimens. J Urol 131:690–693, 1984.

61. Mills SE, Fowler JE: Gleason histologic grading of prostatic carcinoma. Correlations between biopsy and prostatectomy specimens. Cancer 57:346–349, 1986.

62. Spires SE, Cibull ML, Wood D Jr, et al.: Gleason histologic grading in prostatic carcinoma: correlation of 18-gauge core biopsy with prostatectomy. Arch Pathol Lab Med 118:705–708, 1994.

63. Gleason DF: Undergrading of prostate cancer biopsies: A paradox inherent in all biologic bivariate distributions. Urology 47:289–291, 1996.

64. Kubota Y, Kondo I, Harada M, et al.: The worst histological elements in needle biopsy specimens of prostate cancer: Do they predict the prognosis? Lancet ii:822–823, 1996.

65. Narayan P, Jajodia P, Stein R, et al.: A comparison of fine needle aspiration and core biopsy in diagnosis and preoperative grading of prostate cancer. J Urol 141:560–563, 1989.

66. Mohler JL, Erozan YS, Walsh PC, et al.: Fine needle core and aspiration biopsy. A new method for diagnosis of prostatic carcinoma. Cancer 63:1846–1855, 1989.

67. Gaeta JF, Asirwatham JE, Miller G, et al.: Histologic grading of primary prostatic cancer: A new approach to an old problem. J Urol 123:689–693, 1980.

68. Fan K, Peng CF, Geta J, et al.: Predicting the probability of bone metastasis through histopathological grading of prostatic carcinoma: A retrospective correlative analysis of 81 autopsy cases with antemortem transurethral resection specimens. J Urol 130:708–711, 1983.

69. Foulds L: Neoplastic Development. New York: Academic Press, 1975.

70. Fidler IJ, Hart R: Biologic diversity in metastatic neoplasms: Origins and implications. Science 217:998–1003, 1982.

71. Poste G, Grieg R: On the genesis and regulation of cellular heterogeneity in malignant tumors. Invasion Metastasis 2:137–176, 1982.

72. Bashir I, Sikora K, Foster CS: Multidrug resistance and behavioural phenotype of cancer cells. Cell Biol Int 17:907–917, 1993.

73. McNeal JE, Bostwick DG, Kindrachuk RA, et al.: Patterns of progression in prostate cancer. Lancet 1:60–63, 1986.

74. McNeal JE: Morphologic indices of progression in prostatic carcinoma. In Coffey DS, Gardner WA, Bruchovsky N, et al. (eds): Current Concepts and Approaches to the Study of Prostate Cancer. New York: Alan R Liss, 1987.

75. Partin AW, Epstein JI, Cho KR, et al.: Morphometric measurement of tumor volume and per cent of gland involvement as predictors of pathological stage in clinical stage B prostate cancer. J Urol 141:341–345, 1989.

76. Humphrey P, Vollmer RT: The ratio of prostate chips with cancer: A new measure of tumor extent and its relationship to grade and prognosis. Hum Pathol 19:411–418, 1988.

77. Foucar E, Haake G, Dalton L, et al.: The area of cancer in transurethral resection specimens as a prognostic indicator in carcinoma of the prostate: A computer-assisted morphometric study. Hum Pathol 21:586–592, 1990.

78. Diamond DA, Berry SJ, Jewett HJ, et al.: A new method to assess metastatic potential of human prostate cancer: Relative nuclear roundness. J Urol 128:729–734, 1982.

79. Epstein JI, Berry SJ, Eggleston JC: Nuclear roundness factor. A predictor of progression in untreated stage A2 prostate cancer. Cancer 54:1666–1671, 1984.

80. Tannenbaum M, Tannenbaum S, DeSanctis PN, et al.: Prognostic significance of nucleolar surface area in prostate cancer. Urology 19:546–551, 1982.

81. Myers RP, Neves RJ, Farrow GM, et al.: Nucleolar grading of prostatic adenocarcinoma: Light microscopic correlation with disease progression. Prostate 3:423–432, 1982.

82. Bain GO, Koch M, Hanson J: Feasibility of grading prostatic carcinomas. Arch Pathol Lab Med 106:265–267, 1982.

83. Di Loreto C, Fitzpatrick B, Underhill S, et al.: Correlation between visual clues, objective architectural features and interobserver agreement in prostate cancer. Am J Clin Pathol 96:70–75, 1991.

84. De Las Morenas A, Siroky MB, Merriam J, et al.: Prostatic adenocarcinoma: Reproducibility and correlation with clinical stages of four grading systems. Hum Pathol 19:595–597, 1988.

85. Cintra ML, Billis A: Histologic grading of prostatic adenocarcinoma: Intraobserver reproducibility of the Mostofi, Gleason and Böcking grading systems. Int Urol Nephrol 23:449–454, 1991.

86. Neilsen K, Overgaard J, Bentzen SM, et al.: Histological grade, DNA ploidy and mean nuclear volume as prognostic factors in prostatic cancer. APMIS 101:614–620, 1993.

87. Humphrey PA, Walther PJ, Currin SM, et al.: Histologic grade, DNA ploidy and intraglandular tumor extent as indicators of tumor progression of clinical stage B prostatic carcinoma. Am J Surg Pathol 15:1165–1170, 1991.

88. Anscher MS, Prosnitz LR: Multivariate analysis of factors predicting local relapse after radical prostatectomy—possible indications for postoperative radiotherapy. Int J Radiat Oncol 21:941–947, 1991.

89. Wirth MP, Muller HA, Manseck A, et al.: Value of nuclear DNA ploidy patterns in patients with prostate cancer after radical prostatectomy. Eur Urol 20:248–252, 1991.

90. Voges GE, Eigner EB, Ross W, et al.: Pathologic parameters and flow cytometric ploidy analysis in predicting recurrence in carcinoma of the prostate. Eur Urol 24:132–139, 1993.

91. Epstein JI, Pizov G, Walsh PC: Correlation of pathologic findings with progression after radical retropubic prostatectomy. Cancer 71:3582–3593, 1993.

92. Cheng WS, Frydenberg M, Bergstralh EJ, et al.: Radical prostatectomy for pathologic stage C prostate cancer: Influence of pathologic variables and adjuvant treatment on disease outcome. Urology 42:283–291, 1993.

93. Pisansky TM, Cha SS, Earle JD, et al.: Prostate-specific antigen as a pretherapy prognostic factor in patients treated with radiation therapy for clinically localized prostate cancer. J Clin Oncol 11:2158–2166, 1993.

94. Zagars GK, von Eschenback AC, Ayala AG: Prognostic factors in prostate cancer. Analysis of 874 patients treated with radiation therapy. Cancer 72:1709–1725, 1993.

95. Van den Ouden D, Tribukait B, Blom JH, et al.: Deoxyribonucleic acid ploidy of core biopsies and metastatic lymph nodes of prostate cancer patients: Impact on time to progression. The European Organization for Research and Treatment of Cancer Genitourinary Group. J Urol 150:400–406, 1993.

96. Irinopoulou T, Rigaut JP, Benson MC: Toward objective prognostic grading of prostatic carcinoma using image analysis. Anal Quant Cytol Histol 15:341–344, 1993.

97. Chodak GW, Thisted RA, Gerber GS, et al.: Results of conservative management of clinically localized prostate cancer. N Engl J Med 330:242–248, 1994.

98. Brawn P, Kuhl D, Johnson C, et al.: Stage D1 prostate carcinoma. The histologic appearance of nodal metastases and its relationship to survival. Cancer 65:538–543, 1990.

99. Forsslund G, Esposti PL, Nilsson B, et al.: The prognostic significance of nuclear DNA content in prostatic carcinoma. Cancer 69:1432–1439, 1992.

100. Visakorpi T, Kallioniemi OP, Heikkinen A, et al.: Small subgroup of aggressive, highly proliferative prostatic carcinomas defined by p53 accumulation. J Natl Cancer Inst 84:883–887, 1992.

101. Ritter MA, Messing EM, Shanahan TG, et al.: Prostate-specific antigen as a predictor of radiotherapy response and patterns of failure in localized prostate cancer. J Clin Oncol 10:1208–1217, 1992.

102. Partin AW, Steinberg GD, Pitcock RV, et al.: Use of nuclear morphometry. Gleason histologic scoring, clinical stage, and age to predict disease-free survival among patients with prostate cancer. Cancer 70:161–168, 1992.

103. Bagshaw MA, Kaplan ID, Cox RC: Prostate cancer. Radiation therapy for localized disease. Cancer 71:939–952, 1993.

104. Egawa S, Go M, Kuwao S, et al.: Long-term impact of conservative management on localized prostate cancer. A twenty-year experience in Japan. Urology 42:520–527, 1993.

105. Tribukait B: Nuclear deoxyribonucleic acid determination in patients with prostate carcinomas: Clinical research and application. Eur Urol 23:64–76, 1993.

106. Cadeddu JA, Pearson JD, Partin AW, et al.: Relationship between changes in prostate-specific antigen and prognosis of prostate cancer. Urology 42:383–389, 1993.

107. Schmid HP, McNeal JE, Stamey TA: Clinical observations on the doubling time of prostate cancer. Eur Urol 23:60–63, 1993.

108. Schmid HP, McNeal JE, Stamey TA: Observations on the doubling time of prostate cancer. The use of seriel prostate-specific antigen in patients with untreated disease as a measure of increasing cancer volume. Cancer 71:2031–2040, 1993.

109. Hanks GE, D'Amico A, Epstein BE, et al.: Prostatic-specific antigen doubling times in patients with prostate cancer: A potentially useful reflection of tumour doubling time. Int J Radiat Oncol Biol Phys 27:125–127, 1993.

110. Humphrey PA, Frazier HA, Vollmer RT, et al.: Stratification of pathologic features in radical prostatectomy specimens that are predictive of elevated initial postoperative serum prostate-specific antigen levels. Cancer 71:1821–1827, 1993.

111. McNeal JE, Villers EA, Redwine EA, et al.: Histologic differentiation. Cancer volume and pelvic lymph node metastasis in adenocarcinoma of the prostate. Cancer 66:1225–1233, 1990.

112. Bostwick DG: Significance of tumor volume in prostate cancer. In Rous S (ed): Urology Annual. Philadelphia: Norton, 1994.

113. Gaffney EF, O'Sullivan SN, O'Brien A: A major solid undifferentiated carcinoma pattern correlates with tumor progression in locally advanced prostatic carcinoma. Histopathology 21:249–255, 1992.

114. Blackwell KL, Bostwick DG, Myers RP, et al.: Combining prostate specific antigen with cancer and gland volume to predict more reliably pathological stage: The influence of prostate specific antigen cancer density. J Urol 151:1565–1570, 1994.

115. Partin AW, Carter HB, Chan DW, et al.: Prostate specific antigen in the staging of localized prostate cancer: Influence of tumor differentiation, tumor volume, and benign hyperplasia. J Urol 143:747–752, 1990.

116. Ravenna L, Lubrano C, Di-Silverio F, et al.: Androgenic and antiandrogenic control on epidermal growth factor, epidermal growth factor receptor, and

androgen receptor expression in human prostate cancer cell line LNCap. Prostate 26:290–298, 1995.

117. Janssen T, Kiss R, Dedecker R, et al.: Influence of dihydrotestosterone, epidermal growth factor, and basic fibroblastic growth factor on the cell kinetics of the PC3, DU145, and LNCap prostatic cancer cell lines: Relationship with DNA ploidy level. Prostate 27:277–286, 1995.

118. Liu DF, Rabbani SA: Induction of urinary plasminogen activator by retinoic acid results in increased invasiveness of human prostate cancer cells PC-3. Prostate 27:269–276, 1995.

119. Sharpe JC, Abel PD, Gilbertson JA, et al.: Modulated expression of human leukocyte antigen class I and class II determinants in hyperplastic and malignant human prostatic epithelium. Br J Urol 74:609–616, 1994.

120. Jarrard DF, Blitz BF, Smith RC, et al.: Effect of epidermal growth factor on prostate cancer cell line PC3 growth and invasion. Prostate 24:46–53, 1994.

121. Maddy SQ, Chisholm GD, Busuttil A, et al.: Epidermal growth factor receptors in human prostate cancer: Correlation with histological differentiation of the tumour. Br J Cancer 60:41–44, 1989.

122. Sherwood ER, Lee C: Epidermal growth factor-related peptides and the epidermal growth factor receptor in normal and malignant prostate. World J Urol 13:290–296, 1995.

123. Benson RC, Gorman PA, O'Brien PC, et al.: Relationship between androgen receptor binding activity in human prostate cancer and clinical response to endocrine therapy. Cancer 59:1599–1606, 1987.

124. Tarle M, Culig Z, Kokic I: Unoccupied prolactin binding components of the benign and malignant human prostate in a subclinical and clinical procedure. Int J Rad Appl Instrum B 16:461–467, 1989.

125. Wolf JS Jr, Shinohara K, Narayan P: Staging of prostate cancer. Accuracy of transrectal ultrasound enhanced by prostate-specific antigen. Br J Urol 70:534–541, 1992.

126. Foster CS, Mostofi FK: Prostate cancer: Present status. Hum Pathol 23:209–210, 1992.

127. Foster CS, Mostofi FK: Prostate cancer—Quo vadis? Hum Pathol 23:402–406, 1992.

12

PATHOLOGIC FEATURES THAT PREDICT PROGRESSION OF DISEASE FOLLOWING RADICAL PROSTATECTOMY

Jonathan I. Epstein

In recent years, radical prostatectomy has become the therapy of choice for clinically localized adenocarcinoma of the prostate, particularly in the United States, although this policy has not received general acceptance in the United Kingdom and in much of continental Europe. In the past, a 10- to 15-year follow-up was necessary to determine progression following radical prostatectomy, with the use of postoperative serum prostate-specific antigen (PSA) levels, a more rapid means of determining progression is now available. This immunologically based diagnostic test is now being supported by the molecular technique of reverse transcriptase–polymerase chain reaction (RT-PCR) to detect PSA-secreting cells (possible metastatic prostatic carcinoma cells) in the peripheral circulation. The ability to predict progression following radical prostatectomy has implications for therapy and for prognosis. Many institutions employ postoperative radiotherapy for men whose chances for progression following radical prostatectomy are high. On the horizon are newer treatment strategies, such as gene therapy, that will also be used to treat men at high risk of progression after surgery. In this chapter I present the important pathologic parameters of radical prostatectomy specimens that should be assessed and how the findings correlate with progression following surgery.

PATIENT POPULATION

Most of the data presented in this chapter reflect follow-up of men who have undergone radical prostatectomy at the Johns Hopkins Hospital in Baltimore, Maryland.[1-4] In part, this concentration on our own patient population is meant to reflect our personal experience. More importantly, we have available the largest number of patients with the longest follow-up who have been well-characterized pathologically to correlate with progression following surgery. The data presented here reflect an update of our previously published series. They reflect study of 721 men who underwent radical prostatectomy with a mean follow-up of 6.5 years. None of these patients had any form of preoperative hormone therapy. Furthermore, no patient received postoperative radiotherapy or hormone therapy until progression occurred. Consequently, these data demonstrate the natural history of pros-

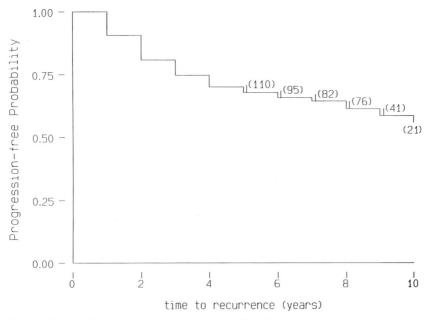

Figure 12–1. Overall progression rate for prostate carcinoma. Numbers in parentheses represent censored patients.

tate cancer following radical prostatectomy as it relates to various pathologic parameters.

DEFINITION OF PROGRESSION

Progression following radical prostatectomy can be measured by a postoperative serum (PSA) level above the female range, local recurrence, or distant failure. Although distant failure and death will ultimately be the most important end points to evaluate after radical prostatectomy, there is not sufficient follow-up in enough patients to provide accurate assessment of these parameters. After radical prostatectomy, a PSA serum level above the female range is the most sensitive and earliest means of detecting progression.[5, 6] Unless specified, progression in this paper is defined as a serum PSA level greater than 0.2 ng/ml, as measured by the Hybritech assay.

OVERALL PROGRESSION

During recent years there has been a marked shift in the clinical stage of prostate cancer at diagnosis and of the men who are candidates for radical prostatectomy. More men are now diagnosed with impalpable prostate cancer, owing to an elevated serum PSA blood value. These tumors typically have a

lower pathologic stage and smaller volume and less frequently have positive margins.[7] Consequently, the overall progression rates reported later are expected to be higher than for patients operated on today. Despite this shift toward more favorable pathologic stage, the findings from this study are applicable to today's practice. It is expected that, for example, the finding of a positive margin stratified by Gleason grade and status of capsular penetration will have the same effect on progression, regardless of the clinical stage.

Overall, 68% and 52% of patients are predicted to be free of progression following radical prostatectomy at 5 and 10 years, respectively (Fig. 12–1). At 5 years after radical prostatectomy, 4% are estimated to have local recurrence, 5% distant metastases, and 2% local and distant failure; the remainder experience only biochemical failure (i.e., PSA elevation).

GRADE

The vast majority of patients who undergo radical prostatectomy have a Gleason score of 5 to 7. Only 6% of our patients have a Gleason score of 2 to 4, and 14% a score of 8 or 9. Most low-grade tumors are small transition zone lesions that are not detected by PSA or needle biopsy, so these men usually do not come to radical prostatectomy. At the other end of the grading spectrum, most patients with Gleason 8 to 10 tumors present with advanced disease and are not candidates for surgical cure. Of all patients who have undergone radical prostatectomy in our population, 48% have Gleason scores of 5 or 6 and 32% score 7. In our series Gleason grade was the most powerful predictor of progression after radical prostatectomy. Gleason score 7 tumors had significantly higher progression rates than tumors with Gleason score 5 or 6 (Fig. 12–2). This finding emphasizes that Gleason tumor scores of 5 to 7 should not be considered together as intermediate-grade tumors. Although Gleason score 7 cancers behave aggressively, score 8 and 9 tumors are associated with even worse prognosis (Fig. 12–2).

LYMPH NODE METASTASES

In our institution, approximately 13% of patients with clinical stage T2 tumors are found to have lymph node metastases. Nonpalpable tumors detected by elevated serum PSA levels have only a 6% risk of nodal metastases.[7] Radical prostatectomy performed for stage T1a disease (less than 5% cancer on transurethral resection of the prostate [TURP]) is not associated with nodal metastases.[8] It is difficult to determine the current incidence of nodal

metastases for stage T1b disease. In the past a sizable number of extensive high-grade tumors were detected incidentally on TURP and were associated with a significant risk of nodal metastases.[9] Currently, before TURP serum PSA level is measured and if the value is elevated disproportionately to the size of the gland, needle biopsy is performed. Consequently, many lesions that would have been extensive T1b tumors are now diagnosed by needle biopsy without TURP being performed. Tumors with nodal metastases invariably progress following radical prostatectomy (Fig. 12–3).

SEMINAL VESICLE INVASION

The incidence of seminal vesicle involvement is 14% for clinical stage T2 (palpable) prostate cancer.[1] Seminal vesicle invasion is seen in 4% to 10% of radical prostatectomy specimens performed for stage T1b disease (at least 5% cancer on TURP)[9] and is virtually absent in stage T1a disease (less than 5% cancer on TURP).[8] Seminal vesicle invasion is defined as tumor invading the muscular wall of the seminal vesicle. When tumor infiltrates the periseminal vesicle tissue the prognosis is not as dim.[10]

Although both seminal vesicle invasion and capsular penetration are pathologic stage T3 disease, seminal vesicle invasion is a much

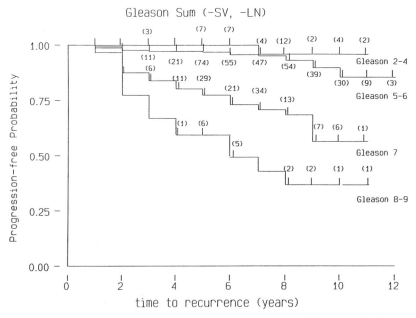

Figure 12–2. Relationship of prostatectomy Gleason sum to progression following radical prostatectomy.

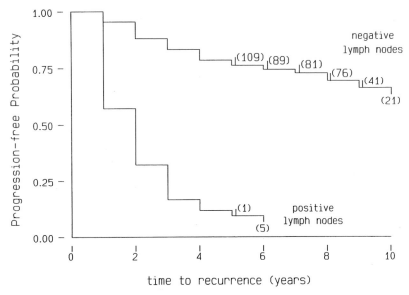

Figure 12–3. Correlation of lymph node metastases with progression following radical prostatectomy.

more dire prognostic finding (Fig. 12–4). In our most recent analysis of 47 men with positive seminal vesicles and negative lymph nodes, the 5- and 10-year progression-free rates were 40% and 27%, respectively.[4] Seminal vesicle invasion most often occurs when tumor penetrates the prostatic capsule at the base of the gland, extends into periseminal vesicle soft tissue, and eventually grows into the seminal vesicles. Less often the tumor spreads through the ejaculatory ducts into the seminal vesicles, or directly from the base of the prostate into the wall of the seminal vesicles. Least common are discrete metastases to the seminal vesicle. Seminal vesicle invasion may be identified by examining the base of the seminal vesicles, almost always the first area of the vesicles to be invaded.

Recently, Villiers and colleagues showed seminal vesicle invasion to correlate with in-

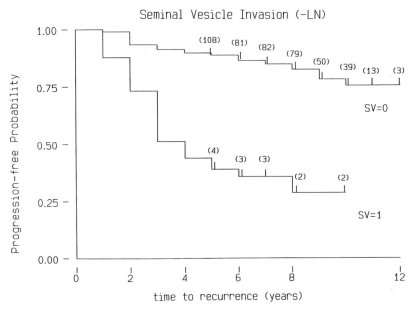

Figure 12–4. Correlation of seminal vesicle invasion with progression following radical prostatectomy.

creased tumor volume and higher Gleason grade tumor.[11] They found seminal vesicle invasion to be only a weak predictor of lymph node metastases, once the grade and tumor volume were known. They conclude that, independently of tumor grade and tumor volume, seminal vesicle invasion may not predict tumor aggressiveness; however, their work indirectly measured tumor aggressiveness by the presence of lymph node metastases. In a recent study we demonstrated that seminal vesicle invasion was a significant independent predictor of progression following radical prostatectomy; progression in these cases occurred over a wide range of tumor volumes.[10]

EXTRAPROSTATIC EXTENSION

Definition

Despite the use of the term *capsular penetration,* the prostate lacks a well-defined capsule.[12, 13] In some areas there appears to be a separation between the most peripheral nonneoplastic acini and the edge of the prostate, giving the appearance of a fibromuscular capsule. Elsewhere nonneoplastic glands extend right up to the edge of the prostate. Anteriorly, the edge of the gland is less defined; the anterior fibromuscular stroma of the prostate merges with smooth muscle that extends to the pubic bone. Because one cannot distinguish where the prostatic capsule begins and the normal prostatic stroma ends, it makes no sense to classify tumors as invading into but not through the prostatic capsule. Furthermore, the majority of studies have demonstrated that prognosis is adversely affected only when tumor penetrates the full thickness of the prostatic capsule to extend into adjacent periprostatic soft tissue.[14] Consequently, tumors should be categorized as either being confined to the gland or extending out of the prostate. Since some authors differentiate between capsular penetration and capsular perforation, pathologists should define their use of these terms until nomenclature is standardized. Recognizing that the prostate lacks a true discrete fibrous or fibromuscular capsule, the term *prostatic capsule* nevertheless conveniently denotes the edge of the gland. Despite the absence of a true histologic capsule, the edge of the prostate nevertheless provides a barrier to the spread of carcinoma; not uncommonly, one sees a front of tumor extending to the edge of the gland yet not out into the periprostatic soft tissue.

The term *perforation* indicates unquestionable extension of carcinoma from the substance of the gland across the capsular margin and into periprostatic tissue. Capsular penetration tends to be underdiagnosed by pathologists. Tumor spreads into the periprostatic soft tissue and induces a desmoplastic stromal response, so it is uncommon to see extraprostatic tumor situated within adipose tissue. Rather, diagnosis of capsular penetration rests on identification of a protuberance to the normal contour of the edge of the prostate as seen at low magnification (Fig. 12–5). The best demarcation for the edge of the prostate is the point where the compact smooth muscle of the gland ends.

Incidence, Pathways, Location

The prevalence of capsular penetration for palpable clinically confined tumors is 20% to 38% and 40% to 66%, depending on whether on rectal examination the tumor is unilateral or bilateral.[15, 16] The incidences of capsular penetration for stages T1a (≤ 5% low or intermediate-grade incidental cancer found on TURP) and T1b disease (> 5% or high-grade incidental cancer found on TURP) are 8% and 26%, respectively.[8, 9] Peripherally located adenocarcinomas of the prostate tend to extend out of the prostate via perineural space invasion.[17] Perineural invasion by itself does not worsen prognosis, since perineural invasion merely represents extension of tumor along a plane of decreased resistance, not invasion into lymphatics.[18] Capsular penetration preferentially occurs posteriorly and posterolaterally, paralleling the location of most palpable adenocarcinomas.

Extent

Only a few institutions measure the extent of capsular penetration. Stamey and colleagues quantify capsular penetration as the sum of the length of capsular penetration along different slides.[19] Because prostate cancer often spreads along nerves parallel to the prostatic capsule, one can see tumor barely out of the gland skimming along for significant distances, so this method tends to overestimate capsular penetration. In our institution we

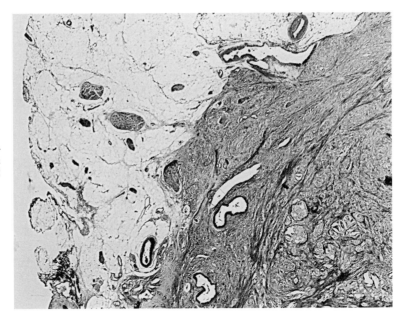

Figure 12–5. Established capsular penetration characterized by a bulge in the normally rounded contour of the prostate.

have classified cases of capsular penetration as showing focal capsular penetration when only a few neoplastic glands are present in periprostatic soft tissue. These glands are barely exterior to the prostate and tend to grow horizontally, parallel to the prostate, rather than extending away from the gland. Tumors with a greater degree of extracapsular spread are designated as having established or extensive capsular penetration. In a series of 514 men with "negative" seminal vesicles and negative lymph nodes, 23% had focal capsular penetration and 35%, established capsular penetration.

Correlation with Progression

Studies have demonstrated that capsular penetration is related to other adverse variables, such as increased tumor volume, seminal vesicle invasion, lymph node metastases, and high histologic grade[19]; however, only a few studies assess the relationship between capsular penetration and recurrence following radical prostatectomy.[20–24] Because disease with either lymph node metastases or seminal vesicle invasion almost invariably progresses after radical prostatectomy, we have analyzed men without these findings to determine the effect of capsular penetration. In an update of our previous work, we studied 617 men with negative seminal vesicles and negative lymph nodes followed for an average of 6½ years.[4] Tumors

with established capsular penetration were associated with a higher risk of progression than those that showed focal capsular penetration (Table 12–1, Fig. 12–6). Organ-confined disease uncommonly progresses: 5- and 10-year progression-free rates are 98% and 85%, respectively (see Table 12–1).

MARGINS OF RESECTION

The first careful pathologic consideration of the resection margins in radical prostatectomy specimens with prostate carcinoma was published only in 1983.[25] At that time the impetus for studying resection margins related to the

Table 12–1. Postoperative Risk of Progression in Tumors with Negative Seminal Vesicles and Negative Lymph Nodes

Findings at Radical Prostatectomy	Progression-free Risk (%)	
	5-Year	**10-Year**
Organ-confined	97.8	84.7
Focal capsular penetration	91.2	67.7
Established capsular penetration	77.8	58.4
Negative margins	94.6	79.4
Positive margins	74.0	54.9
Gleason sum 2–4	100	95.6
Gleason sum 5–6	96.9	81.9
Gleason sum 7	76.9	51.5
Gleason sum 8–9	59.1	34.9

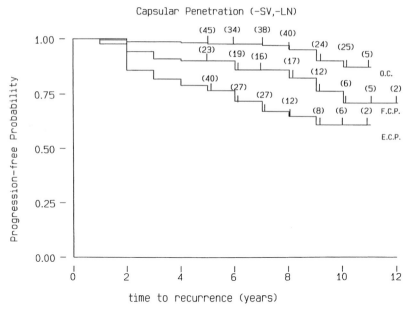

Figure 12–6. Correlation of extent of capsular penetration with progression. Key: OC, organ-confined; FCP, focal capsular penetration; ECP, established capsular penetration.

description of a new modification of the surgical protocol for radical prostatectomy for prostate carcinoma to preserve potency. In this anatomic approach to modified radical prostatectomy by Walsh and associates,[25] the neurovascular bundle was selectively spared (i.e., left within the patient) thus leaving less soft tissue surrounding the excised prostate specimen than had the neurovascular bundle been sacrificed and included with the specimen. This paper, and a subsequent follow-up study by Eggleston and Walsh,[26] carefully assessed the margins in 100 radical prostatectomy specimens removed by the modified technique and demonstrated that the nerve-sparing modification did not compromise tumor removal in these cases. During the same period of time, some institutions were recommending post–radical prostatectomy radiotherapy for advanced pathologic stage and/or margin-positive prostate carcinoma.[27-29]

In large part because of the urologists' interest in margins following the anatomic approach to radical prostatectomy for potency preservation, and radiotherapists' interest in margins to decide whether any postoperative therapy should be instituted, pathologists in turn began paying more attention to the histologic assessment of margins in these radical prostatectomy specimens.

Radical removal of the prostate is limited because the prostate is located deep within the pelvis and is surrounded by vulnerable structures such as the urogenital diaphragm, pelvic side wall, rectum, bladder neck, and trigone.[30] Whereas in cancer surgery the term *radical* usually refers to an operation in which several centimeters of clinically uninvolved tissue surrounding a tumor is removed, radical prostatectomy often provides only 1 or 2 mm of such tissue. This scant tissue may easily be disrupted either intraoperatively or during postoperative handling of the specimen. In such cases, tumor approaches the inked edge of the gland, where it is unclear for the pathologist whether the surgical resection margins do or do not contain invasive cancer.

Recently, it has been suggested that wider margins of resection are necessary in radical prostatectomy specimens in the region of the neurovascular bundle since tumor often extends within 1 mm of the margin, and in other organ systems such a margin would be inadequate.[14] Because of a unique population of patients, we were able to evaluate the margins of resection on the removed prostate in the area of the neurovascular bundle, and then because the neurovascular bundle was removed separately at a later stage during the same operation, we had immediate feedback on whether any residual tumor would have been left in the patient if the neurovascular bundle had not been removed.[31] In 22 cases the distance between the inked margin of resection and the most peripheral tumor gland in the region of the neurovascular bundle was minimal: in only two cases was the distance between ink and tumor greater than 1.0 mm (Fig. 12–7). All of these cases were shown to be truly negative margins, since none showed tumor in the subsequently resected neurovascular bundle. The presence of minimal soft tissue surrounding prostate cancer is sufficient to result in truly negative margins. Margins should be called "positive" when tumor extends to the inked edge of the gland, and when there is an irregular appearance corresponding to the surgeon's cut across tumor (Fig. 12–8). There are several different methods of assessing the distal margin of resection.

We have shown in another study that, if one takes a very thin shave of the distal margin, tumor within this section is associated with the same rate of tumor progression after radical prostatectomy as positive margins elsewhere in the gland.[1] When performing this procedure, care must be taken not to cut deeply into the prostate to obtain urothelium in this distal margin sample, or else false-positive margins will result. Alternatively, one can amputate the distal few millimeters of the prostate and section this tissue parallel to the urethra to obtain perpendicular sections. In the first technique it is important that accurate orientation of the specimen be maintained in the cassette before processing so that sections are taken from the

outermost aspect of the marginal tissue without excessive "trimming" into the block. To date, no studies have shown a correlation between positive distal margins processed with the second technique and tumor progression.

In our material of predominantly stage T2 (palpable) prostate cancer, a total of 298 men (59%) had negative margins, 190 (37%) had focally positive margins, and 19 prostates (4%) demonstrated extensive positive margins.[1] It is difficult to compare our findings with those cited in the literature because of differences in patient selection, pathologic criteria for designating margins of resection, and methods of processing radical prostatectomy specimens. Recognizing these differences, the incidence of positive margins in radical prostatectomy specimens has ranged from 23% to 48%, according to some of the larger series in the literature in which adjuvant therapy was not administered routinely.[21, 32–35]

Stages T1a and T1b are associated with positive margins in 3% and 15% of cases, respectively.[8, 9] The incidence of positive margins is 17% for nonpalpable tumors diagnosed by needle biopsy.[7]

Sites of Positive Margins

In stage T2 cancers with single-site margin involvement, the following sites are most frequently involved: distal margin of resection (22% of positive margins), posterior margin

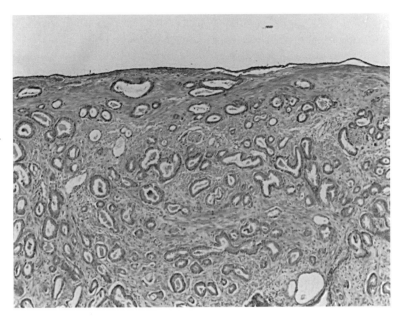

Figure 12–7. Margins are negative, with tumor separated from the ink by a limited amount of non-neoplastic tissue. (From Epstein JI: Prostate and seminal vesicles. In Sternberg SS, et al. (eds): Diagnostic Surgical Pathology, ed 2. New York: Raven Press, 1993, p 1833.)

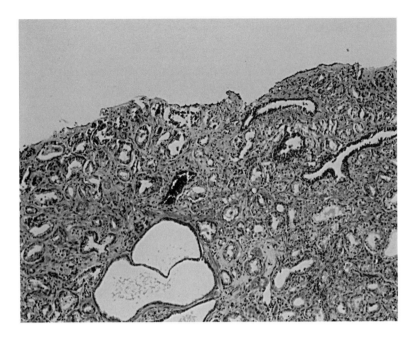

Figure 12–8. Margins are positive with tumor extending to a ragged inked edge of the specimen. (From Epstein JI: The evaluation of radical prostatectomy specimens performed for carcinoma of the prostate. Pathol Ann 26:159, 1991.)

(17% of positive margins), and posterolateral margin (14% of positive margins).[1] The presence of a positive distal margin in conjunction with a positive margin at one other site is also frequent—12% of positive margins. This proclivity for tumor involvement of the apical margin has also been noted by others.[32] Most tumors with positive proximal urethral margins are extensive: 65% of cases also show positive margins at other sites.[1]

In our recent study, of the 28 men who had positive margins only posterolaterally in the region of the neurovascular bundle, 4 had undergone wide resection of the neurovascular bundle at the site of the positive margin.[1] Consequently, of the 507 men in this series, 24 (4.7%) potentially had positive margins owing to attempts to preserve the neurovascular bundle. Of these 24 patients, 4 progressed after radical prostatectomy; the 20 without evidence of disease had follow-ups ranging from 3 to 8 years (mean and median, 5.5 years). Of these 4 patients, 3 manifested elevated serum PSA levels as the only evidence of progression and 1 has a proven local recurrence. These four patients represent 0.8% of the total population who underwent radical prostatectomy. These figures reinforce the advantage of the anatomic approach to radical prostatectomy for potency preservation in which the neurovascular bundle is preserved (or widely excised when necessary). Other studies have found no difference in margin positivity in nerve-sparing versus non–nerve-sparing operations.[33–36]

Because they are often centrally located, tumors diagnosed on TURP are more likely than palpable tumors diagnosed by needle biopsy to demonstrate positive margins anteriorly.[8, 9] In nonpalpable tumors diagnosed by needle biopsy, positive margins occur with almost equal frequency anteriorly, posteriorly, and at the distal margin.[7]

Reasons for Positive Margins

There are several potential explanations for positive margins in radical prostatectomy specimens. One is that the surgeon may inadvertently cut into the prostate, which has been termed "capsular incision." This may occur in the region of the neurovascular bundle, where the surgeon may attempt to preserve the bundle and cut too close and into the prostate. Although this occasionally occurs, there is also a tendency for pathologists to "over-call" capsular incision. Prostate cancer that extends out of the prostate into periprostatic soft tissue induces a desmoplastic stromal response so that extraprostatic tumor is often embedded in fibrous tissue. However, to render the diagnosis of capsular penetration, many pathologists require that tumor be present in adipose tissue. Therefore, when a positive margin occurs in the setting of capsular penetration, the lesion may be misdiagnosed as organ-confined cancer with positive margins (capsular incision).

The other explanation for positive margins is that the surgeon did not go wide enough around the gland in certain areas. By sacrificing the neurovascular bundle, an additional several millimeters of soft tissue may be removed with the gland. As described above, it is uncommon for a patient to have a positive margin solely as a result of the anatomic approach to radical prostatectomy.

The other explanation is that the tumors are so extensive and/or high grade that the tumor, rather than the surgery, dictates the positive margins. Although in some cases this is true, many tumors that are relatively low grade or limited still have positive margins.

The final explanation for positive margins is, we believe, one of the most frequent. Because the prostate is surrounded by vital structures, there is a limit to what the urologist can remove in certain sites—posteriorly, up against the rectum; laterally, against the pelvic sidewall; and apically, at the urogenital diaphragm. In these areas small amounts of tumor just reaching the inked edge of the gland are not uncommon. Although one cannot ascertain with certainty how much tumor is on the other side of the ink left within the patient, in many cases it appears that, had only a small amount of additional soft tissue been removed, the margins might have been negative. Unfortunately, in many sites this additional soft tissue cannot be removed without causing significant morbidity.

Prognostic Significance of Margin Status

Figure 12–9 reflects data on 617 men with negative seminal vesicles and negative lymph nodes with mean follow-up of 6.5 years. The difference in progression between patients with negative and positive margins was highly significant (p<.0001). The low progression rate in patients with negative margins of resection is consistent with our earlier study, in which we found that close margins of resection in the region of the neurovascular bundle were not associated with residual tumor left within the patient.[31] This earlier report and a more recent study support conservative assessment of capsule margins of resection when the

tumor extends close to the inked edge of the gland but does not appear to be cut across.[37]

Discrepancies Between Positive Margins and Progression

Only 45% of patients with positive margins exhibit disease progression 10 years after prostatectomy (see Table 12–1). There are several possible explanations for this phenomenon. First, it could be that, with longer follow-up, most of these patients demonstrate progression; however, because after radical prostatectomy an elevated serum PSA level is such a sensitive indicator of residual tumor, one would anticipate that if residual tumor were left at the time of surgery most cases would be detectable serologically 10 years later.

A second explanation is that in a sizable number of cases, despite the margins' being called positive by the pathologist, no residual tumor is left in the patient. The potential for an artifactually positive margin in radical prostatectomy specimens is great, given the flimsy amount of periprostatic soft tissue surrounding the prostate, which may be easily disrupted either intraoperatively or postoperatively in the handling of the specimen. Support for this theory again comes from our study, in which we analyzed prostate margins of resection in the region of the neurovascular bundle and compared them with additional soft tissue removed from this area. Of the 10 prostates in which the margins of resection were thought to be positive in the region of the neurovascular bundle, 6 (60%) showed residual tumor in the separately resected neurovascular bundle specimen.[31]

Another explanation for histologically positive margins in patients whose disease did not recur is that these were truly positive margins where only a few neoplastic glands reached the inked cut surface but the postoperative granulation tissue and local ischemia destroyed the few tumor cells left in the patient.

TUMOR VOLUME

Accurate measurement of tumor volume is technically much more difficult in the prostate than in most other organ systems. Other tumors such as breast or lung cancers tend to be roughly spherical. In other organs tumor can readily be distinguished from surrounding

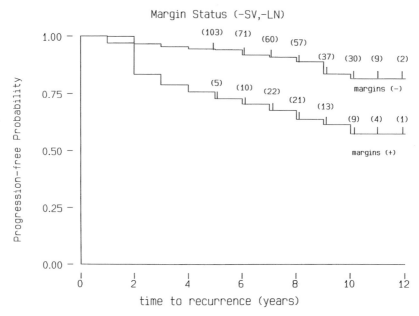

Figure 12–9. Relation of margins to progression.

benign tissue on gross examination. One can therefore easily and accurately measure the maximum diameter of the tumor and calculate the tumor volume based on the gross appearance of the tumor. In contrast, prostate cancers are macroscopically often difficult to delineate from surrounding benign prostate tissue. Even when a prostate tumor is grossly visible its volume is consistently underestimated as compared with volumes determined by microscopic examination. Given the problems of recognizing macroscopic tumor, studies calculating tumor volume on "subtotally submitted prostates" are potentially flawed. In addition, prostate cancers assume a multitude of irregular shapes that do not conform to any known geometric configuration. Consequently, calculations of tumor volume based on the anteroposterior, transverse, and cephalocaudal dimensions of the tumor do not correlate well with actual tumor volume measurements. Previous investigations of prostate cancer tumor volume have in general studied totally submitted prostates whose tumor volume was determined by computer-assisted calculation.[14, 38] Because of the difficulties in accurately quantifying prostate cancer tumor volume as previously mentioned, only a few institutions have actively investigated tumor volume as it relates to prognosis for prostate cancer.

Tumor volume has been shown to be pro-

portional to Gleason grade, capsular penetration, seminal vesicle invasion, lymph node metastases, and capsular margins of resection.[39] While Gleason grade, pathologic stage, and margins of resection are associated with more aggressive tumors, prognosis is measured more directly by long-term follow-up studies. Tumor volume, Gleason grade, pathologic stage, and margins of resection are interrelated variables, so it becomes critical to determine which one provides independent prediction of prognosis of prostate cancer.

The only study to address this issue evaluated 185 men following radical prostatectomy for stage T2 disease in which patients either were free of disease at 5 years or experienced progression.[40] Because tumors with positive lymph nodes or seminal vesicles almost invariably have progressed 5 years after surgery, these are not cases in which one would look for tumor volume to provide predictive information.[1] Consequently, this study analyzed only cases with negative pelvic lymph nodes and seminal vesicles. The distribution of tumor volume according to progression, illustrated in Figure 12–10, shows significant overlap between those with and without progression. In a stepwise regression analysis, tumor volume did not provide independent prognostic information beyond that provided by Gleason score and surgical margins. Once Gleason score and margins of resection were

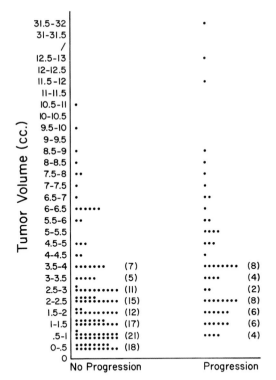

Figure 12–10. Distribution of tumor volume in cases according to presence or absence of tumor progression. (From Epstein JI, Carmichael M, Partin AW, et al.: Is tumor volume an independent predictor of progression following radical prostatectomy? A multivariate analysis of 185 clinical stage B adenocarcinomas of the prostate with 5 years followup. J Urol 149:1478–1481, 1993.)

accounted for, tumor volume was not helpful in further predicting progression after radical prostatectomy. Because an accurate assessment of Gleason score and margins of resection can be performed using a sampling technique, it is not necessary, for clinical purposes, to submit the entire prostate and calculate the tumor volume.[41] A semiquantitative assessment of tumor volume should be part of the pathologic assessment of radical prostatectomy specimens. In particular, tumor volume at either extreme should be commented on. As more radical prostatectomies are being performed for tumor detected by screening techniques, we are noting an increased percentage of small tumors removed by radical prostatectomy.[7, 42] Small low- to intermediate-grade tumors confined to the prostate are undoubtedly cured by the procedure. In these cases, the presence of minimal tumor volume (approximately 0.5 ml or less) should be conveyed to the urologist. At the other extreme, cases with extensive

tumor throughout the prostate should also be noted. For the remaining cases, moderate amounts of tumor may be reported.

Tumor volume has also been studied in patients with adenocarcinoma of the prostate discovered incidentally on TURP. It has been shown that the relationship between tumor volume and both grade and pathologic stage is weaker in these cancers than in palpable prostate cancer.[8] Cancers found on TURP often arise centrally and anteriorly, where they may grow large before extending out of the prostate. In addition, TURP cancers are disproportionately of lower grade; again, large tumor volume does not necessarily translate into aggressive tumors. Accordingly, tumor volume calculations for cancers discovered on TURP most likely would be even less predictive of tumor progression after radical prostatectomy than they are for palpable prostate cancer.

PREDICTION OF PROGRESSION USING A COMBINATION OF GRADE, MARGINS, AND CAPSULAR PENETRATION

Gleason grade, margins of resection, and capsular penetration are interrelated variables. For example, high-grade tumors commonly show capsular penetration, and capsular penetration is frequently associated with positive margins. Consequently, it is important to determine which variables are independent predictors of progression. If there are multiple independent predictors of progression, can these variables be combined in such a way to provide an accurate risk of progression to the individual patient? In multivariate analysis on 617 men with a minimum of 5-year follow-up and negative seminal vesicles and lymph nodes, Gleason grade, capsular penetration, and surgical margins were all highly significant. Gleason score was the most predictive ($p < .0001$), and capsular penetration ($p = .007$) and surgical margins ($p = .004$) added significant prognostic information to the model. The overall model combining all of these variables to predict progression was significant at a P value of .00001.[4]

Only 7% of patients have Gleason scores of 2 to 4 in the radical prostatectomy specimen. As Figure 12–2 shows, these patients have a uniformly excellent prognosis. All of these patients have organ-confined tumor with nega-

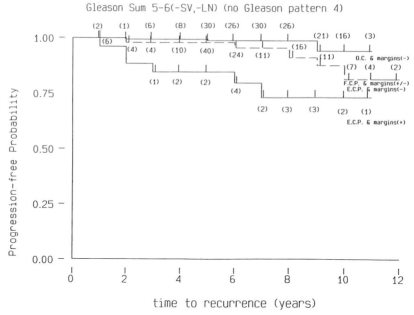

Figure 12–11. Correlation of capsular penetration and margins with progression in men with Gleason sum 5–6 tumors and negative seminal vesicles and lymph nodes.

tive margins. On the other hand, only 5% of patients with negative seminal vesicles and negative lymph nodes have Gleason 8 or 9 tumors. These patients have a poor outcome (see Fig. 12–2): 86% have capsular penetration and 55%, positive margins. Consequently, for these two smaller subgroups the grade is so dominant that a model employing capsular penetration and margins of resection is not as critical.

Table 12–2. Postoperative Risk of Progression in Gleason Sum 5 to 7 Tumors with Negative Seminal Vesicles and Negative Lymph Nodes

Findings at Radical Prostatectomy	Progression-free Risk (%)	
	5-Year	10-Year
Gleason sum 5–6 (OC, MAR−)*	98.7	92.4
Gleason sum 5–6 (FCP, MAR+/−) or (ECP, MAR−)*	97.9	77.2
Gleason sum 5–6 (ECP, MAR+)*	84.5	71.7
Gleason sum 7 (OC, MAR−)	96.6	67.6
Gleason sum 7 (FCP, MAR+/−) or (ECP, MAR−)	82.8	47.9
Gleason sum 7 (ECP, MAR+)	50.0	41.6

*Excluding tumors with Gleason pattern 4.
Key: OC, organ-confined; FCP, focal capsular penetration; ECP, established capsular penetration; MAR−, margins negative; MAR+, margins positive; MAR+/−, margins positive or negative.

In the largest groups of patients, those with Gleason 5 to 7 scores, we have been able to stratify them further based on the status of the margins and on capsular penetration. Men with Gleason tumor sums of 5 or 6 with negative seminal vesicles and negative lymph nodes and no Gleason pattern 4 tumor could be stratified into three groups with different progression curves (Fig. 12–11; Table 12–2). Group 1 consists of 156 men with organ-confined tumors and negative surgical margins. These patients almost invariably are progression free after 10 years. Group 2 consists of 157 men with focal capsular penetration (margins positive or negative) and patients with established capsular penetration and negative surgical margins. The 23 men in group 3 with the worst prognosis had both established capsular penetration and positive surgical margins. These three curves in Figure 12–11 are parallel and appear to be plateauing past 7 years, so with even longer follow-up the differences between these curves should be maintained. We then analyzed men with Gleason score 7 tumors and negative seminal vesicles and negative lymph nodes. As Figure 12–12 shows, one could also stratify progression into the same three groups (see Table 12–2). The number of men in the three groups, from best prognosis to worst, were 32, 119, and 51, respectively.

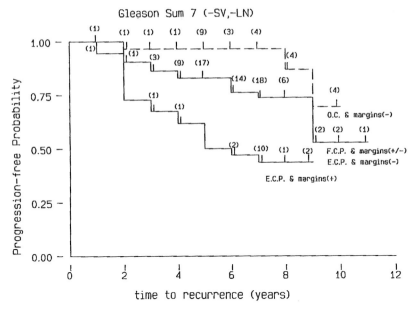

Figure 12–12. Correlation of capsular penetration and margins with progression in men with Gleason sum 7 tumors and negative seminal vesicles and lymph nodes.

For cases with Gleason score 7 tumor, the curves in Figure 12–11 appear to be converging after 7 years; however, relatively few men with this grade are followed beyond 7 years. It is necessary to follow a larger number of men longer to see whether the high-grade tumor dictates the adverse prognosis regardless of margin and capular penetration status or whether the early differences in prognosis persist over time.

A somewhat surprising finding was the virtually identical progression rates for cancers with focal capsular penetration, regardless of whether capsular margins were positive or negative. There are two potential explanations for this disparity. First, many of the margins designated as positive in patients with focal capsular penetration represent artifactually positive margins. Cases with focal capsular penetration appear to the urologist to be organ confined, and less soft tissue may be removed with the prostate, especially around the neurovascular bundle, in an attempt to preserve potency. This minimal extraprostatic soft tissue is easily disrupted, and this may lead to false-positive margins.[31] The other explanation is that tumors with focal capsular penetration are inherently less aggressive, so that, even if tumor is focally cut across by the surgeon, there may be little potential for tumor regrowth.

CLINICAL SIGNIFICANCE OF ISOLATED ELEVATION OF SERUM PROSTATE-SPECIFIC ANTIGEN FOLLOWING RADICAL PROSTATECTOMY

Recognizing that some men with isolated elevation of serum PSA after surgery harbor occult local tumor, one might expect radiation therapy to the prostatic bed to eliminate the tumor cells and render some men disease free. Thus, a method for distinguishing local recurrence from distant metastases for men with isolated elevations of serum PSA only after surgery would be very useful clinically. We recently followed a group of men expectantly without therapy until there was evidence of clinical recurrence.[43] Of 51 such men, local recurrence occurred in 16 and distant metastases in 35. A combination of Gleason score within the radical prostatectomy specimen, pathologic stage, and PSA "velocity" (rate of change of PSA) 1 year after surgery best predicted the likelihood that postoperative isolated elevation of serum PSA represents local recurrence. Figure 12–13 demonstrates the probability of local recurrence for men with elevated PSA following radical prostatectomy. These men had negative seminal vesicles and negative lymph nodes. With higher-grade tu-

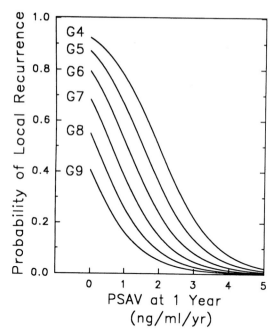

Figure 12–13. Prediction of local recurrence in men with negative seminal vesicles and negative lymph nodes who have elevated postoperative serum PSA values after radical prostatectomy. Parameters include prostatectomy Gleason sum and PSA velocity 1 year after surgery.

mor and increased PSA velocity at 1 year, the probability of local recurrence is lower and the risk of distant metastases correspondingly higher.

MARGIN STATUS AND POSTOPERATIVE ADJUVANT THERAPY

Based on the aforementioned findings, a rational strategy can be developed as to whether to administer postoperative adjuvant therapy in men whose tumors are likely to progress following radical prostatectomy. Whether capsular margins are positive or negative should not influence the decision to administer postoperative therapy for tumors with focal capsular penetration. The following groups are at very low risk of progression, and it is difficult to justify adjuvant therapy: (1) Gleason 2 to 4 tumors; (2) Gleason 5 or 6 tumors with organ-confined disease; (3) Gleason 5 or 6 tumors with focal capsular penetration (margins positive or negative); and (4) Gleason 5 or 6 tumors with established capsular penetration and negative surgical margins.

Approximately 50% of patients with Gleason score 7 non–organ-confined tumor progress 10 years after radical prostatectomy. For this group, postoperative adjuvant therapy might be recommended. Longer follow-up is needed to determine whether those with Gleason score 7 organ-confined tumor may fare better and may not need adjuvant therapy. The dismal prognosis for men with positive seminal vesicles or positive lymph nodes or Gleason score 8 or 9 is presumed to be due to distant failure, so local adjuvant therapy would be of no benefit.

SUMMARY

At first appraisal radical prostatectomy does not seem to be such an effective method of treating clinically localized prostate cancer; approximately 50% of men experience progression 10 years after surgery. However, to date, the vast majority of these patients have manifested recurrence solely by elevated serum PSA level. It is not clear whether isolated elevations in serum PSA represent local tumor recurrence or occult distant metastases. Serum PSA levels may indicate small foci of residual tumor in the region of the prostatectomy; however, given prostate cancer's relatively indolent growth, these small foci may be totally silent clinically. The key issue is not whether these patients are experiencing biochemical failure after radical prostatectomy but whether biochemical failure progresses to clinical failure over the lifetime of the patients. Long-term follow-up of patients with elevated serum PSA levels without the confounding effect of adjuvant therapy is critical to evaluate the long-term efficacy of radical prostatectomy for adenocarcinoma of the prostate.

REFERENCES

1. Epstein JI, Pizov G, Walsh PC: Correlation of pathologic findings with progression following radical prostatectomy. Cancer 71:3582–3593, 1993.
2. Morton RA, Steiner MS, Walsh PC: Cancer control following anatomical radical prostatectomy: An interim report. J Urol 146:1197–1200, 1991.
3. Partin AW, Pound CR, Clemens JQ, et al.: Serum PSA after anatomic radical prostatectomy: The Johns Hopkins experience after 10 years. Urol Clin North Am 20:713–725, 1993.
4. Epstein JI, Partin AW, Sauvageot J, et al.: Prediction of progression following radical prostatectomy: A mul-

tivariate analysis of 721 men with long-term follow-up. Am J Surg Pathol 20:286–292, 1996.

5. Oesterling JE: Prostate specific antigen: A critical assessment of the most useful tumor marker for adenocarcinoma of the prostate. J Urol 145:907–923, 1991.

6. Lightener DJ, Lange PH, Reddy PK, et al.: Prostate specific antigen and local recurrence after radical prostatectomy. J Urol 144:921–926, 1990.

7. Epstein JI, Brendler CB, Carmichael M, et al.: Pathological and clinical findings to predict tumor extent of non-palpable (stage T1c) prostate cancer. JAMA 271:368–374, 1994.

8. Larsen MP, Carter HB, Epstein JI: Can stage A1 tumor extent be predicted by transurethral resection tumor volume, per cent, or grade? A study of 64 stage A1 radical prostatectomies with comparison to prostates removed for stage A2 and B disease. J Urol 146:1059–1063, 1991.

9. Christensen WN, Partin AW, Walsh PC, et al: Pathologic findings in clinical stage A2 prostate cancer: Relation of tumor volume, grade, and location to pathologic stage. Cancer 65:1021–1027, 1990.

10. Epstein JI, Carmichael M, Walsh, PC: Adenocarcinoma of the prostate invading the seminal vesicle: Definition and relation of tumor volume, grade, and margins of resection to prognosis. J Urol 149: 1040–1045, 1993.

11. Villers AA, McNeal JE, Redwine EA, et al.: Pathogenesis and biological significance of seminal vesicle invasion in prostatic adenocarcinoma. J Urol 143:1183–1187, 1990.

12. Ayala AG, Ro JY, Babaian R, et al.: The prostatic capsule: Does it exist? Its importance in the staging and treatment of prostatic carcinoma. Am J Surg Pathol 13:21–27, 1989.

13. Epstein JI: The evaluation of radical prostatectomy specimens performed for carcinoma of the prostate. Therapeutic and prognostic implications. Pathol Ann 26(1):159–210, 1991.

14. Stamey TA, McNeal JE, Freiha FS, et al.: Morphometric and clinical studies on 68 consecutive radical prostatectomies. J Urol 139:1235–1241, 1988.

15. Oesterling JE, Brendler CB, Epstein JI, et al.: Correlation of clinical stage, serum prostatic acid phosphatase, and preoperative Gleason grade with final pathologic stage in 275 patients with clinically localized adenocarcinoma of the prostate. J Urol 138:92–98, 1987.

16. Fowler JE, Mills SE: Operable prostatic carcinoma: Correlations among clinical stage, pathological stage, Gleason histological score, and early disease-free survival. J Urol 133:49–52, 1985.

17. Villers A, McNeal JE, Redwine EA, et al.: The role of perineural space invasion in the local spread of prostatic adenocarcinoma. J Urol 142:763–768, 1989.

18. Hassan MO, Maksem J: The prostatic perineural space and its relation to tumor spread. Am J Surg Pathol 4:143–148, 1980.

19. McNeal JE, Villers AA, Redwine EA, et al.: Capsular penetration in prostate cancer: Significance for natural history and treatment. Am J Surg Pathol 14:240–247, 1990.

20. Schellhammer PF: Radical prostatectomy: Patterns of local failure and survival in 67 patients. Urology 31:191–197, 1988.

21. Paulson DF, Moul JW, Walther PJ: Radical prostatectomy for clinical stage T1-2N0M0 prostatic adenocarcinoma: Long-term results. J Urol 144:1180–1184, 1990.

22. Stein A, DeKernion JB, Smith RB, et al.: Prostate specific antigen levels after radical prostatectomy in patients with organ confined and locally extensive prostate cancer. J Urol 147:942–946, 1992.

23. Epstein JI, Carmichael M, Pizov G, et al.: Influence of capsular penetration on progression following radical prostatectomy: A study of 196 cases with long-term follow-up. J Urol 150:135–141, 1993.

24. Martin AW, Borland RN, Epstein JI, et. al.: Impact of capsular penetration on prognosis in men with clinically localized prostate cancer. J Urol 150:142–148, 1993.

25. Walsh PC, Lepor H, Eggleston JC: Radical prostatectomy with preservation of sexual function: Anatomical and pathological considerations. Prostate 4:473–485, 1983.

26. Eggleston JC, Walsh PC: Radical prostatectomy with preservation of sexual function: Pathological findings in the first 100 cases. J Urol 134:1146–1148, 1985.

27. Anscher MS, Prosnitz LR: Post-operative radiotherapy for patients with carcinoma of the prostate undergoing radical prostatectomy with positive surgical margin, seminal vesicle involvement and/or penetration through the capsule. J Urol 138:1407–1412, 1987.

28. Gibbons RP, Cole BS, Richardson RG, et al.: Adjuvant radiotherapy following radical prostatectomy: Results and complications. J Urol 135:65–68, 1986.

29. Pilepich MV, Walz BJ, Baglan RJ: Post-operative irradiation in carcinoma of the prostate. Int J Radiat Oncol Biol Phys 10:1869–1873, 1984.

30. Lepor H, Gregerman M, Crosby R, et al.: Precise localization of the autonomic nerves from the pelvic plexus to the corpora cavernosa: A detailed anatomical study of the adult male pelvis. J Urol 133:207–212, 1985.

31. Epstein JI: Evaluation of radical prostatectomy capsular margins of resection: The significance of margins designated as negative, closely approaching, and positive. Am J Surg Pathol 14:626–632, 1990.

32. Stamey TA, Viller AA, McNeal JE, et al.: Positive surgical margins at radical prostatectomy: Importance of the apical dissection. J Urol 143:1166–1173, 1990.

33. Catalona WJ, Bigg SW: Nerve-sparing radical prostatectomy: Evaluation of results after 250 patients. J Urol 143:538–544, 1990.

34. Jones EC: Resection margin status in radical retropubic prostatectomy specimens: Relationship to type of operation, tumor size, tumor grade and local tumor extension. J Urol 144:89–93, 1990.

35. Rosen MA, Goldstone L, Lapin S, et al.: Frequency and location of extracapsular extension and positive surgical margins in radical prostatectomy specimens. J Urol 148:331–337, 1992.

36. Killeen KP, Libertino JA, Sughayer MA, et al.: Pathologic review of consecutive radical prostatectomy specimens: Nerve sparing versus nonnerve sparing. Urology 38:212–215, 1991.

37. Epstein JI, Sauvageot J: Do close but negative margins in radical prostatectomy specimens increase the risk of postoperative progression? J Urol 157:241–243, 1997.

38. Partin AW, Epstein JI, Cho KR, et al.: Morphometric measurement of tumor volume and per cent of gland involvement as predictors of pathological stage in clinical stage B prostate cancer. J Urol 141:341–345, 1989.

39. McNeal JE: Cancer volume and site of origin of adeno-

carcinoma in the prostate: Relationship to local and distant spread. Hum Pathol 23:258–266, 1992.

40. Epstein JI, Carmichael M, Partin AW, et al.: Is tumor volume an independent predictor of progression following radical prostatectomy? A multivariate analysis of 185 clinical stage B adenocarcinomas of the prostate with 5 years followup. J Urol 149:1478–1481, 1993.

41. Hall GS, Kramer CE, Epstein JI: Evaluation of radical prostatectomy specimens: A comparative analysis of various sampling methods. Am J Surg Pathol 16:315–324, 1992.

42. DiGiuseppe JA, Sauvageot J, Epstein JI: Increasing incidence of minimal residual cancer in radical prostatectomy specimens. Am J Surg Pathol 21:174–178, 1997.

43. Partin AW, Pearson JD, et al.: Evaluation of serum-prostate specific antigen velocity after radical prostatectomy to distinguish local recurrence from distant metastases. Urology 43:649–659, 1994.

13

HISTOLOGIC FEATURES OF METASTATIC PROSTATE CANCER

PETER N. BRAWN

The histologic features of metastatic prostate carcinoma were discussed by this author in a symposium.[1] A short summary follows:

1. Carcinoma of the prostate usually begins as a small, well-differentiated lesion. Some prostate cancers remain small and well-differentiated; others increase in size and dedifferentiate into moderately or poorly differentiated lesions.

2. Prostate cancers that remain small and well-differentiated rarely metastasize. They usually do not metastasize until they have grown to at least 1 cm^3 and have dedifferentiated into moderately or poorly differentiated carcinoma.

3. The initial metastases from prostatic carcinomas are usually moderately differentiated; fewer are poorly differentiated. Very few metastases are well-differentiated.

4. Metastases are usually found first in regional lymph nodes or bone. Widespread metastases (beyond lymph node and bone) usually originate from other metastases, not from the primary tumor.

5. The histologic appearance of metastases in staging lymphadenectomies has prognostic significance; patients with moderately differentiated metastases have 5- and 10-year survival rates of 79% and 34%, respectively, whereas those with poorly differentiated metastases have 5- and 10-year rates of 13% and 0%.

6. Metastases disseminate as they dedifferentiate. Most initial metastases are moderately differentiated; however, as the metastases dedifferentiate into undifferentiated (non–gland-forming) patterns they disseminate. Rapid dedifferentiation is associated with rapid dissemination and vice versa.

7. "Prostate-specific" immunohistochemical techniques such as prostate-specific antigen (PSA) and prostate-specific acid phosphatase (PAP) are often helpful in determining whether metastases are from the prostate; however, these techniques should be evaluated with appropriate caution since interpretation is subjective and the techniques are not 100% specific or 100% sensitive for prostatic carcinoma.

8. Metastases of unknown origin should rarely, if ever, be attributed to the prostate solely on the basis of immunohistochemical findings or serum PSA levels without confirmation that the patient has prostate cancer with histologic features capable of metastasizing.

In this chapter prostate cancer refers to prostatic adenocarcinoma, which may be either differentiated or undifferentiated, as defined by Mostofi[2]; that is, differentiated prostate cancer forms glands while undifferentiated prostate cancer does not. Furthermore, prostatic adenocarcinoma is considered to consist of three prognostically significant grades: well-differentiated, moderately differentiated, and poorly differentiated. The three grades are defined using a slight modification of the M.D. Anderson Cancer Center Grading System. Well-differentiated prostatic adenocarcinoma is composed of 75% to 100% single, separate, malignant glands. Poorly differentiated cancers are 75% to 100% *un*differentiated (non–gland-forming). All other patterns are moderately differentiated. Patterns that appear to be borderline between well-differentiated and moderately differentiated or borderline between poorly differentiated and moderately differentiated are classified as moderately differentiated to maintain the distinctive prognostic significance of well-differentiated and poorly differentiated prostate cancers.

IS IT IMPORTANT TO DETERMINE WHETHER METASTASES ARE FROM THE PROSTATE?

Yes. The correct identification of the source of metastases may determine the effectiveness of therapeutic intervention. For example, hormone therapy may afford patients with disseminated metastatic prostate carcinoma dramatic symptomatic relief. On the other hand, hormone therapy may have adverse side effects and no therapeutic benefit if the metastases are not from the prostate. Finally, even if no therapy is capable of interrupting the course of the disease, each patient deserves our best assessment of the extent of his disease.

WHICH HISTOLOGIC PATTERNS OF PROSTATE CARCINOMA ARE CAPABLE OF METASTASIZING?

There are three histologic patterns of prostatic adenocarcinoma: (1) single, separate malignant glands; (2) cribriform/papillary or fused glands; and (3) undifferentiated (non–gland-forming). Most prostate cancers begin as single, separate malignant glands, and such glands rarely metastasize. With time, however, some cancers increase in size and dedifferentiate into cribriform/papillary glands, fused glands, or undifferentiated morphologies— all of which have metastatic potential. I consider all prostate tissue with cribriform/papillary glands, fused glands, or undifferentiated cancer as being capable of metastasizing. In all probability, a significant amount (perhaps 25%) of the primary tumor must consist of

these histologic patterns before metastases are likely; however since prostate biopsies are subject to sampling error the identification of cribriform/papillary glands, fused glands, or undifferentiated cancer is the only requirement for documenting metastatic potential.

WHICH STAGES OF PROSTATE CARCINOMA ARE CAPABLE OF METASTASIZING?

Presumably all prostatic adenocarcinomas begin as "latent," or clinically undetectable, (stage A). A few of these cancers progress to stage B, C, or D, although the majority do not. Stage D prostate cancer, by definition, has metastases and stages B and C may have undetected metastases. Very few stage A prostate cancers have undetected metastases. The idea that stage A carcinoma rarely metastasizes is supported by a study of more than 200 autopsies that included 79 latent prostate cancers. Since, after gross and microscopic examination of regional lymph nodes, none of these latent cancers were found to have metastases, it is doubtful that many patients with a normal prostate on digital examination have unsuspected metastases.[3]

WHAT IS THE LIKELIHOOD THAT STAGE A1 PROSTATE CARCINOMA WILL EVER METASTASIZE?

A study compared long-term survival (up to 20 years) of patients with histologically proven benign hyperplasia, atypical hyperplasia/adenosis, stage A1 prostate cancer, and stage A2 prostate cancer.[4] Stage A1 cancer was defined as well-differentiated, regardless of amount, found unexpectedly in transurethral resection (TURP) specimens. Stage A2 was defined as moderately or poorly differentiated, regardless of amount, found unexpectedly at TURP. Survival of patients with histologically proven benign hyperplasia, atypical hyperplasia/adenosis, and stage A1 prostate cancer was almost identical, whereas stage A2 tumors had a worse prognosis (Fig. 13–1). The reason for the first 3 groups' similar survivals is probably threefold. First, few patients with Stage A1 cancers develop metastatic disease. Second, patients with benign hyperplasia or atypical hyperplasia/adenosis are not without risk of developing metastatic cancer (i.e., they may have

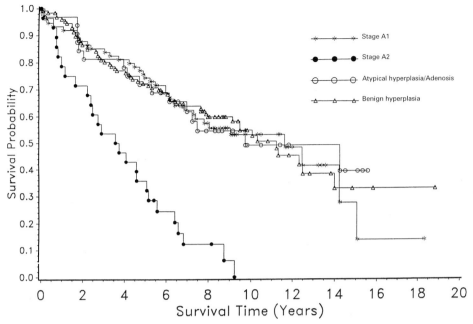

Figure 13–1. Survival of patients with stage A1 prostate cancer, stage A2 prostate cancer, atypical hyperplasia/adenosis, and histologically proven benign hyperplasia. All patients were from a single medical center. (From Brawn PN, Johnson EH, Speights VO, et al.: Long-term survival of Stage A prostate carcinoma, atypical hyperplasia/adenosis and BPH. Br J Cancer 69:1098–1101, 1994.)

undetected prostate cancer at the time of TURP or they may develop cancer after the transurethral resection). Third, our present understanding of well-differentiated prostate cancer may include lesions more properly classified as dysplastic, that is, rather than invariably progressing and, given time, metastasizing, some well-differentiated prostate cancers may be stable lesions or occasionally regress.

WHAT IS THE HISTOLOGIC APPEARANCE OF THE INITIAL METASTASES FROM PROSTATE CARCINOMA?

The initial metastases from prostatic adenocarcinoma usually have a cribriform/papillary or fused gland pattern (Fig. 13–2). Foci of single, separate malignant glands may be present but are rarely the predominant pattern. Undifferentiated patterns are often present but, again, are not usually the predominant pattern. If the metastases are predominantly undifferentiated it is likely the patient already has disseminated, rather than regional, metastases.

WHAT IS THE HISTOLOGIC APPEARANCE OF WIDELY DISSEMINATED METASTATIC PROSTATE CARCINOMA?

Metastases dedifferentiate with time.[5] As they dedifferentiate from cribriform/papillary or fused glands into undifferentiated carcinoma the metastases disseminate. With widespread dissemination, undifferentiated histologic patterns often predominate and only foci of residual cribriform/papillary patterns remain (Fig. 13–3). Some widely disseminated metastases are completely undifferentiated, and it is virtually impossible on histologic grounds alone to determine whether the metastases are from the prostate (Fig. 13–4).

WHAT ARE THE HISTOLOGIC FEATURES OF "OCCULT" PROSTATE CARCINOMA?

Occult prostatic adenocarcinoma refers to those cancers in which metastases are diagnosed before the primary tumor has been identified. Although many metastatic sites have been reported, the most common sites of occult pros-

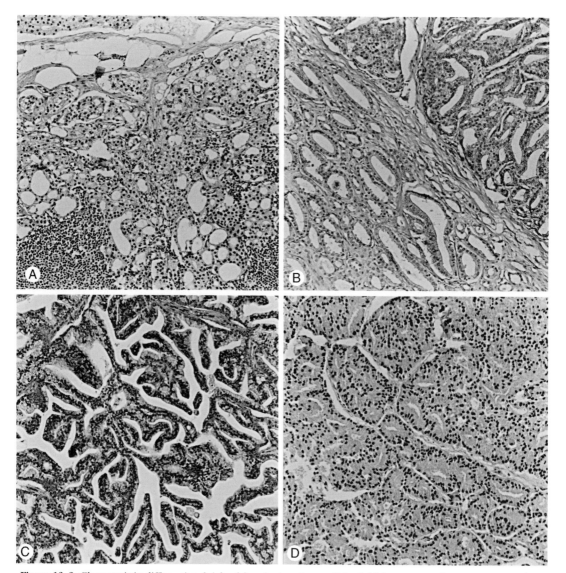

Figure 13–2. Characteristic differentiated (gland-forming) patterns of the initial metastases from prostate carcinoma. *A,* Cribriform patterns. *B,* Single, separate glands (lower left) may be present but are rarely the predominant pattern. *C,* Cribriform/papillary patterns. *D,* Fused glands. As these metastases dedifferentiate into undifferentiated (non–gland-forming) patterns they disseminate. (H&E ×100.)

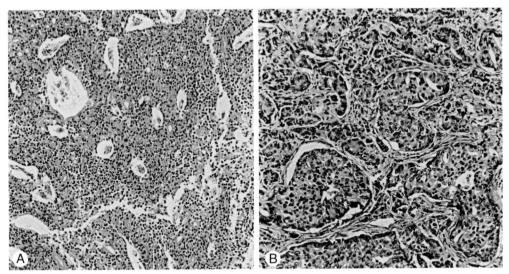

Figure 13–3. *A*, Metastases with residual glandular patterns. These are characteristic of metastases that have dissemin-ated. *B*, With time, these metastases continue to dedifferentiate into completely undifferentiated (non–gland-forming) patterns and become more widely disseminated. (H&E ×100.)

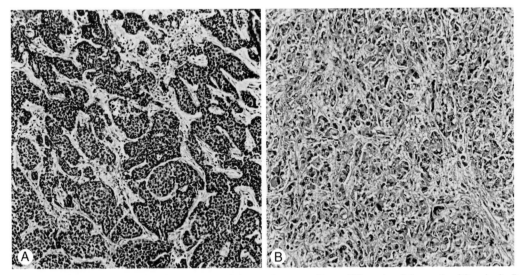

Figure 13–4. *A*, Widely disseminated metastases often are almost totally undifferentiated (non–gland-forming). *B*, On histologic grounds alone, it is often impossible to identify these metastases as being from the prostate. (H&E ×100.)

tate cancer are cervical lymph nodes and bone.[6, 7] Affected patients usually have an abnormal prostate on digital examination, and the metastases are detected before the primary tumor only because the prostate had not been adequately examined.

Patients with occult metastases usually do not have widely disseminated or terminal metastases. If they did, their survival would be measured in months rather than the observed years. Although occult metastases usually are not widely disseminated, the patient probably has other metastases—to regional lymph nodes or bone.

Occult tumors usually have a predominantly cribriform/papillary appearance, similar to that of the initial metastases from prostate cancer. There may be fewer single, separate malignant glands and more undifferentiated cancer than in metastases limited to regional lymph nodes, but a cribriform/papillary pattern is almost always identifiable.

DO METASTASES RESEMBLE THE PRIMARY TUMOR?

The primary tumor usually has more histologic heterogeneity than the metastases, and the metastases do not always resemble the least differentiated areas of the primary tumor. For example, the primary tumor may be largely undifferentiated, but the metastases may be primarily cribriform/papillary. Furthermore, the metastases may vary in appearance from metastatic site to metastatic site, one site being cribriform/papillary and another undifferentiated.

HOW DOES ONE DETERMINE WHETHER METASTASES OF UNKNOWN ORIGIN ARE FROM THE PROSTATE?

First and foremost, it must be ascertained that the patient has histologically proven prostate cancer. If prostate biopsy shows well-differentiated prostatic adenocarcinoma (which rarely metastasizes), the patient could still have metastases (i.e., the biopsy specimen may represent sampling errors, or the prostate may have been biopsied years earlier and the tumor has subsequently dedifferentiated into moderately or poorly differentiated disease).

Second, if the patient does not have histo-logically proven prostate cancer an examination of the prostate and biopsy of abnormal areas is necessary. If the prostate does not have abnormal areas but there is great clinical suspicion that the metastases are from the prostate, blind biopsy of the prostate should be considered. Metastases of unknown origin should not be attributed to the prostate if specimens of the prostate are negative.

Last, if the metastases are histologically characteristic of metastatic prostatic malignancy and the patient has histologically proven prostate cancer, metastatic prostatic adenocarcinoma is likely, even if the primary tumor appears to be well-differentiated (see above). If the patient has histologically proven prostate cancer and there is a high degree of clinical suspicion that the metastases are from the prostate although they are not characteristic of prostate cancer, additional studies may be helpful (see following sections).

ARE IMMUNOHISTOCHEMICAL TECHNIQUES HELPFUL IN IDENTIFYING PROSTATE METASTASES?

These techniques refer to prostate-specific stains such as PSA and PAP. (For a more complete discussion of these techniques the reader is referred to Chapter 15.) The techniques may be invaluable in identifying metastases of unknown origin, especially when the tissue volume from the metastases is limited or when the metastases are completely undifferentiated and not recognizable as metastatic prostatic adenocarcinoma. Unfortunately these techniques more often yield strongly positive results with moderately differentiated metastases than with poorly differentiated ones. This is unfortunate because it is often possible to identify moderately differentiated metastases as being of prostatic origin without additional studies whereas identifying poorly differentiated metastases without additional studies may be difficult.

Limitations to immunohistochemical techniques are the possibility that hormone therapy, including orchiectomy, and possibly antiandrogen therapy, may interfere with the intensity of a positive stain.[8, 9] Furthermore, equivocal or faintly positive staining should be interpreted with caution because these stains may be the result of faulty staining procedures or be over- or underinterpretted by pathologists who have already decided whether the prostate is or is not the source of the metastases. The limitations of immunohistochemical techniques have been recognized by reviewing bodies (Food and Drug Administration in the United States, for example), who have not categorized any immunohistochemical technique as diagnostic. Elgamal and associates have demonstrated a consistently positive reaction for PSA and prostatic acid phosphatase using immunohistochemical techniques in ductal cells of normal pancreas and normal salivary glands, as well as pleomorphic adenoma, adenocarcinoma, and all oncocytic epithelial cells of Warthin's tumor. Further studies will undoubtedly identify additional tissues far from the prostate that react positively for PSA and prostatic acid phosphatase.[10] Finally, an immunohistochemical stain thought to be characteristic of another tumor should not be interpreted as ruling out the prostate as the source of the metastases unless it has been demonstrated that the stain is never positive in prostate carcinoma.

ARE PROSTATE-SPECIFIC ANTIGEN LEVELS HELPFUL IN IDENTIFYING METASTASES OF UNKNOWN ORIGIN?

Elevated—even markedly elevated—serum PSA levels occur in numerous clinical settings and are not diagnostic of metastatic prostate cancer.[11] Elevated serum PSA levels may be used as supporting evidence that metastases are from the prostate but should rarely be used as the only evidence for their conclusion. An exception is rising serum PSA values after radical prostatectomy, which can indicate either local tumor recurrence or metastatic disease.

ARE OTHER STAINS HELPFUL IN IDENTIFYING PROSTATIC METASTASES?

Other stains, such as mucicarmine, periodic acid-Schiff (PAS), or Alcian blue, are rarely diagnostic, principally because prostate carcinomas usually have a heterogeneity of patterns and the staining varies, depending on which part of the cancer has been biopsied. Furthermore, the histologic and staining characteristics of the metastases may vary from site to site.

Attempting to match the staining characteristics of metastases with the corresponding prostatic cancer may prove difficult. Although it is usually stated in jest, "Special stains make what you don't know a different color" has merit when attempting to identify metastases from the prostate.

IN PATIENTS WITH MULTIPLE PRIMARY TUMORS, HOW DOES ONE DETERMINE WHETHER METASTASES ARE FROM THE PROSTATE?

Histologic examination of the metastases and primary tumors is necessary. If the patient has a prostatic adenocarcinoma with histologic features suggesting that the cancer is capable of metastasizing, and the metastases have histologic features characteristic of metastatic prostate cancer, then the metastases are likely to have originated from the prostate. Elevated serum PSA levels and strongly positive immunohistochemical staining are supporting evidence that the metastases are from the prostate. Conversely, if the metastases are histologically similar to another of the patient's tumors, the metastases probably are not from the prostate, even if serum PSA levels are elevated or immunohistochemical staining is equivocal or slightly positive. In this setting strongly positive immunohistochemical staining does not necessarily support a primary prostate tumor because tumors far from the prostate may react positively for PSA and prostatic acid phosphatase in immunohistochemical studies.[10]

IS IT POSSIBLE TO HAVE METASTATIC PROSTATE CANCER IF THE SERUM PSA VALUE IS NORMAL AND IMMUNOHISTOCHEMICAL STAINS ARE NEGATIVE?

Yes. Serum PSA levels and immunohistochemical stains may be influenced by hormone therapy, including orchiectomy and antiandrogen therapy.[8, 9] If the patient has prostate cancer with histologic features capable of metastasizing and the metastases are characteristic of metastatic prostate cancer, the patient should be assumed to have metastatic prostatic adenocarcinoma until a more plausible primary tumor is identified, even without supporting immunohistochemical studies and elevated PSA level.

ARE STRONGLY POSITIVE IMMUNOHISTOCHEMICAL STAINS DIAGNOSTIC OF METASTATIC PROSTATE CANCER REGARDLESS OF THE HISTOLOGY OF THE METASTASES?

This picture may occur when the amount of tissue from the metastases is limited or distorted or when the carcinoma is undifferentiated and not easily identifiable as metastatic prostatic adenocarcinoma. As a general principle, it is foolish not to take seriously strongly positive immunohistochemical staining, especially if the patient has prostatic carcinoma with histologic features capable of metastasizing. However, several tumors far from prostate have been shown to react positively with PSA and prostatic acid phosphatase immunohistochemical staining, and future studies will undoubtedly identify additional tumors with these staining characteristics.[10]

Pathologists must be cautious of equivocal or faint positive immunohistochemical staining: it should not be used *to support or reject* the prostate as the source of metastases of unknown origin. Equivocal or faintly positive staining may be the result of faulty staining technique or be over- or underinterpretted by pathologists who have already decided that the prostate is (or is not) the source of the metastases.

ARE THERE CASES IN WHICH IT IS IMPOSSIBLE TO DETERMINE WHETHER THE METASTASES ARE FROM THE PROSTATE?

Yes. In some clinical settings (primary tumor with histologic features capable of metastasizing, metastases characteristic of prostatic adenocarcinoma, strongly positive immunohistochemical staining, and elevated serum PSA level) the pathologist may, for all practical purposes, be certain that the metastases are from the prostate. Other cases require evaluation of the entire clinical setting to determine whether the metastases are from the prostate.

Different pathologists reviewing the same clinical data may arrive at different conclusions. For example, we reviewed a case in which poorly differentiated metastases were observed during staging lymphadenectomy. Five years later this patient had widespread metastatic prostate cancer (treated with bilateral orchiectomy), Barrett's esophagus, and esophageal biopsy findings of poorly differentiated adenocarcinoma with equivocal PSA immunostaining. Some pathologists would have no difficulty convincing themselves—one way or the other—whether the esophageal biopsy findings represented metastatic prostatic adenocarcinoma or esophageal adenocarcinoma. When it comes to diagnosing such cases it is probably true that, as in all pathology, the less the pathologist knows the more dogmatic the pathologist is likely to be.

REFERENCES

1. Brawn PN: Histologic features of metastatic prostate cancer. Hum Pathol 23:267–272, 1992.
2. Mostofi FK: Grading of prostate carcinoma. Cancer Chemother Rep 59:111–117, 1975.
3. Brawn PN, Kuhl D, Speights VO, et al.: The incidence of unsuspected metastases from clinically benign prostates with latent prostate carcinoma. Arch Pathol Lab Med 119:731–733, 1995.
4. Brawn PN, Johnson EH, Speights VO, et al.: Long-term survival of Stage A prostate carcinoma, atypical hyperplasia/adenosis and BPH. Br J Cancer 69:1098–1101, 1994.
5. Brawn PN, Speights VO: The dedifferentiation of metastatic prostate carcinoma. Br J Cancer 59:85–88, 1989.
6. Butler JJ, Howe CD, Johnson DE: Enlargement of the supraclavicular lymph nodes as the initial sign of prostatic carcinoma. Cancer 27:1055–1058, 1971.
7. Warren MM, Furlow WL: Carcinoma of the prostate presenting as a mass in the neck. JAMA 213:620–622, 1970.
8. Murphy WM, Soloway MS, Barrows GH: Pathologic changes associated with androgen deprivation therapy for prostate cancer. Cancer 68:821–828, 1991.
9. Grignon D, Troster M: Changes in the immunohistochemical staining in prostatic adenocarcinoma following diethylstilbestrol therapy. Prostate 7:195–202, 1985.
10. Elgamal AA, Ectors NL, Sunardhi-Widyaputra S, et al.: Detection of prostate specific antigen in pancreas and salivary glands: a potential impact on prostate cancer overestimation. J Urol 156:464–468, 1996.
11. Brawn PN, Speights VO, Kuhl D, et al.: Prostate-specific antigen levels from completely sectioned, clinically benign, whole prostates. Cancer 68:1592–1599, 1991.

14

RELATIONSHIPS BETWEEN SERUM PROSTATE-SPECIFIC ANTIGEN AND HISTOPATHOLOGIC APPEARANCES OF PROSTATE CARCINOMA

PETER A. HUMPHREY and ROBIN T. VOLLMER

Serum prostate-specific antigen (PSA) is the most important tumor marker for adenocarcinoma of the prostate. Serum PSA is currently in wide clinical use for prostate cancer screening and for following response to treatment. The rapid increase in utilization of serum PSA for detecting prostate cancer is highlighted by a comparison of clinical diagnostic modalities used to diagnose prostate cancer in 1984 and in 1990. In this comparison,[1] in 1984 only 5.8% of patients with prostate cancer had a serum PSA determination as part of the initial evaluation for prostate cancer; in 1990 68.4% did. Indeed, serum PSA is now widely accepted in the United States as part of the annual physical examination, where serum PSA is used in conjunction with the traditional digital rectal examination (DRE) in efforts to detect prostate cancer early. Both the American Cancer Society and the American Urological Association recommend DRE with serum PSA as part of the annual physical examination for all men older than 50 years.[2,3] For African-American men and for men with a family history of prostate cancer, annual screening with DRE and serum PSA is recommended beginning at age 40 years. Not all medical professional societies in the United States support this screening approach, and prostate cancer screening has not been widely implemented in Canada and Europe.

As a result of serum PSA utilization, the aging of the American population—and, possibly, a true increase in incidence (as opposed to increased detection in a population increasingly at risk), the number of cases of prostate cancer diagnosed in the United States has increased more than sixfold over the last decade (1985 to 1995).[4,5] In 1995, it is estimated that 240,000 new cases of prostate cancer will be diagnosed in the United States and 40,400 men will die of this disease.[5]

It is clear that serum PSA has had a profound impact on prostate cancer diagnosis and on management of the disease. In this chapter, we present the current state of knowledge on relationships between serum PSA and histopathologic appearances of prostate cancer. It is beyond the scope of this chapter to consider either serum PSA or histopathologic appearances of prostate carcinoma in isolation as prognosticators; rather, the focus of this text is on the histopathologic basis for serum PSA elevation, the nature of prostate cancers detected by serum PSA testing, and the utilization of the combined information provided by serum PSA testing and morphologic aspects of prostatic carcinoma in the management of patients with prostate cancer. As an introduction, an overview is given of serum PSA as a tumor marker. In the second section the pathologic features of prostatic carcinomas detected in this era of PSA utilization are discussed. Segments three through six are segregated by tissue specimen type. Thus, the third segment delineates pathologic attributes of needle biopsy prostate specimens that, when combined with serum PSA, allow prediction of cancer presence, extent, and response to therapy. Next, morphologic studies of carcinoma in chips from transurethral resections of the prostate (TURP chips) are briefly summarized in relation to serum PSA levels. The fifth part of this chapter addresses the histopathologic characteristics of prostate carcinoma in radical prostatectomy tissue that are potentially useful (in conjunction with postoperative serum PSA measurements) in patient management. The sixth segment describes those appearances of prostate carcinoma after treatment that are helpful, with serum PSA, in posttherapy management of patients with prostate cancer. The seventh part relates PSA kinetics to pathologic conditions in the prostate. Finally, consideration is given to potential future directions in the use of morphologic features of prostatic carcinoma and serum PSA in the care of patients with prostate cancer.

PROSTATE-SPECIFIC ANTIGEN AS A TUMOR MARKER

PSA is a 33-kd glycoprotein that is currently the most important tumor marker for adenocarcinoma of the prostate.[6–14] Previously, serum prostatic acid phosphatase (PAP) was a tumor marker that had been used extensively for diagnosing, staging, and monitoring patients with prostate cancer; however, serum PSA has largely supplanted serum PAP for detection and monitoring of prostate cancer. Currently, the main application of serum PAP is in preoperative staging of patients with biopsy-proven prostate cancer, but even here its accuracy is low, since, while its prostate cancer–related elevation is relatively specific for spread outside the gland, its sensitivity is low.[15]

PSA was identified and characterized from 1966 to 1978.[16] The 6-kb PSA gene,[17,18] which is located on chromosome 19, codes for a single-chain 33-kd glycoprotein.[19] PSA is an enzyme that belongs to the kallikrein family of serine proteases (and, indeed, is also known as *human kallikrein 3*).[14] Its physiologic function is to liquefy seminal coagulum by cleaving the protein semenogelin into small peptides[16]; this results in increased sperm motility.

PSA expression was initially thought to be absolutely specific for the prostate; however, PSA expression, while highly restricted and confined mainly to benign and malignant prostatic luminal epithelial cells, has also been documented in male and female periurethral glands,[20–24] urachal remnants,[25] cystitis cystica and glandularis,[26] Cowper's glands,[24] male anal glands,[21] endometrium,[27] periurethral gland carcinomas, (reviewed in Ref 28), rare bladder adenocarcinomas (reviewed in Ref 28), salivary gland neoplasms,[29] and 30% of breast carcinomas.[30] It has not been established whether PSA expression by extraprostatic cells contributes to serum PSA levels, but urethral sources (i.e., from periurethral glands) do account for elevated urinary PSA levels.[31,32]

PSA is normally secreted from prostatic epithelial cells into the lumina of prostatic acini and ducts and is found in seminal fluids in concentrations nearly a millionfold greater than those in serum. In seminal fluid, PSA concentrations range from 0.24 to 5.50 mg/mL[33] whereas in serum the PSA concentration is normally less than 4.0 ng/mL, as determined by the Tandem-E immunoassay (Hybritech Inc., San Diego, CA). It is beyond the scope of this chapter to discuss assays for PSA in the blood, but it is important to know which assay is being used because reference ranges for normal do vary with assays. Many vital issues related to PSA assay performance and standardization are currently being addressed,[34,35] and new developments in measurement of PSA, such as free versus complexed circulating PSA forms and ultrasensitive assays, have the potential to provide new information for management of prostate cancer.[34]

Conditions that disrupt the barrier(s) for PSA access into the vasculature result in elevation of serum PSA. Such serum elevations may be caused by benign or malignant prostate disease and by prostate manipulations. Benign prostatic hyperplasia (BPH; Fig. 14–1) is a common cause of serum PSA elevation and, indeed, likely accounts for 60% to 70% of

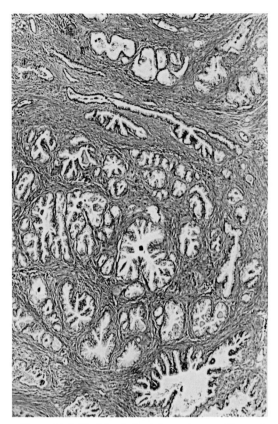

Figure 14–1. Nodule of glandular and stromal hyperplasia of the prostate (BPH). This is the most common cause of an elevated pretreatment serum PSA. (H&E ×40.)

cases with elevated serum PSA. Studies of patients with histologically confirmed BPH have shown that 21% to 86% have an elevated serum PSA value.[10,16,36] Of the patients with an elevated level, the degree of elevation is usually modest (4.1 to 10.0 ng/mL).[16] Additional benign entities that may cause an elevated serum PSA include prostatic inflammation[37–40] (Figs. 14–2, 14–3) and infarction[41] (Fig. 14–4). In our experience, ultrasound-determined prostate volume (most likely reflective of BPH) and inflammation, as identified on needle biopsy, were the most important factors contributing to serum PSA elevation in men without clinically detectable prostate cancer.[37]

In needle biopsies, we found that acute inflammation (see Fig. 14–2) was present in 63% of men with high serum PSA levels, as compared with 27% of men with normal PSA (p = 0.001). Chronic inflammation (see Fig. 14–3) was found more often in needle biopsies from men with elevated serum PSA (99%) but was also common in prostate needle biop-

sies of men with normal PSA (77%). Prostatic infarcts (see Fig. 14–4) have also been shown to elevate serum PSA, although only a few cases have been reported to date.[41] Finally, prostatic manipulations, including cystoscopy, needle biopsy, and TURP, are known to elevate serum PSA levels.[6,10,42] In a small percentage of men, DRE (9%), prostatic massage (6%), and transrectal ultrasound scanning (11%) result in elevation of serum PSA.[42] Acute urinary retention also elevates the PSA value.[43]

Prostatic intraepithelial neoplasia (PIN), a putative preneoplastic epithelial proliferation in the prostate, was initially felt to generate PSA levels intermediate between those associated with hyperplasia and carcinoma, but this observation was based on a diagnosis of PIN in needle biopsy and likely was due to PSA production by adjacent unsampled carcinoma. Currently, it is felt that high-grade PIN by itself does not account for an elevated serum PSA

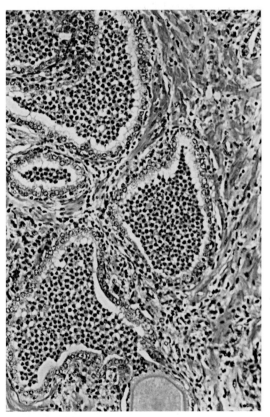

Figure 14–2. Acute inflammatory cell infiltrate in prostatic glands, with microabscess formation. In the absence of carcinoma, acute inflammation is associated with elevated serum PSA. (H&E ×200.)

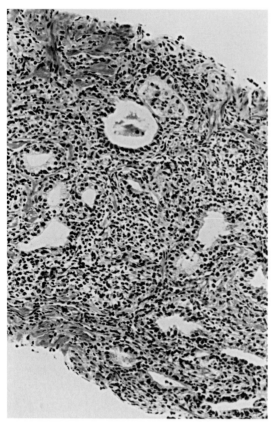

Figure 14–3. Chronic inflammatory cell infiltrate in 18-gauge needle biopsy specimen from the prostate. Inflammation in the prostate is an important cause of elevated serum PSA. (H&E ×200.)

level.[44] This may be due in part to the typically small portion of the prostate gland involved by PIN.[45,46]

Serum PSA as a tumor marker for prostate cancer is currently used for early detection of prostate cancer and for staging and posttreatment follow-up of patients. Serum PSA is being employed both in formal screening programs and in regular physical examinations, in efforts to detect "early" prostate cancer that would be most amenable to cure.[47–49]

Serum PSA has clearly been shown to be the single best predictor of detection of adenocarcinoma in needle biopsy. This is substantiated by the findings of recent prospective studies at six University centers of 6630 male volunteers over 50 years of age.[47] In this investigation the efficacy of DRE and serum PSA values in early detection of prostate cancer was compared. Of the 6630 men, 15% had an elevated serum PSA level, 15% had a suspicious DRE, and 26% had suspicious findings on one or both

tests. The cancer detection rate (with carcinoma diagnosed on quadrant-based needle biopsy) was 3.2% for DRE, 4.6% for PSA, and 5.8% for a combination of the two methods. Thus, serum PSA should be combined with DRE in evaluation for prostate cancer.[47–49] By themselves, DRE and transrectal ultrasonography have limited accuracy in identifying and localizing prostate cancer.[50] Moreover, DRE is subject to examiner variability,[51] and screening by the medically traditional annual DRE alone may be insufficiently frequent and/or sensitive to reduce the morbidity and mortality rates from this disease.[52]

The positive predictive value of a PSA level above 4 ng/mL in the histologic detection of carcinoma in needle biopsy specimens has ranged from 31% to 51%, most reports indicating that with a serum PSA value above 4 ng/mL the chance of identifying carcinoma is 30% to 40%.[9] Thus, for most patients with an elevated serum PSA value the cause for the elevated level is not carcinoma, but most likely

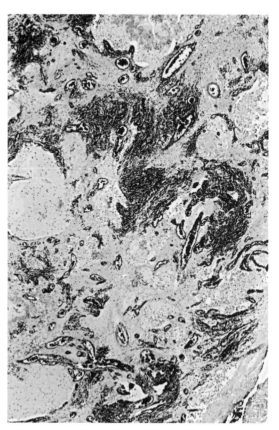

Figure 14–4. Hemorrhagic infarct of hyperplastic prostate tissue. Infarcts may elevate the serum PSA level. (H&E ×40.)

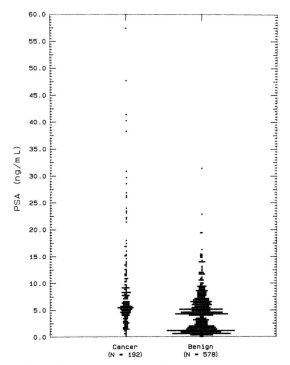

Figure 14–5. Distribution of PSA levels for untreated patients according to a malignant versus benign histopathologic diagnosis. (From Catalona WJ, Richie JP, Ahmann FR, et al.: Comparison of digital rectal examination and serum prostate specific antigen in the early detection of prostate cancer: Results of a multicenter clinical trial of 6,630 men. J Urol 151:1283, 1994.)

BPH. The overlap of PSA levels between benign and malignant disease is such that it is not possible to predict for an individual patient the findings in the needle biopsy based on the serum PSA level alone (Fig. 14–5); although higher PSA levels are more often associated with a diagnosis of carcinoma. For example, in the study cited above of 6630 men, the positive predictive value for a PSA of 4.1 to 9.9 ng/mL was 26.1%, whereas for 10.0 ng/mL or more the positive predictive value was 52.9%.[47] Unfortunately, most men (82%) with an elevated serum PSA value have an elevation in the 4.1 to 9.9 ng/mL range.[47] In addition to the relatively high false-positive rate for PSA, false-negatives also exist. That is, in some cases the serum PSA is not elevated despite a histologic diagnosis of carcinoma. Specifically, some 18% to 42% of prostate cancers fail to elevate serum PSA.[9,47,53,54]

PSA-based screening programs to detect early prostate cancer have been assembled at several medical centers.[55–58] At Washington University Medical Center, more than 30,000

men have now been enrolled in the PSA-based screening program. The experience of this program was recently summarized.[55] Screening of 24,346 men resulted in detection of 1169 carcinomas by needle biopsy, a detection rate of 4.7%. The importance of PSA in detecting these cancers is substantiated in that 39% were not palpable and were detected only by a elevated serum PSA. Screening with serum PSA has resulted in a clinical and pathologic stage shift[54]: in the screening program 97% of the patients had clinically localized disease, as compared with 65% of patients whose cancer was detected by DRE alone.[59] That PSA has likely detected these cancers earlier in their progression is suggested by lead time estimates of 5 to 6 years provided by studies using archival blood.[60,61] That is, an elevated serum PSA level antedated a clinical diagnosis of prostatic carcinoma by 5 to 6 years. Histopathologic study of radical prostatectomy specimens has revealed an increase in organ-confined carcinomas from 33% of cases detected by DRE[62] to 71% of cases in the PSA screening program.[55] As discussed in the following section, most of these PSA-screening program–detected carcinomas are pathologically significant.[63,64]

Although the American Cancer Society, American Urological Association, and American College of Radiology recommend PSA testing, screening for prostate cancer does remain controversial.[11] What remains to be addressed is whether PSA screening improves prostate cancer–specific mortality in a large-scale, controlled, randomized trial with long-term follow-up. The National Cancer Institute has just initiated such a trial,[65] but it will require two decades to complete and it has been criticized on the basis of study design.[11]

Pretreatment serum PSA is related to clinical stage,[66,67] histologic grade (Gleason grade), tumor volume, and pathologic stage of carcinoma in the whole prostate gland (reviewed in Refs 11, 66). PSA levels do correlate with clinical stage, but there is considerable overlap among the clinical stages (Fig. 14–6).[67] Note that a number of patients with metastatic disease have serum PSA levels greater than 10.0 ng/mL, but some also have a normal PSA level (less than 4.0 ng/mL).[67,70] Conversely, patients with organ-confined carcinoma may (although rarely) have serum PSA levels greater than 100 ng/mL.[69] A similar relationship between serum PSA and pathologic stage has been defined, in which increasing serum PSA corre-

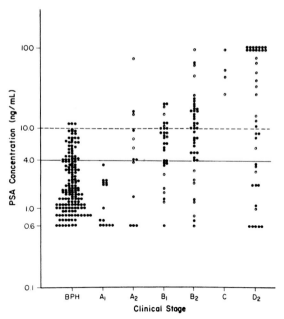

Figure 14–6. Plot of pretreatment serum PSA values for patients with BPH and increasing clinical stage of prostate carcinoma. A PSA level above 4.0 ng/mL is considered elevated. (From Hudson MA, Bahnson RR, Catalona WJ: Clinical use of prostate specific antigen in patients with prostate cancer. J Urol 142:104, 1989.)

lates with advancing pathologic stage (Table 14–1); however, despite this trend, higher PSA levels do not always indicate spread outside the prostate gland, and lower levels do not guarantee that the malignancy will be confined to the gland itself.[67]

Serum PSA levels have been linked directly to a number of important morphologic prognosticators in the whole prostate gland, including tumor volume, histologic grade, and positive surgical margins. The strength of the association between serum PSA and tumor vol-

Table 14–1. Relation of Serum PSA Level to Pathologic Stage of Prostate Cancer in 6630 Men

PSA Level (ng/mL)	Prevalence of Organ-Confined Cancer (%)
0–4	88
4.1–9.9	78
10.0–19.9	52
>20	27

(Data from Catalona WJ, Ritchie JP, Ahmann FR, et al.: Comparison of digital rectal examination and serum prostate-specific antigen in the early detection of prostate cancer. J Urol 151:1283, 1994.)

ume has varied from fair to good, with correlation coefficients ranging from 0.5 (Fig. 14–7) to 0.82.[36,70–73] This lack of a precise correlation is most likely due to multiple factors, including some contribution from BPH and heterogeneity of differentiation and PSA-production within a tumor.[70,73] Indeed, in two studies that found a positive correlation between serum PSA and Gleason grade, upon correction for volume there was actually an inverse relationship between pretreatment serum PSA and Gleason grade.[70,73] This is so because poorly differentiated or higher-grade carcinomas (Gleason primary grades 4 and 5) express less PSA on an individual cell basis but higher-grade tumors have more cells per unit of tumor volume.[73] Not all studies, however, have established an association between serum PSA and histologic grade,[70,71,73–76] and correlation coefficients generally have been weak, ranging from 0.2 to 0.38 (Fig. 14–8).[70,71,73] Finally, the preoperative serum PSA value has been linked to additional features of prostate carcinoma, such as nuclear grade ($r = 0.21$) and the likelihood of positive surgical margins ($r = 0.39$).[71,77]

Given the relationship of pretreatment serum PSA to stage, grade, and volume of prostate carcinoma, it is not surprising that the pretherapy level of this marker is a predictor of response to treatment. For example, in the Johns Hopkins experience with 666 men, the preoperative serum PSA level was directly related to the likelihood of freedom from disease progression after radical prostatectomy.[53] For men with a preoperative PSA level of 0 to 4 ng/mL, 92% were free of disease at 5 years, whereas at 10.1 to 20 ng/mL and more than 20 ng/mL, 56% and 45% of men, respectively, were free of carcinoma at 5 years. Similar results have been reported for radiation therapy and pretreatment serum PSA levels,[78,79] in which postirradiation treatment failure was observed in 6% of patients with a pretreatment PSA of less than 4 ng/mL, but in 66% of patients with a pretreatment value of 10 to 30 ng/mL, and 90% of those whose pretreatment PSA was greater than 30 ng/mL.[79] In contrast, although one study has suggested that a pretreatment PSA greater than 300 ng/mL is predictive of a greater risk of death for men with stage D prostate cancer treated with androgen deprivation hormone therapy,[80] most investigations indicate that pretreatment serum PSA is not useful for predicting response to hormone therapy.[81]

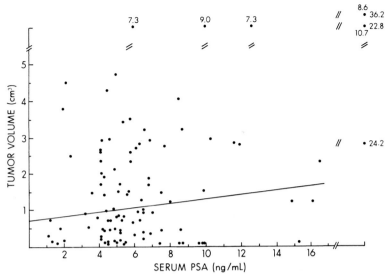

Figure 14–7. Relationship between preoperative serum PSA levels and tumor volume. A modest correlation (r = 0.5) is obtained, with wide scatter of points. Correlation coefficients reported in the literature vary from 0.5 to 0.8.[36,70–73] Presented here are data from the Washington University Medical Center PSA screening program.[64]

Posttreatment serum PSA values have immense clinical utility in following and managing patients after various forms of therapy for carcinoma of the prostate.[11] After radical prostatectomy for clinically localized prostate cancer, a detectable serum PSA is indicative of local disease recurrence or distant metastases.[11,53] (Later in this chapter we explore histologic features of needle biopsy performed to address the issue of local versus distant recurrence in the setting of elevated serum PSA

after radical prostatectomy.) Postoperative PSA elevations are directly related to histopathologic characteristics of the prostate carcinoma, as defined in the radical prostatectomy specimen. When unfavorable histopathologic findings are identified in the radical prostatectomy specimen, there is increased risk of a detectable serum PSA value (greater than 0.2 to 0.6 ng/mL, using the Tandem-E assay) both at initial testing 4 to 6 weeks after surgery[77,82] and in subsequent years.[53] With increasing

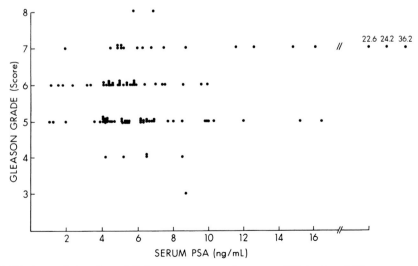

Figure 14–8. Weak correlation (r = 0.2) between preoperative serum PSA level and Gleason score in the radical prostatectomy specimen (n = 100). Data from the Washington University Medical Center PSA screening program.[64]

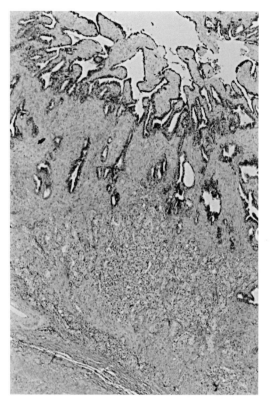

Figure 14–9. Extension of prostate carcinoma outside the confines of the prostate gland is linked to an elevated postoperative serum PSA. Here, seminal vesicle wall invasion by carcinoma is illustrated. This finding is associated with a 58% to 64% chance of the patient's experiencing failure, as defined by an elevated postoperative serum PSA value.[53,77]

stage there is a risk of an elevated postoperative serum PSA,[53,77,82–84] so, 11% of patients with organ-confined disease had a detectable serum PSA value postoperatively, as compared with 66% of patients with positive seminal vesicles or positive pelvic lymph nodes.[67] Gleason's histologic grade and intraglandular tumor extent (quantitated as either tumor volume or percentage of carcinoma) are also significant predictors of an elevated post-surgery PSA level. In multivariate analysis, we found that pathologic stage, percentage of carcinoma, and margin positivity were nearly equivalent in strength in predicting elevated PSA level in the immediate post-surgery period (Figs. 14–9 to 14–11).[82]

Serum PSA has also been used as an end point in the assessment of disease progression after radiation therapy and hormone therapy (reviewed in Refs 11, 79, 81). Briefly, while almost all men treated with radiation therapy

initially experience a significant decrease in serum PSA,[11] long-term follow-up data at 5 to 10 years show that only about 10% of men have undetectable serum PSA levels.[85,86] Serum PSA may also be used to follow the response of patients to radiation therapy directed at the prostate bed after radical prostatectomy.[11,53,87] (The use of postoperative serum PSA in conjunction with pathologic findings in radical prostatectomy specimens is considered later.) Last, for men treated with androgen deprivation therapy the rapidity of the PSA decline, the nadir level, and duration of the nadir all have prognostic significance.[11,13,81] One caveat about measuring serum PSA after hormone therapy is that for a minority of patients cancer progresses despite a normal PSA concentration. Serial PSA determinations should be obtained for all treated patients and, as rising serum PSA reliably predicts disease progression, it may be used to select patients for alternative therapies.[81]

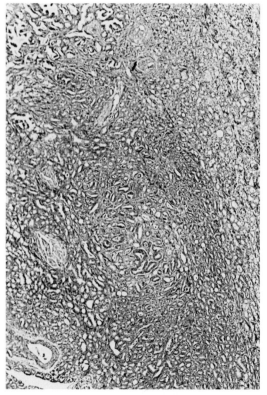

Figure 14–10. Extensive adenocarcinoma of the prostate in radical prostatectomy tissue. (H&E ×20.) Increasing intraglandular tumor extent in radical prostatectomy tissue, as measured using a grid morphometric technique,[193] is associated with an increased risk of elevated postoperative serum PSA.[77,82]

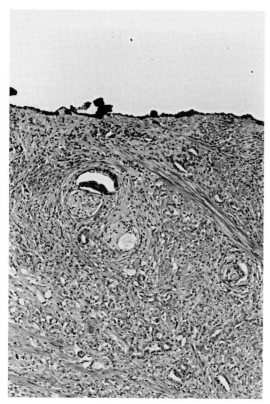

Figure 14–11. A positive peripheral surgical margin in the radical prostatectomy specimen places the patient at risk for elevated postoperative serum PSA,[77,82] which is a marker of clinical failure. (H&E ×100.)

Various modifications and derivatives of the PSA level have recently been utilized in attempts to improve the specificity and/or sensitivity of serum PSA levels.[88] These include PSA density,[89] age-referenced serum PSA cutoffs,[90] PSA velocity,[91] PSA cancer density,[71] measurement of free versus bound PSA,[92] and ultrasensitive PSA assays.[93] The first three parameters are those most widely used. PSA density has been forwarded as a means to reduce the significant false-positive rate of a PSA level over 4.0 ng/ml.[89] PSA density attempts to correct for the contribution of BPH to serum PSA by dividing the serum PSA level by the (ultrasound-determined) volume of the prostate gland. PSA density may increase specificity, but only at the expense of sensitivity.[88,93] Age-referenced serum PSA cutoffs also attempt to control for BPH, which increases with age, by increasing PSA cutoff points with increasing age, at which a level of 2.8 ng/mL is recommended for age 50 and 7.0 ng/mL for age 79.[90] Again, one concern with this approach is

the sacrifice of sensitivity for specificity.[88,94] That is, the biopsy rate may be decreased for older patients, but a certain percentage of cancers may be missed. PSA velocity or slope is the rate of change of PSA over time. The PSA velocity is greater in men with prostate cancer than in men with BPH[91,95]; the recommended slope cutoff is 0.75 ng/mL per year, to maximize sensitivity and specificity in predicting a positive result from needle biopsy. A lower slope cutoff of 0.4 ng/mL per year is optimal for men whose PSA concentration was initially elevated (above 4 ng/mL).[95] A drawback to the use of PSA velocity as a primary diagnostic test is the amount of time required to generate PSA velocity data (2 years).[88] The time is protracted because prostate carcinoma has a low proliferation rate[96]; doubling time for most organ-confined prostate cancers is estimated at more than 2 years.[97]

In this first section we have presented an overview of the remarkable clinical usefulness of serum PSA as an isolated measure of prostate disease. The focus of the sections to follow is the combination of histopathologic features of prostate tissues (particularly those involved with carcinoma) and serum PSA in the management of patients with prostate cancer.

PATHOLOGIC FEATURES OF PSA-DETECTED CARCINOMAS

A primary concern about the use of serum PSA in efforts at early detection of prostate cancer was that a large number of potentially clinically insignificant tumors might be discovered and treated. This concern arose owing to the high prevalence of small, well-differentiated, and noninfiltrative carcinomas that are identified at postmortem examination and in radical cystoprostatectomy specimens when prostate malignancy was not suspected. These cancers, which did not become clinically evident or important for the patient, are often termed "autopsy," "latent," "incidental," or "histologic" cancers. It has been determined that 30% of all men older than 50 years harbor such incidental prostatic carcinomas[98] and that as many as 87% of men in the eighth decade have prostate carcinoma detected at postmortem examination of completely embedded prostate glands.[99]

Thus far, all data suggest that most prostate carcinomas detected in PSA screening programs[55–58,63,64] and in needle biopsy prompted

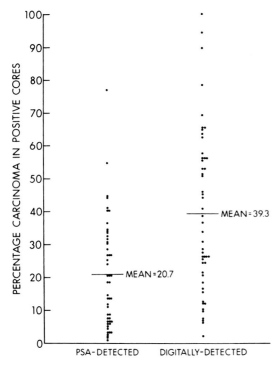

Figure 14–12. Prostatic carcinomas detected in a PSA-based screening program were less extensive in needle biopsy tissue than those detected via the traditional digital rectal examination.[107]

by elevated serum PSA value alone in the absence of a palpable abnormality (a stage T1c lesion) are pathologically significant[56,64,100–106] as judged by analysis of radical prostatectomy specimens. In needle biopsies, prostate carcinomas detected in a PSA-based screening program were of lower histologic grade, were less extensive (Fig. 14–12), and less often exhibited perineural invasion (10%) as compared with digitally detected carcinomas (38%).[107] These findings suggested that PSA-detected carcinoma may be a more difficult histologic diagnosis to establish by needle biopsy.[107] A second needle biopsy–based study[108] found no difference in Gleason scores for prostate cancers detected (1) before and (2) after advent of serum PSA use.

We have performed a prospective study on the characterization of pathologic features of prostate carcinomas in 100 consecutive radical prostatectomy specimens from patients enrolled in the Washington University PSA-based screening program.[63,64] In this program, volunteers older than 50 underwent biopsy if they had an abnormal DRE and/or an elevated serum PSA value (>4 ng/mL). The median

tumor volume was 1.0 cm³. This size is fully 25-fold greater than the median tumor volume (0.04 cm³) of incidental prostate carcinomas identified in cystoprostatectomy specimens.[64] The overwhelming majority of the cancers had Gleason scores of 5 to 8 (median, score 6; Fig. 14–13). Some 22% of the PSA screen–detected carcinomas had a component of high histologic grade (Gleason grade 4 or 5), as compared with a significantly lower (p <0.05) percentage of cases of incidental carcinoma with Gleason 4 or 5 (11%). Whereas almost all (97%) incidental carcinomas were confined to the prostate gland, significantly fewer (61%) of the PSA screen–detected carcinomas were organ confined. Seminal vesicle invasion was uncommon (4%), and pelvic lymph node metastasis rare (1%; Fig. 14–14). In other screening programs,[56–58] 33% to 36% of carcinomas had extended outside the prostate gland and 6% of cases had lymph node metastases.

In the PSA screening era of the last few years, the incidence of prostate carcinoma

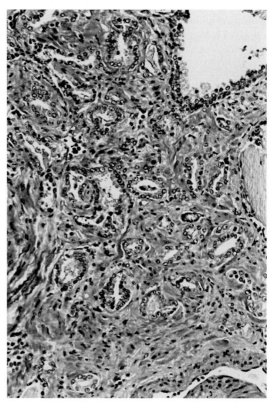

Figure 14–13. Adenocarcinoma of the prostate, Gleason grade 3. The vast majority of carcinomas detected in a PSA-based screening program were of intermediate histologic grade (i.e., Gleason score 5 or 6).[64]

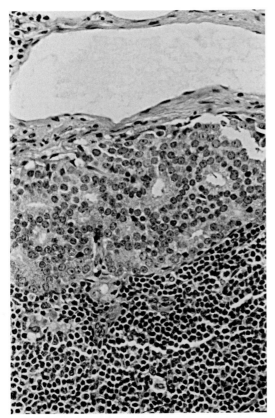

Figure 14–14. Lymph node metastasis of prostate carcinoma detected in a PSA-based screening program.[64] This was the only case of lymph node metastasis in the entire patient population of 100.

lymph node metastasis in patients diagnosed with clinically organ-confined disease decreased significantly. Whereas in the 1970s histopathologists identified metastatic deposits in the lymph nodes of 20% to 40% of patients undergoing pelvic lymphadenectomy, 1% to 6% of patients now have metastatic deposits of prostate cancer in their lymph nodes (see Fig. 14–14).[109]

Impalpable prostate carcinomas detected by needle biopsy because of elevated serum PSA (stage T1c carcinomas)[110] exhibit features similar to those of screen-detected prostate carcinomas (Table 14–2). These tumors are also usually of intermediate grade and organ confined.[56,64,100–106] In a few series,[100,101] the reported mean tumor volumes have been higher at 6.4 to 7.4 cm³, in contrast to 1.7 cm³ in a screening program.[64] The pathologic characteristics of T1c carcinomas in radical prostatectomy tissues have been reported as similar to those of T2 carcinomas[101] or as intermediate

between those of T1a and T2 carcinomas, except that Gleason's histologic grade was similar.[105,111] The impalpability of T1c carcinomas has been attributed to their being located elsewhere than the peripheral zone, their smaller size, and obscuring BPH.[105,112]

Classification schemes have been devised to attempt to define the potential clinical significance of prostate carcinomas identified in screening programs and by serum PSA elevation.[55,102,105,106] These schemes have utilized the pathologic features of histologic Gleason's grade, pathologic stage, and tumor volume to stratify patients into groups based on potential biologic aggressiveness of the malignancy. Such stratifications are not perfect, since morphologic prognosticators do not have the capacity to predict treatment outcome absolutely for individual patients; rather, they indicate trends and the likelihood of outcome.[96] Also, because the definition of these classifications is contingent upon performance of radical prostatectomy, the natural history of the carcinomas in these various categories is obviously unknowable. Thus, it is not possible to know with certainty what constitutes "clinically insignificant" prostate carcinoma. Nevertheless, using different schemes and different groups of patients, all studies have concluded that most carcinomas detected in both PSA screening programs[64] and by serum PSA elevation are medically important. The estimates of so-called clinically insignificant disease have ranged from 5% to 27%.[64,102,105,106] As described in the next section, efforts are currently being directed toward pretreatment identification of these minimal carcinomas.

SERUM PSA PLUS HISTOPATHOLOGIC ATTRIBUTES OF NEEDLE BIOPSY TISSUE AS PREDICTORS OF PRESENCE OF CARCINOMA, EXTENT AND RESPONSE TO THERAPY

Benign Prostate Tissue in Needle Biopsy Specimens

An initial histologic diagnosis of benign prostate tissue on needle biopsy does not exclude carcinoma when the patient has an elevated serum PSA value. In a serial biopsy study of men with an elevated serum PSA level, there was a 34% detection rate of carcinoma on the initial biopsies.[113] After a nonmalignant

Table 14–2. Pathologic Characteristics of Nonpalpable Prostate Carcinomas Detected by Elevated Serum PSA (Stage T1c)

Study	n	Gleason Grade (Mean Score)	Mean Tumor Volume (cm³)	Positive Margins (%)	Organ-Confined (%)	Seminal Vesicle Invasion (%)	Lymph Node Metastasis (%)
Stormont et al.[100]	60	NR	7.4	23	70	5	2
Guthman et al.[104]	20	4.9	3.9	10	70	0	0
Oesterling et al.[101]	208	NR	6.4	44	53	9	3
Mettlin et al.[56]	13	NR	NR	NR	69	NR	8
Epstein et al.[105]	157	6.3	1.9	17	51	6	4
Scaletscky et al.[103]	142	NR	NR	26	68	7	1
Ohori et al.[102]	29	NR	NR*	7	60	0	4
Douglas et al.[106]	71	NR	NR	41	56	8	NR
Humphrey et al.[64]	78	5.6	1.9	35	59	3	0

* Median tumor volume in this study = 1.5 cm³.
NR = Not reported.

diagnosis on the initial set of biopsies, the detection rate was 19% on the second set, 8% on the third, and 7% on the fourth set or later.[113] Elevated serum PSA alone should prompt repeat biopsy in patients with normal or hyperplastic prostate tissue in an initial set of needle biopsies. No histopathologic features in this benign tissue allow for better prediction of a needle biopsy positive for carcinoma in the next set of needle biopsies. As discussed earlier, inflammation in needle biopsies may be associated with increased PSA, but this, of course, does not exclude carcinoma. The detection of carcinoma in serial biopsies after initially negative needle biopsies reflects the sampling error of the 18-gauge needle biopsy, which samples 0.03% of all tissue in the prostate gland.[63] Increasing the number of needle biopsy samples increases the likelihood of detecting carcinoma. Currently, a common practice is to sample the prostate gland systematically with six biopsies,[114] with or without transition zone biopsies.

Prostatic Intraepithelial Neoplasia in Needle Biopsy Specimens

High-grade PIN, when diagnosed in isolated form in needle biopsy, is a powerful predictor of a diagnosis of carcinoma in a subsequent needle biopsy (see Chapter 7). It is not clear whether serum PSA provides additional predictive information to a diagnosis of high-grade PIN.[115,116] In our experience,[115] isolated high-grade PIN was predictive of carcinoma on the next biopsy in 51% (19/37) of cases, and the serum PSA value was not helpful for distinguishing patients who had carcinoma on the next biopsy from those who did not. Other data have been presented to show that serum PSA elevation *was* useful in identifying which PIN patients had carcinoma.[116] Further investigation of large numbers of patients with isolated high-grade PIN will be necessary to better define combined use of high-grade PIN and serum PSA as predictors of carcinoma. At the present time the practical point for patient management purposes is that patients with high-grade PIN on needle biopsy, with or without serum PSA elevation, should undergo repeat biopsy.

Carcinoma in Needle Biopsy Specimens

Carcinoma histologic grade (Gleason grade) and extent in needle biopsy tissue have been utilized in conjunction with serum PSA and PSA density to predict whole gland histologic grade,[117] tumor size and "significance,"[105, 118–120] pathologic stage,[105,118–131] surgical margin status,[132] and response to treatments (including radical prostatectomy[133,134] and radiation therapy[79,135]). Efforts are currently being directed toward pretreatment identification of that subset of 5% to 27% of prostate cancer patients whose tumors have been deemed "clinically insignificant or unimportant." Several approaches have been employed (Table 14–3). One approach applied the total length of cancer on systematic sextant needle biopsies, in combination with prostate volume as measured by ultrasound and serum PSA value, to derive a mathematical equation to predict cancer volume in the whole gland.[120] This model was developed in an attempt to predict tumor volumes of less than 0.5 to 1.0 cm^3, lesions that have been characterized by these investigators as probably being of little clinical significance and requiring no therapy.[136,137] (Note that, while tumor volume by itself is a significant prognosticator,[96,138] it is not a perfect one.[139] We have seen several high-grade, Gleason score 7, prostate carcinomas of less than 0.5 cm^3 in volume that had perforated the prostatic capsule.) While this formula resulted in a good correlation between predicted cancer volume and actual cancer volume ($r^2 = 0.76$), the conclusion was drawn that it was not adequate to predict tumor volume for individual patients.[120] Also, of 15 cancers smaller than 1.0 cm^3, only 10 were accurately identified using the formula. Other models have incorporated PSA density in efforts to distinguish "insignificant" prostate cancers,[105,118] which were defined in different ways (see Table 14–3). In the Johns Hopkins experience,[105] while the individual preoperative parameters of PSA value and density, Gleason grade, and tumor extent in needle biopsies predicted tumor extent in the radical prostatectomy specimen, the best model used a combination of PSA density, grade, and tumor extent by needle biopsy (see Table 14–3). All of the studies cited in Table 14–3 should be considered pilot studies, and these models should be tested for

efficacy in large-scale, prospective trials before they are implemented routinely.

Another important goal is accurate pretreatment staging of patients with biopsy-proven prostate carcinoma. Studies have been performed that utilized, in various combinations, clinical stage, transrectal ultrasonography, serum PSA, PSA density, and Gleason's histologic grade and tumor extent in needle biopsies, to predict pathologic stage (Table 14–4). While it is clear that serum PSA (or PSA density) may be combined with pathologic features from needle biopsy, particularly Gleason grade, to predict pathologic stage, it is also apparent that these data predict trends, rather than being absolutely definitive. This is evident upon examination of published probability tables or nomograms, such as those in one study where only a small percentage (10%) of the 359 categories based on PSA level, Gleason score, and clinical stage were absolutely predictive at 0% or 100%.[130] This does not diminish the practical relevance of pretreatment prediction of pathologic stage. This information allows the physician to inform the patient better about the likelihood of spread of the cancer and of treatment options. In particular, it has been proposed that, with these approaches, cross-sectional imaging—computed tomography (CT) or magnetic resonance imaging (MRI)—and pelvic lymph node dis-

Table 14–3. Pretreatment Prediction of "Insignificant" Prostate Cancer Using Serum PSA and Needle Biopsy Findings

Study	Model	Definition of "Insignificant" Tumor	Number of Patients with Insignificant Tumor	Accuracy (%)
Terris et al.[120]	Log$_{10}$ cancer volume = −0.389 + (0.242) (log PSA) + (0.644 log$_{10}$ step-section planimetry volume) + (0.364) (log$_{10}$ total length of cancer on biopsies)	Tumor volume <1.0 cm^3	15	67
Goto et al.[119]	Normal serum PSA and cancer ≤1 mm of maximum length in biopsy core	Tumor volume ≤0.5 cm^3, organ-confined, no Gleason grade 4 or 5 component	19	86
Epstein et al.[105]	PSA density <0.1 ng/mL/g and good pathologic findings on needle biopsy (no Gleason pattern 4 or 5, fewer than three cores involved, no core with greater than 50% involvement) or PSA density 0.1–0.15 ng/mL/g with cancer <3 mm on one core sample	Tumor volume <0.2 cm^3, organ-confined, no Gleason grade 4 or 5 component	26	73
Irwin et al.[118]	PSA density ≤0.1 ng/mL/g and cancer ≤3 mm of Gleason grade ≤2	Tumor volume ≤0.5 cm^3, organ-confined	23	82

Table 14–4. Pretreatment Prediction of Pathologic Stage Using Serum PSA
and Needle Biopsy Findings

Study	Model	Comment
Ackerman et al.[132]	PSA density >0.230 and number of positive sextant biopsies >2	This combination predicted 59% of positive surgical margins at prostatectomy and was superior to needle biopsy and PSA data alone.
Kleer et al.[121]	Probability plots generated from local clinical stage (determined by DRE), histologic grade, and serum PSA	Predicted probability curves for organ-confined disease, extracapsular disease, and lymph node involvement were presented.
Wolf et al.[122]	Algorithm for staging clinically localized prostate cancer using (in sequence) Gleason score in needle biopsy, serum PSA, and transrectal ultrasound	Staging accuracy achieved in predicting organ-confined disease was 77%.
Arai et al.[123]	Group A: Serum PSA <10 ng/mL and Gleason score 2–7 Group B: Serum PSA >10 ng/mL and Gleason score 8–10	Only 1/18 patients (6%) in group A had lymph node metastasis versus 12/17 (71%) in group B.
Bishoff et al.[124]	Combination of serum PSA, clinical stage, and biopsy Gleason score	It is proposed that, by using these predictive parameters, pelvic lymph node dissection could be avoided in up to 50% of patients with clinically localized prostate cancer.
Bluestein et al.[125]	Combination of local stage, primary Gleason grade, and serum PSA	Table generated showing probabilities that a patient will have positive lymph nodes.
Danella et al.[126]	Serum PSA >15 ng/mL and Gleason score ≥7	Routine laparoscopic node dissection deemed unnecessary unless PSA >40 ng/mL or PSA >15 ng/mL *and* Gleason score ≥7.
Diaz et al.[127]	Risk of positive seminal vesicles (sv): +sv = PSA + (Gleason score −6) × 10	High- and low-risk groups for radiotherapy purposes were defined. Low-risk group may be excluded from seminal vesicle irradiation, thus allowing for higher dose with less rectal toxicity.
Narayan et al.[128]	PSA ≤10 ng/mL and Gleason score ≤6	In this setting, staging pelvic lymphadenectomy may be unnecessary.
Nishiya et al.[129]	PSA density >0.3 ng/mL/mL and Gleason sum >6	These patients had a high probability of having extra-prostatic carcinoma.
Partin et al.[130]	Serum PSA, Gleason score, and clinical stage	Data used to generate nomograms for predicting final pathologic stage. A combination of all three variables predicted more accurately than any single variable the final pathologic stage.
Roach et al.[131]	Risk of positive lymph nodes (N+): N+ = 2/3 (PSA) + (Gleason score −6) × 10	Low-risk group with calculated risk of positive nodes <15% had 6% observed incidence; high-risk group with calculated risk of ≥15% had 40% observed incidence.

section could be avoided in some patients.[123, 124,126,128] If imaging alone were avoided in patients with a low probability of lymph node metastases, it has been established that $50 to $150 million would be saved annually in the United States.[128] Similarly, substantial savings (and potential reduction in patient morbidity) would result by avoiding lymphadenectomy.[128]

Morphologic features in needle biopsy tissue (histologic grade and percentage of positive cores) have been used in conjunction with serum PSA (or PSA density) for pretreatment prediction of response to treatment, including radical prostatectomy[133,134] and radiation therapy.[135] In one report patients had an increasing risk of progression after radical prostatectomy with an increasing number of three

criteria over threshold setpoints.[133] The criteria and setpoints were as follows: percentage of positive biopsies, greater than 66.7%; PSA, greater than 25 ng/mL; PSA density, greater than 0.6 ng/mL. For zero criteria, 24% of patients experienced progression, whereas when thresholds for at least two criteria were exceeded 96% of patients progressed. Unfortunately, in this current PSA-screening era, these thresholds are quite high and are not often attained, thereby potentially limiting use of this technique. (For example, most elevated serum PSA levels are in the 4 to 10 ng/mL range and it is distinctly uncommon for the PSA value to be above 25 ng/mL). The data in Figure 14–5 show that only 11 of 192 patients (6%) with biopsy-proven prostate cancer had a serum PSA greater than 25 ng/mL. Tumor grade (using the less commonly applied Mayo and M.D. Anderson schemes) and pretherapy PSA have been used to stratify patients into risk groups for relapse after radiation therapy.[79,134]

It should be noted that not all investigations have found that PSA and grade together provide more information than grade alone.[63, 140,141] In one evaluation of 569 patients, the gain in predictive accuracy from serum PSA over that obtained from stage and histologic grade was minimal.[140] These researchers forwarded the notion that staging pelvic lymphadenectomy remains the only satisfactory way of determining node status in most patients with carcinoma of the prostate. Similarly, neither serum PSA and grade nor serum PSA, PSA density, and number of needle biopsies with tumor was useful in predicting, respectively, bone metastases[141] and tumor volume.[63]

SERUM PSA WITH HISTOPATHOLOGIC FEATURES OF TURP CHIPS AS PREDICTORS

Glandular and Stromal Hyperplasia in TURP Chips

In healthy men serum PSA levels correlate directly with total volume of the prostate and seem to be linked most closely to volume (and more specifically the epithelial volume[142]) of the transition zone,[143,144] where BPH develops. PSA velocity has also been linked to quantity of epithelium (percentage epithelium) in TURP chips.[145] Based on weights of BPH tissue excised via simple retropubic prostatectomy or TURP and serum PSA, the PSA produced per gram of BPH tissue has been estimated at 0.1 to 0.26 ng/ml.[142,143] (In comparison, on a per weight basis, prostate carcinoma produces a 10-fold greater serum PSA elevation.[83]) Thus, in this setting the weight of the resected tissue is the most important pathologic feature in relation to elevated serum PSA. No histopathologic features of the hyperplastic prostate tissue (with or without serum PSA) have been reported to predict subsequent prostate carcinoma detection. In any case, the long-term risk of patients who underwent TURP for BPH for developing prostate cancer is low: In one study 6.3% of 269 patients developed clinically apparent prostate cancer at a mean interval of 7.0 years.[146]

High-Grade PIN in TURP Chips

Isolated high-grade PIN is uncommon in TURP chips (prevalence 2.3%).[147] This is consistent with the predominant peripheral—as opposed to transition zone—site of high-grade PIN. The identification of high-grade PIN in the transition zone signifies that there is a very high probability that there is carcinoma elsewhere in the prostate gland,[148] but it does not provide any indication of tumor extent within the gland.[149] Only a single study has probed the usefulness for subsequent detection of prostate carcinoma of serum PSA levels in conjunction with a diagnosis of isolated high-grade PIN in TURP chips.[147] Preliminary data show that this combined information does improve predictive capacity.[150]

Carcinoma in TURP Chips

Morphologic features diagnostic of incidental stage A1 (T1a) carcinoma in prostate chips[96] have been used with serum PSA in an attempt to predict significant residual tumor of a volume greater than 0.5 cm³.[151] All nine stage A1 cancer patients with a serum PSA value of 1 ng/mL or less after TURP had residual tumor volume of less than 0.5 cm³ in the radical prostatectomy specimen, whereas those four patients with PSA greater than 10 ng/mL had volumes greater than 0.5 cm³. Based on these findings, the authors suggested that stage A1 (T1a) prostate cancer patients with low serum PSA could be followed with serial PSA measurements.[151] Potential pitfalls in this study include the small number (22) of stage T1a patients studied and the fact that more than half of patients with PSA levels greater than 10 ng/mL have carcinoma outside the prostate gland (see Table 14–1).[47]

In a second study,[152] histologic grade in TURP chips did not provide additional prognostic information once serum PSA was in the multivariate analysis model. In this report, pretreatment serum PSA was the most powerful independent predictor of lymph node metastases.[152]

POSTOPERATIVE SERUM PSA WITH HISTOPATHOLOGIC CHARACTERISTICS OF RADICAL PROSTATECTOMY TISSUES IN PATIENT MANAGEMENT

As isolated factors, both pathologic features of carcinoma in radical prostatectomy specimens and elevated postoperative serum PSA are predictive of clinical progression following surgical treatment by radical prostatectomy.[53] Only limited data exist on prediction of patient outcome after radical prostatectomy using combined histopathologic features and serum PSA. One study developed a logistic regression model that incorporated Gleason score, pathologic stage, and postoperative serum PSA at 1 year *or* PSA velocity; this model distinguished local from distant metastasis in patients with an elevated post–radical prostatectomy serum PSA (more than 0.2 ng/mL).[153] In a second investigation,[154] a multifactor model that incorporated preoperative serum PSA and radical prostatectomy Gleason score and pathologic stage was developed to select men at high risk for cancer recurrence.

Distinguishing local from metastatic disease manifestations is important since men with a local recurrence in the prostate bed may benefit from pelvic irradiation whereas distant metastases require hormone treatment. Most men (about three quarters) with an elevated postoperative serum PSA have metastatic carcinoma whereas roughly a quarter have a local recurrence.[153] Probability plots predicting the likelihood that a postoperative serum PSA elevation represented a local recurrence were generated using logistic regression data for multivariate combinations in two separate but equally predictive models.[153] The first model used Gleason score and pathologic stage in the radical prostatectomy specimen with the serum PSA level 1 year after surgery whereas the second used Gleason score, pathologic stage, and serum PSA velocity 1 year after surgery. These multivariate models provided more information (goodness-of-fit P values 0.954 and 0.972, where 1.0 = perfect fit) than isolated use of time to detectable serum PSA ($P=0.248$), radical prostatectomy Gleason score ($P=0.55$), the PSA value 1 year after surgery ($P=0.427$), the PSA velocity 1 year after surgery ($P=0.624$), and pathologic stage ($P=0.864$). As the number of patients (51) in this investigation was relatively small, additional data should be gathered to confirm and support the use for individual patients of the provided probability plots.

Identification of patients at high risk for recurrence after radical prostatectomy is also an important aim, since these men would comprise an appropriate patient population for efficacy testing of adjuvant therapy.[154] A model for log relative risk (R_W) was devised using serum PSA with a sigmoidal transformation (PSA_{ST}), radical prostatectomy Gleason score (GS), and pathologic stage (PS):

$$R_W = (PSA_{ST} \times 0.06) + (GS \times 0.54) + (PS \times 1.87).$$

This model allowed for stratification of patients into three risk categories—low, intermediate, and high—with corresponding actuarial recurrence rates at 5 years of 8%, 31%, and 79%, respectively. Of significance, this model was validated in a separate cohort of patients. As the authors note, the next step for this model is prospective validation in multiple institutions.[154]

POSTTHERAPY SERUM PSA AND POSTTHERAPY HISTOPATHOLOGIC TRAITS OF PROSTATIC CARCINOMA IN PATIENT MANAGEMENT

After radical prostatectomy, almost all men who have a recurrence have a detectable postoperative serum PSA value.[155–157] In one series of more than 500 radical prostatectomies, no patient had clinical recurrence without elevated postsurgical serum PSA.[157]

For those patients with presumed local recurrence after radical prostatectomy, as detected by elevated serum PSA, in the absence of evidence of metastatic disease, biopsy of the vesicourethral anastomosis or prostatic bed has not always documented carcinoma.[158–160] In a recent study, carcinoma was identified in one biopsy in 39% of cases and in 1 or more biopsies in 59% of patients (Fig. 14–15).[160] A positive DRE or transrectal ultrasound enhances the likelihood of positive biopsy; however, serum PSA and PSA doubling time after surgery were not helpful in predicting negative biopsy findings.[160] Of interest, in a histopathologic study of 14 biopsies, benign prostate tissue was discovered.[159,160] Such a diagnosis on the initial needle biopsy does not rule out recurrence of the malignancy, since repeat biopsy in some of these patients revealed carcinoma.[159,160]

For patients treated with radiation therapy for clinically localized prostate cancer there is no accepted definition of normal or abnormal serum PSA level after irradiation. The trend in PSA levels after radiation therapy may be a more important indicator of disease status

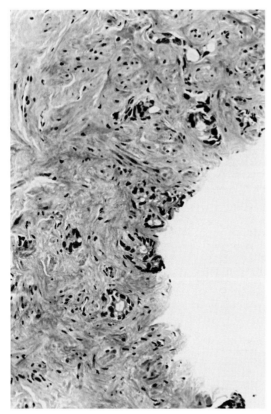

Figure 14–15. Appearance of infiltrating prostate carcinoma in needle biopsy of vesicourethral anastomosis (H& E ×200). Postoperative serum PSA was elevated at 0.6 ng/mL (a normal value is less than 0.6 ng/mL).

than a single PSA measurement.[79,161,162] Since, however, residual prostate carcinoma has been diagnosed in the face of undetectable serum PSA after radiation therapy,[162] a proposal has been made to use both PSA trend (that is, rising level or one that is stable over time) and the histopathologic findings (benign or malignant) in postirradiation needle biopsy to predict disease progression.[78]

KINETICS OF PSA AND PATHOLOGIC CONDITIONS

One of the most interesting things about PSA is its kinetics, and one of the best illustrations of PSA kinetics comes from Carter and associates.[163] Using stored sera from the Baltimore Longitudinal Study of Aging serum bank, these investigators assayed for PSA and plotted the temporal patterns of PSA for four groups of men: one without prostate disease, the second with BPH, the third with localized

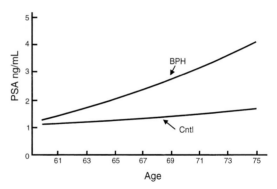

Figure 14–16. Plot of PSA (ng/mL) versus age for an average 75-year-old man without prostatic disease (Cntl) and one with BPH. The curves were obtained from the fitted equations reported by Carter and coworkers.[163]

carcinoma, and the fourth with advanced or metastatic carcinoma. Using their published equations for fitting these curves, we calculated the expected values for all four groups. Figure 14–16 shows the plots of expected PSA versus age from an average control patient (Cntl) and one with BPH. Figure 14–17 shows the plots for the expected PSA versus age for an average man who at age 75 develops localized (Loc) or advanced (Adv) carcinoma. All four curves increase with time, but clearly at different rates and levels; note that the curves for carcinoma—and perhaps even for BPH— look exponential. The Carter group's published curves also demonstrated many temporal peaks for individual patients. These generally had a magnitude of 2 to 5 ng/mL, but since sampling occurred once every 2 years

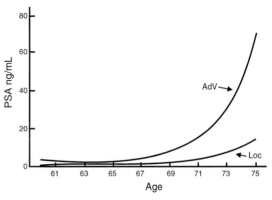

Figure 14–17. Plot of PSA (ng/mL) versus age for an average 75-year-old man with localized prostatic carcinoma (Loc) and one with advanced-stage carcinoma (Adv). The curves were obtained from the fitted equations reported by Carter and coworkers.[163]

Table 14–5. Average Rate Constant b from Equation 1 in units per day^{-1}

Study	Treatment	Category	N	b
Schmid et al.[97]	None	Stages A2 + B1	20	0.000455
Stamey & Kabalin[164]	None	Stage A2	4	0.000589
Schmid et al.[97]	None	Stage B2	8	0.000631
Stamey & Kabalin[164]	None	Stage B2	3	0.000720
Carter et al.[163]	None	Localized	11	0.000789
Hanks et al.[165]	Rad	No deaths	4	0.001033
Carter et al.[163]	None	Advanced	7	0.001052
Pollack et al.[166]	Rad	Grade 2–4	26	0.001109
Schmid et al.[97]	None	Stage D1	5	0.001515
Pollack et al.[166]	Rad	Grades 5,6	40	0.001735
Zagars & Pollack[167]	Rad	All	37	0.001818
Danella et al.[168]	Surg	Localized	39	0.001994
Pollack et al.[166]	Rad	Grade 8–10	12	0.002525
Pollack et al.[166]	Rad	Grade 7	20	0.002583
Stamey & Kabalin[164]	None	Stage D	3	0.002591
Partin et al.[153]	Surg	Local recurrence	9	0.002624
Zagars & Pollack[167]	None	Stage C	2	0.003480
Partin et al.[153]	Surg	Distant recurrence	29	0.003607
Hanks et al.[165]	Rad	10% dead of tumor	11	0.003788
Danella et al.[168]	Surg	Metastasis	11	0.005543
Hanks et al.[165]	Rad	50% dead of tumor	4	0.008417
Kaplan et al.[169]	Rad	All	17	0.009391
Kaplan et al.[169]	Rad	All	5	0.010720
Hanks et al.[165]	Rad	60% dead of tumor	3	0.022726
Schmid et al.[97]	None	Stage D2	4	0.022726

Rad, radiation; Surg, prostatectomy; N, number of patients studied.

both the magnitude and the duration of peaks remains uncertain.

Modeling the Rise in PSA

Carter and colleagues[163] also used an exponential model to fit and describe the rise in PSA for patients with cancer. In a generic formulation this exponential model is given by the equation:

$$y = a * e^{(b*t)} \qquad (1)$$

where y denotes the PSA concentration, e is the natural logarithm base (approximately 2.72), t is time, a is the starting concentration at $t = 0$, and b is the growth rate constant. The investigators found that, on average, those with localized cancer had a b value of 0.29 per year, whereas those with advanced cancer had a higher b value of 0.38 per year. Thus the rate constant b seemed to reflect either stage or aggressiveness of the tumor.

The rate constant b also gives the doubling time (DT) of PSA as follows:

$$DT = ln(2)/b \qquad (2)$$

where ln stands for the natural logarithm, and a number of investigators have reported DT for PSA in either pretreatment or posttreatment situations. For example, Schmid and coworkers[97] reported that PSA followed this exponential model in 43 untreated patients, and Table 14–5 lists the b values from 10 studies over several patient categories and in order of increasing magnitude. It is clear from examining this listing that low values of b tend to occur in tumors of lower stage, lower grade, and longer survival than those with higher values of b. For example, Schmid's group found significantly longer DT (lower b) in patients with organ-confined tumor than in those with tumor outside the organ and significantly shorter DT (higher b) in patients with higher tumor grades.[97] Zagars and associates[167] reported that for patients receiving radiation therapy a shorter DT (higher b) predicted metastasis as opposed to local relapse.

Modeling the Fall in PSA

An exponential function also describes the decline in PSA after surgery, effective radiation, or hormone treatments. For example, both Stamey's and Oesterling's groups reported an exponential decline in PSA after prostatectomy and calculated half-lifes of, respectively, 2.2 days and 3.15 days.[36,170] This decline in PSA follows the generic exponential equation:

$$y = c * e^{(-d*t)} \qquad (3)$$

where c is the initial PSA level at $t = 0$ and d is the rate constant controlling the decline in PSA.

In the hours immediately after prostate surgery for either BPH or carcinoma, PSA rises rapidly before it drops,[36,171] and this produces some of the highest values of d, or even a biphasic exponential decline. For example, Meulemans and colleagues[171] found a sixfold increase in PSA. This more rapid kinetic pattern for PSA in the hours after surgery could result from prostatic and periprostatic tissue necrosis, a phenomenon analogous to the rise in creatine kinase or myoglobin after myocardial infarct[172] or the rise in tumor markers after tumor lysis.[173] It could also be due in part to the free form of PSA, which is thought to have a higher rate of elimination from the blood and via the kidney.[92] On the other hand, since few have measured PSA at hourly intervals after any treatment, surgical or nonsurgi-

cal, we confine our further attention to the slower kinetic decline, which has been found to follow equation 3.

Analogous to the DT for rise in PSA, the rate constant for decline in PSA can be related to a half-life ($T_{1/2}$) with the equation:

$$T_{1/2} = ln(0.5)/d \qquad (4)$$

A number of investigators have measured $T_{1/2}$ of PSA after treatment for prostate cancer. Table 14–6 lists the average d values obtained from each group of patients and by increasing d. The table shows that all of the average values of d for prostatectomy studies were higher than all the averages for radiation treatment studies, which in turn were higher than the averages for hormone treatment studies (excluding the one orchiectomy patient). By inspection this appears far from a random ranking of treatment and d values, and an s test[177] of the order of treatments once sorted by d gave a p value of less than 0.005 that this order could occur by random chance. The overall means of these average values of d, weighted by the number of patients in each study and treatment, were 0.26 for prostatectomy (excluding data from the immediate postoperative hours), 0.014 for radiation and 0.0028 for hormone treatment. On the other hand,

Table 14–6. Average Rate Constant d from Equation 3 in units per day^{-1}

Study	Situation	Therapy	N	d
Apple[172]	Gleason >8	Horm	14	0.00205
Apple[172]	Stage D	Horm	3	0.00234
Apple[172]	Gleason <8	Horm	27	0.00304
Apple[172]	Stage B+C	Horm	13	0.00396
Zagars & Pollack[167]	CA	Rad	5	0.00578
Zagars & Pollack[167]	CA	Rad	17	0.00661
Vogelsang et al.[173]	CA	Rad	32	0.00874
Vogelsang et al.[173]	CA	Rad	15	0.00909
Vogelsang et al.[173]	CA	Rad	7	0.00947
Zagars & Pollack[167]	CA	Rad	25	0.01098
Hanks et al.[165]	CA	Rad	154	0.01196
Arai et al.[174]	CA	Rad	57	0.01337
Arai et al.[174]	CA	Rad	33	0.02841
Arai et al.[174]	CA	Rad	14	0.04132
Kabalin et al.[162]	CA	Orch	1	0.08203
Danella et al.[168]	CA	Surg	30	0.22005
Kaplan et al.[169]	CA	Surg	11	0.27726
Kabalin et al.[162]	CA	Surg	14	0.31507
Kaplan et al.[169]	TCC	Surg	10	0.36101
Kaplan et al.[169]	CA	Surg	7	0.73739
Kaplan et al.[169]	BPH	Surg	10	1.26027
Kabalin et al.[162]	CA	Postop	14	1.30782

CA, adenocarcinoma of the prostate not otherwise specified; TCC, transitional cell carcinoma of the bladder; Horm, hormonal; Rad, radiation; Surg, prostatectomy; Orch, orchiectomy; Postop, immediate postoperative for prostactectomy; N, number of patients.

among irradiated patients alone, neither Ritter and coworkers[175] nor Zagars and Pollack[167] found $T_{1/2}$ related to tumor stage, grade, or outcome in irradiated patients.

Posttreatment Fall and Rise in PSA

Unfortunately, treatment by either surgery or radiation may leave residual tumor (or clinically undetected metastasis may already have occurred), and in this circumstance PSA can first fall and then rise. For example, Stamey and colleagues[85] published curves of PSA like this for patients treated with radiation, and Kaplan and colleagues[169] modeled this pattern with a sum of two exponential functions like those of equations 1 and 3. Although Kaplan and associates used the same rate constant for both the fall and the rise, it seems more realistic to allow for different rates of fall and rise in the PSA curve. Thus, a more general model for this combination of kinetics is the sum of equations 1 and 3 or:

$$y = (y0 - a) * e^{(-d*t)} + a*e^{(b*t)} \quad (5)$$

The first exponential term describes the initial fall in PSA after treatment, and d is defined as before, with a half-life still described by equation 4. Instead of c we have $(y0-a)$ with $y0$ giving the initial concentration of PSA. The second exponential term describes the subsequent rise in PSA due to tumor left untreated, whether because at surgery it was not confined to the prostate or because it was partially insensitive to nonsurgical treatment. The a parameter reflects PSA due to tumor left untreated, and the ratio $a/(y0-a)$ should correlate with the proportion of tumor left untreated. Figure 14–18 demonstrates how well this function can

fit one patient's postradiation PSA levels, published by Stamey and coworkers[85] (the others fit equally well), and we have found that this function accurately describes the posttreatment concentrations of markers of other tumors, such as neuron-specific enolase in small cell lung cancer and of carcinoembryonic antigen (CEA) or alpha-fetoprotein in germ cell tumors, once the initial tumor lysis peak has been passed.[178] Although equation 5 may eventually prove too simplistic to describe all the situations of posttreatment PSA levels, it appears useful for dissecting information from the posttreatment curves. For example, it suggests that in the early posttreatment period a slower fall in PSA could be due to residual tumor rather than a slow half-life. This can be seen in Figure 14–19, which shows what the equation predicts for increasing values of a when d is held constant. We see that, even though increasing values of a suggest longer half-lives, d is actually constant, so that the change is due instead to increasing amounts of residual tumor.

A Compartmental Analysis of PSA Kinetics

We can take another step toward understanding and modeling the kinetics of PSA by using the one-compartment model illustrated in Figure 14–20. Here, PSA comes from the prostate to the blood compartment and is then disposed of through metabolism. A spigot function, labeled f, controls input, and one labeled k controls output. Clearly, what should be of greatest interest is input, because it should most directly reflect the amount of tumor. If PSA is as effective a tumor marker as it appears to be, then the greater the tumor mass, the greater should be the input. Thus if we could somehow monitor the f spigot, we might learn more about the tumor. A look at the mathematics of this model can help.

Mathematically, this compartmental model is expressed as:

$$dy/dt = f(t) - k*y \quad (6)$$

where y again symbolizes PSA level, where dy/dt gives the rate of change of PSA with time (often called PSA velocity), where $f(t)$ denotes the input rate of PSA into the blood compartment, and where k is the rate constant for

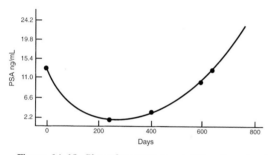

Figure 14–18. Plot of posttreatment PSA values (ng/mL) (*dots*) for one patient published by Stamey and colleagues,[85] together with the fit obtained from equation 5.

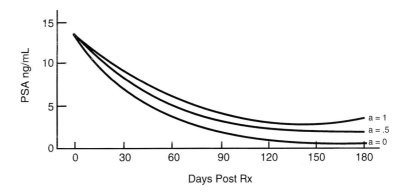

Figure 14–19. Plots of three hypothetical patients' PSA values (ng/mL) after treatment and using equation 5. All three have the same half-life–related d rate constant of 0.0202 per day. The lowest curve has an a value of 0, the next highest an a of 0.5, and the highest an a of 1.

controlling the metabolic loss of PSA from blood. If we solve the equation for $f(t)$, we get:

$$f(t) = dy/dt + k*y, \qquad (7)$$

so that if we know the level of PSA, the rate constant k, and the velocity of PSA, we have enough information to calculate $f(t)$ at any time t.

Perhaps some of the successes and failures of PSA or other serum tumor markers to predict cancer can be understood in terms of this compartmental model. For example, it suggests that neither PSA level nor PSA velocity gives as much information as the sum of these two with y weighted by k. Furthermore, because it is likely that the k value controlling metabolism of PSA is unique for each individual, some of the published noise in the relationships between PSA values and the presence or absence of tumor and between PSA and the volume of tumor may be due to individual variability in k. For example, a false-negative PSA in patients with tumor could be due to higher values of k, because to increase PSA the input rate $f(t)$ must first exceed output. In a similar manner a false-positive result could occur when an unusually low k value is coupled with either age-related or BPH-related increase in $f(t)$.

When we consider the additive effects of different pathologic conditions on PSA level, this compartmental approach suggests that what is added are the f functions, one for each condition. Thus, BPH may have its own $f1(t)$, prostatitis an $f2(t)$, infarct an $f3(t)$, cancer of low grade $f4(t)$, and cancer of high grade an $f5(t)$. The net PSA level we observe then comes from an $f(t)$ that is the sum of these. We suspect that once we gather more kinetic PSA data over different pathologic conditions we may learn that the temporal kinetics of these several f functions will be distinctive, that is, that the amplitudes and time courses of the f for prostatitis will be distinctive from those for BPH, which will be distinctive from those for cancer. Some of the temporal peaks observed in Carter's group's longitudinal data may be due to bursts in one or another of these f functions.[163] Nevertheless, to learn more about these f functions will require more frequent sampling of the blood for PSA.

Considering the success of the exponential model of equation 1 for empirically fitting the temporal pattern of PSA levels, this equation, together with the compartmental model, allows a closer look at both PSA velocity and $f(t)$ for cancer. For example, if the empirical fit is good, then PSA velocity (dy/dt) can be solved by differentiating equation 1 to get:

$$dy/dt = a*e^{(b*t)} * b \qquad (8)$$
$$= b*y$$

Here we see that the PSA velocity is nothing more than the PSA level multiplied by the rate constant b for increase in PSA. Perhaps the similarities in diagnostic sensitivities and specificities for PSA level and PSA velocity[179-181] are due to this proportionality. Another result from the compartmental approach comes

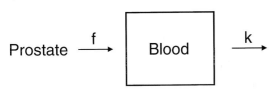

Figure 14–20. One compartmental model for understanding the kinetics of PSA. Input to the blood is from the prostate controlled by the function f, and output is controlled by the metabolic rate constant k.

from substituting equation 8 into equation 7. Now we have one mathematic relationship that shows how $f(t)$ depends on the combination of PSA level (y), the b constant, and the k constant:

$$f(t) = b*y + k*y \\ = (b + k) * y \qquad (9)$$

Since Table 14–5 illustrates that for many prostate cancers b is quite small compared with k, which we presume is approximately 0.26 per day, the contribution of b, and thus of PSA velocity, to $f(t)$ may be outweighed by k. In these circumstances PSA velocity would be expected to add little to PSA level alone in the estimate of $f(t)$, and thus of tumor volume.

Whereas tumor mass in this model is reflected by $f(t)$, the rate of tumor growth should correlate with the rate of change of $f(t)$ or df/dt. We can obtain this by differentiating equation 7 to get:

$$df/dt = d^2y/dt^2 + k*dy/dt \qquad (10)$$

The term d^2y/dt^2 is the change in PSA velocity with time or the acceleration of PSA, and to estimate it requires at least three temporal measures of PSA. Thus, rate of tumor growth should correlate with the PSA acceleration added to the quantity k times the PSA velocity. Once again, if the exponential function of equation 1 fits the PSA curve well, we can use the derivatives of equation 1 to rewrite df/dt as:

$$df/dt = b^2*y + k*b*y \qquad (11)$$

Here, we see the importance of the b rate constant in understanding tumor growth rate, since it multiplies all the terms on the right at

least once. If b is quite small as compared with k, the acceleration term involving b^2 can be ignored and df/dt approximated by:

$$df/dt \approx k*b*y = k*(\text{PSA velocity}) \qquad (12)$$

Thus, this mathematic and compartmental analysis suggests that the greatest importance of PSA velocity may come from its estimate of tumor growth rate. This result in mathematics remains to be tested with data.

Several studies[167,182–184] have found that after treatment, the PSA minimum value or nadir carries important prognostic information. A way to see this in the compartmental model is to recognize that at the nadir, $dy/dt = 0$, so that at this point equation 7 becomes:

$$f(\text{nadir time}) = k*y \qquad (13)$$

In other words, the PSA nadir value (y) at this point is directly proportional to $f(t)$ and thus should directly reflect residual tumor mass.

We see then that, to the degree that input of PSA into the blood reflects tumor mass, the kinetics of PSA levels in the blood provide information about the mass of tumor (including stage), the growth rate of tumor, and the amount of untreated tumor. Specific kinetic parameters are summarized in Table 14–7, which gives their probable associations with cancer based upon either the mathematics of the compartmental model or their associations found from data published previously. The low values of the b rate constant relate to slow tumor growth rates in many prostate cancers and help us understand the limited use of PSA velocity in diagnosis. Nevertheless, the b constant and PSA velocity are likely to provide an estimate of tumor growth rate and could

Table 14–7. Summary of PSA Kinetic Parameters

Parameter	Definition	How Obtained	Probable Relation to CA
k	PSA metabolic rate constant	Rate decrease in PSA	None
$f(t)$	Input function	$dy/dt + k*y$	CA mass
df/dt	Rate of change in $f(t)$	$d^2y/dt^2 + k*dy/dt$	Tumor growth rate
a	Coefficient in exponential growth model	From fit of y vs. t	CA mass-related initial PSA
b	Growth rate constant in exponential fit	From fit of y vs. t	Tumor growth rate, PSA doubling time
$y0$ or c	Coefficients in exponential PSA decline model	From fit of y vs. t	CA mass-related initial PSA
d	Decline rate constant in exponential fit	From fit of y vs. t	Tumor loss rate, PSA half-life
PSA nadir	Minimum posttreatment PSA	As defined	$f(t)$ (& thus CA mass)

help sort tumors into categories of aggressiveness. Perhaps in future studies greater power will come from the combined use of both PSA level and PSA velocity as independent contributors to estimating the biology of prostate cancer.

FUTURE CONSIDERATIONS

Potential future improvements in the joint use of histopathologic appearances of prostate carcinoma and serum PSA in patient management include the use of new measures of PSA, integration of genetic and biologic markers, incorporation of new serum tumor markers, and utilization of new computer modeling systems such as neural networks.

Currently, substantial efforts are being directed toward increasing the sensitivity and specificity of PSA measurements in the serum. As presented in this chapter, a few of these measures, such as PSA density, have already been tested in conjunction with needle biopsy findings in models designed to enhance predictability of tumor behavior. Measurement of free (unbound) serum PSA shows promise in increasing the positive predictive value of single PSA determinations.[185] In the future, newer measures of PSA, such as free PSA and reverse transcriptase–polymerase chain reaction (RT-PCR) assay for PSA mRNA in circulating tumor cells,[186] may assume greater importance in conjunction with the histopathologic appearance of prostate carcinoma in patient management. It is possible that new serum markers for prostate carcinoma may complement or outperform PSA.[6,187] Additionally, new molecular or biologic parameters,[188] such as microvessel density,[189] may be integrated into prognostic indices that incorporate histopathologic appearance of prostatic carcinoma and PSA. Improvement of prognostic indices may be possible in the future with the use of such computer modeling systems as neural networks.[190] It will be important carefully to consider and implement guidelines for evaluation of new prognostic markers and models as they are developed.[191]

Finally, one may speculate that these new developments may be applied to address issues that are critical for patients with prostate cancer.[192] Prominent among these is the need to define pretreatment parameters that will allow for an accurate determination of true (pathologic) stage. Another crucial task is the delineation of those parameters that will allow for a reliable pretreatment distinction between low-risk and high-risk prostate carcinoma. Histopathologic analysis of prostate carcinoma, in conjunction with markers such as PSA, will continue to be a highly significant component in endeavors to address these and other vital issues that affect the clinical management of patients with carcinoma of the prostate.

Acknowledgments

The authors wish to thank Debbie Bahre for typing the manuscript and Dr. David Keetch and Dr. William Catalona, Washington University, for critical reading of this chapter.

REFERENCES

1. Mettlin C, Jones GW, Murphy GP: Trends in prostate cancer care in the United States, 1974–1990: Observations from the patient care evaluation studies of the American College of Surgeons Commission on Cancer. CA Cancer J Clin 43:83–91, 1993.
2. Mettlin C, Jones G, Averette H, et al.: Defining and updating the American Cancer Society guidelines for the cancer-related check-up: Prostate and endometrial cancers. CA Cancer J Clin 43:42–46, 1993.
3. American Urological Association Executive Committee Report, 1992. Baltimore, Md.: American Urological Association, 1992.
4. Steele GD Jr, Osteen RT, Winchester DP, et al.: Clinical highlights from the National Cancer Data Base: 1994. CA Cancer J Clin 44:71–80, 1994.
5. Wingo PA, Tong T, Bolden S: Cancer statistics, 1995. CA Cancer J Clin 45:8–30, 1995.
6. Schellhammer PF, Wright GL Jr: Biomolecular and clinical characteristics of PSA and other candidate prostate tumor markers. Urol Clin North Am 20(4):597–606, 1993.
7. Bostwick DG: Prostate-specific antigen: Current role in diagnostic pathology of prostate cancer. Am J Clin Pathol 102 (Suppl 1):531–537, 1994.
8. Ruckle HC, Klee GG, Oesterling JE: Prostate-specific antigen: Concepts for staging prostate cancer and monitoring response to therapy. Mayo Clin Proc 69:69–79, 1994.
9. Brawer MK: Prostate-specific antigen: Critical issues. Urology 44:9–17, 1994.
10. Oesterling JE: Prostate specific antigen: A critical assessment of the most useful tumor marker for adenocarcinoma of the prostate. J Urol 145:907–923, 1991.
11. Partin AW, Oesterling JE: The clinical usefulness of prostate specific antigen: Update 1994. J Urol 152:1358–1368, 1994.
12. Ploch NR, Brawer MK: How to use prostate-specific antigen. Urology 43 (Suppl):27–35, 1994.
13. Takayama TK, Vessella RL, Lange PH: Newer applications of serum prostate-specific antigen in the management of prostate cancer. Semin Oncol 21:542–553, 1994.

14. McCormack RT, Rittenhouse HG, Finlay JA, et al.: Molecular forms of prostate-specific antigen and the human kallikrein gene family: A new era. Urology 45:729–744, 1995.

15. Lowe FC, Trauzzi SJ: Prostatic acid phosphatase in 1993. Its limited clinical utility. In Oesterling JE (ed): Urol Clin North Am 20(4):589–595, 1993.

16. Armbruster DA: Prostate-specific antigen: Biochemistry, analytical methods, and clinical application. Clin Chem 39:181–195, 1993.

17. Riegman PHJ, Vlietstra RJ, van der Korput JAGM, et al.: Characterization of the prostate-specific antigen gene: A novel human kallikrein-like gene. Biochem Biophys Res Commun 159:95–102, 1989.

18. Lundwall A, Lilja H: Molecular cloning of human prostate specific antigen cDNA. FEBS Lett 214:317–322, 1987.

19. Schaller J, Akiyama K, Tsuda R, et al.: Isolation, characterization and amino-acid sequence of gamma-seminoprotein, a glycoprotein from human seminal plasma. Eur J Biochem 170:111–120, 1987.

20. Frazier HA, Humphrey PA, Burchette JL, et al.: Immunoreactive prostatic specific antigen in male periurethral glands. J Urol 147:246–248, 1990.

21. Kamoshida S, Tsutsumi Y: Extraprostatic localization of prostatic acid phosphatase and prostate-specific antigen: Distribution in cloacogenic glandular epithelium and sex-dependent expression in human anal gland. Hum Pathol 21:1108–1111, 1990.

22. Pollen JJ, Dreilinger A: Immunohistochemical identification of prostatic acid phosphatase and prostate specific antigen in female periurethral glands. Urology 23:303–304, 1984.

23. Tepper SL, Jagirdar J, Heath D, et al.: Homology between female paraurethral (Skene's) glands and the prostate. Immunohistochemical demonstration. Arch Pathol Lab Med 108:423–425, 1984.

24. Elgamal AA, van de Voorde W, van Poppel H, et al.: Immunohistochemical localization of prostate-specific markers within the accessory male sex glands of Cowper, Littre, and Morgagni. Urology 44:84–91, 1994.

25. Golz R, Schubert GE: Prostate specific antigen: immunoreactivity in urachal remnants. J Urol 141:1480–1482, 1989.

26. Nowels K, Kent E, Rinsho K, et al.: Prostate specific antigen and acid phosphatase-reactive cells in cystitis cystica and glandularis. Arch Pathol Lab Med 11:734–737, 1988.

27. Clements J, Mukhtar A: Glandular kallikreins and prostate-specific antigen are expressed in the human endometrium. J Clin Endocrinol Metab 78:1536–1539, 1994.

28. Epstein JI: PSA and PAP as immunohistochemical markers in prostate cancer. In Oesterling JE (ed): Urol Clin North Am 20(4):757–770, 1993.

29. van Krieken JH: Prostate marker immunoreactivity in salivary gland neoplasms. A rare pitfall in immunohistochemistry. Am J Surg Pathol 17:410–414, 1993.

30. Monne M, Croce CM, Yu H, et al.: Molecular characterization of prostate-specific antigen messenger RNA expressed in breast tumors. Cancer Res 54:6344–6347, 1994.

31. Iwakiri J, Grandbois K, Wehner N, et al.: An analysis of urinary prostate specific antigen before and after radical prostatectomy: Evidence for secretion of prostate specific antigen by the periurethral glands. J Urol 149:783–786, 1993.

32. Takayama TK, Vessella RL, Brawer MK, et al.: Urinary prostate specific antigen levels after radical prostatectomy. J Urol 151:82–87, 1994.

33. Sensabaugh GF: Isolation and characterization of a serum-specific protein from human seminal plasma: A potential new marker for serum identification. J Forensic Sci 23:106–115, 1978.

34. Vessella RL, Lange PH: Issues in the assessment of PSA immunoassays. In Oesterling JE, (ed): Urol Clin North Am 20(4):607–619, 1993.

35. Stamey TA: Second Stanford Conference on international standardization of prostate-specific antigen immunoassays. September 1 and 2, 1994. Urology 45:173–184, 1995.

36. Stamey TA, Yang N, Hay AR, et al.: Prostate-specific antigen as a serum marker for adenocarcinoma of the prostate. N Engl J Med 317:909–916, 1987.

37. Nadler RB, Humphrey PA, Smith DS, et al.: Effect of inflammation and benign prostatic hyperplasia on elevated serum prostate specific antigen levels. J Urol 154:409–413, 1995.

38. Bahnson RR: Elevation of prostate specific antigen from bacillus Calmette-Guerin–induced granulomatous prostatis. J Urol 146:1368–1369, 1991.

39. Neal DE Jr, Clejan S, Sarma D, et al.: Prostate specific antigen and prostatitis I: Effect of prostatitis on serum PSA in the human and nonhuman primate. Prostate 20:105–111, 1992.

40. Hasui Y, Marutsuka K, Asada Y, et al.: Relationship between serum prostate specific antigen and histological prostatitis in patients with benign prostatic hyperplasia. Prostate 25:91–96, 1994.

41. Brawn PN, Johnson EH, Foster DM, et al.: Characteristics of prostatic infarcts and their effect on serum prostate-specific antigen and prostatic acid phosphatase. Urology 44:71–75, 1994.

42. Yuan JJ, Coplen DE, Petros JA, et al.: Effects of rectal examination, prostatic massage, ultrasonography and needle biopsy on serum prostate specific antigen levels. J Urol 147:810–814, 1992.

43. Armitage TG, Cooper EH, Newling DW, et al.: The value of the measurement of serum prostate specific antigen in patients with benign prostatic hyperplasia and untreated prostate cancer. Br J Urol 62:584–589, 1988.

44. Ronnett BM, Carmichael MJ, Carter HB, et al.: Does high-grade prostatic intraepithelial neoplasia result in elevated serum prostate specific antigen levels? J Urol 150:386–389, 1993.

45. de la Torre M, Haggman M, Brandstedt S, et al.: Prostatic intraepithelial neoplasia and invasive carcinoma in total prostatectomy specimens: Distribution, volumes and DNA ploidy. Br J Urol 72:207–213, 1993.

46. Humphrey PA, Frazier HA, Paulson DF, et al.: Extent of severe dysplasia in the prostate is inversely related to pathologic stage [Abstr]. Lab Invest 88:54A, 1992.

47. Catalona WJ, Richie JP, Ahmann FR, et al.: Comparison of digital rectal examination and serum prostate specific antigen in the early detection of prostate cancer: Results of a multicenter clinical trial of 6,630 men. J Urol 151:1283–1290, 1994.

48. Catalona WJ, Smith D, Ratliff TL, et al.: Measurement of prostate-specific antigen as a screening test for prostate cancer. N Engl J Med 324:1156–1161, 1991.

49. Cooner WH, Mosley BR, Rutherford CL Jr, et al.: Prostate cancer detection in a clinical urological

practice by ultrasonography, digital rectal examination and prostate specific antigen. J Urol 143:1146–1154, 1990.

50. Flanigan RC, Catalona WJ, Richie JP, et al.: Accuracy of digital rectal examination and transrectal ultrasonography in localizing prostate cancer. J Urol 152:1506–1509, 1994.
51. Smith DS, Catalona WJ: Interexaminer variability of digital rectal examination in detecting prostate cancer. Urology 45:70–74, 1995.
52. Gerber GS, Thompson IM, Thisted R, et al.: Disease-specific survival following routine prostate cancer screening by digital rectal examination. JAMA 269:61–64, 1993.
53. Partin AW, Pound CR, Clemens JQ, et al.: Serum PSA after anatomic radical prostatectomy. The Johns Hopkins experience after 10 years. Urol Clin North Am 20(4):713–725, 1993.
54. Catalona WJ, Smith DS, Ratliff TL, et al.: Detection of organ-confined prostate cancer is increased through prostate-specific antigen-based screening. JAMA 270:948–954, 1993.
55. Smith DS, Catalona WJ: The nature of prostate cancer detected through prostate specific antigen based screening. J Urol 152:1732–1736, 1994.
56. Mettlin C, Murphy GP, Lee F, et al.: Characteristics of prostate cancer detected in the American Cancer Society—National Prostate Cancer Detection Project. J Urol 152:1737–1740, 1994.
57. Brawer MK, Chetner MP, Beatie J, et al.: Screening for prostatic carcinoma with prostate specific antigen. J Urol 147:841–845, 1992.
58. Brawer MK, Beatie J, Wener MH, et al.: Screening for prostatic carcinoma with prostate specific antigen: Results of the second year. J Urol 150:106–109, 1993.
59. Boring CC, Squires TS, Tong T: Cancer statistics, 1993. CA Cancer J Clin 43:7–26, 1993.
60. Gann PH, Hennekens CH, Stampfer MJ: A prospective evaluation of plasma prostate-specific antigen for detection of prostate cancer. JAMA 273:289–294, 1995.
61. Helzlsouer KJ, Newby J, Comstock GW: Prostate-specific antigen levels and subsequent prostate cancer: Potential for screening. Cancer Epi Biomarkers Prevent 1:537–540, 1992.
62. Catalona WJ, Bigg SW: Nerve-sparing radical prostatectomy: Evaluation of results after 250 patients. J Urol 143:538–543, 1990.
63. Humphrey PA, Baty J, Keetch D: Relationship between serum prostate-specific antigen, needle biopsy findings, and histopathologic features of prostate carcinoma in radical prostatectomy tissues. Cancer 75:1842–1849, 1995.
64. Humphrey PA, Keetch DW, Smith DS, et al.: Prospective characterization of pathologic features of prostatic carcinomas detected via serum prostate specific antigen-based screening. J Urol 155:816–820, 1996.
65. Gohagan JK, Prorok PC, Kramer BS, et al.: Prostate cancer screening in the prostate, lung, colorectal and ovarian cancer screening trial of the National Cancer Institute. J Urol 152:1905–1909, 1994.
66. Kleer E, Oesterling JE: PSA and staging of localized prostate cancer. Urol Clin North Am 20(4):695–704, 1993.
67. Hudson MA, Bahnson RR, Catalona WJ: Clinical use of prostate specific antigen in patients with prostate cancer. J Urol 142:1011–1017, 1989.
68. Cohen RJ, Haffejee Z, Steele GS, et al.: Advanced prostate cancer with normal serum prostate-specific antigen values. Arch Pathol Lab Med 118:1123–1126, 1994.
69. Stamey TA, Dietrick DD, Issa MM: Large organ confined, impalpable transition zone prostate cancer: Association with metastatic levels of prostatic specific antigen. J Urol 149:510–515, 1993.
70. Partin AW, Carter HB, Chan PW, et al.: Prostate specific antigen in the staging of localized prostate cancer: Influence of tumor differentiation, tumor volume and benign hyperplasia. J Urol 143:747–752, 1990.
71. Blackwell KL, Bostwick DG, Myers RP, et al.: Combining prostate specific antigen with cancer and gland volume to predict more reliably pathological stage: The influence of prostate specific antigen cancer density. J Urol 151:1565–1570, 1994.
72. Palken M, Cobb OE, Warren BH, et al.: Prostate cancer: Correlation of digital rectal examination, transrectal ultrasound and prostate specific antigen levels with tumor volumes in radical prostatectomy specimens. J Urol 151:1155–1162, 1990.
73. Aihara M, Lebovitz RM, Wheeler TM, et al.: Prostate specific antigen and Gleason grade: An immunohistochemical study of prostate cancer. J Urol 151:1558–1564, 1994.
74. Greskovich FJ III, Johnson DE, Tenney DM, et al.: Prostate specific antigen in patients with clinical stage C prostate cancer: Relation to lymph node status and grade. J Urol 145:798–801, 1991.
75. Zagars GK, Sherman NE, Babaian RJ: Prostate-specific antigen and external beam radiation therapy in prostate cancer. Cancer 67:412–420, 1991.
76. Babaian RJ, Camps JL, Frangos DN, et al.: Monoclonal prostate-specific antigen in untreated prostate cancer. Relationship to clinical stage and grade. Cancer 67:2200–2206, 1991.
77. Frazier HA, Robertson JE, Humphrey PA, et al.: Is prostate specific antigen of clinical importance in evaluating outcome after radical prostatectomy? J Urol 149:516–518, 1993.
78. Goad JR, Chang S-J, Ohori M, et al.: PSA after definitive radiotherapy for clinically localized prostate cancer. Urol Clin North Am 20(4):727–736, 1993.
79. Zagars GK: Serum PSA as a tumor marker for patients undergoing definitive radiation therapy. Urol Clin North Am 20(4):737–747, 1993.
80. Cooper EH, Armitage TG, Robinson MR, et al.: Prostatic specific antigen and the prediction of prognosis in metastatic prostatic cancer. Cancer 66:1025–1028, 1990.
81. Petros JA, Andriole GL: Serum PSA after antiandrogen therapy. Urol Clin North Am 20(4):749–756, 1993.
82. Humphrey PA, Frazier HA, Vollmer RT, et al.: Stratification of pathologic features in radical prostatectomy specimens that are predictive of elevated initial postoperative serum prostate-specific antigen levels. Cancer 71:1821–1827, 1993.
83. Stamey TA, Kabalin JN, McNeal JE, et al.: Prostate specific antigen in the diagnosis and treatment of adenocarcinoma of the prostate. II. Radical prostatectomy treated patients. J Urol 141:1076–1083, 1989.
84. Stein A, deKernion JB, Smith RB, et al.: Prostate specific antigen levels after radical prostatectomy in patients with organ-confined and locally extensive prostate cancer. J Urol 147:942–946, 1992.

85. Stamey TA, Kabalin JN, Ferrari M: Prostate specific antigen in the diagnosis and treatment of adenocarcinoma of the prostate. III. Radiation treated patients. J Urol 141:1084–1087, 1989.

86. Schellhammer PF, el-Mahdi AM, Wright GL Jr, et al.: Prostate-specific antigen to determine progression-free survival after radiation therapy for localized carcinoma of prostate. Urology 42:13–20, 1993.

87. McCarthy JF, Catalona WJ, Hudson MA: Effect of radiation therapy on detectable serum prostate specific antigen levels following radical prostatectomy: Early versus delayed treatment. J Urol 151:1575–1578, 1994.

88. Catalona WJ, Smith DS: Comparison of different serum prostate specific antigen measures for early prostate cancer detection. Cancer 74:1516–1518, 1994.

89. Seaman E, Whang M, Olsson CA, et al.: PSA density (PSAD): Role in patient evaluation and management. Urol Clin North Am 20(4):653–663, 1993.

90. Oesterling JE, Cooner WH, Jacobson SJ, et al.: Influence of patient age on serum PSA concentration: An important clinical observation. Urol Clin North Am 20(4):671–680, 1993.

91. Carter HB, Pearson JD: PSA velocity for the diagnosis of early prostate cancer. Urol Clin North Am 20(4):665–670, 1993.

92. Lilja H: Significance of different molecular forms of serum PSA. The free, noncomplexed form of PSA versus that complexed to alpha-1-antichymotrypsin. Urol Clin North Am 20(4):681–686, 1993.

93. Prestigiacomo AF, Stamey TA: A comparison of 4 ultrasensitive prostate specific antigen assays for early detection of residual cancer after radical prostatectomy. J Urol 152:1515–1519, 1994.

94. Catalona WJ, Richie JP, deKernion JB, et al.: Comparison of prostate specific antigen concentration versus prostate specific antigen density in the early detection of prostate cancer: Receiver operating characteristic curves. J Urol 152:2031–2036, 1994.

95. Smith DS, Catalona WJ: Rate of change in serum prostate specific antigen levels as a method for prostate cancer detection. J Urol 152:1163–1167, 1994.

96. Humphrey PA, Walther PJ: Adenocarcinoma of the prostate. Part II. Tissue prognosticators. Am J Clin Pathol 100:256–259, 1993.

97. Schmid H-P, McNeal JE, Stamey TA: Observations on the doubling time of prostate cancer. The use of serial prostate-specific antigen in patients with untreated disease as a measure of increasing cancer volume. Cancer 71:2031–2040, 1993.

98. Scardino PT, Weaver R, Hudson MA: Early detection of prostate cancer. Hum Pathol 23:211–222, 1992.

99. Haas GP, Sakr WA, Heilbrun LK, et al.: Prevalence of prostatic intraepithelial neoplasia and cancer in black and white men: Update of the Wayne State University Autopsy Study [Abstr]. J Urol 153:313A, 1995.

100. Stormont TJ, Farrow GM, Myers RP, et al.: Clinical stage BO or Tlc prostate cancer: Nonpalpable disease identified by elevated serum prostate-specific antigen concentration. Urology 41:3–8, 1993.

101. Oesterling JE, Suman VJ, Zincke H, et al.: PSA-detected (clinical stage Tlc or BO) prostate cancer: Pathologically significant tumors. Urol Clin North Am 20(4):687–693, 1993.

102. Ohori M, Wheeler TM, Dunn JK, et al.: The pathological features and prognosis of prostate cancer de-

tectable with current diagnostic tests. J Urol 152:1714–1720, 1994.

103. Scaletscky R, Koch MO, Eckstein CW, et al.: Tumor volume and stage in carcinoma of the prostate detected by elevations in prostate specific antigen. J Urol 152:129–131, 1994.

104. Guthman DA, Wilson TM, Blute ML, et al.: Biopsy-proved prostate cancer in 100 consecutive men with benign digital rectal examination and elevated serum prostate-specific antigen level. Prevalence and pathologic characteristics. Urology 42:150–154, 1993.

105. Epstein JI, Walsh PC, Carmichael M, et al.: Pathologic and clinical findings to predict tumor extent of nonpalpable (stage Tlc) prostate cancer. JAMA 271:368–374, 1994.

106. Douglas TH, Sesterhenn IA, Moul JW, et al.: The significance of PSA-detected, nonpalpable adenocarcinoma of the prostate (stage Tlc) [Abstr]. J Urol 153:251A, 1995.

107. Humphrey PA, Geary WA, Catalona WJ: Prostate specific antigen–detected versus digitally detected prostatic adenocarcinoma: Comparative pathologic features in needle biopsies [Abstr]. Mod Pathol 6:61A, 1993.

108. Berman JJ, Moore GW, Alonsozana ELC, et al.: Prostate-specific antigen screening for prostate cancer: No reduction in Gleason scores. Mod Pathol 7:487–489, 1994.

109. Petros JA, Catalona WJ: Lower incidence of unsuspected lymph node metastases in 521 consecutive patients with clinically localized prostate cancer. J Urol 147:1574–1575, 1992.

110. Schroder FH, Hermanek P, Denis L, et al.: The TNM classification of prostate cancer. Prostate 4(Suppl): 129–138, 1992.

111. Ohori M, Wheeler TM, Scardino PT: The New American Joint Committee on Cancer and International Union Against Cancer TNM classification of prostate cancer. Clinicopathologic correlations. Cancer 74:104–114, 1994.

112. Aihara M, Goto Y, Song S, et al.: What makes a cancer palpable—a comparison of the pathologic features of Tlc and T2 prostate cancers [Abstr]. J Urol 153:517A, 1994.

113. Keetch DW, Catalona WJ, Smith DS: Serial prostatic biopsies in men with persistently elevated serum prostate specific antigen values. J Urol 151:1571–1574, 1994.

114. Stamey TA: Making the most out of six systematic sextant biopsies. Urology 45:2–12, 1995.

115. Keetch DW, Humphrey P, Stahl D, et al.: Morphometric analysis and clinical follow-up of isolated prostatic intraepithelial neoplasia in needle biopsy of the prostate. J Urol 154:347–351, 1995.

116. Weinstein MH, Epstein JI: Significance of high-grade prostatic intraepithelial neoplasia on needle biopsy. Hum Pathol 24:624–629, 1993.

117. Kojima M, Troncoso P, Babaian RJ: Use of prostate-specific antigen and tumor volume in predicting needle biopsy grading error. Urology 45:807–812, 1995.

118. Irwin MB, Trapasso JG: Identification of insignificant prostate cancers: Analysis of preoperative parameters. Urology 44:862–868, 1994.

119. Goto Y, Ohori M, Arakawa A, et al.: Distinguishing clinically unimportant prostate cancers before treatment: Preliminary report [Abstr]. J Urol 151:289A, 1994.

120. Terris MK, Haney DJ, Johnstone IM, et al.: Prediction

of prostate cancer volume using prostate-specific antigen levels, transrectal ultrasound, and systematic sextant biopsies. Urology 45:75–80, 1995.

121. Kleer E, Larson-Keller JJ, Zincke H, et al.: Ability of preoperative serum prostate-specific antigen value to predict pathologic stage and DNA ploidy. Influence of clinical stage and tumor grade. Urology 41:207–216, 1993.

122. Wolf JS Jr, Shirohara K, Carroll PR, et al.: Combined role of transrectal ultrasonography, Gleason score, and prostate-specific antigen in predicting organ-confined prostate cancer. Urology 42:131–137, 1993.

123. Arai Y, Yoshiki T, Yamabe H, et al.: Value of prostate-specific antigen measurements in predicting lymph node involvement in prostatic cancer. Urol Int 45:356–360, 1990.

124. Bishoff JT, St. Clair SR, Reyes A, et al.: Pelvic lymph-adenectomy can be omitted in selected patients with carcinoma of the prostate: Development of a system of patient selection. Urology 45:270–274, 1995.

125. Bluestein DL, Bostwick DG, Bergstralh EJ, et al.: Eliminating the need for bilateral pelvic lymphade-nopathy in select patients with prostate cancer. J Urol 151:1315–1320, 1994.

126. Danella JF, deKernion JB, Smith RB, et al.: The contemporary incidence of lymph node metastases in prostate cancer: Implications for laparoscopic lymph node dissection. J Urol 149:1488–1491, 1993.

127. Diaz A, Rouch M III, Marquez C, et al.: Indications for and the significance of seminal vesicle irradiation during 3D conformal radiotherapy for localized prostate cancer. Int J Radiat Oncol Biol Phys 30:323–329, 1994.

128. Narayan P, Fournier G, Gajendran V, et al.: Utility of preoperative serum prostate-specific antigen concentration and biopsy Gleason score in predicting risk of pelvic lymph node metastases in prostate cancer. Urology 44:519–524, 1994.

129. Nishiya M, Miller GJ, Lookner DH, et al.: Prostate specific antigen density in patients with histologically proven prostate carcinoma. Cancer 74:3002–3009, 1994.

130. Partin AW, Yoo J, Carter HB, et al.: The use of prostate specific antigen, clinical stage and Gleason score to predict pathological stage in men with localized prostate cancer. J Urol 150:110–114, 1993.

131. Roach M III, Marquez C, Yuo H-S, et al.: Predicting the risk of lymph node involvement using the pre-treatment prostate specific antigen and Gleason score in men with clinically localized prostate cancer. Int J Radiat Oncol Biol Phys 28:33–37, 1993.

132. Ackerman DA, Barry JM, Wickland RA, et al.: Analysis of risk factors associated with prostate cancer extension to the surgical margin and pelvic node metastases at radical prostatectomy. J Urol 150:1845–1850, 1993.

133. Ravery V, Boccon-Gibod LA, Dauge-Geffroy MC, et al.: Systematic biopsies accurately predict extracapsular extension of prostate cancer and persistent/recurrent detectable PSA after radical prostatectomy. Urology 44:371–376, 1994.

134. D'Amico AV, Whittington R, Malkowicz SB, et al.: A multivariate analysis of clinical and pathological factors which predict for prostate specific antigen failure after radical prostatectomy for prostate cancer [Abstr]. J Urol 153:430A, 1995.

135. Pisansky TM, Cha SS, Earle JD, et al.: Prostate-specific antigen as a pretherapy prognostic factor in patients treated with radiation therapy for clinically localized prostate cancer. J Clin Oncol 11:2158–2166, 1993.

136. Stamey TA, McNeal JE: Adenocarcinoma of the prostate. In Walsh PC, Retik AB, Stamey TA, et al. (eds): Campbell's Urology, 6th ed. Philadelphia: W.B. Saunders, 1992, pp 1159–1160.

137. Stamey TA, Freiha FS, McNeal JE, et al.: Relationship of tumor volume to clinical significance for treatment in prostate cancer. Cancer 71:933–940, 1993.

138. McNeal JE: Cancer volume and site of origin of adenocarcinoma in the prostate: Relationship to local and distant spread. Hum Pathol 23:258–266, 1992.

139. Epstein JI, Carmichael M, Partin AW, et al.: Is tumor volume an independent predictor of progression following radical prostatectomy? A multivariate analysis of 185 clinical stage B adenocarcinomas of the prostate with 5 years of follow-up. J Urol 149:1478–1481, 1993.

140. Sands ME, Zagars GK, Pollack A, et al.: Serum prostate-specific antigen, clinical stage, pathologic grade, and the incidence of nodal metastases in prostate cancer. Urology 44:215–220, 1994.

141. Vijayakumar V, Vijayakumar S, Quadri SF, et al.: Can prostate-specific antigen levels predict bone scan evidence of metastases in newly diagnosed prostate cancer? Am J Clin Oncol 17:432–436, 1994.

142. Lepor H, Wang B, Shapiro E: Relationship between prostatic epithelial volume and serum prostate-specific antigen levels. Urology 44:199–205, 1994.

143. Hammerer PG, McNeal JE, Stamey TA: Correlation between serum prostate specific antigen levels and the volume of the individual glandular zones of the human prostate. J Urol 153:111–114, 1995.

144. Lloyd SN, Collins GN, McKelvie GB, et al.: Predicted and actual change in serum PSA following prostatectomy for BPH. Urology 43:472–479, 1994.

145. Caddedu JA, Pearson JD, Lee BR, et al.: Relationship between changes in prostate-specific antigen and the percent of prostatic epithelium in men with benign prostatic hyperplasia. Urology 45:795–800, 1995.

146. Kearse WS Jr, Seay TM, Thompson IM: The long-term risk of development of prostate cancer in patients with benign prostatic hyperplasia: Correlation with stage A1 disease. J Urol 150:1746–1748, 1993.

147. Gaudin PB, Wojno KJ, Sesterhenn IA, et al.: High-grade PIN in TURP specimens [Abstr]. Mod Pathol 8:76A, 1995.

148. McNeal JE, Bostwick DG: Intraductal dysplasia: A premalignant lesion of the prostate. Hum Pathol 17:64–71, 1986.

149. Epstein JI, Cho KR, Quinn BD: Relationship of severe dysplasia to stage A (incidental) carcinoma of the prostate. Cancer 65:2321–2327, 1990.

150. Epstein JI: Personal communication, April 1995.

151. Carter HB, Partin AW, Epstein JI, et al.: The relationship of prostate specific antigen levels and residual tumor volume in stage A prostate cancer. J Urol 144:1167–1171, 1990.

152. Berner A, Waere H, Nesland JM, et al.: DNA ploidy, serum prostate specific antigen, histological grade and immunohistochemistry as prediction parameters of lymph node metastases in T1-T3/NO prostatic adenocarcinoma. Br J Urol 75:26–32, 1995.

153. Partin AW, Pound CR, Pearson JD, et al.: Evaluation of serum prostate-specific antigen velocity after radical prostatectomy to distinguish local recurrence from distant metastases. Urology 43:649–659, 1994.

154. Partin AW, Piantadosi S, Sanda MG, et al.: Selection of men at high risk for disease recurrence for experimental adjuvant therapy following radical prostatectomy. Urology 45:831–838, 1995.

155. Goldrath DE, Messing EM: Prostate-specific antigen not detectable despite tumor progression after radical prostatectomy. J Urol 142:1082–1084, 1989.

156. Takayama TK, Krieger JN, True LD, et al.: Recurrent prostate cancer despite undetectable prostate-specific antigen. J Urol 148:1541–1542, 1992.

157. Goad JR, Kassahian VS, Weaver RL, et al.: PSA as measure of recurrent prostate cancer after radical prostatectomy [Abstr]. J Urol 149:447A, 1993.

158. Abi-Aad AS, MacFarlane MT, Stein A, et al.: Detection of local recurrence after radical prostatectomy by prostate specific antigen and transrectal ultrasound. J Urol 147:952–955, 1992.

159. Foster LS, Jojodia P, Fournier G Jr, et al.: The value of prostate specific antigen and transrectal ultrasound guided biopsy in detecting prostatic fossa recurrences following radical prostatectomy. J Urol 149:1024–1028, 1993.

160. Fowler JE Jr, Brooks J, Dandey P, et al.: Variable histology of anastomotic biopsies with detectable prostate specific antigen after radical prostatectomy. J Urol 153:1011–1014, 1995.

161. Carter HB: Current status of PSA in the management of prostate cancer. In Cameron JL, Balch CM, Langer B, et al. (eds): Advances in Surgery, vol 27. Chicago: Mosby-Year Book, 1994, pp 81–95.

162. Kabalin JN, Hodge KK, McNeal JE, et al.: Identification of residual cancer in the prostate following radiation therapy: Role of transrectal ultrasound guided biopsy and prostate specific antigen. J Urol 142:326–331, 1989.

163. Carter HB, Morrell CH, Pearson JD, et al.: Estimation of prostatic growth using serial prostate-specific antigen measurements in men with and without prostate disease. Cancer Res 52:3323–3328, 1992.

164. Stamey TA, Kabalin JN: Prostate specific antigen in the diagnosis and treatment of adenocarcinoma of the prostate. I. Untreated patients. J Urol 141:1070–1075, 1989.

165. Hanks GE, D'Amico A, Epstein EE, et al.: Prostatic-specific antigen doubling times in patients with prostate cancer: A potentially useful reflection of tumor doubling time. Int J Radiat Oncol Biol Phys 27:135–137, 1993.

166. Pollack A, Zagars GK, Kavadi VS: Prostate specific antigen doubling time and disease relapse after radiotherapy for prostate cancer. Cancer 74:670–678, 1994.

167. Zagars GK, Pollack A: The fall and rise of prostate-specific antigen. Kinetics of serum prostate-specific antigen levels after radiation therapy for prostate cancer. Cancer 72:832–842, 1993.

168. Danella J, Steckel J, Dorey F, et al.: Detectable prostate specific antigen levels following radical prostatectomy: relationship of doubling time to clinical outcome [Abstr]. J Urol 149:447A, 1993.

169. Kaplan ID, Cox RS, Bagshaw MA: A model of prostatic carcinoma tumor kinetics based on prostate specific antigen levels after radiation therapy. Cancer 68:400–405, 1991.

170. Oesterling JE, Chan DW, Epstein JI, et al.: Prostate specific antigen in the preoperative and postoperative evaluation of localized prostatic cancer treated with radical prostatectomy. J Urol 139:766–772, 1988.

171. Meulemans A, Haab F, Boccon-Gibod L: Clearance of serum PSA after open surgery for BPH, radical prostatectomy and cystoprostatectomy: A comparative prospective study [Abstr]. J Urol 149:402A, 1994.

172. Apple FS: Acute myocardial infarction and coronary reperfusion. Serum cardiac markers for the 1990's. Am J Clin Pathol 97:217–226, 1992.

173. Vogelsang NJ, Lange PH, Goldman A, et al.: Acute changes of alpha-fetoprotein and human chorionic gonadotropin during induction chemotherapy of germ cell tumors. Cancer Res 42:4855–4861, 1982.

174. Arai Y, Yoshiki T, Yoshida O: Prognostic significance of prostate specific antigen in endocrine treatment for prostate cancer. J Urol 144:1415–1419, 1990.

175. Ritter MA, Messing EM, Shanahan TG, et al.: Prostate-specific antigen as a predictor of radiotherapy response and patterns of failure in localized prostate cancer. J Clin Oncol 10:1208–1217, 1992.

176. Dundas GS, Porter AT, Venner PM: Prostate-specific antigen. Monitoring the response of carcinoma of the prostate to radiotherapy with a new tumor marker. Cancer 66:45–48, 1990.

177. Noether GE: Introduction to Statistics, a Nonparametric Approach. Boston: Houghton Mifflin, 1976, pp 192–193.

178. Vollmer RT: Unpublished results.

179. Carter HB, Pearson JD: Evaluation of changes in PSA in the management of men with prostate cancer. Semin Oncol 21:554–559, 1994.

180. Mettlin C, Littrup PJ, Kane RA, et al.: Relative sensitivity and specificity of serum prostate specific antigen (PSA) level compared with age-referenced PSA, PSA density, and PSA change. Cancer 74:1615–1620, 1994.

181. Littrup PJ, Kane RA, Mettlin C, et al.: Cost-effective prostate cancer detection. Cancer 74:3146–3158, 1994.

182. Stamey TA, Kabalin JN, Ferrari M, et al.: Prostate specific antigen in the diagnosis and treatment of adenocarcinoma of the prostate. IV. Anti-androgen treated patients. J Urol 141:1088–1090, 1989.

183. Babaian RJ, Kojima M, Saitoh M, et al.: Detection of residual prostate cancer after external radiotherapy. Role of prostate specific antigen and transrectal ultrasonography. Cancer 75:2153–2158, 1995.

184. Critz FA, Tarlton RS, Holladay DA: Prostate specific antigen-monitored combination radiotherapy for patients with prostate cancer. Cancer 75:2383–2391, 1995.

185. Catalona WJ, Smith DS, Wolfert RL, et al.: Evaluation of percentage of free serum prostate-specific antigen to improve specificity of prostate cancer screening. JAMA 274:1214–1220, 1995.

186. Katz AE, Vries GM, Begg MD, et al.: Enhanced reverse transcriptase-polymerase chain reaction for prostate specific antigen as an indicator of true pathologic stage in patients with prostate cancer. Cancer 75:1642–1648, 1995.

187. Su SL, Huang I-P, Fair WR, et al.: Alternatively spliced variants of prostate-specific membrane antigen RNA: Ratio of expression as a potential measurement of progression. Cancer Res 55:1441–1443, 1995.

188. Netto GJ, Humphrey PA: Molecular biologic aspects of human prostatic carcinoma. Am J Clin Pathol 102(Suppl):559–564, 1994.

189. Bostwick DG, Wheeler TM, Blule M, et al: Optimized microvessel density analysis improves prediction of

cancer stage from prostate needle biopsies. Urology 48:47–57, 1996.
190. Snow PD, Smith DS, Catalona WJ: Artificial neural networks in the diagnosis and prognosis of prostate cancer: A pilot study. J Urol 152:1923–1926, 1994.
191. Clark GM: Integrating prognostic features. Br Cancer Res Treat 22:187–191, 1992.

192. Lange PH: Future studies in localized prostate cancer. What should we think? J Urol 152:1932–1938, 1994.
193. Humphrey PA, Vollmer RT: Intraglandular tumor extent and prognosis in prostatic carcinoma: Application of a grid method to prostatectomy specimens. Hum Pathol 21:779–804, 1990.

15

HISTOCHEMISTRY OF THE PROSTATE

William C. Allsbrook, Jr., and Eric A. Pfeifer

Practically every day diseases of the prostate present problems for the pathologist. The single most difficult problem is, of course, the diagnosis of prostate carcinoma; however, other areas are also difficult. In addition to making a diagnosis of malignancy, pathologists must determine, at times, whether a metastatic tumor represents prostate carcinoma. Further, they may be called upon to decide whether a tumor involving tissue adjacent to the prostate, particularly the bladder, represents prostate carcinoma or a primary tumor. Alternatively, secondary involvement of the prostate by carcinoma must also be diagnosed. Recognition of histologic variants of prostate carcinoma, as well as identification of residual carcinoma following treatment, are very important. Finally, pathologic parameters for predicting behavior of prostate carcinoma are being refined, and the pathologist must be familiar with them.

In addition to these routine problems, the basic biology and pathobiology of the prostate are poorly understood. Neuroendocrine cells of the prostate, programmed cell death, growth factors, hormone receptors, oncogenes, and tumor suppressor genes, among others, are being studied intensively and efforts are being made to apply the results of these studies to clinical prostate diseases.

Histochemical studies are very important, often indispensable, for practicing pathologists and basic scientists. In this chapter we review both established techniques and more recent developments in histochemistry of the prostate.

PRELIMINARY CONSIDERATIONS

To perform a histochemical study is not simply to order a "special stain." First, adequate clinical history must be available. Second, adequately fixed tissue or, increasingly commonly, fresh tissue must be obtained and processed appropriately. Third, excellent hematoxylin and eosin (H & E)–stained slides must be prepared. A decision to order histochemical stains is made only after histologic evaluation of the H & E slides. Fourth, the pathologist should be familiar and experienced with the stain that is ordered. Finally, histochemical stains should always be interpreted in their histologic context. The critical importance of each of these steps, particularly the last one, cannot be overstated.

A number of problems are associated with immunohistochemistry.[1] First, standardization in immunohistochemistry, including fixatives, antibodies, and chromogens, has not been achieved. Second, there is little standardization in interpretation of "positivity" or of degree and/or extent of positivity. Fixation, including delay in fixation and time in fixative, are major variables that must be considered in deciding whether a "negative" stain is truly negative or is a false-negative result. Third, it is now apparent that there are few, if any, monospecific immunohistochemical stains. Reports of false-positive staining are increasing in the literature. Finally, a variety of antigen retrieval techniques have been introduced recently, with variable results.[2] These, too, have not been standardized. The pathologist must be conversant with all of these issues.

Histochemistry,[3] including histochemistry of the prostate, was recently reviewed.[4]

PROSTATE-SPECIFIC ANTIGEN AND PROSTATIC ACID PHOSPHATASE

Although prostate-specific antigen (PSA) and prostatic acid phosphatase (PAP) are distinct entities, they are usually employed concurrently in histochemical studies of the prostate and will be considered together. Both have been the subject of review articles containing extensive references.[4,5]

PAP was reported in the prostate, urine, and seminal fluid by Demuth in 1925, and by Kutscher and Wolbergs in 1935 (reviewed by Allsbrook and Simms, 1992[4]). It was subsequently shown to be present in skeletal metastases of prostate carcinoma and in the serum of patients with metastatic prostate carcinoma. Until recently, it was widely used as a serum marker for prostate carcinoma. PAP is a sialoglycoprotein composed of two identical subunits and has a molecular weight of approximately 100 kd. It is produced by benign and malignant prostatic epithelial cells, and its production is regulated by androgens. PAP has been demonstrated by electron microscopy, principally in lysosomes. It has also been demonstrated in secreting vesicles, autophagic vesicles, and Golgi cisternae. The cDNA encoding human PAP has been cloned and sequenced. Serum levels of PAP can be measured by enzymatic, counterimmunoelectrophoretic, or radioimmunologic techniques.

PSA was first characterized and purified to homogeneity from prostate tissue in 1979 by Wang and coworkers (see Allsbrook et al[4,6]). It has been claimed that PSA had been demonstrated earlier and independently under the names *gamma seminoprotein, semen El antigen,* and *p30*; however, Wang and coworkers[7] recently pointed out that these, as originally reported, apparently were not truly PSA and that their reported chemical composition has changed over the years. Gamma seminoprotein and p30, as now reported, are virtually identical to PSA.

PSA,[4] a 33-kd glycoprotein, is a kallikrein-like serine protease. The cDNA for PSA has been cloned and sequenced. PSA rapidly cleaves the structural protein of human seminal coagulum, leading to coagulum liquefac-

tion. It is produced by both benign and malignant prostatic epithelial cells, and its production is androgen related. Ultrastructurally, PSA has been demonstrated in rough endoplasmic reticulum, cytoplasmic vesicles and granules, and occasionally in lysosomal dense bodies. It has also been demonstrated ultrastructurally in stromal macrophages and neutrophils, and this may help to explain how PSA enters the blood.[8]

There are, in the United States, a number of commercially available assays for the detection of serum PSA. The two that have been used most commonly account for most of the clinical data in the literature. One is a radioimmunoassay (RIA) employing a polyclonal antibody, and the other is an immunometric assay employing a monoclonal antibody. Both are accurate and have a close linear correlation, but the values obtained with the former are roughly 1.4 to 1.9 times greater than those for the latter. It has been shown that these differences are due to different calibration standards employed in the assays. A recent international conference has adopted national and international standards for PSA calibrators, and hopefully uniform results will be reported in the future.[9]

It was recently shown that PSA exists in serum in "free" (f-PSA) and bound forms, the latter most commonly bound to alpha-1 antichymotrypsin (PSA-ACT), a major serine protease inhibitor found in the serum and produced by the liver. Immunohistochemical and in situ hybridization studies have shown that ACT is also produced by prostatic epithelial cells. Determination of ratios of serum f-PSA–total PSA and PSA-ACT–total PSA appears to be helpful in distinguishing early prostate cancer from benign prostatic hypertrophy (BPH), the two ratios being low and high, respectively, in persons with prostate cancer. In one study little or no ACT was produced in BPH but striking ACT production was observed with prostate carcinoma.[10] These molecular forms of PSA are currently under intensive study.

For a number of reasons, including stability and sensitivity, PSA has replaced PAP as the preferred serum marker for prostate carcinoma. PSA plays an important role in prostate cancer screening, although the issue of screening has not yet been completely resolved.

EARLY HISTOCHEMICAL STUDIES

Acid phosphatase was first demonstrated histochemically in normal and neoplastic prostate tissue more than 50 years ago by Gomori, who used an enzymatic technique.[4] In 1964, Parkin and colleagues, using another enzymatic technique, studied acid phosphatase in prostate carcinoma and noted decreased intensity of staining in carcinoma as compared with normal tissue and in carcinomas in association with decreasing differentiation (see Allsbrook and Simms, 1992[4]). Pontes and coworkers[11] in 1977 reported an indirect immunofluorescence technique for detection of PAP. Burns,[12] also in 1977, was the first to use immunoperoxidase staining of formalin-fixed paraffin-embedded tissue to demonstrate PAP in two cases of BPH, two cases of prostate carcinoma, and one case of metastatic prostate carcinoma. Jobsis and coworkers subsequently reported a large group of cases that showed positive indirect immunoperoxidase staining for PAP in 29 of 30 primary prostate carcinomas, all of 20 metastatic prostate carcinomas, and none of 55 extraprostatic carcinomas.[4]

The first report of immunoperoxidase staining for PSA appeared in 1981,[4] when Papsidero and coworkers demonstrated positive staining in benign and malignant prostate epithelium but negative staining in a number of extraprostatic tissues. Nadji and associates subsequently demonstrated PSA staining in normal and hyperplastic prostate epithelium and in all 110 primary and metastatic prostate carcinomas, but no staining in 78 nonprostatic malignancies.[4]

STAINING OF NORMAL AND NONNEOPLASTIC PROSTATE TISSUE

There are three major cellular components of normal prostatic ducts and acini: luminal epithelial cells, basal cells, and neuroendocrine cells. The latter are the subject of another chapter in this book. Staining of basal cells is discussed later in this chapter.

PAP and PSA staining of normal luminal cells, as well as those in BPH, have, with few exceptions, been reported as relatively uniform and strong. Coexpression of PAP and PSA in prostatic neuroendocrine cells has been reported. In general, basal cells have not been shown to stain with either PAP or PSA and basal cell–specific cytokeratin staining has been negative in luminal epithelial cells. Bonkhoff and colleagues,[13] using microwave antigen retrieval and double labeling techniques, re-

cently reported co-expression of PSA and basal cell–specific cytokeratin in basal cells, albeit a great minority, of normal and hyperplastic prostate tissue. In addition, they demonstrated rare focal basal cell cytokeratin staining in neuroendocrine cells but no staining in luminal cells. Most, but not all, neuroendocrine cells were negative for PSA staining. They concluded that the basal cell layer contains a population of stem cells, of endodermal origin, that have the ability to form luminal cells, basal cells, or neuroendocrine cells. This has yet to be proved conclusively. Other recent studies, employing cytokeratin staining, have also suggested that the basal cell layer contains a population of stem cells.[14] Cells with a cytokeratin phenotype intermediate between those of basal cells and of luminal cells were recently demonstrated in normal prostate and in prostatic carcinoma.[14]

Normal transitional and squamous epithelium do not stain with PAP or PSA. Metaplastic squamous epithelium occasionally stains with PAP, but not with PSA.[5]

Goldfarb and coworkers[15] have shown a bimodal staining distribution for PAP and PSA that is related to age. Staining was strong from birth to age 6 months, decreased from age 6 months to 10 years (PSA staining was virtually absent in this group), and increasing again from age 10 until puberty. These changes suggest a hormonal influence on staining in children similar to that in adults.

A number of monoclonal and polyclonal antibodies to PSA and PAP have been reported in the literature, and a number of immunohistochemical staining kits employing either monoclonal or polyclonal antibodies are commercially available. It is difficult to compare studies of histochemical staining because antibodies are often to different antigenic determinants, from different tissue sources, and raised in different animals. Some have shown that polyclonal antibodies to PAP are more sensitive than monoclonal antibodies tested, the former apparently recognizing multiple antigenic sites. Epstein[5] has recommended that monoclonal antibodies for PAP not be used for routine studies.

PSA and PAP antigenicities are well-preserved even after prolonged (3 to 7 days) fixation in formalin[16] and after most methods of decalcification. Decreased staining for PAP has been noted, however, following decalcification of bony metastases with nitric acid or with formic acid and sodium citrate. In a study employing formic acid and sodium citrate decalcification, 86% of metastatic prostate carcinomas were positive for PSA but only 36% were positive for PAP.[17] The role of the Zenker's fixation in the decreased PAP in this study is not certain. Prostate tissue fixed in Zenker's fixative has been shown to exhibit decreased PAP and PSA staining.[4]

STAINING OF NEOPLASTIC PROSTATE TISSUE

PSA and PAP staining of prostate carcinoma tissue is generally less intense than that seen in normal or hyperplastic prostate tissue.[4] In contrast to benign tissue, the great majority of reports of prostate carcinoma have demonstrated cell-to-cell and/or field-to-field staining variability for both PSA and PAP. In addition to variability of staining with a specific stain, there may also be interstain variability between PAP and PSA from cell to cell and/or area to area within the same tumor. Decreased PAP and PSA expression in carcinoma, or trends in that direction, have been demonstrated in immunoassays and molecular studies. These studies indicate that the elevated serum levels of PAP and PSA seen in prostate carcinoma reflect, not increased production of PAP and PSA by carcinoma cells, but increased volume of carcinoma and/or increased entry into the circulation. The mechanisms of increased entry have yet to be defined.

In most studies,[4] there appears to be at least a tendency toward correlation of staining variability with increasing tumor grade, and a specific correlation has been noted in several reports. Recently, Zhou and coworkers,[18] employing an image analysis technique, demonstrated no correlation between quantitative PAP extent, or intensity, and grade and suggested that tumor cells' ability to produce PAP is not related exclusively to their ability to form glands. Results of additional studies, again employing immunoassays and molecular techniques, have not been conclusive, although some suggest an inverse relation between tumor grade and tissue PAP and PSA levels. Additional studies are needed to clarify this issue.

A few studies[4] of either PAP or PSA staining alone have shown occasional false-negative staining of prostate carcinoma tissue. A large percentage of these cases were high-grade carcinomas or tumors from which only a small amount of tissue was available for study. One in situ hybridization study of PSA mRNA has shown that, even in cases with negative histochemical stains, PSA mRNA is present. No stain is consistently "best." While the great majority of prostate carcinomas stain with both PAP and PSA, a few stain with only one or the other, and, occasionally with neither. Consequently, it is recommended that both PAP and PSA stains be performed or, certainly, if only one is performed and the result is negative that the other be performed. It is also recommended that, in the case of negative staining of a tumor suspected to be prostate carcinoma, the stain be repeated with increased antibody concentration or incubation time or, if applicable, polyclonal antibodies.

Sesterhenn and colleagues[19] have reported negative PAP and PSA staining of squamous cell carcinoma and transitional cell carcinoma. Prostate carcinomas with areas of either spontaneous or therapy-induced squamous change can have PAP or PSA positivity in some of the cells with squamous features.[19]

CROSS-REACTIVITY OF PAP AND PSA STAINS IN NORMAL AND NEOPLASTIC PROSTATE AND IN EXTRAPROSTATIC TISSUES

Cross-reactivity, or false-positive staining, for PAP has been reported in a variety of normal and neoplastic extraprostatic tissues (Table 15–1, see all Cross-Reactivity references). Occasional staining of urachal remnants, cystitis cystica, cystitis glandularis, or periurethral glands (including Cowper's glands) has been reported and could conceivably be misinterpreted as prostate carcinoma. With the exception of staining of neuroendocrine tumors, particularly carcinoid tumors of hindgut origin, bladder adenocarcinoma, and salivary gland tumors, false-positive PAP staining of tumors has not been a significant potential diagnostic problem.

False-positive staining for PSA has been even less of a problem. Occasional staining of urachal remnants, cystitis cystica, cystitis glandularis, and periurethral glands (including Cowper's glands) has also been reported with PSA; however, extraprostatic neuroendocrine tumors have consistently been negative. Rare PSA-positive tumor cells have been reported in bladder adenocarcinoma. Salivary gland tumors have also been shown to stain with PSA.

Table 15–1. Immunohistochemical Staining for PSA and PAP in Extraprostatic Tissue: Literature Review

Site	Cell or Tumor Type	PSA	PAP
Neuroendocrine (NE)			
Nonneoplastic	Normal gastrointestinal NE cells		Positive[a]
	Crypts of Lieberkuhn, adjacent to carcinoid		Positive[b]
	Rectum/anus, endocrine type	Negative[c]	9/17 Positive, focally[c]
	Pancreatic islets		Positive, often weak, focal[d-g]
Neoplastic	Medullary carcinoma		3/20 Positive[a]
	Islet cell tumor		Positive[a,g,h]
	Carcinoid tumors	Negative[l-q] Negative[j]	Negative[b,i,j] Positive[b,f,g,k-q] Negative[j]
Urinary bladder			
Nonneoplastic	Urothelium	Negative[c,r]	Negative[c,g,r,s]
	Brunn's nests, cystitis cystica, cystitis glandularis	Positive CC + CG[t]	Positive CC + CG[t,u]
	Nephrogenic adenoma	Negative[c,v-x]	Negative[c,g,s,v]
	Urachal remnants	Negative[y]	Negative[y]
Neoplastic	Adenocarcinoma	Positive 4/25[z] Positive, rare, focal 2/14[u] Positive, 3/22 polyclonal 0/22 monoclonal[aa] Negative, 16 cases[bb]	5/14 Positive[u]
Periurethral glands			
Nonneoplastic	Littre, Morgagni	Positive, majority, including focal urethral lining[c,cc,ff,gg]	Positive, majority, including focal urethral lining[c,cc,ff]
Paraurethral (Skene's) glands	Cowper's	3/15 Positive focal,[cc] 0/13 negative[dd,ee]	3/15 Positive focal,[cc] 0/13 negative[dd,ee]
Nonneoplastic	Skene's	Positive, most[c,hh-jj,yy]	Positive, most[c,hh-jj,yy]
Neoplastic	Adenocarcinoma	Positive[ll,yy]	Positive[ll,yy]
Seminal vesicle			
Nonneoplastic	Epithelium	Negative[r]	Negative[d,f,g,n,mm]
Neoplastic	Carcinoma		Positive, focal, faint[i,s,nn]
Rectum and anus			
Nonneoplastic	Anal glands	Negative[oo]	Negative[oo]
Neoplastic	Cloacogenic carcinoma	Positive 11/25 males, 0/20 females[c]	Positive 11/25 males, 0/20 females[c] Positive, 2 cases[pp]
Breast			
Nonneoplastic	Duct cells		Positive, few cells[f]
Neoplastic	Carcinoma		Positive, weak 5/14 bone marrow[d] 7/25 primary[e]

Salivary glands			
Nonneoplastic	Ducts	Positive, luminal surface[qq]	Negative[qq]
Neoplastic	Adenomas, carcinomas	Positive, 15/22 males & females[qq,rr]	Positive 15/22 males & females[qq,rr]
Kidney			
Nonneoplastic	Tubules		Positive, focal faint[d,e,mm,ss]
Neoplastic	Renal cell carcinoma		Positive, weak 1 case[f]
Liver			
Nonneoplastic	Hepatocytes		Positive, faint, occasional[d,e]
Blood, bone marrow			
Nonneoplastic	Granulocytes	Positive, weak, immature, bone marrow[uuu]	Positive, weak[d,e,tt]
Penis			
Neoplastic	Extramammary Paget's disease, associated with prostate carcinoma	Positive[vv]	
Stomach			
Nonneoplastic	Parietal cells		Positive, occasional, weak[d,e]
Lung			
Neoplastic	Carcinoma, metastatic to mediastinal lymph node	Positive, weak focal[ww]	Negative[ww]
Ovary			
Neoplastic	Mature teratoma	Positive[rr,xx]	Positive[xx]

References: [a]Uribe M, Grimes M, Fenoglio-Preiser C, et al.: Am J Surg Pathol 9:577, 1985; [b]Kimura N, Sasano N: Virchows Arch [A] 410:247,1986; [c]Kamoshida S, Tsutsumi Y: Hum Pathol 21:1108,1990; [d]Li C, Lam K, Yam L: Cancer 46:706, 1980; [e]Yam L, Janckila A, Lam W, et al.: Prostate 2:97, 1981; [f]Fishleder A, Tubbs R, Levin H: Cleve Clin Q 48:331, 1981; [g]Jobsis A, De Vries G, Meijer A, et al.: Histochem J 13:961, 1981; [h]Choe B, Pontes E, Rose N, et al.: Invest Urol, 15:312, 1978; [i]Mahan D, Bruce A, Manley P, et al.: J Urol 124:488, 1980; [j]Cohen C, Benz M, Budgeon L: Arch Pathol Lab Med 107:277, 1983; [k]Kimura N, Sasano N, Namiki T: Int J Gynecol Pathol 5:269, 1986; [l]Sobin L, Hjermstad B, Sesterhenn I, et al.: Cancer 58:136, 1986; [m]Federspiel B, Burke A, Sobin L, et al.: Cancer 65:135, 1990; [n]Azumi N, Traweek T, Batifora H: Am J Surg Pathol 15:785, 1991; [o]Goldblum J, Lloyd R: Arch Pathol Lab Med 117:855, 1993; [p]Stagno P, Petras R, Hart W: Arch Pathol Lab Med 111:440, 1987; [q]Sidhu J, Sanchez R: Cancer 72:1673, 1993; [r]Sesterhenn I, Mostofi F, Davis C: In Immunocytochemistry in Tumor Diagnosis, S. Russo, ed. Boston, Martinius Nijhoff, 337, 1985; [s]Jobsis A, De Vries G, Anholt R, et al.: Cancer 41:1788, 1978; [t]Nowels K, Kent E, Rinsho K, et al.: Arch Pathol Lab Med 112:734, 1988; [u]Epstein J, Kuhajda F, Lieberman P: Hum Pathol 17:939, 1986; [v]Kiernan M, Gaffney E: J Urol 137:877, 1987; [w]Nadji M, Tabei S, Castro A, et al.: Cancer 48:1229, 1981; [x]Remick D, Kumar N: Am J Surg Pathol 8:833, 1984; [y]Malpica A, Ro J, Troncoso P, et al.: Hum Pathol 25:390, 1994; [z]Golz R, Schubert G: J Urol 141:1480, 1989; [aa]Grignon D, Ro J, Ayala A, et al.: Cancer 67:2165, 1991; [bb]Abenoza P, Manivel C, Fraley E: Urology 29:9, 1987; [cc]ElGamal A, Van De Voorde W, Van Poppel H, et al.: Urology 44:84, 1994; [dd]Shiraishi T, Kusano I, Watanabe M, et al.: Am J Surg Pathol 17:618, 1993; [ee]Huffman H, Saboorian M, Ashfaq R, et al.: Mod Pathol 8:77A, 1995; [ff]Frazier H, Humphrey P, Burchette J, et al.: J Urol 147:246, 1992; [gg]Takayoff T, Vessella R, Brawer M, et al.: J Urol 151:82, 1994; [hh]Pollen J, Dreilinger A: Urology 23:303, 1984; [ii]Tepper S, Jagirdar J, Heath D, et al.: Arch Pathol Lab Med 108:423, 1984; [jj]Spencer J, Brodin A, Ignatoff J: J Urol 143:122, 1990; [kk]Zaviacic M, Sidlo J, Borovsky M: Virchows Arch [A] 423:523, 1993; [ll]Svanholm H, Andersen O, Rohl H: Virchows Arch [A] 411:395, 1987; [mm]Bentz M, Cohen C, Demers L, et al.: Urology 19:584, 1982; [nn]Lippert M, Bensimon H, Javadpour N: J Urology 128:1114, 1982; [oo]Benson R, Clark W, Farrow G: J Urol 132:483, 1984; [pp]Fernandez P, Gomez M, Caballero T, et al.: Am J Surg Pathol 16:526, 1992; [qq]Van Krieken J: Am J Surg Pathol 17:410, 1993; [rr]Feiner H, Gonzalez R: Am J Surg Pathol 10:765, 1986; [ss]Shaw L, Yang N, Brooks J, et al.: Clin Chem 9:1505, 1981; [tt]Yam L, Janckila, A, Li C, et al.: Invest Urol 19:34, 1981; [uu]Lam K, Li C, Yam L, et al.: Prostate 15:13, 1989; [vv]Cho K, Epstein J: Am J Surg Pathol 11:457, 1987; [ww]Sleater J, Ford M, Beers B: Hum Pathol 25:615, 1994; [xx]Cote R, Taylor C: In Immunomicroscopy: A Diagnostic Tool for the Surgical Pathologist, 2nd ed. Taylor C, Cote R, eds. Philadelphia, W.B. Saunders, pp 256–276, 1994; [yy]Wernert N, Albrech M, Sesterhenn I, et al.: Eur Urol 22:64, 1992.

It is of interest that most paraurethral (Skene's) glands, the female homologue of the prostate, have been shown to stain positively with both PAP and PSA. Many carcinomas of Skene's gland origin have also been reported to be positive for both PAP and PSA.

Recently, more sensitive techniques have demonstrated PSA in a variety of extraprostatic tumors, including tumor cell lines, and in the serum of patients with extraprostatic tumors.[20] These studies demonstrate that PSA is not as "specific" as originally was thought. Staining for PSA in these tissues and tumors has generally been reported to be negative. This disparity probably reflects the inability of routine immunohistochemistry to detect very low levels of PSA.

Literature reports of cross-reactivity of PAP and PSA immunohistochemical staining in nonneoplastic and neoplastic extraprostatic tissue are reviewed in Table 15–1. In a number of instances staining was noted to be weak. Epstein[5] and others believe that weak staining should not be considered to be diagnostic. Great care should be taken in interpreting this finding. A few comments will be made on selected sites and tumors.

All references to cross-reactivity are included with Table 15–1.

Neuroendocrine Cells and Tumors

As noted above, the normal prostate gland contains neuroendocrine cells. Both neuroendocrine tumors and neuroendocrine expression in typical prostate carcinoma can be demonstrated by immunohistochemical studies. This topic has been studied extensively by di Sant'Agnese and others and is the subject of another chapter in this book. PAP and PSA staining of prostate carcinomas with neuroendocrine differentiation are discussed briefly below.

Normal gastrointestinal neuroendocrine cells, including neuroendocrine cells of the rectum and anus, have been reported to stain positively for PAP, as have pancreatic islet cells. PSA staining has been uniformly negative in these sites.

More than 250 cases of carcinoid tumors, mostly involving the gut, have been studied for PAP- and usually PSA-staining characteristics. Roughly 83% of 120 cases of anorectal carcinoids have been positive for PAP, whereas only 15% of 80 midgut carcinoids and 9% of 20 foregut carcinoids have been positive. More than 40 carcinoids from a number of other sites have been studied, and four—1 of 28 lung, 1 of 1 ovary, and 2 of 2 kidney carcinoids—have been positive. As in benign extraprostatic neuroendocrine tissue, PSA staining has been uniformly negative.

A significant percentage of islet cell tumors have also been reported to be PAP positive, as have 3 of 20 cases of medullary carcinoma of the thyroid and the great majority of stromal carcinoids of the ovary. Again, PSA staining has been negative.

Urinary Bladder

With rare exceptions, transitional epithelium has been consistently reported as having staining negative for PAP and PSA. In general, proliferative cystitis has been negative for PAP and PSA; however, one study of cystitis cystica and cystitis glandularis has demonstrated PAP and/or PSA staining in 14 of 40 lesions, including lesions from five female patients. Nephrogenic adenoma was recently shown to be negative for both PAP and PSA. Four of 25 urachal remnants, three in males and one in a female, were shown to be focally positive for PSA.

In 1986, Epstein reported positive polyclonal PAP staining in 5 of 14 primary bladder adenocarcinomas, including 2 from women, and in 3 of 9 transitional cell carcinomas with glandular change, including 2 from women. In two of the primary adenocarcinoma cases, there were rare polyclonal PSA-positive cells. Epstein noted that the distribution of the PAP-positive cells was similar to that of chromogranin-positive cells in the bladder tumors. A subsequent series of 16 cases of adenocarcinoma failed to stain with PSA. Finally, in a more recent report, 3 of 22 adenocarcinomas stained with PSA using a polyclonal antibody, but there was no staining when a monoclonal antibody was employed.

Periurethral Glands

Periurethral glands in males were recently shown to stain for PAP and PSA. The staining has been variable from gland to gland. In two reports there were scattered positive cells over the entire membranous and penile urethra. It has been suggested that these findings might help to explain elevated urine PSA levels in postprostatectomy prostate cancer patients with no evidence of residual carcinoma and that elevated urinary PSA levels do not necessarily reflect early recurrence of disease. Scattered positive PAP and PSA staining in three of three Cowper's glands was reported in one study; however, in most cases reported, PAP and PSA staining have been negative in Cowper's glands.

Seminal Vesicles

PAP staining of seminal vesicles has, with the exception of a couple of early articles, been reported as negative. The early reports note faint focal PAP positivity in seminal vesicles, but another from the same laboratory but using a different antibody showed negative PAP staining. PSA staining of seminal vesicle has been consistently negative. Seminal vesicle epithelium normally contains brown granular pigment, and this should not be misinterpreted as positive immunohistochemical staining.

Rectum and Anus

PAP and PSA positivity was recently reported in perianal glands of 11 of 25 males but in none of 20 females. Two cases of cloacogenic carcinoma of the anorectum have been shown to stain positively for PAP. These two cases were specifically noted *not* to be carcinoid tumors.

Breast

An early report noted PAP staining in a few duct cells of normal breast tissue, and there have been a couple of reports of weak staining of breast carcinoma in 7 of 25 primary tumors and 5 of 14 metastatic ones. Others have reported negative PAP staining in breast carcinoma. In spite of the reports of PSA in breast carcinoma cytosols noted above, PSA staining has been generally negative. It is apparent that the levels of PSA, if it is present at all in breast tissue, are too low to be detected by routine immunohistochemistry. We are not aware of any studies that employed in situ hybridization to study this issue.

Salivary Glands

There was a recent report of positive PAP and PSA staining in 11 of 27 adenomas and carcinomas of the salivary gland. Five and two, respectively, additional tumors were positive only for PSA or PAP. The positive tumors included pleomorphic, but not monomorphic, adenoma, mucoepidermoid carcinoma, adenoid cystic carcinoma, and adenocarcinoma not otherwise specified (NOS). Earlier a Warthin's tumor was reported in vendor literature to be PSA positive.

Other

The early literature contains occasional reports of PAP positivity in renal tubules, hepatocytes, polymorphonuclear leukocytes, and parietal cells of the stomach. There is a report of focal positivity in a renal cell carcinoma. In these reports, the staining has, in general, been faint and focal. There is a report of weak PSA staining of immature granulocytes in bone marrow and of mast cells. Finally, there is a report of faint PSA positivity in a lung cancer metastasis in a mediastinal lymph node.

There is one other aspect of cross-reactivity that should be mentioned. There are four reports of PSA positivity in normal epithelial cells and carcinomas from a wide variety of sites, and these are not in agreement with the remainder of the literature. One of these studies employed a commercial PSA antibody that was subsequently shown to cross-react with a number of epithelial tissues and with mucin secretions.[21] These antibody lots were subsequently withdrawn by the company, and a letter acknowledging this and the possibility of spurious results was published. Another study, again using the same antibody lot and published as an abstract, showed PSA staining in extraprostatic tumors.[22] An attempt was made to withdraw the abstract, but it had already gone to press (DC Wilbur, Personal communication). A third study, published in 1989, apparently using a different antibody lot from the same commercial vendor showed weak PSA staining in 5 of 10 breast cancers, a large cell carcinoma of lung, a cylindroma of lung, and a squamous cell carcinoma of skin.[23] In bone marrow biopsies, there was faint staining of 13 cases of metastatic breast cancer, 1 case of metastatic squamous cell carcinoma, 2 cases of medulloblastoma and 1 case of adenoid cystic carcinoma. The significance of the weak staining of primary and metastatic breast cancer is interesting in the light of the demonstration of PSA in cytosols of breast cancer noted previously. It should be noted that all of the staining was "weak" or "faint." A final study, published as an abstract in 1990 also reported significant false-positive staining for PSA.[24] The antibody source was not noted, and the results have yet to be published in a referred journal.

These latter cases emphasize the importance of including the source of antibodies, together with lot number, in reports of immunohistochemical studies.

We recently performed stains for PSA (Polyclonal PSA, Lot #DC4148, Signet, Dedham, MA) on 8 cases of moderately differentiated lung carcinoma, 10 cases of moderately differentiated colon carcinoma, and 9 cases of grade II breast carcinoma. All of these could conceivably have been confused with prostate carcinoma. Staining was uniformly negative.

USES OF IMMUNOHISTOCHEMICAL STAINING FOR PAP AND PSA

Immunohistochemical staining for PAP and PSA has been particularly useful to the practicing pathologist in three major settings: (1) identification of metastatic prostate carcinoma, (2) identification of primary prostate carcinoma secondarily involving the bladder or periprostatic tissue or, alternatively, differentiating urothelial or other carcinomas involving the prostate secondarily, from primary prostate carcinoma, and (3) identification of benign mimics of prostate carcinoma. Staining may also be helpful in identifying variants of prostate carcinoma, and may aid recognition of residual carcinoma following radiation or androgen deprivation therapy. Recently, there have been attempts to correlate the degree of staining for PAP and PSA with prognosis for prostate carcinoma.

Evaluation of the histologic features of these lesions is, by far, the single most important tool available to pathologists. Immunohistochemical stains in these settings are ancillary procedures.

Identification of Metastatic Prostate Carcinoma

Identification of metastatic prostate carcinoma is well established as a major application for PAP and PSA staining. Before ordering stains for PAP and PSA, it should be recalled that it is very uncommon for metastatic prostate carcinoma to form well-differentiated acini: most lesions are poorly or moderately differentiated. Further, nuclear pleomorphism is not a feature of prostate carcinoma. Consequently, in a metastatic site, a very well-differentiated adenocarcinoma or an adenocarcinoma with marked nuclear pleomorphism probably is not prostate carcinoma.

We recommend (for reasons discussed earlier) that both PAP and PSA stains be studied. Decreased PAP staining of prostate carcinoma in bony metastases decalcified with nitric acid or formic acid and sodium citrate, and in tissue fixed in Zenker's fixative should be kept in mind. PSA staining has not been shown to be affected by decalcification procedures. With the exception of possible false-positive staining noted above, a positive PAP or PSA stain "rules in" the diagnosis of metastatic prostate carcinoma. On the other hand, negative PAP and PSA stains do not completely rule out the diagnosis of metastatic prostate carcinoma, particularly when the carcinoma is poorly differentiated. Furthermore, a small percentage of known prostate carcinomas treated with a variety of methods of androgen deprivation have decreased PAP and/or PSA staining, at times to a negative result. When both PAP and PSA stains are negative and the suspicion of prostate carcinoma is still strong, consideration should be given to increasing the antibody concentrations and incubation times or, if applicable, employing a polyclonal antibody. Finally, Sesterhenn and colleagues[19] have pointed out that in those cases when prostate carcinoma is the suspected primary lesion, negatively stained metastatic carcinomas should be carefully compared with stained sections of the primary tumor to rule out the possibility that the metastasis represents a nonstaining clone of cells from the primary tumor.

PSA and cytokeratin staining have also been employed to detect occult micrometastases in lymph nodes and bone marrow. In one study employing double staining for PSA and cytokeratin, several cases contained cells that were PSA negative and cytokeratin positive.[25] The significance of this finding is not certain, but certainly the use of cytokeratin staining in this setting warrants caution. PSA staining appears to add little to routine H & E examination of lymph nodes. More recently, molecular assays of PSA and of PSA and prostate-specific membrane antigen (PSM), employing reverse transcriptase polymerase chain reaction (RT-PCR),[26] have been used to detect prostate carcinoma cells in peripheral blood, bone marrow, and lymph nodes. Certainly, circulating tumor cells do not necessarily equate with the development of metastases; however, some studies have shown a correlation between the presence of tumor cells detected by molecular techniques and outcome.[27] On the other hand, as noted above, the sensitivity of these techniques may lead to false-positive results.[20] These findings are currently under intensive investigation.

Identification of Primary Prostate Carcinoma Involving Bladder or Periprostatic Tissue and of Carcinoma Secondarily Involving the Prostate

The most common problem encountered in this setting is differentiating prostate carcinoma secondarily involving the bladder or bladder neck from primary transitional cell carcinoma, transitional cell carcinoma with glandular change, or urothelial adenocarcinoma. While prostate carcinoma involving the bladder can often be well- or moderately-differentiated (or poorly differentiated) there is, in general, more nuclear monotony in prostate carcinoma than in bladder carcinoma. Alternatively, urothelial carcinoma involving the prostate is usually a high-grade in situ or infiltrating tumor characterized by marked nuclear pleomorphism. In the case of urothelial carcinoma with glandular change or urothelial adenocarcinoma invading the prostate, there will also usually be considerable nuclear pleomorphism. In these settings, prostate carcinoma should be PAP and PSA positive, whereas most of the others should usually be PAP- and especially PSA-negative. Obviously, the possibility of a false-positive PAP result—and, rarely, focal PSA positivity—noted earlier, should be considered; however, in our experience, combining histologic features with PAP and PSA staining usually resolves difficult cases.

Two benign lesions involving the bladder and prostatic urethra should also be considered here. PAP and PSA staining have been reported in cystitis glandularis, but the histologic features of that lesion are not generally confused with those of prostate cancer. Finally, nephrogenic adenoma, which might be confused with prostate cancer in the bladder or prostatic urethra, has characteristic histologic features and has recently been shown to stain negatively for both PAP and PSA.

Carcinoid tumors of the anorectal region can be confused histologically with prostate carcinoma. Further, PAP staining is positive in the majority of these tumors; however, PSA staining has been uniformly negative. Rectal adenocarcinomas, are, in general, more pleomorphic than prostate carcinoma. In addition, they do not stain for PAP and PSA.

Identification of Benign Mimics of Prostate Carcinoma

Identification of benign mimics of prostate carcinoma is discussed in detail elsewhere in this book. PAP and PSA staining can often be used as ancillary studies in difficult cases. Again, the histology is by far the most important factor in identifying these lesions.

Seminal vesicle tissue in a needle biopsy can be misdiagnosed as prostate carcinoma; however, in addition to the histologic features of seminal vesicle, including the epithelial brown granular cytoplasmic pigment and nuclear pleomorphism, stains for PAP and PSA are negative. Care should be taken not to misinterpret the brown granular cytoplasmic pigment as a positive finding on immunohistochemical stains. At times, PAP and PSA stains are helpful in identifying seminal vesicle involvement by prostate carcinoma.

Granulomatous prostatitis[28] and malakoplakia can be confused, clinically and histologically, with prostate carcinoma. This is particularly true when most of the lesion is composed of histiocytes with relatively few other inflammatory cells and when the histiocytes have a reactive appearance. In malakoplakia, characteristic Michaelis-Gutman inclusions are present. PAP, PSA, and also low–molecular weight cytokeratin stains of the histiocytes in these lesions are negative; however, PAP and PSA stains of poorly differentiated prostate carcinoma may also be negative. Stains for macrophages, which are negative in prostate carcinoma, should therefore also be obtained, and these will be positive.

Occasionally in chronic prostatitis the individual chronic inflammatory cells have artifactual perinuclear clearing, which at times can be confused with poorly differentiated prostate carcinoma or signet ring cell prostate carcinoma.[29] Most examples of this change are believed to represent artifact encountered in transurethral resection of the prostate (TURP) specimens. Recognition of the inflammatory pattern of these cells, when they are present, is important. In addition, the cells are PAP and PSA negative. While poorly differentiated prostate carcinoma can be PAP and PSA negative, the inflammatory cells will stain positively with leukocyte common antigen (LCA). Stromal cells may also occasionally have artifactual perinuclear clearing,[29] and occasionally capillaries and tiny vessels can be confused with carcinoma; however, PSA and PAP would be negative and, in the case of stromal cells, stains for actin or desmin would be positive; endothelial cells would be positive for endothelial markers. Signet ring cell prostate carcinoma cells are positive for PAP and PSA.

Recently, seven cases of prostate xanthoma,[30] a lesion that can mimic prostate carcinoma, have been reported. PAP and PSA stains are negative in prostate xanthoma, and macrophage markers are positive.

Staining of Histologic Variants of Prostate Carcinoma

Histologic variants of prostate carcinoma are also discussed in detail elsewhere in this book. PAP and PSA staining may be helpful for classifying these variants appropriately. Prostate duct carcinoma is uncommon.[31] It is usually associated with typical acinar prostate carcinoma, and, indeed, some observers believe that prostate duct carcinoma is simply acinar prostate carcinoma with intraductal spread. When duct carcinoma involves periurethral ducts, it often extends into the urethra in an exophytic papillary and/or cribriform growth pattern. Duct carcinomas are generally positive for both PAP and PSA. These tumors appear to have a more aggressive course than typical prostate carcinoma. Duct carcinomas can occasionally be confused with transitional cell carcinoma, transitional cell carcinoma with glandular change, or urothelial adenocarcinoma. Use of immunohistochemical staining to differentiate these urothelial lesions from prostate carcinoma was discussed earlier in the section on Urinary Bladder.

Mucinous ("colloid") carcinoma of the prostate is discussed in the section on mucins. Since these tumors are similar histologically to colloid carcinoma in other sites, distinguishing primary tumors from secondary involvement, particularly by rectal or bladder carcinomas, can be exceedingly difficult; however, PAP and PSA stains of mucinous prostate carcinoma are positive. Carcinoembryonic antigen (CEA) staining has been reported to be negative in mucinous prostate carcinoma.

Neuroendocrine differentiation in prostate carcinoma can include small cell (oat cell) carcinoma, carcinoid and carcinoid-like tumors, and neuroendocrine differentiation in typical prostate carcinoma.[32] This topic is extensively reviewed in Chapter 20. Small cell carcinoma of the prostate is usually seen as the only histologic pattern in a tumor, but often it is seen in combination with typical prostate carcinoma. In general, small cell carcinomas that are positive for neuroendocrine markers are negative for PAP and PSA staining. Only rare carcinoid tumors of the prostate have been stained for PAP and PSA, and most are positive. It is well-known that neuroendocrine cells can be demonstrated, at least focally, in most, if not all, typical prostate carcinomas. Co-expression of PSA and PAP and neuroendocrine markers has been demonstrated in these tumors. In roughly 10% of these carcinomas, neuroendocrine differentiation is extensive.

Signet ring cell prostate carcinoma[33] is a poorly differentiated lesion composed of mucin-negative signet ring cells. These cells have nuclear abnormalities and are PAP and PSA positive. This tumor is frequently associated with other patterns of high-grade prostate carcinoma. It should not be confused with clear cell or signet ring changes seen in treated prostate carcinoma, or with artifactual changes noted previously.

PAP and PSA staining have been reported in some cases of spindle cell carcinoma of the prostate.[19] The spindle cell carcinoma is always a component of pleomorphic prostate carcinomas. PAP and PSA staining in sarcomas is uniformly negative. Prostate and bladder neck postoperative spindle cell nodules, which may be confused with sarcoma or spindled prostate carcinoma, are also negative for PAP and PSA staining. Finally, comedocarcinoma of the prostate is positive for both PAP and PSA.

Identification of Prostate Carcinoma After Treatment

The histopathologic changes in benign and malignant prostate tissue following radiation therapy and androgen ablation therapy are discussed in Chapter 17. At times, treatment causes marked "shrinking" of acini and cells, and it may be difficult to recognize them as prostate epithelium. PAP and PSA stains may be helpful in this setting. Cytokeratin stains for luminal epithelial cells are also helpful, since they stain most prostate carcinomas; however, poorly differentiated prostate carcinomas and some carcinomas that have been treated, particularly those treated with androgen ablation, may show little or no PAP and PSA staining.[5] Luminal epithelial cytokeratin staining appears to be less affected by treatment. Sesterhenn (I. Sesterhenn, Personal communication) has demonstrated cells that were PAP and PSA negative but broad-spectrum cytokeratin positive in irradiated prostates. Finally, the presence of PAP, PSA, or cytokeratin staining in this setting only identifies prostatic epithelium and does not distinguish between benign and malignant cells. Basal cell–specific cytokeratin stains (see below) are helpful in differentiating benign ducts and acini from carcinoma following treatment.

PAP and PSA Staining and Prognosis of Prostate Carcinoma

There have been a few reports of positive correlation of PAP (and, at times, PSA) staining with prognosis. As early as 1981, Pontes and colleagues[34] suggested that, since PAP production is related to androgens, immunohistochemical demonstration of PAP in carcinoma should identify carcinomas that would be responsive to androgen ablation. Another way of explaining this correlation is that tumors with decreased staining are, histochemically, less differentiated tumors and should, therefore, have a worse prognosis. In 1984, Epstein and Eggleston[35] reported on 19 patients with stage A2 prostate carcinoma and showed a statistically significant correlation between progression of disease and negative to weak staining for PSA. A similar, but not statistically significant, trend was found for PAP. Subsequently, however, Ito and coworkers[36] were unable to demonstrate a correlation between PAP or PSA staining and responsiveness to endocrine therapy in 72 patients with prostate carcinomas of various histologic grades. In 1989, Hammond and associates[37] reported PAP staining in three groups of patients, one with

matched pairs of patients free of disease or dead of disease, and two Radiation Therapy Oncology Group (RTOG) cohorts treated with radiation therapy. They demonstrated a relationship between intensity or intensity and extent of staining and survival. In a subsequent study,[38] these investigators used image analysis to quantitate PAP staining in the RTOG cases that they had previously studied, along with an additional RTOG cohort. There was a correlation between quantitative measures of intensity and extent of staining and overall survival. Additional studies of PAP and PSA have also shown trends or a positive correlation between staining and survival. Carefully controlled studies of this issue are clearly needed.

HISTOCHEMICAL AND IMMUNOHISTOCHEMICAL STAINS IN THE DIAGNOSIS OF PROSTATE CARCINOMA

The diagnosis of well-differentiated prostate carcinoma can be one of the most difficult problems faced by pathologists and is reviewed in another chapter in this book. The diagnosis of prostate carcinoma is a subjective evaluation of a number of histologic criteria,[39] and each pathologist has a subjective threshold for rendering that diagnosis. Obviously, expertise in diagnosing prostate carcinoma varies from pathologist to pathologist and depends on multiple factors, especially experience. For example, a pathologist who sees 20 prostate biopsies or TURP specimens per week will be able to maintain keener diagnostic skills than if she or he saw only one or two specimens per week. Consequently, in difficult cases, pathologists' use of ancillary studies, including step sections and special stains, as well as seeking outside consultation, is highly variable. Obviously then, there are no clear-cut rules for the use of histochemistry in the diagnosis of prostate carcinoma. Unfortunately, there is no "cancer stain." Certainly, pathologists must always consider whether attempts at histochemistry would be truly helpful or whether the "facing up" of the block and staining of slides for histochemistry simply destroy important sections that would otherwise be available for evaluation by a consultant.

A final point, particularly relating to diagnostic evaluation of needle biopsies of the prostate, should be made. Most pathology laboratories initially prepare multiple levels of prostate biopsy for histologic evaluation. Since areas of concern are often present in only a few of the total number of sections, it is recommended that, in addition to the H & E slide, at least one unstained, positively charged slide be prepared at each level and retained for possible histochemical studies, or an additional H & E-stained slide. If additional step sections are performed for H & E or histochemical stains, great care must be taken to ensure that the area in question is not cut through during preliminary facing up of the block. We recommend that at least one unstained, positively charged slide, for possible histochemical study, be retained at each of the step section levels. Unstained, positively charged slides decrease the possibility of losing the tissue from the slide during pretreatment for immunohistochemical staining or during the staining itself.

Three types of histochemistry approaches have been suggested to be helpful in the diagnosis of prostate carcinoma: basal cell–specific cytokeratin stains, acid mucin stains, and intraluminal crystalloids. Although the latter is not truly a "stain," it is discussed in this section. The most useful of these three is basal cell–specific cytokeratin staining. Finally, we reiterate that these procedures are ancillary studies and that the cornerstone of the diagnosis of prostate carcinoma is evaluation of a well-prepared H & E slide.

BASAL CELL–SPECIFIC CYTOKERATIN

Cytokeratins are a type of intermediate filament that make up part of the cell cytoskeleton[40] and characteristically are found in epithelial cells. They are a complex group of polypeptides that can be separated by two-dimensional gel electrophoresis based on isoelectric pH values ranging from acidic to alkaline and of molecular weights from 40 to 68 kd. Each polypeptide has been assigned a sequential arabic number beginning with 1. At least 20 have been identified. Different combinations of polypeptides can be divided into subgroups, and these subgroups are expressed in different epithelia. The expression of these subgroups is retained in carcinomas arising in the various epithelia. Immunohistochemical staining for cytokeratins is now used routinely to help pathologists identify tumors as carcinomas.

Cytokeratin expression in the prostate has been studied extensively. Luminal epithelial cells and basal cells have characteristic cytokeratin phenotypes, and immunohistochemical stains can be used to distinguish them. In addition, as noted previously, it was recently shown that there are also cells in the prostate, including prostate carcinoma tissue, that have keratin phenotypes intermediate between those of basal cells and luminal cells.

It has been known for many years that the absence of basal cells is an important criterion for the diagnosis of infiltrating prostate carcinoma, the absence of basal cells reflecting the clonal proliferation of the carcinomatous cells without concomitant proliferation of basal cells.[41] Basal cells, however, particularly in cases of prostatic hyperplasia or atypical adenomatous hyperplasia (AAH), are often difficult to identify on routine H & E sections. Consequently, there is a significant chance that such areas will be found to have no basal cells, which could lead to an incorrect diagnosis of carcinoma. Alternatively, stromal cells adjacent to well-differentiated carcinoma can, at times, be interpreted incorrectly as basal cells, leading to an incorrect diagnosis of benignity. Antibodies, usually monoclonal, that are specific for the basal cell cytokeratin phenotype can be used to accurately identify the presence or absence of basal cells in these cases. Although these antibodies recognize the basal cell phenotype, some recognize different combinations of cytokeratins. The antibody most often employed in the literature is 34β-E12, also known as EAB 903 (Enzo Biochemical, New York, NY).

In 1983, Barwick and Mardi,[42] employing a polyclonal antibody to keratin proteins, were the first to draw attention to the importance of an immunohistochemical stain for prostatic basal cells in the diagnosis of prostate carcinoma. Subsequently, Brawer and coworkers[43] studied benign and malignant prostate tissue employing two commercial monoclonal antibodies, one that stained only basal cells and another that stained both luminal cells and basal cells. They noted that basal cells were absent in all cases of prostate carcinoma, confirming the observations of Barwick and Mardi. Several additional studies have confirmed the importance of this stain.[4,44] Only one study has shown disparate results. In 1992, McMahon and coworkers[45] demonstrated basal cell–specific cytokeratin staining to be positive in 11 of 33 prostate carcinomas; however, they also demonstrated luminal epithelial staining in a number of noncancerous prostates, and we tend to discount these results. Two additional cases of prostate carcinoma with positive staining, these with luminal epithelial staining near the cell surface, have been reported. Wojno and Epstein[46] recently published a detailed study of their experience with basal cell–specific cytokeratin. In addition to finding the stain to be very helpful, they also showed it to be cost effective. A recent abstract from a large commercial laboratory[47] noted that use of basal cell–specific cytokeratin stains in difficult diagnostic cases led to a striking decrease in the number of ultimately equivocal cases.

Basal cell–specific cytokeratin staining (Fig. 15–1) is usually employed in two settings: (1) distinguishing AAH from well-differentiated prostate carcinoma, usually in TURP specimens, and (2) evaluating atypical acini in needle biopsy specimens. A few caveats should be remembered in using this stain. First, it is well known that there is variability in staining of basal cells of normal and hyperplastic acini, much of it is due to formalin fixation and routine processing. In some acini, the staining is focally discontinuous, in others the disruption is greater, and some acini stain not at all.

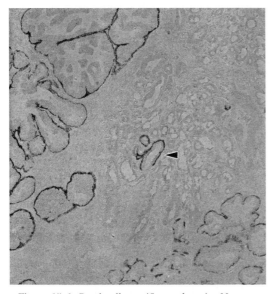

Figure 15–1. Basal cell–specific cytokeratin. Note negative acini of prostate carcinoma in central portion. There is also an entrapped benign acinus (*arrowhead*). At upper left, there is high-grade PIN, and at lower right there is benign prostate, both of which retain basal cell–specific cytokeratin staining. (Basal cell specific cytokeratin stain ×100)

This variability increases from normal prostate tissue to hyperplasia to AAH. Basal cells in atrophic acini generally stain strongly and uniformly. If negative-staining acini are present but histologically similar acini in the same area stain positive, the negative acini probably represent examples of staining variability and should not be interpreted as evidence of carcinoma. Second, prostate carcinoma often infiltrates around preexisting benign ducts and acini, which, of course, contain basal cells. When this is the case, the benign structures are usually recognizable histologically as being different from the carcinoma, the latter having no basal cells. Third, cribriform prostatic intraepithelial neoplasia (PIN) and cribriform hyperplasia have basal cells, although the basal cell staining is often discontinuous. Given this discontinuous staining, a diagnosis of infiltrating cribriform carcinoma should not be made on only a couple of cribriform foci that lack basal cell staining. Fourth, some, at times many, duct-like areas of prostatic duct carcinoma may have basal cells but others are devoid of basal cells. Fifth, Cowper's glands do not contain basal cells, and great care should be taken not to misinterpret these as carcinoma. Cowper's glands have a characteristic histologic appearance and usually, but not always, have been reported to be negative for PAP and PSA. Finally, in our hands, reliable staining is technically more difficult to achieve and maintain with basal cell–specific cytokeratin than with most other immunohistochemical stains.

In summary, in the appropriate histologic setting and given the caveats discussed above, negative staining by basal cell–specific cytokeratin is very helpful in the diagnosis of infiltrating prostate carcinoma. The number of negatively stained acini required to be of help in the diagnosis of carcinoma varies with each case and from pathologist to pathologist. Certainly, as the number of negatively stained acini in question decreases, the diagnostic weight the pathologist gives to the negative staining decreases as well. On the other hand, demonstration of basal cells in acini in question is strong evidence against a diagnosis of carcinoma. The pathologist can be much more confident in interpreting basal cell–positive lesions as benign than in interpreting basal cell–negative ones as malignant. Finally, basal cell–specific cytokeratin staining is also helpful in differentiating benign acini from carcinoma in prostates that were previously irradiated or treated with androgen ablation for prostate carcinoma: The presence of basal cells identifies benign acini.

Basal cell cytokeratin staining is also positive in basal cell hyperplasia and atypical basal cell hyperplasia. The latter may have atypical features, most commonly prominent nucleoli. Basal cell adenoma and adenoid basal cell tumor of the prostate also stain positively with basal cell–specific cytokeratin.[48] Sclerosing adenosis[49] of the prostate also has basal cell–specific cytokeratin staining along with positive actin and S-100 stains in some of the basal cell–specific cytokeratin–positive cells, including staining of mesenchymal appearing cells in the stroma.

MUCINS

"Mucin" is a term used to describe a chemically complex and heterogeneous group of hexosamine-containing polysaccharides that are covalently bound to variable amounts of protein. They are produced by several types of epithelial and connective tissue cells. Although mucins are heterogeneous compounds, they have been broadly categorized on the basis of their reactions with a variety of histochemical stains. Mucin-staining techniques have shown variation from normal staining patterns in a number of atypical and neoplastic lesions throughout the body, including the prostate.

Pilcher, in 1938 (Table 15–2, including all mucin references), reported the first extensive study of mucin production in prostate carcinomas in the American literature. He performed mucicarmine stains, demonstrating a slight trace of mucin in 4 of 10 normal prostates, in 13 of 13 cases of BPH (9 of which had only small amounts), and in 50 of 73 (69%) prostate carcinomas. He noted that a greater percentage of well-differentiated tumors (as compared with poorly differentiated ones) contained mucin. Foster and Levine, also using mucicarmine stains, subsequently confirmed these results. Franks and colleagues employed a battery of stains to study mucins in 155 autopsy prostates, some normal and others containing latent or clinical prostate carcinoma (see Table 15–2). Forty biopsies of clinical prostate carcinoma from living patients were also studied. They demonstrated neutral mucins in both benign and malignant prostatic acini. In addition, they used Alcian blue staining to demonstrate acid mucins

"very frequently" in both latent and clinical prostate carcinomas but only rarely in benign prostatic acini. They also suggested that acid mucin staining might be helpful in the diagnosis of prostate carcinomas, particularly well-differentiated lesions.

Since that time, a number of additional articles on mucin stains in prostate carcinoma have appeared in the literature. In general, most well-differentiated prostate carcinomas contain intraacinar acid mucins. Further, acid mucin staining in benign acini is uncommon, and when present it is often described as being present in only "occasional," "focal," or "rare" acini and in "faint" or "minute" amounts. Consequently, demonstration of acid mucins in the appropriate histologic setting is believed by many, but not all, to be helpful in the diagnosis of prostate carcinoma. No one believes that a diagnosis of carcinoma should be based on the presence of acid mucin or blue-tinged secretions alone (see below).

One other aspect of this issue should be noted. In 1992, Epstein and Fynheer, employed high iron diamine–Alcian blue staining to study acid mucin in 28 cases of adenosis (AAH) in TURP specimens (see Table 15–2). They demonstrated acid mucin in 15 cases, 11 having acid mucin in the majority of acini, 4 in focal acini, and 2 additional cases with equivocal staining. They concluded that acid mucin staining is not helpful in differentiating adenosis from well-differentiated prostate carcinoma. Consequently, when atypical adenomatous hyperplasia is a consideration in the differential diagnosis of a particular lesion, acid mucin stains certainly should not be used. This underscores the critical importance of interpreting acid mucin stains in the appropriate histologic context. We do not employ acid mucin staining in the diagnosis of prostate carcinoma.

Acid mucin staining has also been reported in sclerosing adenosis and in basal cell hyperplasia of the prostate, but these lesions have other characteristic features that should prevent misdiagnosis of prostate carcinoma. Acid mucin–secreting cells (mucinous metaplasia)[50] in the "benign prostate" have also been recently reported and could be confused with prostate carcinoma. These cells are negative for PAP and PSA stains, however, and basal cells are present beneath them.

In a number of the papers on mucin staining of prostate carcinoma (see Table 15–2), the presence of characteristic ("stringy,"

Table 15-2. Acid Mucins in Benign Prostate Tissue and Prostate Carcinoma

Source	Benign Prostate		Prostate Carcinoma	
	Positive Acid Mucin Stains	Mucin (H & E)	Positive Acid Mucin Stains	Mucin (H & E)
Pilcher, 1938[a]	4/10 normal 13/13 BPH	N/A	50/73 (69%)	N/A
Foster & Levine, 1963[b]	N/A	N/A	75/125 (63%) (S)* / 8/22 (36%) (A)*	N/A
Levine & Foster, 1964[c]	"Roughly half" of 25 cases	N/A	53/122 (43%)	N/A
Franks et al., 1964[d]	"Few cases" of 61 (A)	"Some"	94 (A) 40 (S) "very frequently"	"Some" (A) / 12/40 (S)
Hukill & Vidone, 1967[e]	"Occasional" in "a number of normal and pathologic prostates without tumor"	N/A	33/50 (66%)	N/A
Schaefer et al., 1969[f]	11 "Stringy" of 57 normal / 25 "Non-stringy" of 57 normal "minute amounts"	36/125 (29%) / 22/66 normal areas in carcinoma cases (33%)	45/47 (96%)	62/66 (94%)
Taylor, 1979[g]	N/A	N/A	17/27 (63%) (A) (S)	17/27 (63%)
Dollberg, 1980[h]	1/1 case BPH	N/A	N/A	N/A
Ro et al., 1986,1988[i,j]	0/343 (S)	No	200/343 (61.2%)	70/343 (20%)
Srigley, 1988[k]	No staining "many cases" with normal areas	Rare in AAH	N/A	Often in CaP
Pinder & McMahon,[l] 1990	No staining "many cases" with normal areas	No	20/53 (38%) >5% tumor	N/A
McNeal et al., 1991[m]	N/A	N/A	33/100 (33%)	23/100 (23%)
Humphrey, 1991[n]	"Rarely" in "many" of 17 cases	N/A	8/17 (PIN III), focal / 2/17 (PIN III), prominent / 13/17 CaP	N/A
McMahon et al., 1992[o]	5/33 (15%) only weakly	N/A	17/34 (50%)	N/A
Epstein & Fynheer, 1992[p]	15/28 (54%) "adenosis", 11 majority, 4 focal, 2/28 adenosis, equivocal; "occasional" atrophic gland, "occasional" small acinar foci in BPH	"Rarely seen"	N/A	N/A
Sentinelli, 1993[q]	None in 20 sections	N/A	19/27 (70%) CaP / 7/20 (35%) PIN II / 5/20 (25%) PIN III	N/A
Bostwick et al., 1993[r]	38 AAH Basophilic luminal mucinous secretions more frequent in carcinoma than in AAH			8 Carcinomas Basophilic luminal mucinous secretions more frequent in carcinoma than in AAH
Gaudin & Epstein, 1994[s]	N/A	3/145 foci "adenosis"	N/A	2/6 (33%)
Epstein, 1995[t]	N/A	0/134	N/A	102/300 (34%)

AAH, atypical adenomatous hyperplasia, synonymous with "adenosis"; N/A, not applicable or not noted specifically; BPH, benign prostatic hypertrophy; CaP, carcinoma of prostate.

*All surgical (S) cases unless autopsy (A) noted.

Note. References, including those cited in text: [a]Pilcher F: Am J Clin Pathol 8:366, 1938; [b]Foster E, Levine A: Cancer 16:506, 1963; [c]Levine A, Foster E: Cancer 17:21, 1964; [d]Franks L, O'Shea J, Thomson A: Cancer 17:983, 1964; [e]Hukill P, Vidone R: Lab Invest 16:395, 1967; [f]Schaefer J, Lilien O, Sandler M: Invest Urol 6:493, 1969; [g]Taylor N: Hum Pathol 10:513, 1979; [h]Dollberg L: Hum Pathol 11:688, 1980; [i]Ro J, Ayala A, Ordonez N, et al.: Cancer 57:2397, 1986; [j]Ro J, Grignon D, Troncoso P, et al.: Semin Diag Pathol 5:273, 1988; [k]Srigley J: Semin Diag Pathol 5:254, 1988; [l]Pinder S, McMahon R: Histopathology 16:43, 1990; [m]McNeal J, Alroy J, Villers A, et al.: Hum Pathol 22:979, 1991; [n]Humphrey P, Surg Pathol 4:137, 1991; [o]McMahon R, McWilliam L, Mosley S: J Clin Pathol 45:1094, 1992; [p]Epstein J, Fynheer J: Hum Pathol 23:1321, 1992; [q]Sentinelli S: Histopathology 22:271, 1993; [r]Bostwick D, Srigley J, Grignon D, et al.: Hum Pathol 24:819, 1993; [s]Gaudin P, Epstein J: Am J Surg Pathol 18:863, 1994; [t]Epstein J: Hum Pathol 26:233, 1995.

"blue-tinged," "fibrillar," or "basophilic") H & E-stained intraacinar mucin similar to intraacinar mucins in benign and malignant acini in other areas was specifically noted. These stain with acid mucin stains and account for a significant percentage (in the largest study, 20%) of cases of carcinoma with acid mucin–positive acini. The reasons for their presence are not known, and both qualitative and quantitative explanations, including fixation and processing techniques, have been suggested but never proved. While these blue-tinged secretions can occasionally be seen in foci of AAH or benign prostate tissue, they are much more common in prostate carcinoma, and it is currently believed that their presence in the appropriate histologic setting (for example, in a few atypical acini infiltrating around benign ones), is helpful in the diagnosis of prostate carcinoma. They are also helpful in differentiating AAH from well-differentiated prostate carcinoma. However, in 1969 Schaefer and colleagues[69] published a study of mucins in prostate carcinoma that we have never seen cited in the literature(see Table 15–2). They noted "thick and stringy" mucin in 94% of 66 cases of prostate carcinoma. In addition, they noted similar mucin in roughly one third of 57 normal prostates and in normal acini of a third of the 66 cases of prostate carcinoma. In the former, at least, there were apparently usually only small amounts in occasional acini. The reasons for these disparate results are not clear. It is noteworthy that the 94% prevalence of blue-tinged secretions in carcinoma reported by these authors is, by far, the highest in the literature. This study further points out the importance of being careful in using the presence of blue-tinged secretions to help in the diagnosis of prostate carcinoma.

Epstein[39] recently noted that pink acellular intraluminal secretions are helpful in the diagnosis of prostate carcinoma. They are apparently seen "only occasionally" in benign acini. In a recent study he demonstrated these secretions in 55% of 300 cases of prostate carcinoma but noted that these did not appear to be as specific as blue-tinged secretions. We have no experience with these secretions in prostate carcinoma.

Mucinous adenocarcinoma of the prostate, defined by Epstein and Lieberman,[51] as a primary tumor containing more than 25% mucin lakes, is rare. By this definition, mucinous carcinomas are as aggressive as, or likely more aggressive than, usual prostatic carcinomas.

Many do not respond well to hormone therapy, but some do.

INTRALUMINAL CRYSTALLOIDS

Holmes in 1977 (Table 15–3, including all "crystalloid" references) reported the presence of intraluminal crystalloids in 23% of 335 cases of clinical prostate carcinoma and (rarely), in hyperplastic acini adjacent to prostatic carcinoma. She suggested that the presence of crystalloids might be helpful in

Table 15–3. Crystalloids in Benign and Malignant Prostate Tissue

Source	Prevalence (%)	Lesion
Holmes, 1977[a]	23	335 clin. CaP
Jensen et al., 1980[b]	10	393 clin. CaP
Bennett & Gardner, 1980[c]	3.6	456 BPH
Ro et al., 1986[d]	10.2	343 clin. CaP
Ro et al., 1988[e]	100	9 clin. CaP (4-mm ser. sect.) rad. prostatect.
	64.5	31 incid. CaP, Prost/cystect. for TCC (4-mm ser. sect.)
Furusato et al., 1989[f]	62	108 latent CaP (3-mm ser. sect.)
Bostwick et al., 1993[g]	16	38 AAH
	75	8 CaP, well-differentiated
del Rosario et al., 1993[h]	0	50 BPH
	2	50 AAH
	17	150 clin. CaP
Gaudin & Epstein, 1994[i]	40	145 AAH, foci (TUR)
Tressera & Barastegui, 1995[j]	22	302 CaP
Epstein, 1995[k]	25	300 CaP
Gaudin & Epstein, 1995[l]	24	75 AAH, foci (NB)

CaP, carcinoma of prostate; BPH, benign prostatic hypertrophy; ser. sect., serial sections; TCC, transitional cell carcinoma; AAH, atypical adenomatous hyperplasia, synonymous with "adenosis"; TUR, transurethral resection; NB, needle biopsy; clin., clinical; rad. prostatect., radical prostatectomy; incid., incidental.

References, including those cited in the text: [a]Holmes E: Cancer 39:2073, 1977; [b]Jensen P, Gardner W, Piserchia P: Prostate 1:25, 1980; [c]Bennett B, Gardner W: Prostate 1:31, 1980; [d]Ro J, Ayala A, Ordonez N, et al.: Cancer 57:2397, 1986; [e]Ro J, Grignon D, Troncoso P: Prostate 13:233, 1988; [f]Furusato M, Kato H, Takahashi H, et al.: Prostate 15:259, 1989; [g]Bostwick D, Srigley J, Grignon D, et al.: Hum Pathol 24:819, 1993; [h]del Rosario A, Bui H, Abdulla M, et al.: Hum Pathol 24:1159, 1993; [i]Gaudin P, Epstein J: Am J Surg Pathol 18:863, 1994; [j]Tresserra F, Barastegui C: Am J Clin Pathol 103:665, 1995; [k]Epstein J: Hum Pathol 26:223, 1995; [l]Gaudin P, Epstein J: Am J Surg Pathol 19:737, 1995.

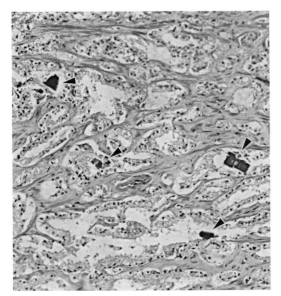

Figure 15–2. Well-differentiated prostate carcinoma. Several intraluminal crystalloids are present (*arrowheads*). (H&E, ×200.)

diagnosing prostate carcinoma. Subsequent reports, employing a variety of study methods on both surgical and autopsy specimens (see Table 15–3), have demonstrated crystalloids in 10% to 100% of prostate carcinomas, the wide prevalence discrepancy reflects the thoroughness of sampling of the tissue. Routine pathologic studies of prostate carcinoma generally demonstrate a prevalence of 10% to 25%.

The bright eosinophilic crystalloids are angular and vary in size and shape. They are easily recognized in routine H & E sections (Fig. 15–2). Their composition has not been completely elucidated. Ultrastructurally, they do not have characteristic features of a true crystal; however, occasional foci of linear periodicity have been reported. By electron probe x-ray microanalysis, the crystalloids have been found to contain much inorganic sulfur. Their significance in the pathobiology of prostate carcinoma is not known. They are usually seen in small, localized areas in prostate carcinomas, often at the periphery, and are usually seen in well-differentiated acini. Only rarely are they seen in metastatic prostate carcinoma. Furusato and coworkers have suggested that intraluminal crystalloids are related to early development of prostate carcinoma.

Intraluminal crystalloids are not often seen in benign prostate tissue (prevalence, not greater than 3.6%). In the study with 3.6% prevalence, most were seen in areas of AAH.

Crystalloids are seen occasionally in benign, often atypical, acini adjacent to prostate carcinoma, and in a couple of cases where crystalloids were present in benign acini, repeat biopsies have demonstrated prostate carcinoma. Crystalloids have also been seen occasionally in sclerosing adenosis of the prostate.

It is generally believed that the presence of intraluminal crystalloids is helpful in arriving at a diagnosis of prostate carcinoma. It has also been suggested that, when needle biopsy specimens contain crystalloids in benign acini, repeat biopsy should be requested. Three recent studies of AAH, two in TURP specimens and one in needle biopsy tissue, have demonstrated crystalloids in 16%, 40%, and 24% of cases, respectively. In the first, it was concluded that crystalloids were helpful in differentiating AAH from well-differentiated carcinoma. In the latter two, they were found not to be helpful. Consequently, until these differences are resolved, in cases where AAH is part of the differential diagnosis, the presence of crystalloids should be used advisedly as a diagnostic indicator. We believe, however, that when AAH is not a consideration, (for example, when a few atypical acini infiltrate between preexisting benign acini), the presence of crystalloids is a helpful finding.

IMMUNOHISTOCHEMICAL STAINING FOR p53 PROTEIN

Tumor suppressor gene p53, located on the short arm of chromosome 17 (17p13.1), is the gene most often mutated in human malignancies. The gene codes for a nuclear phosphoprotein involved in regulation of the cell cycle. Normal p53 protein is not detectable by routine immunohistochemistry because, owing principally to its short half-life, detectable quantities do not accumulate in the nucleus. Abnormal p53 protein, which generally reflects p53 mutations and has a longer half-life than normal p53 protein, does collect in quantities sufficient for immunohistochemical demonstration. It is detectable in a large percentage of most types of malignancies. It is not detected as frequently in prostate carcinomas.[52]

The p53 mutation was first demonstrated in a prostate carcinoma cell line in 1991 by Rubin and coworkers[53] and subsequently in prostate carcinoma cell lines and clinical carcinomas by Isaacs and associates.[54] Abnormal p53 protein was first demonstrated immunohisto-chemically in prostate carcinoma in 1992 by Thompson and associates,[55] who reported strong staining in 5 of 29 cases but in none of 34 cases of BPH. Since that time, a number of immunohistochemical studies of p53 in prostate carcinoma have been reported. Most were performed on formalin-fixed, paraffin-embedded tissue and, more recently, some employed antigen retrieval techniques, which appear to be helpful. Both monoclonal and polyclonal antibodies have been used, and there are a variety of criteria for positivity. Staining is generally variable and often focal. Although it is well-known that abnormal p53 protein staining does not detect all p53 gene abnormalities and that formalin fixation itself decreases p53 staining, abnormal p53 protein staining has generally correlated reasonably well with concurrent molecular studies demonstrating p53 mutations. In a recent extensive molecular study,[56] however, 20 of 48 (42%) cases of prostate carcinoma had p53 gene mutations and several had more than one. Of a total of 32 reported mutations, 12 were "silent" and alone would not have produced abnormal protein.

In most studies, abnormal p53 protein expression is related to increasing tumor grade and stage. In some studies, the relationship has been shown to be statistically significant, at times strongly significant.[57–61] Although there is much variability in reports in the literature, relatively few low-grade and low-stage tumors and roughly at least half of high-stage and high-grade tumors exhibit abnormal p53 protein staining. It is generally believed that these abnormal proteins might represent markers of progressive disease. Whether these p53 mutations are primary or secondary events is not known at this time. On the other hand, in the extensive molecular study[56] previously noted, mutations were present in 42% of cases of prostate carcinoma, and a substantial fraction were in low-grade and low-stage tumors. There was no correlation with grade or stage. These same authors had previously reported p53 mutations in five of nine cases of BPH. They hypothesized that, contrary to most reports, p53 changes appear to occur relatively early in prostate carcinoma.

Finally, some, but not all, studies of abnormal p53 protein staining have shown a significant correlation between staining and decreased survival, disease progression (including development of metastases), decreased dis-ease-free interval, and hormone-refractory tumors.[59,62,63] In some of these studies staining was an independent variable. These results must be confirmed with standardized studies. One problem that would seem difficult to overcome with needle biopsy specimens is the focal and variable nature of staining of abnormal p53 protein, which could lead to false-negative results.

IMMUNOHISTOCHEMICAL STAINING FOR ANDROGEN RECEPTOR

For more than 50 years androgen ablation has been the cornerstone of treatment of high-stage prostate carcinoma. The majority of patients treated with androgen ablation respond initially, but they are not cured. Ultimately, androgen-independent clones of cells emerge and the tumor progresses.

Androgen activity depends largely on the presence of androgen-binding components or "receptors," which are present in the nucleus of prostatic epithelial, basal, stromal, and, according to some, neuroendocrine cells. A number of studies of androgen receptors (AR) in the prostate, including prostate carcinoma tissue, have been published.[4] These studies employ both biochemical and histochemical techniques, the former having a number of disadvantages, including radioactive reagents (usually), expensive equipment, and specially trained technical personnel. A major disadvantage of biochemical assays is that tissue homogenates are generally utilized, thus precluding histologic evaluation. Initial histochemical studies of AR required frozen tissue, but, recently, microwave antigen retrieval techniques have made possible immunohistochemical studies of AR[64] in formalin-fixed, paraffin-embedded tissues as well. These studies have employed both monoclonal and polyclonal antibodies, at times to different epitopes. As in p53 studies, AR staining is often only focal and, consequently, could lead to false-negative results in needle biopsies.

Studies of AR in prostate carcinoma have often been contradictory, and currently there is no consensus on the usefulness of AR staining in prostate carcinoma. AR staining does not necessarily reflect a structurally intact, functionally active receptor. Correlations of staining with grade have been noted by some, but not by others.[65] One study showed greater variability in AR staining in tumors with poor response to androgen ablation.[66] Another showed no correlation between staining and time to progression of disease.[67] Finally, a recent study employing image analysis techniques showed that mean concentration of AR in tumor cells is the principal predictor of outcome in patients undergoing hormonal ablation therapy for stage D2 diseases.[68]

Acknowledgments

This chapter is dedicated to the memory of Dr. Charles W. Hooker (1910–1994), Emeritus Professor of Anatomy, University of North Carolina School of Medicine. He was truly a gentleman and a scholar.

Dr. Wesley Simms and the senior author (WCA) of this chapter co-authored a review of histochemistry of the prostate.[4] Dr. Simms' contributions to this chapter are gratefully acknowledged. Dr. Kathy Mangold reviewed the manuscript and offered valuable suggestions. Ms. Michelle Page provided excellent secretarial and computer assistance.

Conversations with Dr. Jonathan Epstein were very helpful in preparation of this chapter.

A portion of this work was supported by a grant from AFLAC, Columbus, Georgia.

REFERENCES

1. Taylor CR: An exaltation of experts: Concerted efforts in the standardization of immunohistochemistry. Hum Pathol 25:2–11, 1994.
2. Brown RW, Chirala R: Utility of microwave-citrate antigen retrieval in diagnostic immunohistochemistry. Mod Pathol 8:515–520, 1995.
3. Taylor CR, Cote RJ, (eds): Immunomicroscopy: A Diagnostic Tool for the Surgical Pathologist, 2nd ed. Philadelphia: W.B. Saunders, 1993.
4. Allsbrook WC, Simms WW: Histochemistry of the prostate. Hum Pathol 23:297–305, 1992.
5. Epstein JI: PSA and PAP as immunohistochemical markers in prostate cancer. Urol Clin North Am 20:757–770, 1993.
6. Allsbrook WC, Simms WW, Steinsapir J: On the identification and characterization of prostate specific antigen. Hum Pathol 24:811–812, 1993.
7. Wang MC, Papsidero LD, Chu TM: Prostate specific antigen, p30, gamma-seminoprotein, and E1. Prostate 24:107–108, 1994.
8. Sinha AA, Wilson MJ, Gleason DF: Immunoelectron microscopic localization of prostatic specific antigen in human prostate by the protein A gold complex. Cancer 60:1288–1293, 1987.
9. Murphy GP: The Second Stanford Conference on International Standardization of Prostate Specific Antigen Assays. Cancer 75:122–128, 1995.
10. Bjork T, Bjartell A, Abrahamsson P, et al.: Alpha-1-antichymotrypsin production in PSA producing cells is common in prostate cancer but rare in hyperplasia. Urology 43:427–433, 1994.
11. Pontes JE, Choe B, Rose N, et al.: Indirect immunofluorescence for identification of prostatic epithelial cells. J Urol 117:459–463, 1977.
12. Burns J: Prostatic acid phosphatase in tissue sections revealed by the unlabelled antibody peroxidase-antiperoxidase method. Biomedicine 27:7–10, 1977.
13. Bonkhoff H, Stein U, Remberger K: Multidirectional differentiation in the normal, hyperplastic, and neoplastic human prostate: Simultaneous demonstration of cell-specific epithelial markers. Hum Pathol 25:42–46, 1994.
14. Verhagen APM, Ramaekers FCS, Aalders TW, et al.: Colocalization of basal and luminal cell-type cytokeratins in human prostate cancer. Cancer Res 52:6182–6187, 1992.
15. Goldfarb DA, Stein BS, Shamszadeh M, et al.: Age-related changes in tissue levels of prostatic acid phosphatase and prostate specific antigen. J Urol 136:1266–1269, 1986.
16. Leong AS, Gilham PN: The effects of progressive formaldehyde fixation on the preservation of tissue antigens. Pathology 21:266–268, 1989.
17. Shah NT, Tuttle SE, Strobel SL, et al.: Prostatic carcinoma metastatic to bone: Sensitivity and specificity of prostate-specific antigen and prostatic acid phosphatase in decalcified material. J Surg Oncol 29:265–268, 1985.
18. Zhou R, Hammond EH, Sause WT, et al.: Quantitation of prostate-specific acid phosphatase in prostate cancer: Reproducibility and correlation with subjective grade. Mod Pathol 7:440–448, 1994.
19. Sesterhenn I, Mostofi FK, Davis CJ: Immunopathology of prostate and bladder tumors. In Russo J (ed): Immunocytochemistry in Tumor Diagnosis. Boston: Martinus Nijhoff, 1985, pp 337–361.
20. Smith MR, Biggar S, Hussain M: Prostate specific antigen messenger RNA is expressed in non-prostate cells: Implications for detection of micrometastases. Cancer Res 55:2640–2644, 1995.
21. Herman E, Elfont E, Boenisch T: Prostate specific antigen. Histopathology 12:687–688, 1988.
22. Wilbur DC, Krenzer K, Bonfiglio TA: Prostate specific antigen (PSA) staining in carcinomas of non-prostatic origin. Am J Clin Pathol 88:530A, 1987.
23. Lam K, Li C, Yam LT, et al.: Improved immunohistochemical detection of prostatic acid phosphatase by a monoclonal antibody. Prostate 15:13–21, 1989.
24. Minkowitz G, Peterson P, Godwin TA: A histochemical and immunohistochemical study of adenocarcinomas involving urinary bladder. Mod Pathol 3:68A, 1990.
25. Riesenberg R, Oberneder R, Kriegmair M, et al.: Immunocytochemical double staining of cytokeratin and prostate specific antigen in individual prostatic tumour cells. Histochemistry 99:61–66, 1993.
26. Israeli RS, Miller WH, Su SL, et al.: Sensitive detection of prostatic hematogenous tumor cell dissemination using prostate specific antigen and prostate specific membrane-derived primers in the polymerase chain reaction. J Urol 153:573–577, 1995.
27. Katz AE, de Vries GM, Begg MD, et al.: Enhanced reverse transcriptase-polymerase chain reaction for prostate specific antigen as an indicator of true patho-

logic stage in patients with prostate cancer. Cancer 75:1642–1648, 1995.

28. Presti B, Weidner N: Granulomatous prostatitis and poorly differentiated prostate carcinoma. Their distinction with the use of immunohistochemical methods. Am J Clin Pathol 95:330–334, 1991.

29. Alguacil-Garcia A: Artifactual changes mimicking signet ring cell carcinoma in transurethral prostatectomy specimens. Am J Surg Pathol 10:795–800, 1986.

30. Sebo TJ, Bostwick DG, Farrow GM, et al.: Prostatic xanthoma: A mimic of prostatic adenocarcinoma. Hum Pathol 25:386–389, 1994.

31. Christensen WN, Steinberg G, Walsh PC, et al.: Prostatic duct adenocarcinoma. Findings at radical prostatectomy. Cancer 67:2118–2124, 1991.

32. Di Sant'Agnese PA: Neuroendocrine differentiation in human prostatic carcinoma. Hum Pathol 23:287–296, 1992.

33. Ro JY, El-Naggar A, Ayala AG, et al.: Signet ring cell carcinoma of the prostate. Electron microscopic and immunohistochemical studies of eight cases. Am J Surg Pathol 12:453–460, 1988.

34. Pontes JE, Rose NR, Ercole C, et al.: Immunofluorescence for prostatic acid phosphatase: Clinical implications. J Urol 126:187–189, 1981.

35. Epstein JI, Eggleston JC: Immunohistochemical localization of prostate specific acid phosphatase and prostate specific antigen in stage A2 adenocarcinoma of the prostate. Prognostic implications. Hum Pathol 15:853–859, 1984.

36. Ito H, Yamaguchi K, Sumiya H, et al.: Histochemical study of R1881-binding protein, prostatic acid phosphatase, prostate specific antigen, and gamma-seminoprotein in prostatic cancer. Eur Urol 12:49–53, 1986.

37. Hammond ME, Sause WT, Martz KL, et al.: Correlation of prostate specific acid phosphatase and prostate specific antigen immunocytochemistry with survival in prostate carcinoma. Cancer 63:461–466, 1989.

38. Zhou R, Hammond EH, Sause WT, et al.: Quantitation of prostate specific acid phosphatase in prostate cancer: Reproducibility and correlation with subjective grade. Mod Pathol 7:440–448, 1994.

39. Epstein JI: Diagnostic criteria of limited adenocarcinoma of the prostate on needle biopsy. Hum Pathol 26:223–229, 1995.

40. Moll R, Franke WW, Schiller DL, et al.: The catalog of human cytokeratins: Patterns of expression in normal epithelia, tumors and cultured cells. Cell 31:11–24, 1982.

41. Totten RS, Heinemann MW, Hudson PB, et al.: Microscopic differential diagnosis of latent carcinoma of the prostate. Arch Pathol 55:131–141, 1953.

42. Barwick KW, Mardi JA: An immunohistochemical study of the myoepithelial cell in prostate hyperplasia and neoplasia. Lab Invest 48:7A, 1983.

43. Brawer MK, Peehl DM, Stamey TA, et al.: Keratin immunoreactivity in the benign and neoplastic human prostate. Cancer Res 45:3663–3667, 1985.

44. Hedrick L, Epstein JI: Use of keratin 903 as an adjunct in the diagnosis of prostate carcinoma. Am J Surg Pathol 13:389–396, 1989.

45. McMahon RFT, McWilliam LJ, Mosley S: Evaluation of three techniques for differential diagnosis of prostatic needle biopsy specimens. J Clin Pathol 45:1094–1098, 1994.

46. Wojno KJ, Epstein JI: The utility of basal cell specific anti-cytokeratin antibody (34betaE12) in the diagnosis

of prostate cancer. A review of 228 cases. Am J Surg Pathol 19:251–260, 1995.

47. Kahane H, Sharpe JW, Schuman GB, et al.: Utilization of high molecular weight cytokeratin (hmwCK) on prostate needle biopsies in a reference laboratory. Mod Pathol 8:78A, 1995.

48. Devaraj LT, Bostwick DG: Atypical basal cell hyperplasia of the prostate. Immunophenotypic profile and proposed classification of basal cell proliferations. Am J Surg Pathol 17:645–659, 1993.

49. Grignon DJ, Ro JY, Srigley JR, et al.: Sclerosing adenosis of the prostate gland. A lesion showing myoepithelial differentiation. Am J Surg Pathol 16:383–391, 1992.

50. Grignon DJ, O'Malley FP: Mucinous metaplasia in the prostate gland. Am J Surg Pathol 17:287–290, 1993.

51. Epstein JI, Lieberman PH: Mucinous adenocarcinoma of the prostate gland. Am J Surg Pathol 9:299–308, 1985.

52. Soussi T, Legros Y, Lubin R, et al.: Multifactorial analysis of p53 alteration in human cancer: A review. Int J Cancer 57:1–9, 1994.

53. Rubin SJ, Hallahan DE, Ashman CR, et al.: Two prostate carcinoma cell lines demonstrate abnormalities in tumor suppressor genes. J Surg Oncol 46:31–36, 1991.

54. Isaacs WB, Carter BS, Ewing CM: Wild type p53 suppresses growth of human prostate cancer cells containing mutant p53 alleles. Cancer Res 51:4716–4720, 1991.

55. Thompson SJ, Mellon K, Charlton RG, et al.: p53 and Ki-67 immunoreactivity in human prostate cancer and benign hyperplasia. Br J Urol 69:609–613, 1992.

56. Chi S, deVere White R, Meyers FJ, et al.: p53 in prostate cancer: Frequent expressed transition mutations. JNCI 86:926–933, 1994.

57. Navone NM, Troncoso P, Pisters LL, et al.: p53 protein accumulation and gene mutation in the progression of human prostate carcinoma. JNCI 85:1657–1669, 1993.

58. Henke R, Kruger E, Ayhan N, et al.: Immunohistochemical detection of p53 protein in human prostatic cancer. J Urol 152:1297–1301, 1994.

59. Aprikian AG, Sarkis AS, Fair WR, et al.: Immunohistochemical determination of p53 protein nuclear accumulation in prostatic adenocarcinoma. J Urol 141:1276–1280, 1994.

60. Kallakury BVS, Figge J, Ross JS, et al.: Association of p53 immunoreactivity with high gleason tumor grade in prostatic adenocarcinoma. Hum Pathol 25:92–97, 1994.

61. Hughes JH, Cohen MB, Robinson RA: p53 immunoreactivity in primary and metastatic prostatic adenocarcinoma. Mod Pathol 8:462–466, 1995.

62. Thomas DJ, Robinson M, King P, et al.: p53 expression and clinical outcome in prostate cancer. Br J Urol 72:778–781, 1993.

63. Grignon D, Caplan R, Sarkar F, et al.: p53 suppressor gene status as a predictor of outcome in patients with locally advanced prostatic adenocarcinoma (PCa) treated by radiation therapy with and without androgen ablation pre-treatment: A study based on RTOG protocol 8610. Mod Pathol 8:77A, 1995.

64. Loda M, Fogt F, French FS, et al.: Androgen receptor immunohistochemistry on paraffin-embedded tissue. Mod Pathol 7:388–391, 1994.

65. Chodak GW, Kranc DM, Puy LA, et al.: Nuclear local-

ization of androgen receptor in heterogeneous samples of normal, hyperplastic and neoplastic human prostate. J Urol 147:798–803, 1992.

66. Sadi M, Barrack ER: Image analysis of androgen receptor immunostaining in metastatic prostate cancer. Heterogeneity as a predictor of response to hormonal therapy. Cancer 71:2574–2580, 1993.

67. Sadi MV, Walsh PC, Barrack ER: Immunohistochemical study of androgen receptors in metastatic prostate cancer. Comparison of receptor content and response to hormonal therapy. Cancer 67:3057–3064, 1991.

68. Tilley WD, Lim-Tio SS, Horsfall DJ, et al.: Detection of discrete androgen receptor epitopes in prostate cancer by immunostaining: Measurement by color video image analysis. Cancer Res 54:4096–4102, 1994.

69. Schaefer J, Lilien O, Sandler M: Frozen section diagnosis and mucin production in prostatic carcinoma. Invest Urol 6:493–504, 1969.

16

ULTRASONOGRAPHY IN THE DIAGNOSIS OF PROSTATE CANCER

MATTHEW D. RIFKIN and JEFFREY S. ROSS

Prostate cancer, now the world's most common malignancy, may, in certain circumstances, be a diagnostic problem. Although routine digital rectal examination (DRE) has for many years been the mainstay of diagnosis, early diagnosis of prostate cancer, essential to ensuring a better chance for cure, often is not possible by DRE alone.

The development of serum markers for prostate cancer has been a major advance in the early diagnosis of this disease. Prostatic acid phosphatase (PAP) was one of the first developed that had potential clinical applications; however, it is not an acceptably accurate tool for determining the presence of small, early, or confined prostate cancers. It is more appropriate in the evaluation of larger, advanced, and nonlocalized tumors. Prostate-specific antigen (PSA) is more reliable in its ability to identify potential, early prostate cancer in the gland.

None of these reagents is acceptable, however, either alone or together, for definitively identifying cancer in the prostate. An abnormal or questionable DRE finding may be due to prostatic calculi, corpora amylacea, cysts, benign enlargement, or the sequelae of inflammation. Elevated levels of PSA may be due to benign prostatic enlargement, prostatic infarct, or prostatitis.[1-3] It is not possible with the DRE or PSA to differentiate any of these cases from cancer. Other tools are needed,

and ultrasonography (US) has the greatest potential at the lowest cost.

Early studies suggested that US, particularly, endorectal or transrectal (ERU or TRUS), had the potential to identify many prostate cancers not palpable by DRE.[4-6] Because of the expense of the US examination, however, and the expertise required to obtain a high-quality study, current thinking holds that US should be reserved as an ancillary and not a primary tool. The American Cancer Society (ACS) and the American Urological Association have concurred in the following recommendations:[7]

The American Cancer Society recommends annual examination for early detection of prostate cancer with digital rectal examination (DRE) and serum prostate-specific antigen (PSA) beginning at age 50. However, men in high-risk groups, such as African Americans, or those with strong familial predisposition may start at a younger age. Generally, men with a life expectancy of at least 10 years after detection may benefit from examination.

DRE should be performed by a health care worker skilled in detecting subtle abnormalities, including those of symmetry and consistency as well as the more classic findings of marked induration or nodules. Furthermore, the ACS guidelines for early detection of colorectal cancer recommend DRE, including prostate examination, starting at age 40.

PSA is generally agreed to be significantly abnormal when greater than 4.0 ng/mL (monoclonal). However, abnormal elevation of PSA may be associated with benign prostatic hyperplasia (BPH) or prostatitis, in the absence of cancer.

Transrectal ultrasound (TRUS) is currently used to evaluate patients with abnormal digital rectal and/or PSA examinations. In such circumstances, if the TRUS and/or biopsy are negative, the patient should have follow-up surveillance at intervals specified by his managing physician.

While an examination for prostate carcinoma detects tumors at more favorable stages (anatomically less extensive disease), reduction in mortality from screening has not yet been documented.

Once it has been decided that further evaluation of the prostate is warranted, based on the results of the DRE and/or PSA, endoluminal ultrasound should be employed.[1] The ability of ultrasound to identify potential areas of tumor infiltration has been questioned by a number of investigators, owing in part to the complexity of the study and in part to discrepancies in the scientific data.

When using endoluminal US, appropriate equipment, correct technique, and a clear understanding of the abilities and the deficiencies of the examination are essential. ERU has the ability to identify many prostate cancers. It is essential that, when performing ultrasound, multiplane, or at least biplane, imaging techniques must be utilized. This approach ensures that the entire gland is imaged in its entirety. Different orientations are best used to identify or serve as a guide for various portions of the examination:[8]

- The base of the gland is best appreciated on the longitudinal view.
- The apex of the gland is best appreciated on the longitudinal view.
- The lateral aspects of the gland are best seen on the axial view.
- Obvious asymmetry of the seminal vesicles is best noted on the axial view.
- Subtle seminal vesicle involvement may be best appreciated on longitudinal views.
- The neurovascular bundles are best identified on the axial views.
- The apex of the prostate is best seen on the longitudinal views.
- Most biopsies are most accurately performed using the longitudinal orientation, although, with the development of the end-fire probe, the oblique axial view may better position the biopsy needle into some lateral lesions.

EQUIPMENT

The initial equipment developed for ERU had a 2.25 or 3.5 mHz transducer at the end of a long, thin metal tube slightly thicker than a conventional cystoscope. Depending on the specific equipment, the transducer rotated in a continuous 360-degree rotation at a rate of approximately 1 to 5 rotations per second.[9, 10] Thus, the term *radial scanning* was born. These transducers imaged only in transverse or axial rotation. Modern "real-time" equipment images the prostate with 5–8 mHz transducers.

DIAGNOSTIC ULTRASONOGRAPHY

Most men who will be examined with US for possible prostate cancer are older, since this population is at higher risk. This group of men all have some degree of benign prostatic hyperplasia (BPH). Thus, the US appearance of a cancer-free prostate can vary significantly, depending on the degree of BPH.

Without obvious enlargement, the normal prostate measures approximately 2.5 to 3.0 cm in antero-posterior dimension (thickness), 4.0 to 4.5 cm in lateral or transverse dimension (width), and 3.0 to 4.0 cm in cephalocaudad (height) view. The inner gland (along with the sonographically undifferentiable anterior fibromuscular stroma) is seen as a midline, anterior, superior area, slightly less "echogenic" (or acoustically reflective) than the normal outer gland (Fig. 16–1).

With increasing amounts of inner gland enlargement (BPH), the inner portion of the prostate enlarges and the outer gland becomes compressed.[11] On the endorectal US, the inner gland usually becomes even less echogenic than the outer gland (Fig. 16–2). This is due predominately to a compressed and more ho-

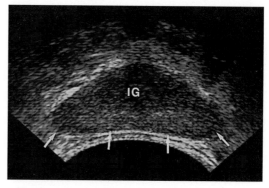

Figure 16–1. Normal prostate. A transverse ERU image in a normal young man demonstrates no obvious enlargement of the inner gland (IG) and poor delineation from the normal outer gland *(arrows).*

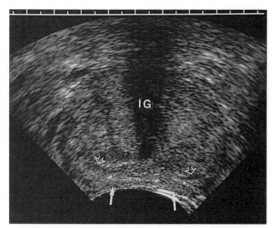

Figure 16–2. Benign prostatic enlargement. The inner gland (IG) is markedly enlarged and slightly less echogenic than the compressed outer gland *(arrows)*. The hypoechogenic surgical capsule *(arrowheads)* separates the inner from the outer gland.

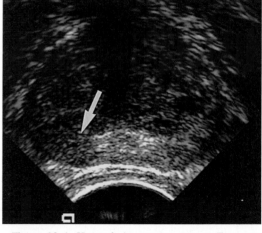

Figure 16–4. Hypoechoic prostate cancer. Transverse ERU looking toward the base of the gland demonstrates a hypoechoic focus *(arrow)* representing cancer in a prostate with a markedly enlarged inner gland from benign prostatic hyperplasia.

mogeneous echogenic appearance of the outer gland. The enlarged inner gland is not necessarily as homogeneous in its US appearance, owing to a number of factors:[12]

- The cellular component of BPH can include muscular, fibrous, acinar, stromal, and other tissue types.
- The amount of each cell type can vary and can be homogeneous, comprising only one variety or a multiple of cell types.
- Some areas of BPH can undergo degenerative change.

With increasing amounts of inner gland en-largement and outer gland compression, the area separating the two regions, the surgical capsule, can become pronounced as a thin, hypoechoic rim of tissue between the inner and outer glands.

The use of the newest high-resolution equipment can define many cancers, the most obvious being the hypoechoic lesion seen in the outer portion of the prostate, where 80% of cancers originate (Figs. 16–3, 16–4). However, not all of even the largest tumors are seen as obvious hypoechoic lesions (Fig. 16–5).[13] Up

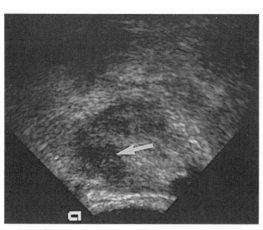

Figure 16–3. Hypoechoic prostate cancer. Transverse ERU image looking toward the apex of the gland demonstrates a hypoechoic focus *(arrow)* representing prostate cancer.

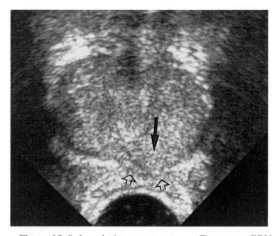

Figure 16–5. Isoechoic prostate cancer. Transverse ERU image looking toward the apex of the gland demonstrates an isoechoic focus *(arrow)* representing prostate cancer. Note that the normal, brightly echogenic periprostatic fat *(arrowheads)* is disrupted allowing this lesion to be identified more readily.

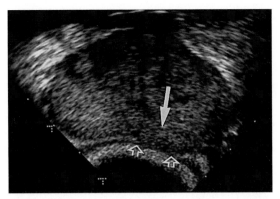

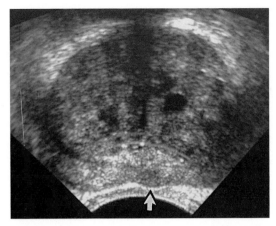

Figure 16–6. Isoechoic prostate cancer. Transverse ERU image looking toward the apex of the gland demonstrates a large, but only subtly hypoechoic, region *(arrow)* representing prostate cancer. Note that the normal brightly echogenic periprostatic fat *(arrowheads)* is disrupted, allowing this lesion to be identified more readily.

Figure 16–7. Prostate cancer. Transverse ERU image looking toward the base of the gland demonstrates periprostatic capsular distortion *(arrow)* owing to infiltrating prostate cancer.

to 40% of cancer may have a different appearance on ERU. Less obvious US-visualized lesions may be identified by distortion of the gland, irregularity, asymmetry, or regions of pericapsular abnormality (Figs. 16–5 to 16–7). A close inspection of the prostate and a specific region of concern may discern the following sonographic characteristics:[11, 14]

Hypoechoic Lesions

Less acoustically reflective lesions are the most obvious lesions and the easiest to identify. They are well-delineated by their obvious echogenic differences from normal tissue. This "acoustic mismatching"—differing echogenic characteristics of two adjacent types of tissue—makes the lesions most obvious. The lesion can be best discerned by comparing the adjacent or contralateral normal tissue to the area of abnormality (Fig. 16–8; see also Figs. 16–3, 16–4). Only about 60% of cancers larger than 5 mm have this appearance.[13] Not all hypoechoic cancers are properly represented by US. Some may appear smaller on US than on pathologic examination, others much smaller (Figs. 16–9, 16–10).

Hyperechoic Lesions

More acoustically reflective lesions are only subtly increased in echogenicity as compared with normal tissue (Fig. 16–11). They are not brightly echogenic with thick foci that are due

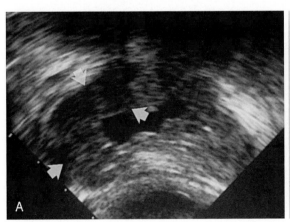

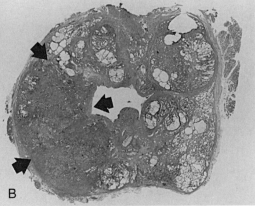

Figure 16–8. Prostate cancer. Transverse ERU image *(A)* and step-section radical prostatectomy specimen *(B)* looking toward the base of the gland demonstrates a hypoechoic focus *(arrows)* correlating to the prostate cancer on the radical prostatectomy specimen. The patient had previously undergone transurethral resection of the prostate.

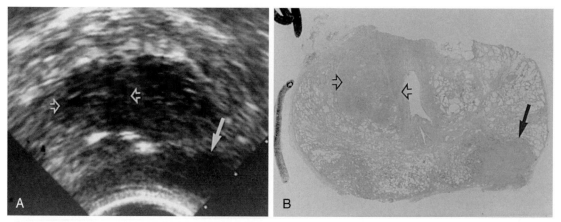

Figure 16–9. Prostate cancer. Transverse ERU image (*A*) and step-section radical prostatectomy specimen (*B*) looking toward the base of the gland demonstrates a hypoechoic focus *(arrows)* in the patient's left posterolateral peripheral zone, correlating to the prostate cancer on the radical prostatectomy specimen. Note that the 2-cm cancer in the right inner gland *(arrowheads)* is not clearly identified on the US study.

to calculi or corpora amylacea, although these processes are also considered hyperechoic. The exact number or percentage of cancers that have this type of appearance is unknown, but is relatively small.

Mixed Echogenic Lesions

Mixed-echogenicity lesions have a mixture of areas of increased and decreased echogenicity. While close inspection demonstrates the heterogeneity of the acoustic pattern, many sonographers still consider these lesions hypoechoic. This appearance may represent as many as 20 percent of cancers identified by US.

Isoechoic Lesions

Isodense lesions can be quite large but may not be seen on high-resolution US because the acoustic reflectivity is similar to that of normal tissue (see Fig. 16–5).

US is technically different from most other imaging tools. The technique of the examination, the technical factors used for the examination, the sophistication of the equipment can alter the sonographic findings, which can be reliably diagnostic or limited. The relative echogenicity of a lesion as compared with that of normal adjacent tissue cannot be altered (Figs. 16–12, 16–13); however, the absolute echogenicity, and more importantly, the con-

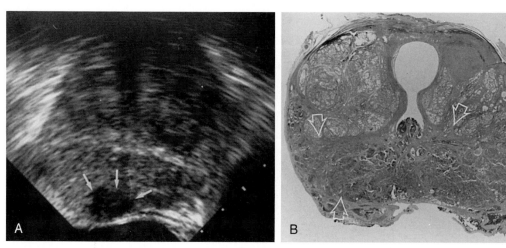

Figure 16–10. Prostate cancer. Transverse ERU image (*A*) and step-section radical prostatectomy specimen (*B*) looking toward the base of the gland demonstrates a small, hypoechoic focus *(arrows)* correlating to only a small segment of a much larger prostate cancer *(arrowheads)* as seen on the radical prostatectomy specimen.

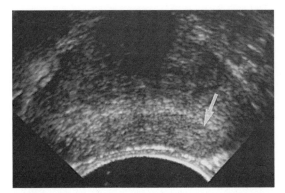

Figure 16–11. Hyperechoic prostate cancer. Transverse ERU image looking toward the base of the gland demonstrates subtle periprostatic, capsular distortion from a slightly hyperechoic lesion *(arrow)*, an infiltrating prostate cancer.

spicuousness of a lesion can be enhanced or diminished, depending on how the equipment is adjusted and tailored for each patient. Each machine and each subject being examined is different. Thus, it is essential to optimize the examination for each subject. Certain technical features should be tailored for each study:[11]

Frequency

The theoretical resolution of an US transducer may increase with the frequency of the transducer; however, the sound beam penetrates tissue less as frequency increases. Thus, the practical resolution of a transducer is not completely dependent on the frequency of the insonating crystal. Some cancers may be seen better with the higher-frequency transducers (i.e., 7.5 mHz) others with lower frequencies (i.e., 5.0 mHz; see Fig. 16–12).

Gain and Time Gain Compensation Curve

The time gain compensation curve (TGC) can be altered for each individual patient to account for the differences that may be observed in absorption and scattering of the sound beam and the subsequent variations that can occur in penetrating and visualizing the deeper structures.,

Postprocessing

Different postprocessing curves can be used to accentuated or diminish the acoustic properties of adjacent structures, so some lesions or regions of interest may be better seen with different settings (see Fig. 16–13).

Appropriate use of these technical features may enhance the area of concern, within the gland or in the pericapsular regions. Unfortunately, even with the image-enhancing features described above, not every lesion seen on US will be cancer. In fact, most are not. Overall, only about one third of lesions identified by the highest-resolution equipment are malignant.

The chance that a lesion is malignant

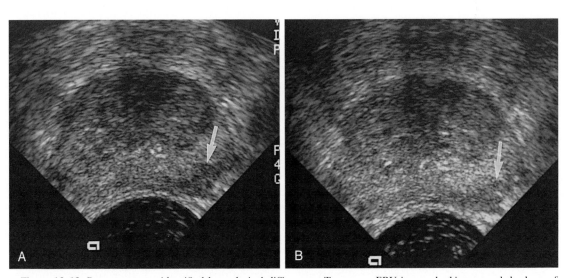

Figure 16–12. Prostate cancer identified by technical differences. Transverse ERU images looking toward the base of a relatively normal-sized gland demonstrates a hypoechoic lesion, a cancer *(arrows)* seen differently by 5.0-mHz *(A)* and 7.5-mHz *(B)* transducers.

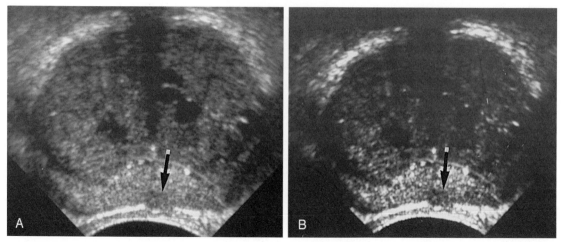

Figure 16–13. Prostate cancer identified by technical differences. Transverse ERU image looking toward the base of an enlarged gland demonstrates a hypoechoic lesion, a cancer *(arrows)* seen with two different postprocessing curves, *A, B.*

depends on a number of factors, including the size and conspicuousness of the lesion, the patient's PSA level, and the findings on DRE.[1, 11, 14]

Even with the greatest attention to maximizing the technical approach to the US examination, not every cancer can be identified by conventional gray-scale ultrasound. Color Doppler, which demonstrates flow, may, theoretically and practically, improve US's capability to delineate cancer. Cancer in general, being a faster-growing process than benign growth, requires an increased supply of nutrients. Thus, an increased amount of blood flow can be by obtained by increasing the number, course, caliber, size, and volume of flow.

By setting the color Doppler and sensitivity controls appropriately, normal flow in the prostate can be visually diminished, so that visibly abnormal flow is enhanced. Many prostate cancers show flow. While early results suggested that as many as 85% of all prostate cancer demonstrated focal flow to the cancer,[15, 16] more recent data have suggested it to be only about 50% of all cancers.[17] Unfortunately, like gray-scale ultrasound, an abnormal area of flow is not pathognomonic for malignancy. Biopsy is still required; however, most important is the use of color Doppler imaging to identify lesions that are more difficult to detect on conventional gray-scale US and, thus, to use US as a guide for biopsy. Many studies have suggested that at least 10 percent of additional cancers can be delineated by color Doppler alone.[15–17] In these cases, US-directed biopsies can utilize color as the guiding tool.[15–18]

ULTRASOUND-GUIDED PROSTATE BIOPSY

Some physicians performing prostate imaging believe that US should be used only as an aid for directed biopsy in specific quadrants of the prostate. If the imager utilizes the equipment correctly, however, many subtle lesions may be seen, and this allows more appropriate directed biopsies and a larger yield of cancers.

The conventional, digitally guided biopsy may still be an acceptable approach to many palpable lesions, but even for palpable lesions, US-guided prostate biopsy is a far more precise technique for ensuring that tissue from the lesion is obtained accurately.[19–22] US must be used to ensure adequate biopsy for subtly palpable or nonpalpable but sonographically visible lesions. US should be used to guide prostate biopsy in all cases, except for digitally palpable but sonographically invisible lesions. US allows accurate placement of the biopsy needle into specific areas of the prostate to obtain tissue for pathologic diagnosis.

In general, prostatic biopsy is simple, safe, rapid, and accurate. The technique varies slightly, depending on what equipment is utilized. Use of an intrarectal probe in which the transducer is positioned so that the line of insonation is perpendicular to the long axis of the probe, requires a transperineal biopsy approach (Fig. 16–14). Those rectal probes

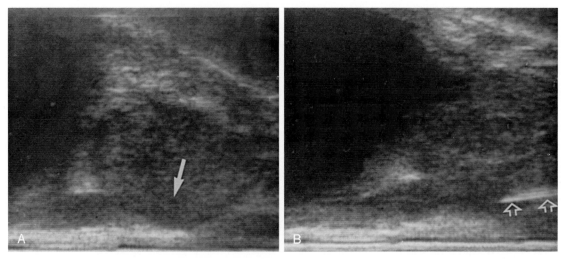

Figure 16–14. Transperineal prostate biopsy. Longitudinal images of the prostate demonstrate a hypoechoic region (*arrow* in *A*), and the highly acoustically reflective biopsy needle (*arrowheads* in *B*) during the biopsy.

that have the transducer insonating in a direction relatively parallel to the length of the probe allow use of a transrectal biopsy (Fig. 16–15). The latter, the transrectal biopsy, is employed most frequently in today's clinical practice. The transperineal biopsy is still used in certain instances and is the approach for needle placement when US-guided percutaneous interstitial radioactive seed implants are used for treatment or cryoablation of the prostate is employed.

Transperineal biopsy is performed under aseptic conditions with the patient in the lithotomy position. No pre- or postbiopsy antibiotics are required if conditions are sterile. A cleansing enema before the study is required only if retained fecal material interferes with the US image. The rectal contents should not be punctured with this approach. The use of extensive local anesthesia and the recently developed spring-loaded biopsy needles have rendered transperineal biopsy relatively painless. This approach allows the entire needle to be identified as it is positioned in the prostate and tissue is extracted.[11, 19]

The transrectal core biopsy, once thought to be associated with unacceptably high risk of urosepsis, is now considered safe and the primary tool for obtaining tissue.[11, 20, 21] Because the biopsy needle traverses the rectal contents and the rectal wall and into the prostate, the risk of urosepsis is increased compared with transperineal biopsy. This risk is reduced by pretreating the patient with a

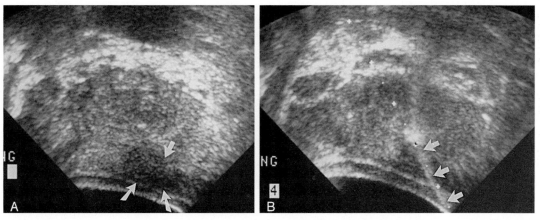

Figure 16–15. Transrectal prostate biopsy. Longitudinal images of the prostate demonstrate a hypoechoic region (*arrows* in *A*) and the highly acoustically reflective needle (*arrowheads* in *B*) during the biopsy.

cleansing enema (Fleet Enema), and a broad-spectrum antibiotic. Postbiopsy administration of antibiotics is also recommended. With the use of the 18-gauge spring-loaded biopsy needle and the pretreatment armamentarium described above, the procedure is safe, quick, and essentially painless. The needle is easily visible during the biopsy, but its orientation is obviously different from that for transperineal biopsy. It is essential, that, when transrectal biopsy is performed, the anal sphincter not be punctured. The rectal wall has virtually no pain fibers sensitive to sharp needles. The anal sphincter has an abundance of these nerve fibers.

In all cases when an obvious or subtle lesion is seen, a number of tissue cores should be obtained from the area. It is advisable to obtain tissue samples in other regions of the gland in addition. For example, if a palpable lesion is identified by US, no other area of concern is identified, and the PSA is normal, then a biopsy of the contralateral, normal-looking side may suffice. However, if the PSA is elevated, regardless of the size and visibility of a focal lesion, systematic quadrant or sextant biopsies may be warranted.[11, 23]

The quadrant biopsy should include, in addition to any specimens obtained from focal areas of concern, tissue sample cores obtained systematically by US guidance of the biopsy needle into the left apex and base and the right apex and base. A sextant biopsy would also include sampling of the apex and base of the middle of the gland, the midportion of the right and left peripheral glands, or the right and left inner gland (transition zone).[11, 23]

Complications of US-guided biopsy of the prostate performed with automatic spring-loaded biopsy needles are unusual. While some 25% to 30% of all men may develop transient hematuria, hematochezia, or hemospermia, clinically significant bleeding is quite unusual. If the pre- and postbiopsy antimicrobial regimen described above is followed, the risk of urosepsis following the procedure is far less than 1% for all men undergoing biopsy.[11]

STAGING OF PROSTATE CANCER WITH ULTRASONOGRAPHY

Initially, there was great hope that ERU imaging would provide accurate staging of prostate cancer; however, very rigorous scientific

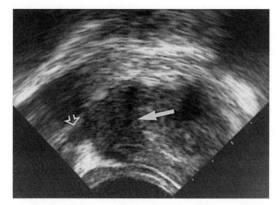

Figure 16–16. Capsular infiltration. Transverse ERU image demonstrates a hypoechoic prostate cancer *(arrows)* directly infiltrating into the periprostatic fat *(arrowhead)*.

studies have shown that it is not an accurate tool for staging of early or small tumors.[13] However, US does on occasion have a place in evaluation for possible extraprostatic extension of prostate cancer. Ultrasound may demonstrate regions of possible abnormality in the prostate capsule (Fig. 16–16), the seminal vesicles, the neurovascular bundles (Fig. 16–17), and other regions prone to infiltration with cancer. As with diagnosis, the delineation of an abnormal area is not definitive; however, if an area of concern is identified, US-guided biopsy of the region can be performed without significant risk to the patient. The results of the biopsy may have enormous implications for treatment of the disease.

SUMMARY

Ultrasound has exceptional capability for identifying many prostate cancers, but it is not

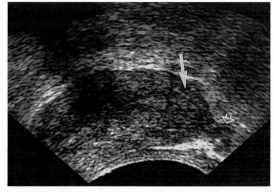

Figure 16–17. Neurovascular bundle infiltration. Transverse endorectal sonogram demonstrates a subtly hypoechoic prostate cancer *(arrow)* and an enlarged infiltrated left neurovascular bundle *(arrowhead)*.

a perfect tool and it has limitations. These limitations must be understood by the clinicians utilizing the examination, but the lack of perfection should not discourage application of ERU for evaluation of possible prostate cancer. Its use has greatly improved the clinician's ability to identify prostate cancer and to more accurately and safely biopsy the prostate. The diagnostic capability of ERU should not be downplayed.

REFERENCES

1. Cooner WH, Mosley BR, Rutherford CL, et al.: Prostate cancer detection in a clinical urological practice by ultrasonography, digital rectal examination and prostate-specific antigen. J Urol 143:1146–1154, 1990.
2. Lee F, Littrup PJ, Loft-Christensen L, et al.: Predicted prostate specific antigen results using transrectal ultrasound gland volume. Cancer 70:211–220, 1992.
3. Benson MC, Whang IS, Pantuck A, et al.: Prostate specific antigen density: A means of distinguishing benign prostatic hypertrophy and prostate cancer. J Urol 147:815–816, 1992.
4. Watanabe H, Kaiho H, Tanaka M, Terasawa Y: Diagnostic applications of ultrasonotomography to the prostate. Invest Urol 8:548–559, 1971.
5. Rifkin M, Kurtz A, Choi H, Goldberg B: Endoscopic ultrasonic investigation of the prostate using a transrectal probe: Prospective evaluation and acoustic characterization. Radiology 149:265–271, 1983.
6. Lee F, Littrup P, Torp-Pederson S, et al.: Prostate cancer: Comparison of transrectal US and digital rectal examination for screening. Radiology 168:389–394, 1988.
7. Mettlin C, Jones G, Averette H, et al.: Defining and updating the American Cancer Society guidelines for cancer-related checkup: Prostate and endometrial cancers. CA Cancer J Clin 43:42–46, 1993.
8. Rifkin MD: Transrectal prostatic ultrasonography: Comparison of linear array and radial scanners. J Ultrasound Med 4:1–5, 1985.
9. Watanabe H: History of transrectal sonography of the prostate. Urol Clin North Am 16:617–622, 1989.
10. Resnick M, Willard J, Boyce W: Recent progress in ultrasonography of the bladder and prostate. J Urol 117:444–446, 1977.
11. Rifkin MD: Ultrasound of the prostate, 2nd ed. Philadelphia: Lippincott-Raven, 1997.
12. Franks L: Benign prostatic hyperplasia: Gross and microscopic anatomy. In Grayhack J, Wilson W, Scherbenske M (eds.): Benign Prostatic Hyperplasia. NIAMDD Workshop Proceedings. Washington: US Government Printing Office, 1976.
13. Rifkin MD, Zerhouni EA, Gatsonis CA, et al.: Comparison of MRI and US in staging early prostate cancer: Results of a multiinstitutional cooperative trial. N Eng J Med 323:621–626, 1990.
14. Rifkin M, McGlynn E, Choi H: Echogenicity of prostate cancer correlated with histologic grade and stromal fibrosis: Endorectal US studies. Radiology 186:549–552, 1993.
15. Rifkin MD, Sudakoff GS, Alexander AA: Color Doppler imaging of the prostate: Techniques, results and potential applications. Radiology 186:509–513, 1993.
16. Kelly IMG, Lees WR, Rickards D: Prostate cancer and the role of color Doppler ultrasound. Radiology 189:153–156, 1993.
17. Cheng SS, Rifkin MD, Bajas MA, et al.: Color Doppler imaging: An important adjunct to endorectal US in the diagnosis of prostate cancer. Radiology 201(P):38, 1996.
18. Littrup PJ, Klein RM, Sparschu RA, et al.: Color Doppler of the prostate: Histologic and racial correlations. Radiology 197(P):365, 1993.
19. Rifkin MD, Kurtz AB, Goldberg BB: Sonographically guided transperineal prostatic biopsy: Preliminary experience with a longitudinal linear array transducer. AJR 139:745–747, 1983.
20. Lee F, Littrup PJ, Kumasaka GH, et al.: Use of transrectal ultrasound in the diagnosis, guided biopsy, staging and screening of prostate cancer. Radiographics 7:617, 1987.
21. Resnick MI: Transrectal ultrasound guided versus digitally directed prostatic biopsy: A comparative study. J Urol 139:754–757, 1988.
22. Rifkin MD, Alexander A, Pisarchick J, Matteucci T: Ultrasound-guided prostate biopsy: Superior accuracy compared to digital guided biopsy of palpable masses. Radiology 179:41–42, 1991.
23. Czerwinskyj CD, Rifkin MD, Bajas MA, et al.: Should US-guided prostate biopsy routinely include the transition zone?: Report of a prospective study. Radiology 201(P):338, 1996.

17

DIAGNOSIS OF PROSTATE CANCER ALTERED BY IONIZING RADIATION WITH AND WITHOUT NEOADJUVANT ANTIANDROGEN HORMONAL ABLATION

DOUGLAS B. SIDERS, FRED LEE, and DANIEL M. MAYMAN

Carcinoma of the prostate gland is the most prevalent and the second most deadly malignant neoplasm of males in the United States.[1] Effective definitive therapy is still unproven, so some authorities question the utility (i.e., cost-effectiveness) of early detection.[2–4] Curative therapeutic options for clinically confined disease are radical prostatectomy or radiation therapy. Both provide long-term local control and equivalent survival times.[5] Combinations thereof—salvage radical prostatectomy after radiation therapy and salvage radiation therapy after definitive prostatectomy—are frequently applied after initial treatment failure.[6,7] The growing use of neoadjuvant total androgen ablation therapy, in any or all therapeutic phases, further complicates the picture for pathologists. Transrectal ultrasound (TRUS)–guided biopsies have detected persistent cancer in 30% to 90% of irradiated prostate glands, and these patients have a high risk of local recurrence.[8–12] Recurrent or persistent cancer may have pathologic and biochemical indicators for increased biologic aggressiveness. This evidence consists of dedifferentiation with increasing Gleason scores,[11] increase of DNA aneuploidy,[13,14] and shortened doubling time of serum prostate-specific antigen (PSA) from postradiation nadir levels.[15,16]

Early diagnosis is essential for detecting these cancers while they are confined to the prostatic fossa. Should the serum PSA increase from nadir, TRUS-guided biopsy 18 to 24 months after radiation therapy may lead to the diagnosis of carcinoma in this high-risk group.

Salvage radical prostatectomy for radiation failures has been attempted, but it is technically challenging, and in patients who have had pelvic lymphadenectomies has resulted in serious technical complications.[17] Cryosurgery after radiation failure, though investigational at this time, has been successful in approximately 89% of cases but is associated with increased morbidity.[18]

Total androgen ablation therapy (i.e., a leuteinizing hormone–releasing hormone [LH-

RH] agonist together with flutamide) in randomized studies has proved that downstaging of prostate cancer is achievable, and its use followed by salvage radical prostatectomy is presented in this paper.[19–23]

Pathologic interpretation of irradiated cancer is particularly difficult; both over- and underdiagnosis are reported. Since patients may have received some form of androgen ablation therapy before biopsy for probable radiation failure, the pathologic effect of the combination of radiation therapy and total androgen ablation, particularly on benign acini, compounds the problem of interpretation of "persistent cancer." In this study, we report on the pathology of 33 patients in whom radiation therapy failed and who subsequently were treated with salvage radical prostatectomy. The majority (28/33, 85%) were given total androgen ablation therapy for a minimum of 3 months.

METHODS AND MANAGEMENT

Between 1985 and 1995, 35 consecutive salvage radical prostatectomies were attempted for persistent cancer in irradiated prostates. One operation was not possible owing to extensive pelvic fibrosis, and another was excluded because pathologic data were lost. A total of 33 patients remained for statistical evaluation.

Age

The mean age at radical prostatectomy was 65.5 ± 5.4 (range, 50.8 to 75.1) years.

Stage of Cancer

All lesions were clinically localized (stages A to C or T1 to T3, NxM0). Bone scans and computed tomography (CT) were negative.

TRUS-Guided Staging Biopsy

All TRUS studies used a Hitachi model EU-450 or EUB-515 scanner with 5.0- and 6.5-MHz transducers and/or color Doppler and spectral analysis. All ultrasound images were obtained in both transverse and longitudinal projections and recorded on multiformat film,

printer paper, or 3/4-inch videotape. An 18-gauge automatic biopsy device (ASAP 19-18TM, Microvasive, Watertown, Mass.) was used to sample the hypoechoic lesions and related sites of tumor escape from the peripheral, central, or transition zones. The primary criterion for biopsy was interval from end of therapy, which was arbitrary (but at least 18 months) and was not necessarily based on clinical or biochemical failure (rising PSA levels).

Total Androgen Ablation Therapy

Total androgen ablation therapy consisted of an LH-RH agonist (Lupron, Tap Pharmaceuticals, Deerfield, IL, or Zoladex, ICI Pharma, Wilmington, DE) and flutamide (Eulexin, Shering, Kenilworth, NJ). In this study group, 85% (28 of 33) of the patients were pretreated for a mean duration of 4.7 ± 1.8 months.

Needle Core Specimens

Needle core specimens were dyed at the proximal (capsular) end with bluing. The entire core was then stained with eosin, fixed in buffered 10% formalin, and step-sectioned at at least two levels for diagnosis, leaving approximately one half of the archival processed paraffin core for further studies. Biopsy material included pre- and postradiation specimens. The Gleason scoring system was applied uniformly.[24]

Radical Prostatectomy Specimens

All specimens (needle core biopsies and radical prostatectomies) were evaluated by one pathologist (DBS). The glands were described, weighed, and measured. Indelible inks were used to mark the gland boundaries (The Davidson Marking System; Bradley Products, Bloomington, MN). The prostate gland was painted on the left side with blue dye, on the right side with gold dye, and with a red dye stripe over the anterior fibromuscular stroma.

Before 1991, the prostate glands were fixed for at least 1 week in 10% buffered formalin and then sectioned. Beginning in 1991, the glands were cut in the fresh state to provide tumor samples for molecular studies. The gland, whether fresh or fixed, was subsequently sectioned at 3- to 4-mm intervals in parasagittal (longitudinal) planes. The slices were then placed on bond paper, and outline tracings were made. At that time, the gland was inspected and palpated to try to delineate tumor extent, and when possible this area was shaded in the outline tracing. After this, register marks were cut through the gland onto the paper to aid in subsequent orientation. The most lateral right- and left-hand slices were cut transversely to evaluate lateral resection margins accurately. The other slices were then processed as whole mounts. All slides were sectioned at 7-μm intervals and stained with hematoxylin and eosin and examined using both dissecting and conventional microscopy. A variation of this approach may be found in Chapter 10: "Examination of Radical Prostatectomy Specimens: Therapeutic and Prognostic Significance."

Average tumor dimensions were calculated using a formula similar to that described for ultrasound measurements: The sum of the gland's dimensions (width + height + length) was divided by 3. Tumor location was noted and correlated with the ultrasound images. Tumor morphology was determined, and multiple tumors were precisely located. Gleason scores were determined for all tumors, and comparisons were made between the prostatectomy samples and the preradiation and postradiation needle cores. Nonconfined cancer (stage C) was defined as complete capsular penetration into periprostatic fat, trapezoid space (apex), or seminal vesicle. A positive surgical margin required that tumor be in contact with the inked margin of the specimen.

RESULTS

Time to Failure

The time to biopsy was approximately 3 years (mean), and time from end of therapy to radical prostatectomy was approximately 3.3 years (mean). Time to biopsy was based more on protocol, at least 18 months from end of irradiation, than on clinical or biochemical failure or rising PSA (Table 17–1).

Androgen Ablation Therapy

Total androgen ablation therapy was given to 85% of the study group and did not yield significant outcome results when compared

Table 17–1. Variables of 33 Men in Study Group

Age (yr)
65.5 ± 5.4 (SD: 50.8–75.1)
Radiation type
External beam ($N = 24$)
Seed implant ($N = 9$; ^{125}I = 8, ^{103}P = 1)
Duration of TAA ($N = 28$)
4.7 ± 1.8 mo 85%
Interval from radiation therapy to SRP (yr)
Mean 3.3 ± 1.4 (range 2.0–7.2)
Median 2.8
Failure rate
External beam ($N = 7$) 29%
Seed implant ($N = 4$) 44%

TAA, total androgen ablation therapy; SRP, salvage radical prostatectomy

with the 15% (5 of 33) in the non-treatment group. This may be due to the small number in the untreated group. There was no significant difference in success or failure in either stage B or C when total androgen ablation therapy was used preoperatively (Table 17–2).

Type of Radiation

External beam radiation was more successful than seed implant for outcome of confined

Table 17–2. Characteristics of Stage B and Stage C Cancers

	Prevalence	
	N	(%)
Prostate cancer, confined, stage B	22/33	66.7
*Radiation type		
External beam	17/24	70.8
Seed implant	5/9	55.6
*TAA (>3 mo)		
Yes	19/28	67.9
No	3/5	60.0
Prostate cancer, nonconfined, stage C	11/33	33.3
*Radiation type		
External beam	7/24	29.2
Seed implant	4/9	44.4
*TAA		
Yes	9/28	32.1
No	2/5	40.0
Extracapsular extension	6/11	54.5
SM negative	3/6	50.0
SM positive	3/6	50.0
Seminal vesicle involvement	5/11	45.5
SM negative	3/5	60.0
SM positive	2/5	40.0

*The results of radiation type and TAA are related to the entire group of n = 33 to assess impact on pathologic stage.

TAA, total androgen ablation

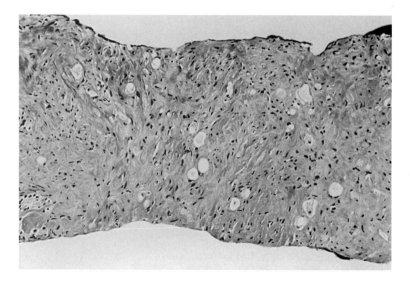

Figure 17–1. Irradiated carcinoma. Note the haphazard pattern and the nucleomegaly and cytomegaly. (H & E, scanning power, needle-core biopsy, total androgen ablation therapy & radiation therapy.)

cancer. For nonconfined cancer, the failure rate for seed implant was also greater than that for external beam (see Table 17–2). These results are statistically significant.

Within the entire group of resected specimens (n = 33), those with negative surgical margins comprise 85% (28/33). Of these latter, 21.4% (6/28) had no extracapsular extension of the tumor. However, these patients remain at risk for future progression of disease. The specimens with positive surgical margins comprised only 15% (5/33). Overall confined cancer occurred in 66.7% (22/33) and nonconfined cancer in 33.3% of the total.

Pathology Results

Architectural and cytologic changes in irradiated and hormonally altered prostate biopsy specimens have been described.[20,25–30] The latter include antiandrogen agents such as estrogen, and more recently total androgen replacement therapy. Even in autopsy or radical prostatectomy specimens, interpretation of tissue subjected to these agents is difficult. Adding to our challenges has been the advent of the fine (18-gauge) needle, ultrasound-guided biopsy cores, which provide even less tissue for inspection. In a recent study of postirradiated prostate biopsy findings, 19.7% were classified as indeterminate.[31] In the irradiated prostate gland the most important single characteristic that helps pathologists diagnose carcinoma is the lack of acinar structure. Enlarged glands or fused glandular elements are broadcast haphazardly within sclerotic stroma (Fig. 17–1, Table 17–3).

Paradoxically, benign irradiated glands exhibit more and varied atypia than do malignant glands. Frequently nuclear "holes" or "windows" are seen in benign irradiated epithelium, which reflect marked nuclear poly-

Table 17–3. Microscopic Features of Irradiated Carcinomas

Changes in carcinomas
　Histologic
　　Loss of ductal acinar configuration
　Cytologic
　　Massive cytomegaly and nucleomegaly with
　　　prominent nucleoli
　　Moderate nuclear atypia
Changes in benign tissue
　Histologic
　　Preservation of acinar configuration
　　Vascular sclerosis
　Cytologic
　　Moderate cytomegaly and nucleomegaly with
　　　prominent nucleoli
　　Squamous metaplasia
　　Endothelial and fibroblastic atypia
　　Nuclear "holes" or "windows"
　　Nuclear folding and lobulation
Changes helpful in distinguishing benign and malignant
irradiated glands
　Significant atypia is more striking in benign glands
　　than in malignant glands.
　Squamous metaplasia is more common in benign
　　glands.
　Intranuclear holes are more striking in benign
　　irradiated cells.
　Nuclear folding and nuclear lobulation are more
　　prominent in benign cells.

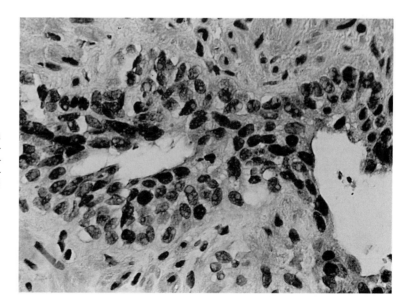

Figure 17-2. Irradiated benign gland. Epithelial cells with intranuclear "holes" and nuclear polyploidy. (H & E, high power, needle-core biopsy, radiation therapy.)

ploidy, usually in the basal (myoepithelial) cells (Fig. 17-2; see Table 17-3). Mitotic figures are found rarely in irradiated carcinoma but more commonly in benign irradiated glands (Fig. 17-3). Squamous metaplasia is more characteristic of benign irradiated cells than of malignant irradiated cells. Nucleoli are of little help in differentiating benign from malignant cells, although they tend to be larger in the malignant cells, and the malignant cells themselves are usually larger than the benign ones (see Table 17-3).

The most prominent changes in glands subjected to antiandrogen therapy are degeneration and apoptosis. The malignant nuclei become smaller and more hyperchromatic and exhibit fewer apparent nucleoli, producing the "nucleoli-poor cell" carcinoma (Fig. 17-4).[32] The cytoplasm becomes shrunken and takes on a clear appearance. Both in the outer and inner gland regions (peripheral, central, or transition zones) the secretory elements become markedly atrophic and relatively inapparent. The basal or myoepithelial cell is little affected by androgen deprivation and remains prominent in benign glands, outlining these structures.

Dysplastic epithelium (prostatic intraepithelial neoplasia [PIN]) has been described as undergoing regression under total androgen

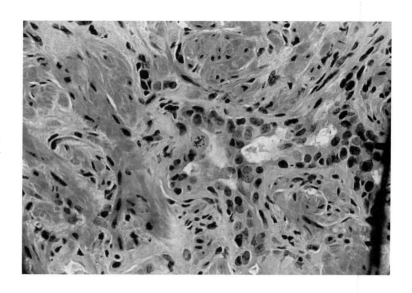

Figure 17-3. Irradiated benign gland with persistent myoepithelial cells and atypical (effete?) mitosis. (H & E, medium power, needle-core biopsy, radiation therapy.)

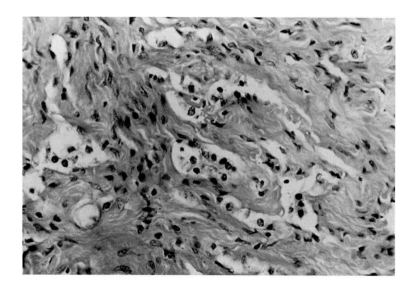

Figure 17–4. Sclerosing "nucleoli-poor" carcinoma. (H & E, high power, whole mount, total androgen ablation therapy and radiation therapy.)

ablation therapy.[26,27,33] In our experience dysplastic epithelium does not undergo significant regression but exhibits the same changes noted in malignant cells, with a prominent decrease in nucleolar size. The secretory cellular stratification persists, however, and nuclear polarity is lost (Figs. 17–5, 17–6).

The dying androgen-deprived tumor cell occasionally induces a lymphocytic or histiocytic inflammatory reaction that may be an immune-mediated component of tumor destruction, in addition to the more important process of apoptosis. The term "apoptosis" has been used in the literature for more than a decade. It has been employed mostly by pathologists to refer to individual cellular changes that mark irreversible degeneration leading to cell death. More recently it has been appropriated in molecular pathology to indicate cellular events that lead to irreversible cell death. It is distinguished from necrotic cell death by the absence of an acute inflammatory reaction. Current molecular studies of carcinoma place increasing emphasis on inducers and inhibitors of apoptosis.[34,35]

Adenocarcinoma of the prostate gland is a paradigm for an androgen-dependent tumor in which apoptosis is inhibited by the presence of androgen.[34] The removal of this apoptotic inhibitor sets into motion the apoptotic death cycle that results in cytoplasmic and nuclear disruption. The nucleus undergoes condensa-

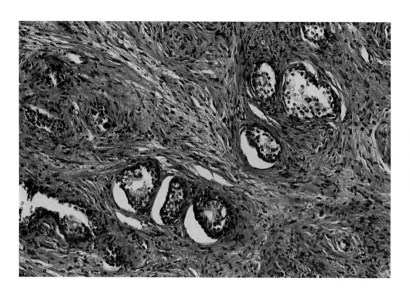

Figure 17–5. Irradiated, dysplastic glands with delimiting myoepithelial cells and multiple layers of secretory cells. (H & E, medium power, whole mount, total androgen ablation therapy and radiation therapy.)

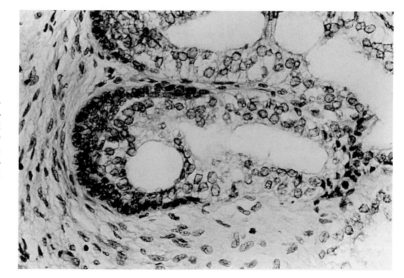

Figure 17–6. Persistent high-grade dysplasia (PIN 3) with enhanced basal or myoepithelial layer. Multiple secretory cell layer with loss of polarity. (H & E, high power, whole mount, total androgen ablation therapy & radiation therapy.)

tion and chromatin clumping. The cytokeratin skeletal disruption causes cellular distortion, but the cell usually maintains to the end its cytoplasmic integrity.

At the light microscopic level apoptotic bodies may be intracytoplasmic or intercytoplasmic.[33] We have noted two more distinct varieties of total androgen ablation–related apoptotic changes.[20] The most common one, mucinous, is usually seen in radical prostatectomy specimens and occasionally in needle core biopsies. The change ranges from shriveled carcinoma cells floating in mucin pools to the most extreme manifestation, where only pools of mucin are present (Fig. 17–7). Less common is hyaline apoptosis, in which tumor cells undergo hyaline change. We have seen this in radical prostatectomy specimens within the gland itself (Fig. 17–8) and in a perineural site outside the gland (Fig. 17–9). Hyaline apoptosis has as its end stage ghost cells similar to those seen in calcifying epithelioma of Malherbe. Since hyaline apoptosis is rarely seen in needle cores, it is probably a later phenomenon than mucinous change and unlikely to be seen except at autopsy or in radical prostatectomy specimens (Table 17–4).

High–molecular weight cytokeratin staining of small acinar lesions of the prostate gland has been suggested as being helpful in distinguishing benign small acini from malignant infiltrative carcinoma, in both irradiated[36] and

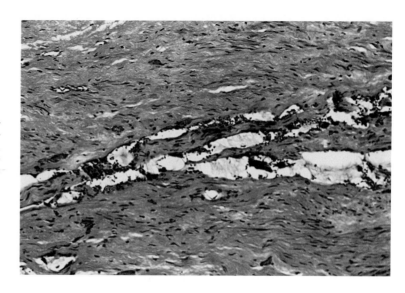

Figure 17–7. Perineural apoptosis with complete absence of tumor cells in mucin pools. (H & E, medium power, whole mount, total androgen ablation therapy & radiation therapy.)

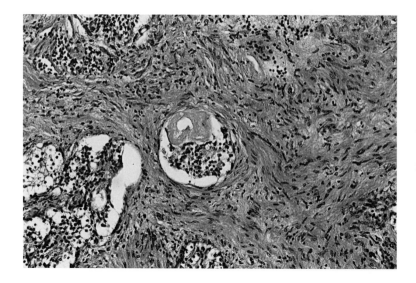

Figure 17–8. Irradiated cribriform carcinoma undergoing hyaline apoptosis. (H & E, medium power, whole mount, total androgen ablation therapy and radiation therapy.)

Table 17–4. Microscopic Changes in Androgen-Deprived Carcinomas

Histologic	Cytologic
Atrophy of secretory cells with preservation of myoepithelial cells	Cytoplasmic vacuolization or clearing
Lymphocytic and histiocytic reaction to apoptotic tumor cells	Nuclear pyknosis
	Nucleolar regression
Mucinous apoptosis, especialy in perineural tumor	Squamous metaplasia
Hyaline apoptosis, especially in perineural tumor	

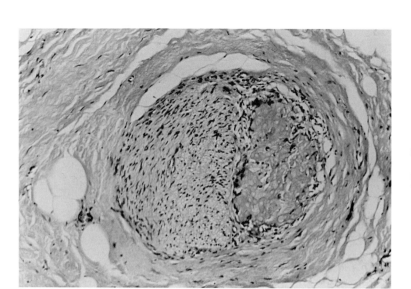

Figure 17–9. Perineural hyaline apoptosis. Note "ghost" cells. (H & E, medium power, whole mount, total androgen ablation therapy and radiation therapy.)

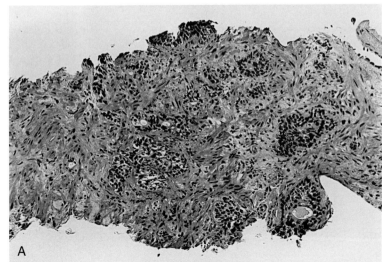

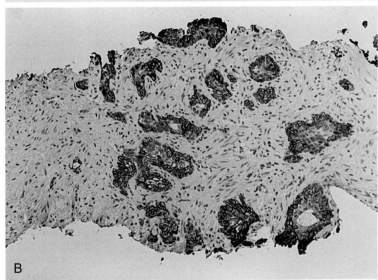

Figure 17–10. *A,* Persistent, irregular glands with a pseudocribriform pattern. (H & E, low power, needle-core biopsy, total androgen ablation therapy [2 years] & radiation therapy.) *B,* Intense staining of layered, atypical-looking basal cells: not PIN, not malignant. (Keratin 903, low power, needle-core biopsy, serial section of same specimen.)

nonirradiated[37] carcinomas. Although this stain is occasionally helpful, we have not used it routinely. Monoclonal antibody 34β-E12 (Enzo Diagnostics, New York) is a useful immunohistochemical reagent for highlighting basal cell hyperplasia (see Chapter 10) and profound atrophy of the secretory acinar element in the irradiated androgen-ablated tissue (Fig. 17–10).

Perhaps the most difficult challenges in our experience have been biopsy cores from patients who have been subjected to both radiation therapy and neoadjuvant hormonal ablation. As in the irradiated gland, architecture is the most important feature, followed by basal cell absence, and apoptotic changes (Table 17–5).

It has been stated that Gleason scoring is not appropriate or is misleading in iatrogenically altered tumors.[25,27] We certainly agree that nuclear-grading systems[38] are inappropriate, but

Table 17–5. Microscopic Changes Helpful in Distinguishing Benign and Malignant Irradiated, Androgen-Deprived Glands

Preservation of ductal and acinar architecture is the most helpful feature.

Accentuation or preservation of the basal or myoepithelial cells is not seen in malignant epithelium.

Mucinous or hyaline apoptosis does not occur in benign glands.

a tumor-grading system based on architectural relationships between tumor and stroma and the shapes and sizes of formed glands with lumina is still valuable as a predictor and should be discredited or discounted only after careful studies with sufficient follow-up.

Our work in the irradiated prostatic cancers indicates that along with Gleason dedifferentiation (increasing Gleason scores) we have noticed increasing DNA ploidy abnormalities. It may then be inferred that the Gleason scoring system has grading merit even in irradiated tumors.

DISCUSSION

This study relates mainly to the effects of radiation therapy and total androgen ablation therapy on prostate cancer. The specimen-confined cancer rate of nearly 67% was almost the same as that for radical prostatectomy without radiation therapy. The surgical margin negative rate of 85% in this series is also nearly equivalent to most standard radical prostatectomy series using pretreatment total androgen ablation therapy.[21,23,39] A comparison, however, with four other recent series of salvage radical prostatectomy for radiation failures without total androgen ablation therapy revealed only 36%, 20%, 29%, and 28%[6,17,40,41] organ-confined cancers and surgical margin positive rate of 43%, 36%, 48%, and 31%, respectively. These pathologic results are considerably less satisfactory than our 67% for confined cancer and 15% for surgical margin positive ones.

Total androgen ablation therapy has been shown to be capable of downstaging prostate cancer. Labrie and colleagues, in a randomized study, had a 21.1% downstaging rate following 3 months of total androgen ablation therapy and a surgical margin positive rate of 7.8%. His control group has a surgical margin positive rate of 33.8%.[22] Had total androgen ablation therapy been utilized in these four reported series, applying Labrie's results would have resulted in confined cancer rates of 55%, 31%, 44%, and 43%, all values more comparable to our 67%. In our series, total androgen ablation therapy appeared to have limited positive results when compared with other series in which the downstaging and surgical margin negative specimens is dramatic. This may be due in part to the few patients (5) not pretreated with total androgen ablation therapy; however, clinical outcomes over time

are needed for correlation of prognosis in the surgical cures (specimen confined). Outcome analysis of this group of patients is the subject of another paper.

In our series the mean time before salvage radical prostatectomy was 3.3 years. This may account in part for our 67% success rate of specimen-confined tumor. Since studies indicate that postirradiated cancer may be of increased biologic aggressiveness, only early diagnosis may prevent extracapsular extension.[11,14]

The pathologic changes associated with radiation therapy have caused uncertainty, with a reported "indeterminate" diagnosis of 19.7%.[31] This further delays definitive therapy and increases the probability of tumor escape. This indeterminate category may be further enlarged with the addition of total androgen ablation therapy. In our series the indeterminate category was not used. Since we had radical prostatectomy–confirmed specimens, the use of the aforestated histologic and cytologic differential diagnostic features was validated as diagnostic for persistent cancer and not an "indeterminate" finding. The importance of proper interpretation is that persistent cancer has been proven to progress.

A more worrisome finding has been the increased biologic aggressiveness of postradiation cancers: tumor doubling times are expected to decrease. Therefore, the earliest clinically significant time for diagnosis would be important. Our series had a mean time from end of radiation therapy to radical prostatectomy of 3 years. Other reports had longer evaluation periods of 5 to 8 years, and this may explain in part our high confined cancer rate. The largest series of 132 salvage radical prostatectomies had a 38-month median interval from irradiation to surgery and only 28% with confined cancer at prostatectomy.[41]

The pathologic changes required for the diagnosis of persistent cancer after radiation therapy and total androgen ablation therapy are significant and should allow one to be more aggressive about appropriate definitive re-treatment.

The new treatment option, cryoablation, is currently utilized for those patients in whom radiation therapy failed to control their disease. Although the results are preliminary, an 85% increased rate of local destruction of cancer has been reported.[18] In our series, severe pelvic fibrosis was common after blind suprapubic iodine-125 brachytherapy. Salvage radical prostatectomy for these patients may necessitate pelvic exenteration and all its morbid sequelae. Cryoablation for these patients is technically possible and may provide a much less invasive approach and hopefully a comparable success rate with decreased surgical morbidity.

Total androgen ablation therapy may be the principal factor that explains our high level of pathologic success (67%) with organ-confined cancers. Only time is now needed to substantiate biochemical correlation with pathology. Presently, randomized studies[21–23] with and without total androgen ablation in standard radical prostatectomy series have found similar pathologic outcomes. Longer follow-up will be needed for confirmation.

REFERENCES

1. Wingo PA, Tong T, Bolder S: Cancer statistics, 1995. Cancer J Clin 45:8, 1995.
2. Krahn MD, Mahoney JE, Eckman MH, et al.: Screening for prostate cancer—a decision analytic view. JAMA 272:773, 1994.
3. Litwin MS, Hays RD, Fink A, et al.: Quality-of-life outcomes in men treated for localized prostate cancer. JAMA 273:129, 1995.
4. Albertson PC, Fryback DG, Storer BE, et al.: Long-term survival among men with conservatively treated localized prostate cancer. JAMA 274:626, 1995.
5. Hanks GE: External beam radiation treatment for prostate cancer: Still the gold standard. Oncology 6:79, 1992.
6. Link P, Freiha FS: Radical prostatectomy after definitive radiation therapy for prostate cancer. Urology 37:189, 1991.
7. Ray GR, Bagshaw A, Freiha F: External beam radiation salvage for residual or recurrent local tumor following radical prostatectomy. J Urol 132:926, 1984.
8. Babaian RJ, Kojima M, Saitoh M, et al.: Detection of residual prostate cancer after external radiotherapy. Cancer 75:2153, 1995.
9. Freiha FS, Bagshaw MA: Carcinoma of the prostate: Results of post-irradiation biopsy. Prostate 5:19, 1984.
10. Kabalin JN, Hodge KK, McNeal JE, et al.: Identification of residual cancer in the prostate following radiation therapy: Role of transrectal ultrasound guided biopsy and prostate specific antigen. J Urol 142:326, 1989.
11. Lee F, Torp-Peterson S, Meiselman L, et al.: Transrectal ultrasound in the diagnosis and staging of local disease after I125 seed implantation for prostate cancer. Int J Radiat Oncol Biol Phys 15:1453, 1988.
12. Kuban DA, El-Mahdi AM, Schellhammer PF: Prognostic significance of post-irradiation prostate biopsies. Oncology 7:29, 1993.
13. deVere White RW, Deitch A, Myer-Haass GM, et al.: DNA ploidy in the irradiated prostate. J Urol 143:201A, 1990.
14. Deitch AD, deVere White RW: Flow cytometry as a predictive modality in prostate cancer. Hum Pathol 23:352, 1992.
15. Kaplan I, Prestidge BR, Cox RS, et al.: Prostate specific antigen after irradiation for prostate carcinoma. J Urol 144:1172, 1990.
16. Stamey TA, Ferrari MK, Schmid HP: The value of serial prostate specific antigen determinations 5 years after radiotherapy: Steeply increasing values characterize 80% of patients. J Urol 150:1856, 1993.
17. Rogers E, Ohori M, Kassabian VS, et al.: Salvage radical prostatectomy: Outcome measured by serum prostate specific antigen levels. J Urol 153:1047, 1995.
18. Bahn DK, Lee F, Solomon MH, et al.: Prostate cancer: US-guided percutaneous cryoablation. Radiology 190:551, 1994.
19. Van Poppel H, De Ridder D, Elgamal AA, et al.: Neoadjuvant hormonal therapy before radical prostatectomy decreases the number of positive surgical margins in stage T2 prostate cancer: Interim results of a prospective randomized trial. J Urol 154:429, 1995.
20. Lee F, Siders DB, Newby J, et al.: The role of transrectal ultrasound-guided staging biopsy and androgen ablation therapy prior to radical prostatectomy. Clin Invest Med 16:458–470, 1993.
21. Fair WR, Aprikian A, Sogani P, et al.: The role of neoadjuvant hormonal manipulation in localized prostatic cancer. Cancer 71(Suppl):1031, 1993.
22. Labrie F, Cusan L, Gomez JL, et al.: Down-staging of early stage prostate cancer before radical prostatectomy: The first randomized trial of neoadjuvant combination therapy with flutamide and a luteinizing hormone–releasing hormone agonist (Symposium). Urology 44:29, 1994.
23. Soloway MS, Sharifi R, Wajsman Z, et al.: Randomized prospective study comparing radical prostatectomy alone versus radical prostatectomy preceded by androgen blockade in clinical stage B2 (T2bNxM0) prostate cancer. J Urol 154:424, 1995.
24. Gleason DF: Histologic grading of prostate cancer: A perspective. Hum Pathol 23:273, 1992.
25. Grignon DJ, Sakr WA: Histologic effects of radiation therapy and total androgen blockade on prostate cancer. Cancer 75(Suppl):1837, 1995.
26. Tetu B, Srigley JR, Boivin JC, et al.: Effect of combination endocrine therapy (LHRH agonist and flutamide) on normal prostate and prostatic adenocarcinoma. Am J Surg Pathol 15(2):111, 1991.
27. Murphy WM, Soloway MS, Barrows GH: Pathologic changes associated with androgen deprivation therapy for prostate cancer. Cancer 68:821, 1991.
28. Siders DB, Lee F: Histologic changes of irradiated prostatic carcinoma diagnosed by transrectal ultrasound. Hum Pathol 23:344, 1993.
29. Bostwick DG, Egbert BM, Fajardo LF: Radiation injury of the normal and neoplastic prostate. Am J Surg Pathol 6:541, 1982.
30. Civantos F, Marcial MA, Banks ER, et al.: Pathology of androgen deprivation therapy in prostate carcinoma. Cancer 75:1634, 1994.
31. Kaye KW, Olson DJ, Payne JT: Detailed preliminary analysis of 125Iodine implantation for localized prostate cancer using percutaneous approach. J Urol 153:1020, 1995.
32. Ellison E, Bostwick DG, Ferguson J, et al.: 'Nucleoli poor' clear cell adenocarcinoma of the prostate: A distinctive histologic pattern following total androgen blockade. Mod Pathol 6:59A, 1993.
33. Bostwick DG: High grade prostatic intraepithelial neoplasia: The most likely precursor of prostate cancer. Cancer 75:1823, 1995.
34. Kyprianou N, English HF, Isaacs JT: Programmed cell

death regression of pc-82 human prostate cancer following androgen ablation. Cancer Res 50:3748, 1990.

35. Kerr JF, Winterford CM, Harmon BV: Apoptosis. Its significance in cancer and cancer therapy. Cancer 73:2013, 1994.

36. Brawer MK, Nagle RB, Pitts W, et al.: Keratin immunoreactivity as an aid to the diagnosis of persistent adenocarcinoma in irradiated human prostates. Cancer 63:454, 1989.

37. Wojno KJ, Epstein JI: The utility of basal cell–specific anti-cytokeratin antibody (34BE12) in the diagnosis of prostate cancer. A review of 228 cases. Am J Surg Pathol 19:251, 1995.

38. Mostofi FK, Sesterhenn IA, Sobin LH: International Histological Classification of Prostatic Tumours. Geneva: World Health Organization, 1980.

39. Solomon MH, McHugh TA, Dorr RP, et al.: Hormone ablation therapy as neoadjuvant treatment to radical prostatectomy. Clin Invest Med 16:6, 1993.

40. Younes E, Haas GP, Montie JE, et al.: Value of preoperative PSA in predicting pathologic stage of patients undergoing salvage prostatectomy. Urology 43:22, 1994.

41. Lerner SE, Blute ML, Zincke H: Critical evaluation of salvage surgery for radio-recurrent/resistant prostate cancer. J Urol 154:1103, 1995.

18

DNA FLOW CYTOMETRY AND IMMUNOHISTOCHEMISTRY OF *p53* PATHWAY GENES AS PREDICTIVE MODALITIES IN LOCALIZED PROSTATE CANCER

ARLINE D. DEITCH AND RALPH W. DEVERE WHITE

Detection of prostate cancer has increased nearly three-fold during the past ten years, making it the most frequently diagnosed male malignancy other than skin cancer in the United States. The treatment of localized prostate cancer is problematic because of the unpredictable behavior of this disease and the fact that the currently accepted markers—tumor stage, histologic grade, and prostate-specific antigen (PSA) levels—offer inadequate guidance for choosing among therapies. While DNA ploidy analysis of archival prostate tissue provides added prognostic information, it does not help to select therapy for the majority of these patients, those with diploid or tetraploid tumors. The authors review DNA ploidy studies and describe three additional markers: S-phase fraction and the immunodetection of the p53 and Bcl-2 gene products, that, when used in conjunction with DNA ploidy, better define subsets of patients who are suitable candidates for the available therapy options: active surveillance, definitive radiation therapy, and radical prostatectomy.

CLINICAL BACKGROUND

The treatment dilemmas posed by prostate cancer have intensified as the result of the increased detection of the disease. Currently 240,000 cases are diagnosed each year in the United States,[1] an increase of 179% over the past 10 years. Having detected these cases, clinicians must decide on appropriate treatment strategies. Prostate cancers vary markedly in malignant potential; however, if the patient with untreated cancer does not die of other causes, he has an increasing chance of dying of his disease. A recent retrospective study from Sweden reported on 149 patients with localized prostate cancer who were treated by surveillance.[2] Mortality due to other causes dominated among patients with short follow-up, while deaths due to prostate cancer increased with increasing observation time. While the risk of dying from prostate cancer thus increases with time, it is possible that some of these patients do not need immediate intervention. Ideally, one would like to postpone intervention until it becomes necessary, without however incurring the risk that these patients will develop metastatic disease during observation. This would require ongoing monitoring with the decision to initiate therapy being based on changes in the malignant potential of the patient's tumor and evaluation of his co-morbidities. However, once the decision is made to initiate therapy, there are few objective guidelines for choosing between radiation therapy and surgical intervention. It is clear that additional markers are needed to inform these decisions. DNA ploidy obtained by flow cytometry has been suggested as an appropriate marker of malignant potential in prostate cancer. This leads us to our first question.

Question 1. Can DNA ploidy be helpful in managing individual prostate cancer patients?

If treatment practice for prostate cancer were to change to ongoing reevaluation of these tumors, would there be a role for repetitive DNA content analyses in the management of individual patients? Furthermore, once the decision is made that treatment has become necessary, could such marker studies help guide us to select the appropriate therapy? It should be recognized at the outset that *if* we could cure metastatic prostate cancer, we would be more willing to use DNA analysis and other markers as reliable guides for selecting therapy. Unfortunately, at this time no treatment is available to cure metastatic prostate cancer. This helps explain the current tendency in the United States to risk overtreatment rather than to undertreat at the time of presentation. We should acknowledge, therefore, that treatment decisions for patients with localized prostate cancer will probably not be made in an ongoing manner in the near future and that the answer to our first question must be postponed. Nevertheless, it makes good sense to learn whether DNA ploidy and other markers of malignant potential can be used to provide information that is additive to tumor stage, histologic grade, and PSA levels, so that we can identify subsets of patients who are suitable for various types of therapy, including active surveillance. This leads to our second question:

Question 2. Can DNA ploidy, together with other markers, help characterize the malignant potential of prostate cancers?

This is a more limited question than question 1. The currently accepted markers, tumor stage, histologic grade, and PSA levels, effect only imperfect separations between favorable and unfavorable prognosis groups. In this setting, DNA ploidy studies would be only one in a series of additional tumor descriptors that would be considered in making treatment decisions. By phrasing the question in this way, we acknowledge that more information needs to be gathered, probably in the form of large clinical trials, to learn whether the chosen marker studies provide additional information that will help us to make appropriate treatment decisions for individual patients. We also need to understand the tumor biology of prostate cancer better, so we can design and test effective new therapies. With this information in hand, we could advance toward our ultimate goal, the prevention of prostate cancer.

DNA Ploidy and Its Relationship to Outcome in Prostate Cancer

Associating DNA ploidy analysis with outcome in prostate cancer has a long history. Thirty years ago, in a study employing static cytometry, Tavares reported that ploidy predicted outcome in prostate cancer.[3] He and his colleagues observed that patients having DNA diploid or tetraploid tumors had survival times that were similar to those found for the population at large, while the survival of those having aneuploid tumors was poor. The authors also observed that patients with diploid or tetraploid tumors responded well to estrogen therapy, whereas those with aneuploid tumors responded poorly. In 1993, Tribukait reported on 287 initially untreated patients[4] whose survival was similar to that of the patients studied earlier by Tavares. While stage and grade provided prognostic information, DNA ploidy was the most powerful predictor of prognosis in low-grade, low-stage prostate cancer. A number of other studies, including many emanating from the Mayo Clinic,[5, 6] have reported similar findings. Nevertheless, the issue is far from settled. The vast majority of clinicians do not obtain DNA ploidy studies prior to initiating therapy, and those who do so seldom use this information to make treatment decisions. To what is this reluctance to use ploidy in the clinical management of prostate cancer attributable?

Conclusions from the World Health Organization Consensus Conference on DNA Ploidy in Prostate Cancer

A consensus conference on the clinical utility of DNA ploidy studies in the management of prostate cancer was convened by the World Health Organization (WHO) in 1993.[6] The consensus group concluded that knowledge of the DNA content of localized prostate tumors is important for appropriately stratifying patients for clinical trials; however, except in a limited number of cases, DNA ploidy was not found to provide sufficient information to help select treatment for individual patients.

The WHO consensus conference concluded that patients with aneuploid tumors should not be considered for long-term surveillance. In the United States, patients probably would not be considered to be candidates for surveillance if their Gleason scores are higher than 6. In a series of 74 radical prostatectomies performed at the University of California Davis, only 7% of tumors having Gleason scores of 6 or less were aneuploid. If diagnostic biopsies had been used, because of sampling problems we probably would have found only 4% to 5% of such samples to be aneuploid. This prediction is based on information from Duke University, the University of California Los Angeles, and Sweden. Let us assume that the decision would be that those having diploid or tetraploid Gleason 2 to 6 tumors would be observed while only those having aneuploid tumors would receive conventional therapy. Considering that using biopsies we would miss 2% to 3% of the aneuploid tumors, we can ask if it would be cost effective to examine 100 tumors to find four or five that would be detectably aneuploid. Moreover, it is well documented that 15% of diploid cases exhibit disease progression within 5 years after radical prostatectomy.[7] This figure will be at least that high if active surveillance is used. In addition, the definition of what constitutes tetraploidy varies among studies, ranging from a lower threshold of 6% to 20% G2 cells. As a result, there is no general agreement about the prognostic significance of tetraploidy. Should tetraploid cases be included with the diploid cases, as suggested above, or with the aneuploid cases, as has been done in several studies, or

do they have an intermediate prognostic significance? These considerations make the reluctance to use active surveillance for those with low-grade, diploid or tetraploid tumors understandable. Clearly, additional tumor markers are needed to subclassify prostate cancers to better characterize the malignant potential of individual tumors.

The WHO consensus conference predicted that outcome after radiation therapy for those with aneuploid tumors would be poor. This conclusion was based largely on a single report from the Mayo Clinic in which ploidy determinations were performed using image analysis on the preradiation therapy biopsy.[8] The 10-year post-therapy survival rate was found to be only 20% for those with nondiploid and 75% for those with diploid or near diploid lesions. A recent flow cytometric study of localized prostate cancer treated by external-beam radiation therapy confirmed these findings.[9] These authors defined radiation failure as either rising serum PSA levels or clinical relapse. Their study had a mean follow-up of 36 months. In that time, only 16% of those with diploid tumors failed therapy, as compared to 52% with near-diploid and 77% with aneuploid tumors. To date, as in the treatment of localized prostate cancer by surgery, this information has had little impact on clinical practice.

The WHO consensus conference also concluded that aneuploid lesions respond poorly to hormonal ablation. While this information may be useful in clinical trials, the unfortunate fact is that we have no other therapy available for patients with metastatic disease.

Rather than reviewing all the previous literature on the DNA ploidy of prostate cancer, the reader is referred to the published WHO consensus conference,[6] which covers much of this literature, and to our previous publication in *Human Pathology,* since it contains our interpretation of the literature and summarizes our experience in this field.[7] We continue to believe that DNA ploidy information is valuable in studying prostate cancer, whether obtained from image analysis or flow cytometry; however, we have become convinced that to understand the biology of prostate cancer better and to make DNA ploidy useful in the management of individual patients, additional predictive markers are needed. We do not anticipate that such markers will replace ploidy; rather we expect that they will add information that will help choose between therapies and more accurately predict the risk and timing of treatment failure. Such assessments would be particularly valuable for patients who have the large majority of prostate cancers, those that are localized and either diploid or tetraploid. At this time, the most valuable potential markers appear to be tumor proliferation and the expression of tumor suppressor genes and oncogenes. The former can be obtained, together with DNA ploidy, by flow cytometric analysis of fresh or archival prostate tissue; the latter can be obtained from histochemical staining of adjacent sections of the same tissues.

Flow Cytometry of Archival Tissue

The introduction in 1983 of a successful method for enzymatically dissociating paraffin-embedded tissue by Hedley and coworkers[10] opened the possibility of performing retrospective flow cytometric studies on large cohorts of patients who have long-term follow-up. Hundreds of papers have been published using modifications of this method, but only a small fraction of these have employed cell cycle analysis. Hedley, reviewing 10 years of breast cancer research, notes that the impact of DNA aneuploidy on the prognosis of early breast cancer has been small.[11] The percentage of cells in the DNA synthetic portion of the cell cycle (S-phase) has, however, emerged as an important prognostic factor in axillary lymph node–negative and node-positive breast cancer. He remarks that the magnitude of the effect varies considerably between series, primarily because of technical differences in the way the tests were performed. Moreover, he notes that reliable S-phase estimates are jeopardized more by the presence of debris from sectioning archival tissue than is the detection of DNA aneuploidy. While the earlier published studies used primitive methods for calculating the percentage of cells in S-phase, the recent publication of sophisticated computer-based programs for debris correction have significantly improved the predictive power of S-phase estimates. The newer flow cytometers are usually equipped with these sophisticated computer programs.

Hedley's comments are also appropriate for studying the proliferation of prostate cancer. In addition, our experience has led us to believe that the process of dissociation and staining of archival prostate tissue requires special maneuvers to obtain DNA histograms of quality comparable to those obtained from fresh

or frozen tissue. Many reports have noted that the DNA histograms from archival tissue give broader peaks (i.e., they have larger coefficients of variation [CV]) and show more low channel debris than do fresh tissue. As far as CV is concerned, our group has not found this to be the case. Our recent study of DNA histograms from 74 archival stage T2 and T3 prostate cancers that were analyzed by the Multicycle software program gave a mean CV of the diploid G1 peak of 4.2% ± 0.8% with a range of 2.7% to 7.7%. The comparable mean CV for DNA histograms from 27 similarly analyzed fresh prostate aspirates (from BPH and diploid prostate cancers) was 5.5% ± 2.1% with a range of 2.7% to 9.9% (unpublished observations). Details of our tissue dissociation and staining technique for archival tissue have been published.[12] In general, we and others have found that using 50-μm sections results in better histogram quality than does using thinner sections. Furthermore, the enzymatic dissociation of the tissue to obtain isolated nuclei should be prolonged until the tissue flakes disappear. This may require 1½ to 2 hours of treatment at 37°C. Moreover, we have found that the use of tris/magnesium buffer for propidium iodide gives the best CVs for archival tissue as well as permitting long-term storage of fresh samples, as we had reported previously.[13] The importance of these technical details is that histograms having poor CVs may give estimates of percent S-phase which may not be entirely corrected for by the computer programs currently in use.

Computer Modeling of Debris Subtraction and Calculation of the S-Phase Fraction

The use of computer programs to model cell cycle data from flow cytometric histograms dates back more than 25 years to the studies of Dean and Jett.[14] These authors assumed that DNA histogram distributions obtained by flow cytometry of cultured cells resulted from Gaussian broadening of the theoretical distributions. They developed models for "deconvoluting" DNA histograms to obtain estimates of the fraction of cells in G0/G1, S, and G2/M (for detailed discussions, see Rabinovitch[15] and Weaver[16]). Dean and Jett presented experiments in which the fraction of cultured cells labeled with tritiated thymidine during DNA synthesis was compared to flow cytometric estimates of S-phase using their curve-fitting routines. These comparisons were in close agreement[14] and became a major impetus to using flow cytometry for cell cycle analysis. However, when archival tissue is studied there is increased debris that not only shows up at lower channels than the diploid G1 peak but also underlies the G1 and S-phase regions of the histogram and thereby causes spurious increases in the S-phase fraction.[17] Bagwell and colleagues published a method that models the shape of the debris peak of individual histograms.[18] This debris is assumed to result primarily from slicing nuclei during sectioning. In newer computer modeling programs, debris subtraction is accompanied by a nonlinear, least squares method of curve fitting to obtain the predicted cell cycle distributions. Similar methods of computer-driven debris subtraction and cell cycle analysis are employed in two of the major commercially available cell cycle programs, Modfit (Verity Software House) and Multicycle (Phoenix Flow Systems). In interinstutional comparisons, Silvestrini and associates noted that when different groups employ the same or closely similar mathematical models for histogram curve fitting, highly reproducible results for S-phase were obtained, while the use of different models gave markedly different results.[19] These factors, taken together with our observations that the composition of the propidium iodide reagent and other details of tissue preparation and staining affect histogram quality, make it necessary to determine the cutoff point between low and high S-phase fractions in individual laboratories.

It should also be recognized that, for similar reasons, definitions of DNA diploidy, tetraploidy, and aneuploidy currently differ in different laboratories. In Figures 18–1 to 18–3, we present DNA histograms obtained from nuclei isolated from formalin-fixed, paraffin-embedded prostate cancers. The DNA histograms were obtained on a Coulter Epics V flow cytometer. The two DNA histograms presented in Figure 18–1 fit our laboratory's definition of DNA diploidy. Those in Figure 18–2 are classified as tetraploid and those in Figure 18–3 as aneuploid. The Multicycle analysis of the histograms shown in these figures permits us to subclassify them as having low S-phase (Figs. 18–1A to 18–3A) or high S-phase (Figs. 18–1B through 18–3B). We believe that there is a considerable need to perform interlaboratory studies to standardize DNA flow cytometric

analysis of archival tissues to gain consensus on ploidy definitions and to elucidate what constitutes low and high S-phase fractions in prostate cancer.

Our study of localized prostate cancers treated by radical surgery, referred to above, using Kaplan-Meier estimates of mean time to failure, found that either aneuploidy or a high-percent S-phase ($\geq 4.5\%$, fourth quartile) predicted post-prostatectomy failure. In that study, this was defined as rising PSA levels, positive bone scans, or other evidence of metastatic disease, or death due to prostate cancer (manuscript in preparation). Several published flow cytometric studies have used computer modeling to obtain estimates of S-phase. Romics and coworkers found a significant correlation between abnormal ploidy, high S-phase fraction, advanced tumor stage, and less differentiated morphology in prostate cancer.[20] Tinari and colleagues analyzed factors that contribute to failure of radical prostatectomy.[21] Among patients in different risk categories (tumor T stage, Gleason score, positive or negative lymph nodes), ploidy improved the identification of patients with stage T3 or T4 disease who had poor survival. Using Cox regression analysis, these authors found that DNA ploidy was significantly related to survival. Of interest, bivariate models containing only DNA ploidy and either S-phase or Gleason score had a predictive value similar to that of including all the study variables.[21] In an interinstitutional study by van den Ouden and colleagues comprising 87 patients, most of whom had T2 or T3 prostate cancer and lymph node metastases, the percent of cells in S phase correlated significantly with time to progression.[22] Visakorpi and coworkers found that above median S-phase and DNA aneuploidy indicated shorter progression-free survival after hormone therapy.[23] Finally, a study of radiation therapy for prostate cancer[24] found that the histologic differentiation of the tumor was an independent predictor of overall and disease-free survival. Unlike the two radiation therapy studies referred to earlier,[8, 9] neither DNA ploidy nor proliferation predicted these end points for the group as a whole; however, a favorable subgroup of patients was identified for whom local control was achieved. These patients had well- or moderately well-differentiated diploid tumors with low proliferation. There was no comparably favorable subgroup among those who had poorly differentiated tumors.

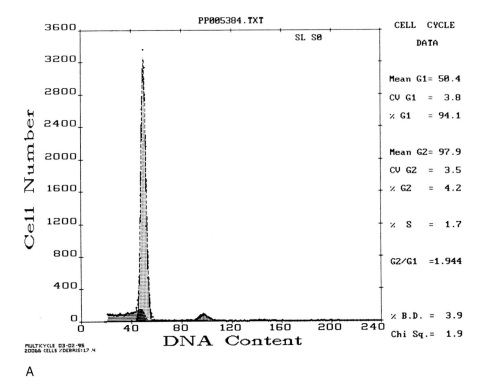

A

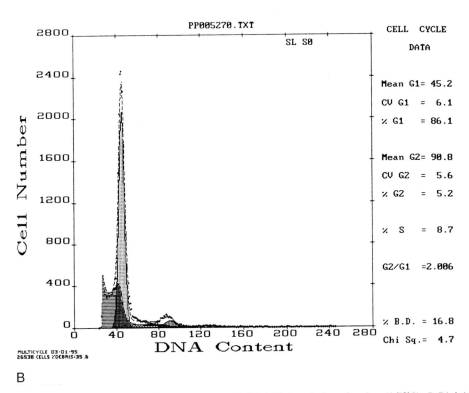

B

Figure 18–1. Histograms of DNA-diploid prostate cancers. *A*, Diploid, low–S-phase fraction (1.7%S). *B*, Diploid, high–S-phase fraction (8.7%S).

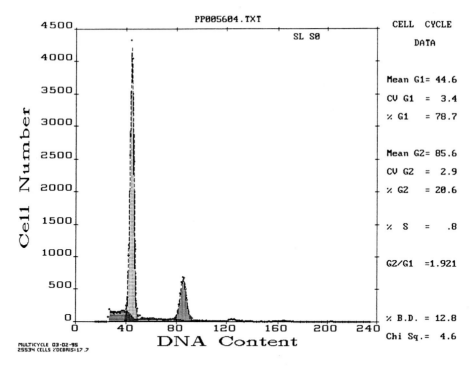

A

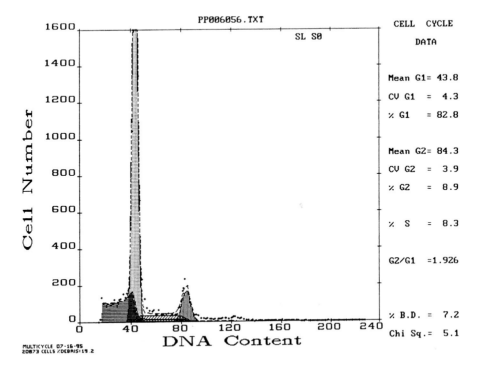

B

Figure 18–2. Histograms of tetraploid prostate cancers. *A,* Tetraploid, low–S-phase fraction (0.8%S). *B,* Tetraploid, high–S-phase fraction (8.3%S).

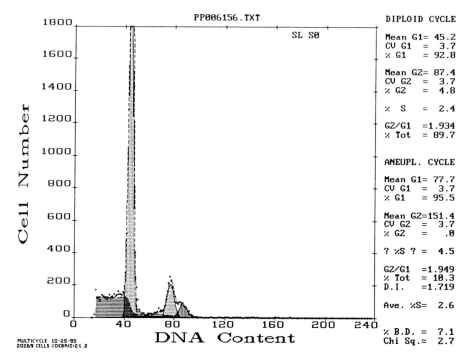

A

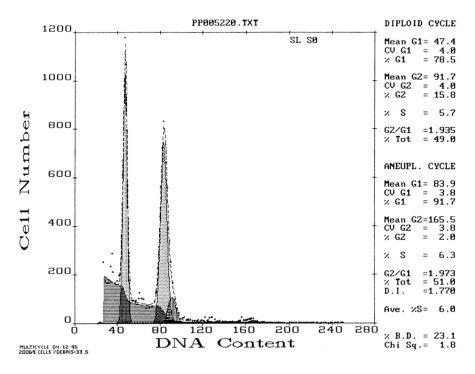

B

Figure 18–3. Histograms of aneuploid prostate cancers. *A*, Aneuploid, low–S-phase fraction (2.6% average %S). *B*, Aneuploid, high–S-phase fraction (6.0% average %S).

It appears from this brief review of recent flow cytometric studies, which include S-phase analysis of archival tissue, that a combination of factors, including ploidy, proliferation, and histologic differentiation, may improve the characterization of the malignant potential of prostate cancers. It seems unlikely, however, that this combination of tumor features will be sufficiently predictive of outcome for individual patients. Furthermore, little information is available in the studies cited that would allow clinicians to choose the appropriate therapy for localized prostate cancer. For these reasons, we are currently exploring additional markers that may be especially useful in predicting response to radiation therapy.

Immunohistochemical Analysis of the Tumor Suppressor Gene *p53* and the *bcl-2* Oncogene

The wild-type *p53* tumor suppressor gene product (p53) has been shown to arrest cells in G1 or induce apoptosis (programmed cell death) after genotoxic damage. A recent review is presented in Chang.[25] Cell-cycle arrest in G1 permits time for DNA repair, whereas apoptosis eliminates cells that are damaged beyond repair. These mechanisms are responsible for the tumor suppressor activity of the *p53* gene, which is the gene most commonly mutated in many types of cancer.[26–28] The most frequent genetic changes are point mutations leading to amino acid substitutions in *p53* exons 5 through 8. The most common result of such missense mutations is the production of nonfunctional p53 protein. Cells having such *p53* mutations are genetically unstable and will develop further mutations, leading to tumor progression. Many clinical studies have reported that the presence of mutated *p53* in various types of tumors is an independent predictor of unfavorable prognosis.[25]

Wild-type p53 has a short half-life and is normally expressed at low levels in G0/G1 cells. Exposure to x-rays or other ionizing radiation leads to transient cell cycle arrest in G1 that is accompanied by an increase in expression of wild-type p53.[28, 29] In contrast to these cell cycle–related changes, most *p53* missense mutations result in marked cell cycle–independent increases in p53 levels that can be detected by immunohistochemical staining. It is widely recognized, however, that immunohistochemical detection of p53 protein does

not necessarily indicate that *p53* is mutated.[30] Details of the immunohistochemical protocol, such as the choice of the primary antibody and its concentration, as well as whether an epitope-unmasking procedure has been employed, markedly influence the sensitivity of p53 detection in archival clinical samples.[30, 31] Furthermore, the type of *p53* mutation also affects whether the mutant form is immunopositive. For lung cancer, 16 of 17 cell lines (94%) having missense mutations in *p53* exons 5 through 8 were immunopositive (i.e., they expressed p53 at high levels) while cell lines having deletions, splicing errors, nonsense mutations, or mutations outside of exons 5 through 8 either had low staining intensity or were immunonegative.[32] While the prognostic value of *p53* is well-established for a number of cancers, its importance in prostate cancer is problematic, since the frequency of *p53* mutations in localized prostate cancer reported in different studies ranges from 6% to 50%.[33–37] Several of these reports have found only wild-type *p53* in benign prostatic hyperplasia (BPH), whereas our group has found *p53* mutations to be common in both BPH and localized prostate cancer.[37, 38] Since reports on the frequency of p53 immunopositivity in prostate cancer have also shown a wide range of positivity (from 6% to 79%) and since several different immunohistochemical protocols were employed in those studies, we attempted to resolve these discrepancies by evaluating four commercially available p53 antibodies by testing them on a panel of cell lines and patient samples for which our group had already determined the *p53* status by molecular genetic analysis.[39] The mutational status of these samples was characterized by single-strand conformational polymorphism (SSCP) analysis of *p53* messenger RNA (mRNA) using reverse transcriptase polymerase chain analysis (RT-PCR) and DNA sequencing.[37, 38] We first optimized staining conditions to get the best possible accord between the molecular genetic *p53* status of the samples and their staining with each antibody. We used sections of two formalin-fixed, paraffin-embedded prostate cancer cell lines as positive and negative controls: DU-145, a cell line that is heterozygous for two *p53* missense mutations in exons 5 and 6, and LNCaP, which has wild-type *p53* protein. The staining of these cell lines also served to set thresholds for assaying the immunopositivity of comparably fixed and processed archival patient samples. We then investigated the p53 staining of additional kidney and prostate cancer cell lines and patient samples from BPH, localized stage T2-T4 prostate cancers, and lymph node metastases. We found the number of positively stained cells and the intensity of their staining in these samples to be markedly dependent on epitope unmasking by microwave heating. Maximal nuclear staining was achieved using a cocktail of two monoclonal antibodies, DO-1 and DO-7. This approach correctly identified all four kidney cancer cell lines and 10 of 11 patient samples that had exon 5 through 8 *p53* missense mutations (14 of 15, 93%). The remaining cell lines and patient samples that were either normal by SSCP or had mutations or deletions that were not expected to stain[32] were mainly immunonegative, with only 3 of 21 (14%) considered to be immunopositive.[39] We illustrate p53 immunopositivity in localized prostate cancer in Figure 18–4.

For the radical prostatectomy samples discussed above that were studied by DNA ploidy and S-phase analysis, approximately half were p53 immunopositive. The proportion of p53-positive cases was greater among Gleason 7 through 9 tumors than in Gleason 4 through 6 cases (61% versus 35%, $P = .034$) and in stage C as compared with stage B samples (59% vs 33%, $P = .036$, manuscript in preparation). This study currently has a mean follow-up of only 2 years, and p53 immunopositivity was not significantly associated with time to failure in Kaplan-Meier analyses. A recent p53 immunohistochemical study of prostate cancer using a different p53 antibody and having longer follow-up found that p53 positivity was significantly associated with progressive disease.[40] The 139 patients in that study had a mean follow-up of 4 years. One third experienced disease progression, usually detected as rising PSA levels. Overall, 61% had p53-positive tumors. While 85% of those with progressive disease had p53-positive tumors, so did 49% of those who did not experience disease progression. For those with p53-immunonegative tumors, 87% did not experience disease progression. The p53 status was positively associated with rising grade and stage, and in multivariate analysis it was found to be an independent predictor of disease-free survival. Nevertheless, in view of the high rate of p53 positivity in those who did not experience progressive disease, one can question the clinical utility of these observations.

A second study from this group found an increasing incidence of p53-positive tumors as prostate cancer progresses from localized to hormone-refractory metastatic disease.[41] While our methods differ, our studies agree with the latter findings. Furthermore, they are also in accord with many previously published molecular, genetic, and immunohistochemical studies of prostate cancer.[33–36, 42–46]

The *bcl-2* gene is known to oppose wild-type p53 by blocking apoptosis after genotoxic damage.[47] The *bcl-2* gene is the prototype of a newly described class of oncogenes that modu-

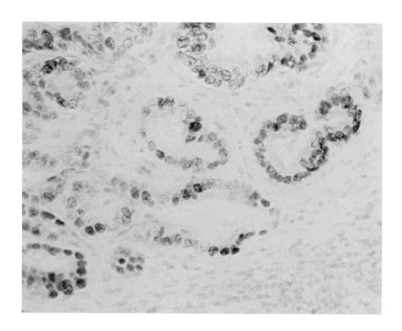

Figure 18–4. Gleason score 6 prostate cancer, p53 immunopositive ($\times$ 400).

late apoptosis.[48, 49] Furthermore, *bcl-2* functions in both *p53*-dependent and -independent pathways to programmed cell death.[50, 51] This is particularly interesting, since Bcl-2 immunopositivity has been linked to the emergence of androgen independence in metastatic prostate cancer.[52–54] While the relationship of p53 to androgen independence is currently in doubt,[50, 55] if Bcl-2 expression proves to be a major player in the development of androgen independence, it may help explain why hormone withdrawal fails to kill all prostate cancer cells.

There is general agreement that the cellular response to the genotoxicity of radiation and chemotherapy involves the *p53* pathway. We developed an immunohistochemical method for detecting high Bcl-2 expression that utilizes a commercially available anti-Bcl-2 monoclonal antibody (Clone 124, Dako) and illustrate Bcl-2 immunopositivity in prostate cancer in Figure 18–5. Immunohistochemical evidence for *p53* and Bcl-2 accumulation was examined for a group of patients who failed radiation therapy by having persistent prostate cancer 2 years after treatment. The staining of pre- and posttreatment cancers was compared to the cancers of patients who underwent radical retropubic prostatectomy without prior therapy (manuscript in preparation). While the p53 immunopositivity of the prostate cancers in the two treatment groups were similarly high, there were striking differences in Bcl-2 immunopositivity in the radiation failure group as compared with those who were treated surgi-

cally. Only approximately 10% of those treated by radical surgery had Bcl-2–positive cancers. In contrast, 40% of the pre-radiation cancers and 60% of the post-radiation cancers stained positively for bcl-2 (*P* <.0001). This high rate of immunopositivity for both p53 and Bcl-2 among the radiation failures may help explain why radiation therapy can fail to eradicate prostate cancer and why this form of cancer is also chemoresistant.

Question 2 Revisited: Can flow cytometric and immunohistochemical marker studies help manage treatment decisions for individual prostate cancer patients?

While it is undoubtedly true that the definitive answer to this question will require study of larger cohorts of patients, some progress has already been made. Immunopositivity for Bcl-2 and p53 together with aneuploidy help to define groups of patients with localized prostate cancers who are not good candidates for radiation therapy. Rapidly proliferating diploid cancers may be a subset of localized prostate cancers that radical prostatectomy is destined to fail. At present, the most stringent criteria we could adopt for selecting patients for active surveillance is that the Gleason score should be less than 7, the PSA level low, and the tumor diploid with low proliferation. Furthermore, since mutant *p53* is known to induce genetic instability, it would be preferable

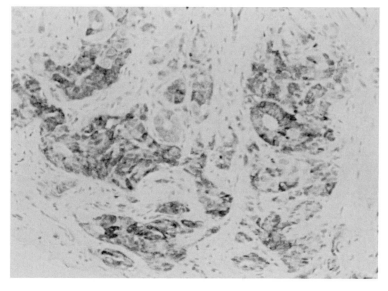

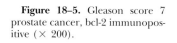

Figure 18–5. Gleason score 7 prostate cancer, bcl-2 immunopositive (× 200).

that cancers selected for surveillance should be p53-immunonegative as well. It is obvious that much remains to be learned. We hope, however, that this review will serve to point the way toward answering some of these questions.

Acknowledgments

Supported in part by PHS grant PO1-CA55792 awarded by the National Cancer Institute, DHHS and by the Robert J. Mathews Foundation for Prostate Cancer Research.
The authors thank Jennine Lunetta, Ingrid Wertz and Salvador Toscaro for their careful reading of this review and for their helpful suggestions.

REFERENCES

1. Wingo PA, Tong T, Bolden S: Cancer statistics, 1995. CA: Cancer J Clin 45:8–30, 1995.
2. Aus G: Prostate cancer. Mortality and morbidity after non-curative treatment with aspects on diagnosis and treatment. Scand J Urol Nephrol (Suppl) 167:1–41, 1994.
3. Tavares AS, Costa J, de Carvalho A, et al.: Tumor ploidy and prognosis in carcinomas of the bladder and prostate. Br J Cancer 20:438–441, 1966.
4. Tribukait B: Nuclear deoxyribonucleic acid determination in patients with prostate carcinomas: Clinical research and application. Eur Urol 23 (Suppl 2): 64–76, 1993.
5. Lieber MM: Prognostic importance of nuclear DNA content as measured by flow cytometry for patients with adenocarcinoma of the prostate. Urol Int 47 (Suppl 1):74–76, 1991.
6. Schröder F, Tribukait B, Böcking A, et al.: Clinical utility of cellular DNA measurements in prostate carcinoma. Consensus conference on diagnosis and prognostic parameters in localized prostate cancer. Scand J Urol Nephrol (Suppl) 162:51–63, 1994; discussion 15–27.
7. Deitch AD, deVere White RW: Flow cytometry as a predictive modality in prostate cancer. Hum Pathol 23:352–359, 1992.
8. Song J, Cheng WS, Cupps RE, et al.: Nuclear deoxyribonucleic acid content measured by static cytometry: important prognostic association for patients with clinically localized prostate carcinoma treated by external beam radiotherapy. J Urol 147:794–797, 1992.
9. Pollack A, Zagars GK, El-Naggar AK, et al.: Near-diploidy: a new prognostic factor for clinically localized prostate cancer treated with external beam radiation therapy. Cancer 73:1895–1903, 1994.
10. Hedley DW, Friedlander ML, Taylor IW, et al: Methods for analysis of cellular DNA content of paraffin-embedded pathological material using flow cytometry. J Histochem Cytochem 31:1333–1335, 1983.
11. Hedley DW: DNA Cytometry Consensus Conference. DNA flow cytometry and breast cancer. Breast Cancer Res Treat 28:51–53, 1993.
12. Deitch AD, Miller GJ, deVere White RW: Significance of abnormal diploid DNA histograms in localized prostate cancer and adjacent benign prostatic tissue. Cancer 72:1692–1700, 1993.
13. Deitch AD, Law H, deVere White R: A stable propidium iodide staining procedure for flow cytometry. J Histochem Cytochem 30:967–972, 1982.
14. Dean PN, Jett JH: Mathematical analysis of DNA distributions derived from flow microfluorometry. J Cell Biol 60:523–527, 1974.
15. Rabinovitch PS: DNA content histogram and cell cycle analysis. Methods Cell Biol 41:263–296, 1994.
16. Weaver DL, Bagwell CB, Hitchcox SA, et al: Improved flow cytometric determination of proliferative activity (S-phase fraction) from paraffin-embedded tissue. Am J Clin Pathol 94:576–584, 1990.
17. Kallioniemi O-P: Comparison of fresh and paraffin-embedded tissue as starting material for DNA flow cytometry and evaluation of intratumor heterogeneity. Cytometry 9:164–169, 1988.
18. Bagwell CB, Mayo SW, Whetstone SD, et al.: DNA histogram debris theory and compensation. Cytometry 12:107–118, 1991.
19. Silvestrini R and the SICCAB Group for Quality Control of Cell Kinetic Determinations: Quality control for evaluation of the S-phase fraction by flow cytometry. A multicentric study. Cytometry (Communications in Clinical Cytometry) 18:11–16, 1994.
20. Romics I, Boesi J, Bach D, et al: DNA content of prostatic cancer measured by flow cytometry in patients undergoing radical prostatectomy. Anticancer Res 15:1131–1134, 1995.
21. Tinari N, Natoli C, Angelucci D, et al.: DNA and S-phase analysis by flow cytometry in prostate cancer. Clinicopathologic implications. Cancer 71:1289–1296, 1993.
22. van den Ouden D, Tribukait B, Blom JHM, et al.: Deoxyribonucleic acid ploidy of core biopsies and metastatic lymph nodes of cancer patients: impact on time to progression. J Urol 150:400–406, 1993.
23. Visakorpi T, Kallioniemi O-P, Paronen IYI, et al.: Flow cytometric analysis of DNA ploidy and S-phase fraction from prostatic carcinomas: Implications for prognosis and response to endocrine therapy. Br J Cancer 64:578–582, 1991.
24. Centeno BA, Zietman AL, Shipley WU, et al.: Flow cytometric analysis of DNA ploidy, percent S-phase fraction and total proliferative fraction as prognostic indicators of local control and survival following radiation therapy for prostate carcinoma. Int J Radiat Oncol Biol Physics 30:309–315, 1994.
25. Chang F, Syrjänen S, Syrjänen K: Implications of the p53 tumor-suppressor gene in clinical oncology. J Clin Oncol 13:1009–1022, 1995.
26. Hollstein M, Sidransky D, Vogelstein B, et al.: P53 mutations in human cancer. Science 253:49–53, 1991.
27. Levine AJ, Momand J, Finlay CA: The p53 tumor suppressor gene. Nature 351:453–456, 1991.
28. Kastan MB, Onyekwere O, Sidransky D, et al.: Participation of p53 protein in the cellular response to DNA damage. Cancer Res 51:6304–6311, 1991.
29. Kuerbitz SJ, Plunkett BS, Walsh WV, et al.: Wild-type p53 is a cell cycle checkpoint determinant following irradiation. Proc Natl Acad Sci USA 89:7491–7495, 1992.
30. Hall PA, Lane DP: P53 in tumor pathology: Can we trust immunohistochemistry?—Revisited! J Pathol 172:1–4, 1994.
31. Baas IO, Mulder J-WR, Offerhaus GJA, et al.: An evaluation of six antibodies for immunohistochemistry of

mutant p53 gene product in archival colorectal neoplasms. J Pathol 172:5–12, 1994.

32. Bodner SM, Minna JD, Jensen SM, et al.: Expression of mutant p53 proteins in lung cancer correlates with the class of p53 mutation. Oncogene 7:743–749, 1992.

33. Voeller JH, Sugars LY, Pretlow T, et al. p53 Oncogene mutations in human prostate cancer specimens. J Urol 151:492–495, 1994.

34. Navone NM, Tronsoso P, Pisters LL, et al.: P53 Protein accumulation and gene mutation in the progression of human prostate carcinoma. J Natl Cancer Inst 85:1657–1669, 1993.

35. Bookstein R, MacGrogan D, Hilsenbeck SG, et al.: P53 is mutated in a subset of advanced-stage prostate cancers. Cancer Res 43:3369–3373, 1993.

36. Visakorpi T, Kallioniemi O-P, Heikkinen A, et al.: Small subgroup of aggressive, highly proliferative prostatic carcinomas defined by p53 accumulation. J Natl Cancer Inst 84:883–887, 1992.

37. Chi S-G, deVere White RW, Meyers FJ, et al.: P53 in prostate cancer: Frequent expressed transition mutations. J Natl Cancer Inst 86:926–933, 1994.

38. Meyers FJ, Chi S-G, Fishman JR, et al.: p53 mutations in benign prostatic hyperplasia. J Natl Cancer Inst 85:1856, 1993.

39. Wertz IE, Deitch AD, Gumerlock PH, et al.: Correlation of genetic and immuno-detection of TP53 mutations in malignant and benign prostate tissue. Hum Pathol 27:573–580, 1996.

40. Bauer JJ, Sesterhenn IA, Mostofi KF, et al.: p53 nuclear protein expression is an independent prognostic marker in clinically localized prostate cancer patients undergoing radical prostatectomy. Clin Cancer Res 1:1295–1300, 1995.

41. Heidenberg HB, Sesterhenn IA, Gaddipati JP, et al.: Alterations of the tumor suppressor gene p53 in a high fraction of hormone refractory prostate cancer. J Urol 154:414–421, 1995.

42. Aprikian AG, Sarkis AS, Fair WR, et al.: Immunohistochemical determination of p53 protein nuclear accumulation in prostatic adenocarcinoma. J Urol 151:1276–1280, 1994.

43. Hall MC, Navone NM, Troncoso P, et al.: Frequency and characterization of p53 mutations in clinically localized prostate cancer. Urology 45:470–475, 1995.

44. Shurbaji MS, Kalbfleisch JH, Thurmond TS: Immunohistochemical detection of p53 protein as a prognostic indicator in prostate cancer. Hum Pathol 26:106–109, 1995.

45. Grizzle WE, Myers RB, Arnold MM, Evaluation of biomarkers in breast and prostate cancer. J Cell Biochem (Suppl) 19:259–266, 1994.

46. Thomas DJ, Robinson M, King P, et al.: P53 expression and clinical outcome in prostate cancer. Br J Urol 72:778–781, 1993.

47. Stewart BW: Mechanisms of apoptosis: integration of genetic, biochemical and cellular indicators. J Natl Cancer Inst 86:1286–1296, 1994.

48. Korsmeyer SJ: Bcl-2 initiates a new category of oncogenes: Regulators of cell death. Blood 80:879–886, 1992.

49. Reed JC: Bcl-2 and the regulation of programmed cell death. J Cell Biol 124:1–6, 1994.

50. Berges RR, Furuya Y, Remington L, et al.: Cell proliferation, DNA repair and p53 function are not required for programmed cell death of prostatic glandular cells induced by androgen ablation. Proc Natl Acad Sci USA 90:8910–8914, 1993.

51. Planchon SM, Wuerzberger S, Frydman B, et al.: β lapachone-mediated apoptosis in human promyelocytic leukemia (HL-60) and human prostate cancer cells: A p53-independent response. Cancer Res 55:3706–3711, 1995.

52. McDonnell TJ, Troncoso P, Brisbay SM, et al.: Expression of the protooncogene bcl-2 in the prostate and its association with emergence of androen-independent prostate cancer. Cancer Res 52:6940–6944, 1992.

53. Colombel M, Symmans F, Gil S, et al.: Detection of the apoptosis-suppressing oncoprotein bcl-2 in hormone-refractory human prostate cancers. Am J Pathol 143:390–400, 1993.

54. Raffo AJ, Perlman H, Chen M-W, et al.: Overexpression of bcl-2 protects prostate cancer cells from apoptosis in vitro and confers resistance to androgen depletion in vivo. Cancer Res 55:4438–4445, 1995.

55. Colombel M, Olsson CA, Ng P-Y, et al.: Hormone-regulated apoptosis results from reentry of differentiated prostate cells onto a defective cell cycle. Cancer Res 52:4313–4319, 1992.

19

MAGNETIC RESONANCE IMAGING OF PROSTATE CARCINOMA

VICTOR WALUCH

Prostate carcinoma is the most common cancer of men in the United States. It is found more frequently in blacks than in Caucasians and less often in Asians.[1, 2] It is the most common cancer of men older than 50 years: a male has about 1 chance in 6 of developing prostate carcinoma within his lifetime. For 1995, it is estimated there will have been 244,000 new cases and more than 40,000 deaths in the United States.[3] The disease, it seems, is also on the rise in the United States and throughout Europe, in part because of the aging male population and in part because of greater use of prostate-specific antigen (PSA) in clinical screening.

Given the alarming nature of the problem, every advanced imaging modality has been thrown into the fray, from computed tomography (CT) to transrectal ultrasound, and, for the past 12 years, to magnetic resonance imaging (MRI). All modalities have enjoyed a modicum of success. Ultrasonography/CT have reached their asymptote in technical development. The book on their usefulness in this disease is nearly closed. MRI, on the other hand, is still undergoing major technical developments, and its future is promising.

RATIONALE

Advanced imaging modalities have little role in mass screening for prostate carcinoma.

They are much too involved and much too expensive. This bailiwick is currently reserved for serum PSA, clinical digital rectal examination, and transrectal ultrasonography (TRUS) together with fine-needle aspiration biopsy, in that order. Once a high level of suspicion is aroused, the existence of the disease may be established by one of these imaging modalities or a combination. When the presence of the disease is established and confirmed by histopathologic examination, a consideration of treatment options requires knowledge of the histology and stage of the disease. The usefulness of imaging modalities is measured by their ability to contribute information to these latter considerations.

TREATMENT CONSIDERATIONS

The treatment options depend much on the clinical stage of the disease—A, B, C, or D (modified Jewitt-Whitmore). In stages A and B, where the cancer is confined to the gland, cure may be attempted through radical prostatectomy. In stage C, when the disease has perforated the capsule, excision may not be warranted, and local control may be attempted with radiation. Distal metastatic disease is often treated by hormone manipulation. The role of MRI, or any imaging modality for that matter, is to improve the accuracy of clinical staging so that appropriate therapy may be

341

instituted. To date, MRI's major clinically useful contribution has been to sort patients into stage B and stage C, as will be discussed. MRI is not reliable in detecting stage A disease and shares the spotlight with plain film x-ray, CT, and nuclear medicine methods in detecting distal metastases.

Although treatment based on this classification is commonly accepted and practiced, some consider it too simplistic. Many believe that therapy should be guided by expected outcomes. For example, a patient with stage B disease whose life expectancy is less than 15 years may simply be treated with radiation therapy and avoid the risks of surgical morbidity.[4] Similarly, patients with microinvasion of the capsule, though technically their disease is stage C, may be better served if it is treated as stage B.

In this review, the current techniques of performing MRI examination of the prostate are presented and the appearance of the normal gland and the features of prostate carcinoma as seen on MRI are discussed. In addition, recent advances in MRI technology will be presented that have already made MRI the examination of choice in the staging of this disease.

TECHNICAL CONSIDERATIONS

Technical advances in MRI have managed to remain several steps ahead of the most recent clinical evaluations of this modality in the imaging of prostate carcinoma. In the mid 1980s, the large whole-body MRI coil was used in an attempt to image this disease. It provided a large field of view (30 to 40 cm) of the pelvis, allowing detection of enlarged lymph nodes, but the images of the prostate were grainy and the resolution was poor. In a typical clinical setting, fine details of the prostate were poorly resolved and staging accuracies were in the range of 50%.[5]

In an effort to overcome the poor image characteristics offered by body coils, researchers turned to endorectal surface coils, which were first used clinically in 1989.[6] These coils are small (3- to 4-cm diameter) and are introduced into the rectum by means of a probe and held there against the dorsal surface of the prostate by balloon. The advantage of these coils is that the signal strength received is much increased, owing to the proximity of the prostate to the coil, and the noise much

decreased, owing to the limited field of view of the coil. This increased wealth of signal permits imaging matrices to be increased to 512 by 512 and slice thickness to less than 3 mm. The primary disadvantage of these coils is that the coil cannot "see" much beyond its diameter, so the central and more ventral zones of the prostate are poorly visualized. Furthermore, the more proximal portion of the prostate and periprostatic and perirectal fat are seen too well, often saturating the image and obscuring details. Nevertheless, compared to the body coil, staging accuracies improved to values as high as 68%.[7, 8] More importantly, the increased resolution allowed for the first time accurate assessment of the seminal vesicles. Accuracy of 91% for seminal vesicles involvement was reported by Chelsky and coworkers.[7]

In part to overcome these deficiencies of the endorectal coil and to enable the examination of the entire pelvis in the same session while maintaining good signal-to-noise ratio, endorectal coils were teamed with phased-array coils. Phased-array technology uses a number of small surface coils (usually four) that have their own electronic data paths through the MRI system, and each produces a separate image simultaneously. These images are then added to form a summed image. This final summed image has a signal-to-noise ratio greater than that of a single coil and at the same time has a field of view of the ensemble, which, if positioned judiciously around the pelvis, can image the entire pelvis in much the same manner as a body coil but with much better resolution. Resolutions of 0.4 mm can readily be obtained.[9]

More recently, this technology was advanced further. Each coil of the phased-array set was replaced by a quadrature arrangement (Siemens, Erlangen, Germany). This configuration further improved the signal-to-noise ratio. The early practitioners found enough improvement in signal-to-noise ratio that the endorectal coil portion of the array could be omitted with no loss of image quality or information.[10] Not only did this permit a high-resolution examination of the prostate and the entire pelvis, but, by eliminating the rectal probe, it reduced the discomfort to the patient, leading to fewer motion artifacts and more successful imaging.

Concurrent progress was made in radiofrequency pulse sequence design. The imaging sequences employed advanced from routine T1- and T2-weighted spin echo to fast spin echo (FSE), with and without fat suppression. These latter techniques increased the dynamic range of the images and allowed for significantly (8 to 16 times) shorter imaging times, which allowed not only time for additional averaging of signals to improve the signal-to-noise ratio but also permitted the obtaining of additional projections necessary for accurate diagnosis.

TECHNIQUE

MRI of the prostate as discussed here can be performed practically only on high–field strength systems; that is, 1.0 T, and preferably 1.5 T. Keeping all else constant, "signal to noise" varies at least linearly with field strength. At 1.5 T, one has 50% more signal to noise than at 1.0 T, and three times as much as at 0.5 T. These numbers are significant. The minimal coil requirement is an endorectal coil which enables the examination of the dorsal aspect of the prostate and immediate periprostatic tissues. A thorough clinical imaging examination generally includes evaluation of the entire pelvis, so that in this scheme the rectal coil would be removed and the examination concluded with a body coil. The use of rectal phased-array or quadrature phased-array coils allows simultaneous examination of the prostate and pelvis, since the pulsing sequences used for prostate imaging are generally the same as those used for pelvic imaging (Figs. 19–1, 19–2). Any additional pelvic sequences or projections may be carried out without the interruption and time penalty of changing coils. This latter approach can bring imaging time down to a clinically acceptable half hour or less.

A typical set of pulsing sequences for prostate carcinoma detection includes a fast spin echo T2-weighted sequence employing repetition times of 3500 to 5000 msec with echo times on the order of 100 msec, and T1-weighted images with repetition times of 350 to 500 msec with short echo times of 10 to 20 msec. Fields of view for the endorectal coil–only configuration vary 10 to 15 cm for a 256 by 256 matrix. If available, fat suppression may be included. For the phased-array configuration, the field of view may be relaxed to 15 to 25 cm (depending on patient size) and the matrix is increased to 512 by 512. Slice thickness should be less than 5 mm; 3 mm commonly is used. The "axial" plane of the slice is usually taken perpendicular to the fat-prostate

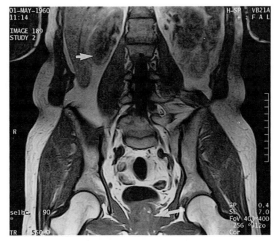

Figure 19–1. Coronal, pelvis, T1-weighted (TR/TE = 550/12 msec). A large–field of view image (40 cm) of the entire pelvis with millimeter resolution can be obtained using a quadrature phased-array coil arrangement wrapped around the patient. The nodal chains can be evaluated to the renal level. Prostate (*long arrow*), kidneys (*short arrow*).

interface posteriorly, and the "coronal" plane is taken parallel to this interface. "Sagittal" planes may be taken parallel to the plane of the seminal vesicles or the neurovascular bundle locus.

CHARACTERISTICS

MRI may properly be called "hydrogen imaging," most of the hydrogen residing in

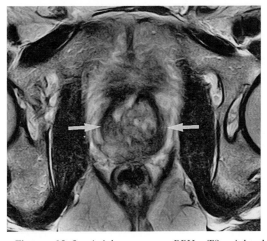

Figure 19–2. Axial, prostate BPH, T2-weighted (TR/TE = 4500/119 msec). The same patient and same coil arrangement as shown in Figure 19–1. By decreasing the field of view to 15 cm, a submillimeter resolution image of the prostate is readily obtained. The prostate (*arrows*) is filled with BPH nodules that obliterate the peripheral zone (PZ).

water and lipids and less in proteins. In the prostate the characteristic histologic feature that gives rise to the MR signal is the secretory product mucus, which traps water. Of the prostatic zones described by McNeal (see Chapter 2), the glandular lumina and ductal structures of the peripheral zone (PZ) of the prostate contain disproportionate shares of mucus; thus they are imaged as high intensity on T2-weighted images (long TR/TE). The periurethral, transitional, and central zones do not differ enough in their water content to be distinguishable by current pulse sequences, and for practical purposes are collectively called the "central gland." On T2-weighted images, this central gland has intermediate signal intensity that is much less than that of the peripheral zone. The two regions have lower intensity on T1-weighted images, although the peripheral zone usually remains somewhat brighter than the central gland. When the central gland becomes involved by benign prostatic hyperplasia (BPH), the signals on T1- (and especially on T2-) weighted images become very heterogeneous, containing areas of both high and low signal intensity (Figs. 19–2 through 19–6). Prostate carcinoma, as a rule, is characterized by high cell density at the expense of extracellular space and lumen mucus. This results in less local water, and, conse-

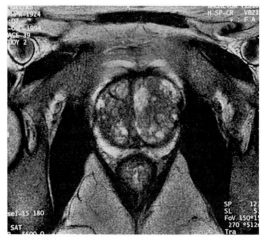

Figure 19–4. Axial, BPH, T2-weighted (TR/TE = 5600/ 119 msec). The two lobes of the prostate contain the heterogeneous signal intensities of BPH. A carcinoma here would be indistinguishable from BPH nodules.

quently, the MRI features of the carcinoma tend to be of low intensity as compared with normal prostate tissue on long TR/TE sequences (Fig. 19–7). That high tissue density correlates with low intensity was recently shown by Quint and coworkers.[11] They demonstrated that fibromuscular hyperplasia and prostate carcinoma have increased optical den-

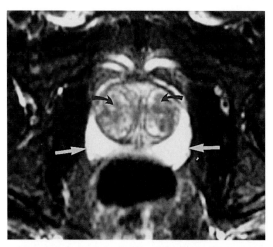

Figure 19–3. Axial, BPH, T2-weighted (TR/TE = 6000/ 120 msec). On heavily T2-weighted images, the peripheral zone of the prostate becomes very high intensity, reflecting the high water content (*white arrows*). The central gland is replaced by two large BPH nodules (*curved arrows*) that contain mixed intensities; the high-intensity signals correspond to areas containing mucus and the low intensity to areas of increased cellular density, scars, and so forth.

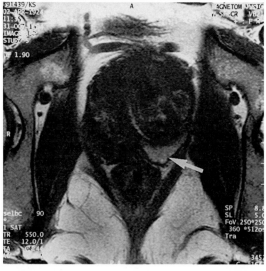

Figure 19–5. Axial, prostate BPH, T1-weighted (TR/TE = 550/12 msec). Most of the central gland has been replaced by BPH, which has low intensity on T1-weighted images, although several high-intensity foci, probably representing mucin collections, are present. The right-hand aspect of the PZ has been effaced; a portion of the left aspect persists (*arrow*).

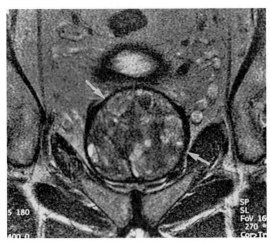

Figure 19–6. Coronal, prostate, BPH, T2-weighted (TR/TE = 4400/119 msec). The prostate is nearly completely replaced by BPH. A carcinoma located here would be difficult to distinguish from BPH nodules. Note the excellent depiction of the prostate capsule (*white arrows*). Its thickness includes subcapsular compressed tissue.

sity. There are exceptions, of course. The so-called signet ring carcinoma that produces copious mucus images with high intensity, and the diffusely infiltrating low-grade carcinoma may not produce enough local density changes and thus go undetected by MRI. Thus, the typical carcinoma located in the peripheral zone would appear as an area of diminished signal as contrasted to the very high signal intensity of the zone. In the central gland, the

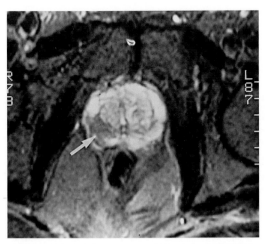

Figure 19–7. Axial, carcinoma, T2-weighted (TR/TE = 4000/20 msec). A small carcinoma near the apex occupying the right PZ (*arrow*) is of low intensity and is easily seen against the high intensity PZ, which is unusually large in this area and blends in with the prostatic venous plexus anteriorly.

contrast between the low-intensity carcinoma and the gland is decreased and the carcinoma is less conspicuous. If the central gland contained modules of BPH, then the conspicuity would be further reduced. Sommer and colleagues reported that carcinomas in the central gland are easily missed.[12]

All low-intensity foci in the prostate do not represent carcinoma. Other prostatic processes that are of low MR intensity and can simulate prostate carcinoma include scars, prostatitis, granulomatous diseases, and calculi. Blood, even when encountered after remote biopsy, can also mimic carcinoma. It is thought that the presence of citrate in prostatic tissues delays coagulation of the blood, keeping the hemoglobin in various states of oxidation and yielding heterogeneous signal intensities.[13, 14]

VOLUMETRIC CONSIDERATIONS

It is well-known that prostate tumor size is a predictor of histologic grade and stage. An accurate assessment of tumor size can play an important role in planning treatment and establishing a prognosis. Sommer and coworkers measured the volume of 20 biopsy-proven prostate cancers using phased-array coils and fat suppression fast spin echo techniques.[12] The sizes of the 17 MRI-detected tumors correlated reasonably with the sizes of the surgical specimens ($r = 0.81$; $P < .001$); however, there was difficulty in establishing the boundaries of tumors in the central gland, where they are obscured, and in misinterpreting as carcinoma benign low–signal intensity processes in the peripheral zone. Kahn and associates, using older MRI technology, reported a mean of 40% underestimation of tumor volume in 43% of their patients, and no tumor size was overestimated.[15] Histologic grade was not taken into account.

EXTRAPROSTATIC SPREAD

The anatomic capsule of the prostate is a thin, fibromuscular layer recognizable as a low-intensity band encircling the prostate. It is usually resolvable by MRI using advanced coils, although if thick imaging sections are used (greater than 3 mm) it may be poorly visualized owing to partial volume averaging, which is most severe at the apex. If signal averaging

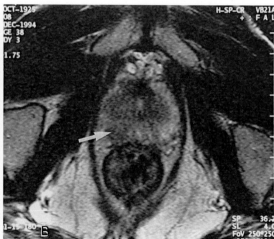

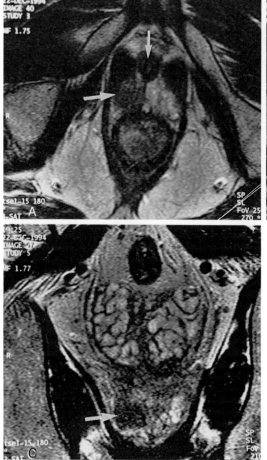

Figure 19–8. Axial (*A* and *B*), coronal (*C*) carcinoma (TR/TE = 5250/120 msec). A small carcinoma (*long arrow*) occupying the right half of the prostate at the apex and bulging outward. *A*, Only the preurethral area (*short arrow*) of the normal prostate is visible. *B*, The carcinoma infiltrates the upper portions of the PZ (*arrow*). *C*, Note the poor visualization of the capsule.

is inadequate so that the images appear grainy, the capsule may be obscured (Fig. 19–8). Gross violation of the capsule by carcinoma with tumors invading the periprostatic fat is readily detected. Less extensive capsular involvement is more problematic for MRI. Small, local, irregular bulging of the capsule may represent capsular invasion or be a consequence of mass effect produced by adjacent but strictly intracapsular tumor.[7, 8] Microinvasion of the capsule cannot be resolved by current MRI techniques (Fig. 19–9). Studies employing gadolinium enhancement showed no improvement in capsule evaluation over routine nonenhanced T2-weighted sequences.[16]

SEMINAL VESICLES

MRI is the only modality that can provide good images of the seminal vesicles. On T2-weighted images the seminal vesicles have a honeycomb appearance, the fluid having high intensity and the stroma low intensity (Figs. 19–10, 19–11). Invasion of the vesicles can occur by transcapsular spread, involvement by contiguity, direct extension along the ejaculatory duct, extension along the neurovascular bundle, or skip metastases.[17] Gross invasion is manifested by architectural disruption and is readily imaged by MRI as regions of low intensity (relative to the fluid; Figs. 19–12, 19–13). Peritubular stromal thickening, though difficult to appreciate, can be an early sign of involvement.[18, 19] Although gadolinium enhancement has been reported to aid in this diagnosis, the results have been mixed.[8, 16] In the aged prostate, with its decreased volume of seminal vesicle fluid, a small carcinoma is more difficult to detect; however, side-to-side comparison of the vesicles may aid in the evaluation. In addition, imaging planes taken parallel to each vesicle aid in the comparison.

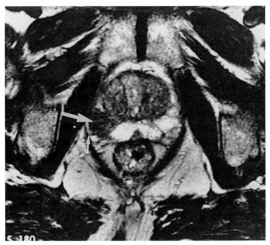

Figure 19–9. Axial, carcinoma, T2-weighted (TR/TE = 5250/119 msec). Large PZ carcinoma (*large arrow*) extends to the capsule. The jagged irregularity of the capsule (*small arrow*) suggests invasion and extension through the capsule. In the surgical specimen the capsule was found to be intact.

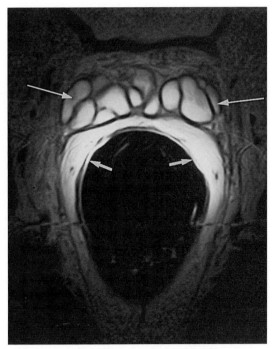

Figure 19–10. Axial, seminal vesicles, endorectal coil, T2-weighted (TR/TE = 5000/119 msec). Highly detailed images of the seminal vesicles (*arrows*) may be obtained with an endorectal coil. The seminal vesicle fluid images with high intensity, whereas the stroma remains dark. Note the high intensity prerectal fact (*small arrows*). Beyond its diameter the coil does not image well, so the prostate located anteriorly to the vesicles would be poorly imaged.

Vesicular disruptions of other causes can mimic carcinoma. False-positive readings may result from protrusion of BPH nodules into the vesicular area, radiation therapy, amyloid deposits, and occasionally calculi.[9]

RESULTS

At this time, an accurate assessment of MRI's ability to detect and stage prostate carcinoma is difficult. Several reported studies are lacking in statistics and can be considered demonstrational or anecdotal at best. Others, though published only recently, are already outdated owing to significant advances in hardware and pulse sequence techniques. The results of other studies suffer from errors introduced by pathologists using random sectioning of the prostate instead of whole-mount sectioning techniques, which would yield some 20% more stage C malignancies.[8, 20] In addition, in an effort to obtain pathologic correla-

tion (i.e., prostatectomy specimens) many of the studies are biased toward minimal (and therefore more subtle) disease, which would underestimate the staging efficacy of MRI. This efficacy is further obscured by a much longer learning curve for image interpretation than is commonly assumed. The recent results of Hricak and coworkers using phased-array coils and advanced pulse sequences are probably representative of the current state of the art.[21] Several of their results of MRI-pathologic correlation are summarized in Table 19–1.

It is clear from the numbers in Table 19–1 that state-of-the-art MRI can have a direct in-

Table 19–1. Correlation of Magnetic Resonance Imaging Data with Pathologic Findings

	Sensitivity %	Specificity %	Accuracy %	Positive Predictive Value %	Negative Predictive Value %
Extraprostatic extension	84	80	81	65	92
Seminal vesicle invasion	83	98	96	77	98

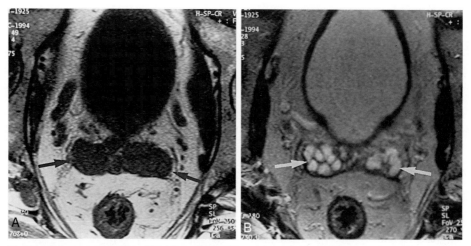

Figure 19–11. Axial, seminal vesicles, T1- (*A*) and T2- (*B*) weighted images (TR/TE = 700/12 and 5250/119 msec, respectively). On T1-weighted images (*A*), the seminal vesicle fluid appears uniformly dark with several bands of even lower-intensity stroma visible. Increasing the T2 weighting intensifies the signal of the fluid. *B*, Note the increased field of view obtained with phased-array coils as compared with the endorectal coil in Figure 19–10.

fluence on current decision making in the clinical management of prostate carcinoma. The negative predictive value of extracapsular and seminal vesicle extension (i.e., that the capsule and vesicles are *not* involved) is reasonably high and should reliably predict which patients may benefit from prostatectomy. Al-

though the positive predictive values are relatively low, targeting staging biopsies by means of endorectal ultrasound may be used when this will make a difference between surgical and other types of management.

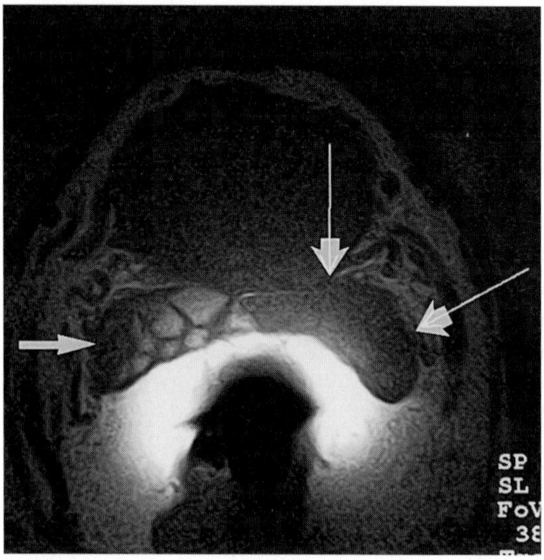

MAGNETIC RESONANCE SPECTROSCOPIC IMAGING (MRSI)

Serum PSA is now commonly used for screening for prostate carcinoma. Levels above 4 mg/ml indicate that something is amiss with the prostate; however, some 20% of patients with clinically localized cancers demonstrate normal PSA levels. In addition, PSA levels may be elevated when no cancer is present.[22, 23] It has been estimated that some two of three patients who undergo biopsy for elevated PSA have negative results.[24] Thus, an elevated PSA value usually leads to other studies.

As discussed above, MRI can contribute much to the localization and staging of this disease, but it is not without its shortcomings. It has difficulty detecting small tumors, is unreliable in detecting even large tumors in the central gland, and cannot consistently yield a reliable estimate of tumor volume.

In vitro spectroscopic methods have long shown that there are significant metabolite differences between prostate cancer, normal tissues, and BPH. Concentrations of many of the phosphorylated compounds—phosphocreatine (PCr), phosphomonoesters (PME),

Figure 19–12. Axial, seminal vesicle carcinoma, T1-weighted (TR/TE = 575/15 msec), endorectal coil. The left seminal vesicle is completely engulfed by carcinoma (*arrowheads*) replacing the high signal of the vesicle fluid by low intensity. Note the peculiar artifact of surface coil field-of-view falloff. The outer aspect of the right vesicle, being beyond the sensitive area of the coil, images as low intensity, simulating a carcinoma (*arrow*).

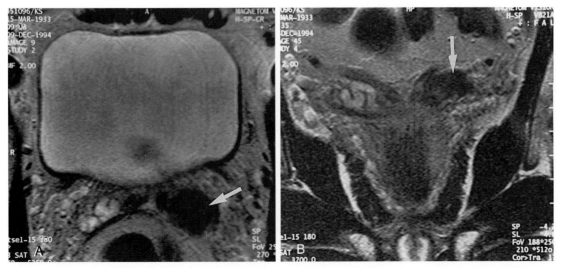

Figure 19–13. Axial (*A*), coronal (*B*) seminal vesicle carcinoma, T2-weighted (TR/TE = 5250/119 msec, 3700/119 msec, respectively). The left seminal vesicle is replaced by carcinoma (*arrows A, B*).

and -diesters (PDE), as well as adenosine triphosphate (ATP)—differ in carcinoma and in normal prostate tissue. BPH exhibits a large increase in citrate, whereas prostate carcinoma demonstrates large decreases. Concentrations of sialic acid and spermidine-spermine ratios also differ in prostate carcinoma.[25–28] In vivo spectroscopic studies with both hydrogen and phosphorus have supported these findings, but exact differences and ratios remain controversial.

Until recently, in vivo magnetic resonance spectroscopy required tumor volumes greater than $2 \times 2 \times 2$ cm³, which allowed for contamination of tumor spectra by other tissue included in the sample volume. However, using the same phased-array coil technology for imaging, three-dimensional phase-encoded spectroscopic studies have now become possible. The entire prostate can be evaluated in one study and excellent spectra obtained from volumes as small as 0.24 ml. Using a variety of metabolite ratios (e.g., citrate-choline ratio, [0.53 ± 0.27 for carcinoma, 1.42 ± 0.51 for BPH, and 1.62 ± 0.41 for normal peripheral zone]) cancers from these small volumes may be detectable by MRSI but not by routine imaging.[29, 30] By superimposing the spectroscopic three-dimensional data set on corresponding images, the exact location of the tumor may be determined and volume estimated.

Clearly, this exciting work carries great promise. Further technical improvements will enable accurate quantification of various spectroscopic peaks, which in turn may lead to estimates of tumor differentiation and possibly predict hormone sensitivity.[31]

Application of MR spectroscopy to the Dunning rat model of prostate cancer has demonstrated the power of this technique in identifying secondary metabolic changes occurring within host hepatic tissues not directly involved by metastatic disease.[32] These studies further revealed that MR spectroscopy could be employed to monitor therapy—in this instance, the use of ω3 fatty acids from fish oil—to inhibit prostate cancer–induced cachexia.[33] Although not yet applied in the human clinical situation, there is no doubt that MR spectroscopic techniques are valuable and powerful modalities with which to assess biochemical changes occurring in prostate cancer–bearing hosts, whether the primary prostatic cancers, their metastases, or the metabolic status of host tissues. It may be anticipated that a role for extracorporeal MR spectroscopy will develop in monitoring the response of prostate cancers to therapy, and analogous to that currently held by MR imaging techniques in the primary diagnosis of the disease.

CONCLUSION

The ability to detect and stage carcinoma of the prostate with MRI is undergoing a revolution that is being driven by technology. Within

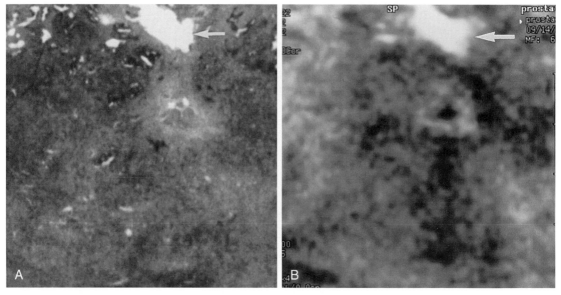

Figure 19–14. Carcinoma. *A*, A low power (80 × 80 × 100 μm³) H & E slide demonstrates prostate carcinoma (basophilic area). Clear area (*arrows [A, B]*) is a collagen scar. *B*, The corresponding MRI section obtained by means of a three-dimensional T2-weighted fast spin echo sequence. The dark areas in *A* and *B* correspond to carcinoma. Resolution and slice thickness are approximately the same in *B* and *A*.

the past several years the technology advanced from the crude body coils to endorectal coils, to endorectal phased-array coils, and now to external quadrature phased-array coils. Pulse sequences evolved from the time-consuming spin echo type to fast spin echo variants that are 8 to 16 times faster. MRI units themselves have also improved. At one time, gradient strengths of 6 mT/m were state-of-the-art; now 25 mT/m are available. Whole-body MR units having field strengths of 4 Tesla are now being marketed. Each technologic advance generated a great improvement in image quality: whereas the prostate was once merely a blur on the pelvic image, now we can examine the lumen of the seminal vesicles in search of millimeter-sized tumors. The end is not yet in sight. It will soon be possible to perform in vivo microscopy using MRI that rivals what the pathologist sees under the microscope (Fig. 19–14). With further technical development and improved tumor metabolite quantification, MRSI will provide the one thing that MRI lacks: a "prostate cancer stain." Perhaps soon another acronym will be added to the MR lexicon: MRH—magnetic resonance histology.

Acknowledgment

The author is grateful for the advice and discussions received from the many researchers in this field. Special thanks to Drs. J. Weinreb, F.G. Sommer, W. Bradley, and Siemens Medical Systems for providing the many interesting cases shown in this review.

REFERENCES

1. Boring CC, Squires TS, Tong T, et al.: Cancer statistics. CA Cancer J Clin 44:7–26, 1994.
2. Dhom G: Epidemiological aspects of latent and clinically manifest carcinoma of the prostate. J Cancer Res Clin Oncol 106:210–218, 1983.
3. Winego PA, Tong T, Bolder S: Cancer statistics. CA Cancer J Clin 45:8–30, 1995.
4. Steinfeld AD: Questions regarding the treatment of localized prostate cancer. Radiology 184:593–598, 1992.
5. Tempany CM, Zhou X, Zerhouni EA, et al.: Staging of prostate cancer: Results of Radiology Diagnostic Oncology Group project comparison of three MR imaging techniques. Radiology 192:47–54, 1994.
6. Schnall MD, Pollack HM: Magnetic resonance imaging of the prostate gland. Urol Radiol 12:109–114, 1990.
7. Chelsky MJ, Schnall MD, Seidmon EJ, et al.: Use of endorectal surface coil magnetic resonance imaging for local staging of prostate cancer. J Urol 150:391–395, 1993.
8. Quinn SF, Franzini DA, Demlow TA, et al.: MR imaging of prostate cancer with an endorectal coil technique: Correlation with whole-mount specimens. Radiology 190:323–327, 1994.
9. Sheibler ML, Schnall MD, Pollack HM, et al.: Current role of MR imaging in the staging of adenocarcinoma of the prostate. Radiology 189:339–352, 1993.

10. Weinreb J: Personal communications.
11. Quint LE, Van Erp JS, Bland PH, et al.: Prostate cancer: Correlation of MR images with tissue optical density at pathologic examination. Radiology 179: 837–842, 1992.
12. Sommer FG, Nghiam HV, Herfkens R, et al.: Determining the volume of prostatic carcinoma: Value of MR imaging with an external array coil. AJR 161:81–86, 1993.
13. Sillerud LO, Halliday KR, Griffey RH, et al.: In-vivo ^{13}C NMR spectroscopy of the human prostate. Magn Reson Med 8:224–230, 1988.
14. Mirowitz SA: Seminal vesicles: Biopsy related hemorrhage simulating tumor invasion at endorectal MR imaging. Radiology 185:373–378, 1992.
15. Kahn T, Burrug K, Schmitz-Drager B, et al.: Prostatic carcinoma and benign prostatic hypertrophy: MR imaging with histopathologic correlation. Radiology 173:847–851, 1989.
16. Mirowitz SA, Brown JJ, Heiken JP: Evaluation of the prostate and prostatic carcinoma with gadolinium-enhanced endorectal coil MR imaging. Radiology 186:153–157, 1993.
17. Wheeler TM: Anatomic considerations in carcinoma of the prostate. Urol Clin North Am 16:623–634, 1989.
18. Schnall MD, Bezzi M, Pollack HM, et al.: Magnetic resonance imaging of the prostate. Magn Reson Q 6:1–16, 1990.
19. Ramchaandani P, Schnall MD: Magnetic resonance imaging of the prostate. Semin Roentgenol 28:74–82, 1993.
20. Donahue RE, Miller GJ: Adenocarcinoma of the prostate: Biopsy of whole mount—Denver VA experience. Urol Clin North Am 18:449–452, 1991.
21. Hricak H, White S, Vigneron D, et al.: Carcinoma of the prostate gland: MR imaging with pelvic phased-array coils versus integrated endorectal-pelvic phased-array coils. Radiology 193:703–709, 1994.
22. Oesterling JE: Prostate specific antigen: A critical assessment of the most useful tumor marker for adenocarcinoma of the prostate. J Urol 145:907–923, 1992.
23. Catalona WJ, Smith DS, Ratliff TL, et al.: Measurement of prostate-specific antigen in serum as a screening test for prostate cancer. N Engl J Med 324:1156–1161, 1991.
24. Oesterling JE, Jacobsen SJ, Chute CG, et al.: Serum prostate-specific antigen in a community-based population of healthy men: Establishment of age-specific reference ranges. JAMA 275:860–864, 1993.
25. Schiebler ML, Miyamoto KK, White M, et al.: In vitro high resolution ^{1}H-spectroscopy of the human prostate: Benign prostatic hyperplasia, normal peripheral zone and adenocarcinoma. Magn Reson Med 29:285–291, 1993.
26. Kurhanewicz J, Dahiya R, MacDonald JM, et al.: Citrate alterations in primary and metastatic human prostatic adenocarcinomas: ^{1}H magnetic resonance spectroscopy and biochemical study. Magn Reson Med 29:149–157, 1993.
27. Cornel EB, Smits GAHJ, Oosterhof GON, et al.: Characterization of human prostate cancer, benign prostatic hyperplasia and normal prostate by in vitro ^{1}H and ^{13}P magnetic resonance spectroscopy. J Urol 150:2019–2024, 1993.
28. Narayan P, Kurhanewicz J: Magnetic resonance spectroscopy in prostate disease: Diagnostic possibilities and future developments. Prostate (Suppl) 4:43–50, 1992.
29. Kurhanewicz J, Vigneron DB, Nelson SJ, et al.: Prostate cancer: Three dimensional spectroscopy with 0.24-cm^3 resolution. Supplement to Radiology—Scientific Program 193(P):196, 1994.
30. Heerschap A, Jager G, Barentsz J, et al.: Functional ^{1}H magnetic resonance in the identification and characterization of localized prostate cancer (Abstract). Proceedings of the Society of Magnetic Resonance 1994; 274.
31. Vigneron DB, Hricak H, James TL, et al.: Androgen sensitivity of rat prostate carcinoma studied by ^{13}P NMR spectroscopy, ^{1}H MR imaging, and ^{23}Na MR imaging. Magn Reson Med 11;152–60, 1989.
32. Dagnelie PC, Bell JD, Williams SCR, et al.: Altered phosphorylation status, phospholipid metabolism and gluconeogenesis in the host liver of rats with prostate cancer: a 31P magnetic resonance spectroscopy study. Br J Cancer 67:1303–1309, 1993.
33. Dagnelie PC, Bell JD, Williams SCR, et al.: Effect of fish oil on cancer cachexia and host liver metabolism in rats with prostate tumors. Lipids 29:195–203, 1994.

20

IDENTIFICATION AND PATHOLOGIC SIGNIFICANCE OF NEUROENDOCRINE DIFFERENTIATION IN HUMAN PROSTATE CARCINOMA

P. Anthony di Sant'Agnese

PROSTATIC NEUROENDOCRINE (ENDOCRINE-PARACRINE) CELLS IN THE NORMAL PROSTATE

Prostatic neuroendocrine (endocrine-paracrine) cells were first described by Pretl in 1944.[1] These cells form part of a diffuse neuroendocrine regulatory system defined by Feyrter in 1938[2] and elaborated upon by Pearse in the 1960s.[3] Neuroendocrine cells in the prostate (Fig. 20–1) are analogous to neuroendocrine cells of the gastrointestinal tract, lungs, thyroid (C cells), and pancreas (islets of Langerhans).

Neuroendocrine cells in the normal prostate are distributed throughout the prostatic urethra, prostatic ducts, and peripheral prostate.[4–6] The largest concentration of neuroendocrine cells is found in the prostatic ducts in the region of the verumontanum. There is great variation in the number of these cells from one prostate to another, and even within a single prostate their density and distribution may be quite variable.

It has been shown that neuroendocrine cells in human prostates are present both in the ducts and in the peripheral prostate, prenatally and at birth, but within a few months the neuroendocrine cells of the peripheral prostate disappear only to reappear again at puberty.[7] Wernert and colleagues[8] studied more than 100 human prostates from 20 weeks' gestational age to 89 years. Applying a variety of generic and more specific immunocytochemical markers they noted that neuroendocrine cells were absent from the utricle until after puberty.

In guinea pigs, neuroendocrine cells in the peripheral prostate increase in number with age, but those in the urethra and prostatic ducts remain constant.[9] It is also of interest that the serotonin levels in guinea pig prostates correlated well with immunohistochemical findings. The ultrastructural neurosecretory granule morphology in guinea pig prostatic neuroendocrine cells showed large pleomorphic granules in the periurethral cells and small round granules in the peripheral prostate, suggesting that cells in different regions of the prostate not only vary with age but probably secrete different neuropeptides

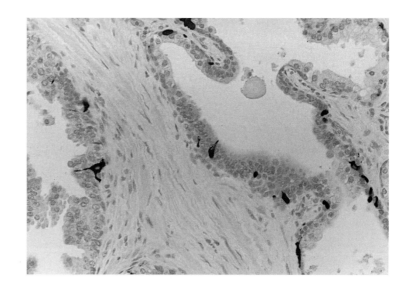

Figure 20–1. Normal prostate gland with scattered open and closed neuroendocrine cells with dendritic processes. (Serotonin immunocytochemistry reduced 40% from ×480.)

and play different roles in the prostate (unpublished observation).

The human and guinea pig findings suggest some differential direct or indirect androgen sensitivity of the cells in the peripheral prostate and utricle, but not of those in the ducts. Androgen receptor is not expressed in human prostatic neuroendocrine cells,[10, 11] so the effect on the peripheral prostatic neuroendocrine cells may be indirect (see below).

Battaglia and colleagues[12] studied the age distribution of prostatic neuroendocrine cells in patients between 14 and 74 years of age (presumably all postpubertal). The largest numbers of neuroendocrine cells were found to peak in the 24- to 54-year-old age group with fewer cells in patients who were younger and older. The mean density of neuroendocrine cells in the 25- to 54-year-old age group was 0.366 neuroendocrine cells per millimeter of epithelium.

Neuroendocrine cells of benign prostatic hyperplasia are markedly decreased in number, except in small early nodules and apparent growth centers of larger nodules. This finding was confirmed when quantitative assays of serotonin concentration in large hyperplastic nodules showed marked decreases in serotonin levels as compared with those in normal control prostates. The areas within the hyperplastic nodules with large numbers of neuroendocrine cells morphologically appeared to be proliferating (i.e., less mature epithelium), and there was a distinct correlation between proliferating cell nuclear antigen staining and the presence of neuroendocrine cells.[13]

The prostatic neuroendocrine cells are of the open (apical extensions to the lumen with specialized surface microvilli) and closed cell types, both of which have complex dendritic processes (Fig. 20–1).[4] Ultrastructural examination of the cells reveals a wide range of neurosecretory granule morphology, suggesting a variety of cell types (Fig. 20–2).[14] Presumably these correspond to the diversity of neurosecretory products that have been found in the cells. These products include serotonin, chromogranin A, and a TSH-like peptide, all of these compounds being found in a large number of prostatic neuroendocrine cells.[4, 5] Subpopulations of neuroendocrine cells are immunoreactive for the calcitonin gene family of peptides, including calcitonin, katacalcin, and calcitonin gene–related peptide.[15, 16] Bombesin/gastrin-releasing peptide[15, 17] and somatostatin[18] immunoreactive cells are rather infrequent. Alpha-human chorionic gonadotropin–like immunoreactivity has also been described in some neuroendocrine cells.[19]

Recently, parathyroid hormone–related protein (PTHrP) has been described in a subpopulation of prostatic neuroendocrine cells using a monoclonal antibody to the 1–34 amino terminal of PTHrP.[20] This was confirmed by in situ hybridization with a cDNA probe complementary to the sequence coding peptides 15 to 120 of PTHrP demonstrating positive staining in the same cells that were immunoreactive for PTHrP. Wu and coworkers, using in situ hybridization with exon-specific probes to PTHrP, studied differential PTHrP gene expression in prostatic neuroendocrine cells.[21]

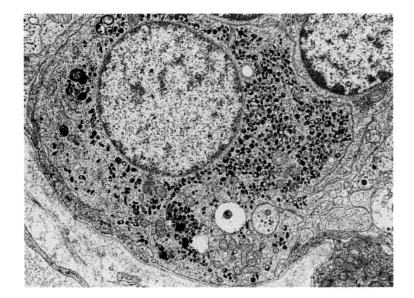

Figure 20–2. Electron photomicrograph of a closed type of prostatic neuroendocrine cell with intermediate-sized pleomorphic secretory granules. Note nerve process invaginating cell at lower right. (Reduced 43% from ×12,500.)

All three forms of PTHrP produced by alternative splicing of gene transcripts were found in subpopulations of neuroendocrine cells.

Chromogranin B and secretogranin II have also recently been described in subpopulations of prostatic neuroendocrine cells.[22] Chromogranin B appears to be expressed more frequently in benign nodular prostatic hyperplasia than in the normal prostate tissue. Calcitonin, bombesin/gastrin-releasing peptide, somatostatin, and PTHrP have all been found in human semen.[6, 23]

How prostatic neuroendocrine cells are regulated is not known; however, these cells do contain receptors for c-erbB-2 and epidermal growth factor.[24] The fact that androgen receptor is not expressed in prostatic neuroendocrine cells suggests that, if there is androgen regulation, it is indirect.[10, 11] Furthermore, prostatic neuroendocrine cells are innervated by autonomic nerves. Prostatic neuroendocrine cells also send out dendritic processes that make connections with each other. Processes from different neuroendocrine cell types often make contact with each other, suggesting that communication and regulation occur. Finally, the open cell types with long microvilli that extend into the glandular lumina may be regulated by luminal contents. Presumably, the prostatic neuroendocrine cells then function through their dendritic

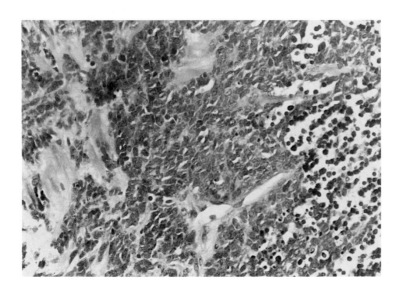

Figure 20–3. Small cell neuroendocrine carcinoma of the prostate. (H&E reduced 40% from ×480.)

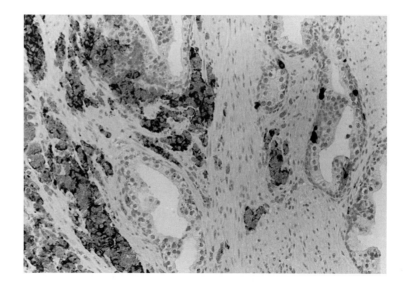

Figure 20–4. Small cell carcinoma of the prostate infiltrating between normal glands showing positive immunostaining for chromogranin A. (Chromogranin A immunocytochemistry reduced 40% from ×240.)

processes to mediate glandular functions via paracrine mechanisms. Autocrine and endocrine regulation may also occur.[6]

A variety of prostatic neuroendocrine products are known to exhibit growth factor activity, including serotonin, bombesin, and calcitonin gene–related peptide. Serotonin is also known to regulate morphogenesis. Prostatic neuroendocrine cells may, therefore, be involved in the regulation of growth and development of the prostate.[6]

NEUROENDOCRINE DIFFERENTIATION IN PROSTATIC CARCINOMA

Prostatic malignancy with neuroendocrine differentiation occurs in several forms, including small cell neuroendocrine carcinoma, carcinoid-like tumors, and adenocarcinoma with focal neuroendocrine differentiation.[6] Small cell carcinoma of the prostate is relatively rare, accounting for approximately 1% to 2% of all prostate malignancies (Fig. 20–3).[25, 26] It usually expresses the neuroendocrine phenotype (Fig. 20–4). Whether or not small cell carcinomas express neuroendocrine markers and/or biogenic amines and neuropeptides, it is usually negative for prostate-specific antigen (PSA) and prostatic acid phosphatase (PAP), both by immunocytochemistry and serum levels (Fig. 20–5). Small cell carcinoma of the prostate may arise de novo but often follows previous therapy, especially hormone therapy, and overgrows conventional adenocarcinoma.

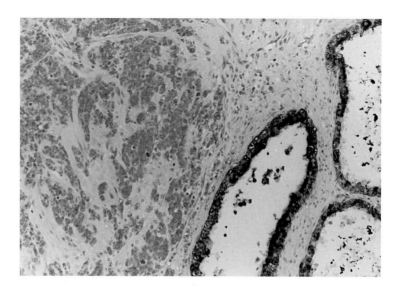

Figure 20–5. Small cell carcinoma of the prostate negative for PSA with normal prostate gland to the right positive for PSA. (PSA immunocytochemistry reduced 40% from ×240.)

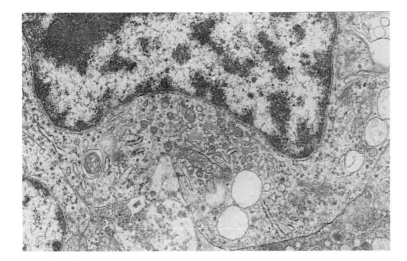

Figure 20–6. Electron photomicrograph of the same small cell carcinoma shown in Figures 20–4 and 20–5 showing small round cytoplasmic neurosecretory granules. (Reduced 43% from ×28,000.)

Small cell carcinoma of the prostate is histologically similar to those of the lung and other organs and demonstrates a high nuclear-cytoplasmic ratio, dispersed chromatin, nuclear molding, and necrosis. In one case we have observed small cell carcinoma in situ adjacent to an invasive small cell carcinoma. The carcinoma in situ appeared to arise in a multinodular fashion within the basal layers of the prostatic epithelium and expanded in other areas to replace the entire epithelium. Ultrastructural analysis of small cell carcinoma of the prostate reveals the presence, at least in some cases, of small, round neurosecretory granules, which are rather sparsely distributed (Fig. 20–6). Small cell carcinoma is very aggressive, tends to metastasize to multiple visceral organs, and responds poorly to hormone ther-

apy. Attempts to utilize chemotherapeutic regimens effective against small cell carcinoma of the lung have met with some limited success in small cell carcinoma of the prostate.

Carcinoid-like tumors have been described in several publications but do not appear to be a well-defined entity.[27–30] Classic carcinoid tumors with typical insular, trabecular, and ribbonlike growth patterns are extremely rare in the prostate, if they exist at all. The carcinoid-like tumors are architecturally poorly differentiated; that is, they grow in sheets and nests with histologic features that include rather uniform small nuclei with a euchromatic nuclear structure and, often, a cleared cytoplasm (Fig. 20–7). Tumors with this histology often express marked neuroendocrine differentiation. They are somewhat carcinoid-like in that

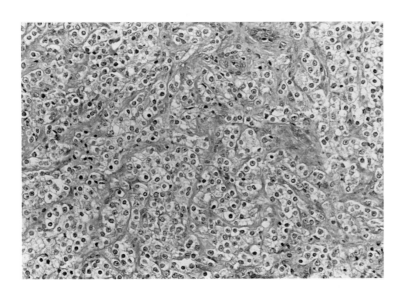

Figure 20–7. Carcinoid-like carcinoma of the prostate. (H&E reduced 40% from ×240.)

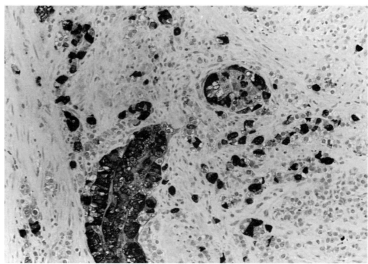

Figure 20–8. The carcinoid-like tumor shown in Figure 20–7 immunostained for serotonin with numerous serotonin-immunoreactive cells with especially pronounced endocrine differentiation surrounding the nerve at lower mid-left. (Serotonin immunocytochemistry reduced 40% from ×240.)

they show neuroendocrine differentiation (Figs. 20–8, 20–9) and are rather bland cytologically, but they are not true carcinoid tumors. In addition, a variety of other poorly differentiated carcinomas with focal neuroendocrine differentiation have, at times, been referred to as "carcinoid-like." Whatever term one uses for these carcinoid-like tumors, they are generally high grade and pursue a rather aggressive course.

The most common pattern of neuroendocrine differentiation in prostate malignancy is conventional prostatic adenocarcinoma with focal neuroendocrine cell differentiation (Figs. 20–10, 20–11). It appears that most, if not all, prostatic carcinomas have at least a rare coproliferating malignant neuroendocrine cell in the tumor.[6, 31]

In some cases, the granules in the malignant cells are large and eosinophilic on hematoxylin and eosin staining. These have been referred to as "Paneth-like cells." In the largest study to date of this phenomenon,[32] it was noted that these larger neuroendocrine granules were present in 10% of cancers (30 of 300) and showed a predilection for a cribriform growth pattern. There was no correlation of Paneth cell–like change with prognostic parameters, but this study did not rule it out as an independent prognostic factor. It should also be noted that in the normal prostate the exocrine secretory epithelium may have large apical eosinophilic granules, and at least theoretically, these could occur in prostatic adenocarcinomas and represent nonneuroendocrine Paneth-like change; however, we have not yet

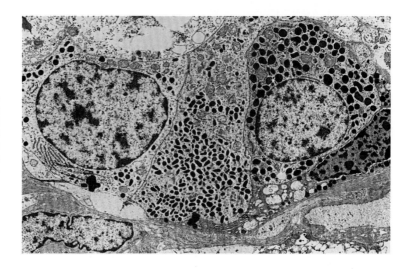

Figure 20–9. Electron photomicrograph of carcinoid-like tumor seen in Figures 20–7 and 20–8 demonstrating neoplastic cells with intermediate pleomorphic neurosecretory granules and large pleomorphic secretory granules. (Reduced 43% from ×7000.)

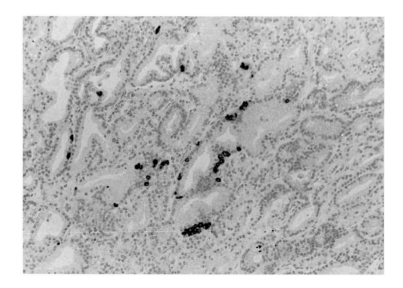

Figure 20–10. Well-differentiated adenocarcinoma with a focus of neuroendocrine differentiation. (Chromogranin A immunocytochemistry reduced 40% from ×240.)

observed this in a carcinoma. The term "Paneth cell–like change" is considered misleading and inappropriate, and we would recommend that these be referred to as neuroendocrine differentiation with large eosinophilic granules.[32, 33]

Neuroendocrine differentiation in prostate carcinoma was originally detected by silver stains and was thought to be present in only about 10% of cases; however, with the advent of immunochemical stains it has been shown that most, if not all, prostatic adenocarcinomas show at least rare neuroendocrine differentiation.[6, 29, 31] Approximately 10% show considerable neuroendocrine differentiation, including multifocal clusters or sheets of neuro-

endocrine cells within the carcinoma. Chromogranin A and serotonin are the best immunostains for detecting neuroendocrine differentiation, chromogranin A being slightly superior in the number of cells detected. It is of interest that in one study chromogranin B was the member of the chromogranin family most often expressed in high-grade tumors. Occasionally, chromogranin A stains normal secretory epithelium and the apical portion of tumor cells, suggesting that it may stain exocrine secretory granules. These areas should not be mistaken for neuroendocrine differentiation. Neuron-specific enolase may be helpful but tends to stain not only focal cells with neuroendocrine differentiation but also some

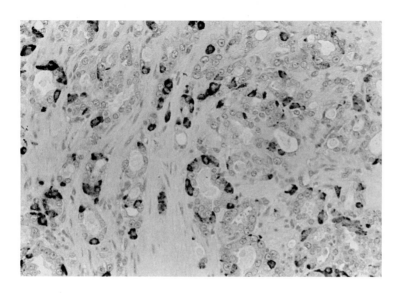

Figure 20–11. Moderately differentiated adenocarcinoma with more diffuse immunostaining for parathyroid hormone–related protein. (Parathyroid hormone–related protein immunocytochemistry reduced 40% from ×120.)

tumors rather more diffusely, which may represent nonspecific staining or a more diffuse neuroendocrine phenotype. In the normal prostate, serotonin and chromogranin appear to be co-expressed in most normal neuroendocrine cells with occasional cells containing chromogranin only. This is often the case in carcinoma, but frequently there is aberrant expression of serotonin-only cells. In some malignancies, double immunostaining for both serotonin and chromogranin reveals a much larger number of cells with neuroendocrine differentiation than either stain alone. Immunocytochemistry for a variety of neuropeptides may detect additional neuroendocrine cells. In addition to eutopic hormone production, ectopic hormone production may occur in prostate carcinoma with focal neuroendocrine differentiation.[6] The most frequent products are adrenocorticotropin (ACTH), beta-endorphin, leu-enkephalin, and glucagon. In summary, the more neuroendocrine immunostains that are performed, the more likely one is to detect neuroendocrine differentiation. Virtually all prostate carcinomas express some degree of neuroendocrine differentiation.

It is useful to distinguish true neuroendocrine differentiation in prostate carcinoma from entrapped normal neuroendocrine cells. The malignant cells with neuroendocrine differentiation show nuclear features identical to those of the other nonneuroendocrine malignant cells, including when present, large nuclei with macronucleoli. Entrapped cells will be associated with benign glandular elements. Neuroendocrine cells in carcinomas exhibit nuclear features similar to adjacent carcinoma cells, thus indicating that they are fully malignant cells. Further support that the neuroendocrine cells in prostatic carcinomas are malignant is the observation that identical lines of divergent differentiation are found both within the primary carcinoma and within the metastases.

Neuroendocrine differentiation in prostate carcinoma recapitulates normal lines of differentiation. In well-differentiated adenocarcinoma, the neoplastic neuroendocrine cells tend to resemble those of the normal prostate, with open and closed cell types and frequent dendritic processes. These cells also tend to occur in clusters with cell bodies and processes of different cell types abutting each other. The neurosecretory granules resemble those of the normal neuroendocrine cells. Nerve processes may be seen adjacent to cells with neuroendo-

crine differentiation, as in the normal prostate. In poorly differentiated tumors, the neuroendocrine cells tend to lose their apical and dendritic processes and occur more randomly throughout the tumors, and their neurosecretory granules are aberrant when compared with those in cells of the normal prostate. PSA and PAP[34-36] may be co-expressed in an abnormal amphicrine manner in malignant cells with neuroendocrine differentiation, suggesting that exocrine and neuroendocrine cells originate from a common stem cell.

We recently observed that foci of perineural carcinoma, within (and particularly outside) the prostate, often express strong, diffuse neuroendocrine differentiation (see Fig. 20–8). While this is not always the case, it is striking when it is present and suggests that factors produced in the nerves may induce neuroendocrine differentiation in prostate carcinoma. This may be of potential significance since extensive perineural invasion correlates well with extracapsular prostatic extension, and high levels of circulating neuroendocrine markers might be an indicator of advanced stage disease.

Paraganglia are present just outside the prostatic capsule and consist of aggregates of small clear cells that can closely resemble prostate carcinoma, particularly the carcinoid-like clear cell type.[37] Neuroendocrine markers may stain these paraganglia, particularly synaptophysin and protein gene product (PGP) 9.5, but they are usually weakly positive to negative for chromogranin A and negative for serotonin. This differential staining pattern helps differentiate them from prostate carcinoma with neuroendocrine differentiation.

Whether neuroendocrine differentiation influences prognosis is not clear, but the weight of evidence at this time suggests there may be an association with a poor prognosis—and in particular resistance to hormone therapy. Cohen and colleagues in 1991 showed[38] a marked prognostic effect for neuroendocrine differentiation in prostate carcinoma. They studied 110 patients with stage B, C, or D carcinoma with a minimum of 4 years' follow-up. Twenty patients were eliminated from the analysis for a variety of reasons. The remaining 90 patients with carcinomas were evaluated, and half showed neuroendocrine differentiation. Only 5 of 44 *without* neuroendocrine differentiation died, whereas 42 of 46 *with* neuroendocrine differentiation died. The authors claimed that neuroendocrine differentiation was an independent variable and was of prognostic significance even for stage-matched disease. In 1993, Berner and colleagues[39] studied 47 patients with prostate cancer who underwent tissue studies before and after hormone therapy. Some 32% were initially positive for neuron-specific enolase, with a trend toward increasing neuroendocrine differentiation in those tumors that had become resistant to hormone manipulation therapy. The findings were not statistically significant. Only one neuroendocrine marker was employed in this study. Aprikian used several neuroendocrine markers to study metastatic, diethylstilbestrol-treated, hormone-refractory tumors.[34] The 77% of the tumors that were not treated showed focal neuroendocrine differentiation, whereas those treated had a somewhat smaller percentage of neuroendocrine differentiation. Neuroendocrine differentiation was not associated with prognostic parameters. Aprikian in 1994 studied 64 metastatic prostate cancers; 46% developed pelvic nodal metastases and 53% bone metastases.[40] Chromogranin A immunostaining showed no correlations with DNA ploidy or disease-specific survival in the stage D1 patients. A rather high level of thyroid stimulating hormone (TSH)-like peptide expression was seen in the metastases. In a study by Van de Voorde and colleagues,[41] prostate cancer patients were treated with estramustine phosphate and flutamide before radical prostatectomy. Chromogranin A was used to detect neuroendocrine differentiation in the radical prostatectomy specimens. It was found that the vast majority of cases were positive for neuroendocrine differentiation, and there were distinct positive correlations between increasing grade, increasing volume, *and* proliferation index, on the one hand, with chromogranin immunostaining, on the other.

Three recent abstracts suggest significant prognostic significance for neuroendocrine differentiation in prostate carcinoma. Epstein and coworkers[42] followed 104 patients who had undergone radical prostatectomy. Forty-eight experienced disease progression (mean time to progression, 3.6 years). Representative sections of the tumors were immunostained for chromogranin. Grade, stage, and neuroendocrine differentiation correlated significantly with prognosis. Multivariate analysis showed grade and neuroendocrine differentiation to be significant. Neuroendocrine differentiation was independent of stage or grade. In patients with Gleason scores less than 7, neuroendocrine differentiation stratified patients according to high and low risk of progression.

Grignon and associates[43] evaluated patients from a prospective trial evaluating the benefit of androgen ablation therapy before definitive external beam radiation therapy for bulky stage T2 and T3 cancer on a Radiation Therapy Oncology Group (RTOG) protocol. Of 471 biopsy specimens, 155 were immunostained for chromogranin A. Overall survival was the end point. Neuroendocrine differentiation (49 of 155 patients) was associated with poor overall survival ($P = 0.02$).

Finally, in a smaller study Schultz and colleagues[44] evaluated 21 stage T2 patients who underwent radical prostatectomy after androgen deprivation therapy. Sections of the prostate were stained for chromogranin and synaptophysin, and they showed that five of six patients that were positive for synaptophysin had rising PSA levels ($P<0.05$). The correlation between chromogranin immunostaining and prognosis was not good.

Tarle and coworkers[45] evaluated neuron-specific enolase serum levels in prostate carcinoma and more frequently found elevations in nonresponders to hormone therapy (10 of 46, 21.7%) than in responders (2 of 89, 2.2%). Untreated patients with local disease were more frequently positive for serum neuron-specific enolase (10 of 35, 28.6%) than were untreated patients with disseminated disease (3 of 28, 10.7%). It was also noted that hormone therapy did not normalize elevated neuron-specific enolase levels. Only surgical treatment reduced neuron-specific enolase levels. In another study by Kadmon and colleagues[46] chromogranin A serum levels were analyzed in 25 patients with node-positive carcinoma and in 25 control patients. All controls had normal levels, whereas 12 of 25 (48%) patients with prostate carcinoma had elevated serum levels of chromogranin A. All patients with chromogranin A had aggressive disease resistant to hormone therapy, and a third also had negative levels of PSA and PAP. Both studies suggest that neuroendocrine differentiation confers resistance to hormone ablation therapy or develops as resistance emerges.

Several lines of experimental evidence suggest mechanisms by which neuroendocrine differentiation may influence prognosis. Neither normal neuroendocrine cells nor malignant cells coproliferating in adenocarcinoma of the prostate express androgen receptor. This may indicate that they are not regulated by androgens. Bang and colleagues have demonstrated that androgen-dependent cell lines

(LNCaP) and androgen-independent cell lines (PC-3-M) can be induced to undergo extensive neuroendocrine differentiation by raising cyclic adenosine monophosphate (cAMP) activity via cAMP analogs or phosphodiesterase inhibitors.[47] Results indicated terminal differentiation, including G-phase synchronization, growth arrest, and loss of clonogenicity. This was suggested as a possible method of treatment for prostate cancer. Since neuroendocrine cells of the prostate and those in neuroendocrine carcinoma appear to be terminally differentiated and nonproliferating, it might be speculated that, rather than overgrowing carcinomas (and the evidence does not particularly suggest an increase in the numbers of neuroendocrine cells in prostate carcinoma in response to escape from hormone therapy), these cells may increase their production of regulatory substances such as growth factors. In fact, an increase in proliferation rates[48] and bcl-2 (antiapoptotic factor)[49] have been shown to be expressed in the vicinity of foci of neuroendocrine differentiation in prostate carcinomas with focal neuroendocrine differentiation. This might account for the poor prognosis for tumors with neuroendocrine differentiation in general and, particularly, those treated by hormone ablation therapy, whereby this effect may become more important or predominant. Sunday and coworkers[50] showed in a hamster tumor model treated with diethylnitrosamine plus hyperoxia that neuroendocrine cell hyperplasia occurs in the lung in the preneoplastic state, but in the latter states when the neoplasm was fully developed, the neoplasm was "nonneuroendocrine." This suggests that neuroendocrine cells differentiate during initial stages of carcinogenesis and then produce factors that stimulate the growth of the nonneuroendocrine cells. This phenomenon may also occur in the prostate.

Prostate cancer cell lines grown in a Matrigel and treated with bombesin increased their penetration of the Matrigel.[51] Cell lines PC3 and D-145 expressed neuroendocrine markers including chromogranin A, neuron-specific enolase, and serotonin. At the time, they expressed a urokinase and a heparinase, which are extracellular matrix degradative enzymes, thus suggesting a mechanism by which neuroendocrine tumors may become more invasive. Prostate cancers that did not exhibit neuroendocrine differentiation were negative for these enzymes. A small cell carcinoma that was positive for neuroendocrine differentiation was also positive for the enzymes.

Several other lines of investigation need to be pursued. For neuroendocrine products to have an effect, receptors for such molecules must be present either on nonneuroendocrine cells or on other neuroendocrine-differentiated cells. Therefore, the presence or absence of specific receptors for neuroendocrine products may be crucial in determining the significance of neuroendocrine differentiation and needs to be investigated further. In addition, neuroendocrine differentiation is defined by the storage of neuroendocrine products detected by immunocytochemistry. The storage of neuroendocrine product does not necessarily indicate active secretion, and, in fact, high levels of constitutive secretion of neuroendocrine products may result in little or no immunocytochemical staining. Therefore, quantitative measurements of tumor levels of neuroendocrine products or serum levels may be more useful. Finally, the types of neuroendocrine products that are produced may be important (i.e., bombesin-like products may have growth factor activity, whereas somatostatin-like expression may actually inhibit tumor growth or secretion). Therefore, a full profile of all known products should be sought in each tumor and correlated with prognosis.

Neuroendocrine differentiation in prostate carcinoma lends itself to potential new therapeutic approaches directed at neuroendocrine differentiation. These include immunotherapy (with interferon, antibodies to growth-promoting peptides or neuropeptides, or antibodies to receptors for such peptides or neuropeptides), endocrine therapy (with antagonist analogs to peptide or neuropeptide growth factors or agonist analogs to secretion- and growth-inhibiting peptides or neuropeptides such as somatostatin), as well as specialized chemotherapeutic agents specifically targeted against neuroendocrine differentiation, such as streptozotocin.

In prostate malignancy, the clinical significance of neuroendocrine differentiation is not known at this time, except for the rare small cell carcinoma that is aggressive and does not respond to hormone manipulation therapy. There are strong theoretical experimental reasons for believing that neuroendocrine differentiation may affect prognosis, particularly in resistance to androgen deprivation therapy. Human clinical studies are few, generally are limited in scope, and, most important, lack a clear definition of neuroendocrine differentiation in conventional adenocarcinoma of the prostate. Some do, however, suggest prognostic significance for neuroendocrine differentiation in prostate carcinoma. No recommendation can be made at this time about how to define significant neuroendocrine differentiation in prostate cancer, how appropriately to diagnose it, or how to treat it. Future studies need to address these issues.

Acknowledgment

The author thanks Ms. Ellen Dee for her dedication and excellent secretarial skills.

REFERENCES

1. Pretl K: Zur Frage der Endokrin der menschlichen Vorsteherdruse. Virchows Arch 32:392–404, 1944.
2. Feyrter F: Uber diffuse endocrine epithelial Organe. Lepzig: J.A. Barth, 1938.
3. Pearse A: The cytochemistry and ultrastructure of polypeptide hormone–producinng cells of the APUD series and the embryologic, physiologic, and pathologic implications of the concepts. J Histochem Cytochem 17:303–313, 1969.
4. di Sant'Agnese, P, de Mesy Jensen K: Human prostatic endocrine-paracrine (APUD) cells: Distributional analysis with a comparison of serotonin and neuron-specific enolase immunoreactivity and silver stains. Arch Pathol Lab Med 109:607–612, 1985.
5. Abrahamsson P-A, Wadstrom L, Alumets J, et al.: Peptide-hormone and serotonin-immunoreactive cells in normal and hyperplastic prostate glands. Pathol Res Pract 181:675–683, 1986.
6. di Sant'Agnese, PA: Neuroendocrine differentiation in carcinoma of the prostate. Diagnostic, prognostic, and therapeutic implications. Cancer 70:254–268, 1992.
7. Cohen R, Glezerson G, Taylor L, et al.: The neuroendocrine cell population of the human prostate gland. J Urol 150:365–368, 1993.
8. Wernert N, Kern L, Heitz H, et al.: Morphological and immunohistochemical investigations of the utriculus prostaticus from the fetal period up to adulthood. Prostate 17:19–30, 1990.
9. di Sant'Agnese PA, Davis N, Chen M, et al.: Age-related changes in the neuroendocrine (endocrine-paracrine) cell population and the serotonin content of the guinea pig prostate. Lab Invest 57:729–736, 1987.
10. Bonkhoff H, Stein U, Remberger K: Androgen receptor status in endocrine-paracrine cell types of the normal, hyperplastic, and neoplastic human prostate. Virchows Arch [A] 423:291–294, 1993.
11. Krijnen J, Janssen P, Ruizveld de Winter J, et al.: Do neuroendocrine cells in human prostate cancer express androgen receptor? Histochemistry 100:393–398, 1993.
12. Battaglia S, Casali A, Botticelli A: Age-related distribution of endocrine cells in the human prostate: A quantitative study. Virchows Arch 424:165–168, 1994.
13. Cockett A, di Sant'Agnese P, Gopinath P, et al.: Rela-
tionship of neuroendocrine cells of prostate and serotonin to benign prostate hyperplasia. Urology 42:512–519, 1993.
14. di Sant'Agnese PA, de Mesy Jensen K: Endocrine-paracrine cells of the prostate and prostatic urethra; an ultrastructural study. Hum Pathol 15:1034–1041, 1984.
15. di Sant'Agnese PA: Calcitonin-like immunoreactive and bombesinlike immunoreactive endocrine-paracrine cells of the human prostate. Arch Pathol Lab Med 110:412–415, 1986.
16. di Sant'Agnese PA, de Mesy Jensen K: Calcitonin, katacalcin and calcitonin gene-related peptide in the human prostate: An immunocytochemical and immunoelectron microscopic study. Arch Pathol Lab Med 113:790–796, 1989.
17. Sunday M, Kaplan L, Motoyama E, et al.: Biology of disease. Gastrin-releasing peptide (mammalian bombesin) gene expression in health and disease. Lab Invest 59:5–24, 1988.
18. di Sant'Agnese PA, de Mesy Jensen KL: Somatostatin and/or somatostatinlike immunoreactive endocrine-paracrine cells in the human prostate gland. Arch Pathol Lab Med 108:693–696, 1984.
19. Fetissof F, Arbeille B, Guilloteau D, et al.: Glycoprotein hormone α-chain–immunoreactive endocrine cells in prostate and cloacal derived tissues. Arch Pathol Lab Med 111:836–840, 1987.
20. Iwamura M, Wu G, Abrahamsson P-A, et al.: Parathyroid hormone–related protein is expressed by prostatic neuroendocrine cells. Urology 43:667–674, 1994.
21. Wu G, Gershagen S, Iwamura M, et al.: Detection of parathyroid hormone–related protein mRNA in neuroendocrine cells of the prostate gland by in situ hybridization with exon specific probes. J Urol 151:296A, 1994.
22. Schmid K, Helpap B, Totsch M, et al.: Immunohistochemical localization of chromogranins A and B and secretogranin II in normal, hyperplastic, and neoplastic prostate. Histopathology 24:233–239, 1994.
23. Schwartz B, Iwamura M, Schoen S, et al.: Prostatic neuroendocrine cell products in human seminal plasma. J Urol 151:299A, 1994.
24. Iwamura M, Benning C, di Sant'Agnese P, et al.: Overexpression of human epidermal growth factor receptor and c-erbB-2 by neuroendocrine cells in normal prostatic tissue. Urology 43:838–843, 1994.
25. Ro JY, Tetu B, Ayala AG, et al.: Small cell carcinoma of the prostate: Immunohistochemical and electron microscopic studies of 18 cases. Cancer 59:977–982, 1987.
26. Tetu B, Ro JY, Ayala AG, et al.: Small cell carcinoma of the prostate part I: A clinicopathologic study of 20 cases. Cancer 59:1803–1809, 1987.
27. Almagro UA, Tieu TM, Remeniuk E, et al.: Argyrophilic, "carcinoid-like" prostatic carcinoma. Arch Pathol Lab Med 110:916–919, 1986.
28. Dauge MC, Delmas V: A.P.U.D. type endocrine tumour of the prostate: Incidence and prognosis in association with adenocarcinoma. In Murphy GP, Khoury S, Kuss R, et al. (eds): Progress in Clinical and Biological Medicine. New York: Alan R. Liss, 1986, pp 529–531.
29. Abrahamsson P-A, Wadstrom LB, Alumets J, et al.: Peptide-hormone- and serotonin-immunoreactive tumour cells in carcinoma of the prostate. Pathol Res Pract 182:298–307, 1987.
30. Turbat-Herrera EA, Herrera GA, Gore I, et al.: Neuro-

endocrine differentiation in prostatic carcinomas: A retrospective autopsy study. Arch Pathol Lab Med 112:1100–1106, 1988.

31. di Sant'Agnese PA, de Mesy Jensen KL: Neuroendocrine differentiation in prostatic carcinoma. Hum Pathol 18:849–856, 1987.

32. Adlakha H, Bostwick D: Paneth cell–like change in prostatic adenocarcinoma represents neuroendocrine differentiation. Report of 30 cases. Hum Pathol 25:135–139, 1994.

33. di Sant'Agnese PA: Neuroendocrine differentiation in prostatic adenocarcinoma does not represent true Paneth cell differentiation. Hum Pathol 25:115–16, 1994.

34. Aprikian A, Cordon-Cardo C, Fair W, et al.: Characterization of neuroendocrine differentiation in human benign prostate and prostatic adenocarcinoma. Cancer 71:3952–3965, 1993.

35. Bonkhoff H, Stein U, Remberger K: Multidirectional differentiation in the normal, hyperplastic, and neoplastic human prostate. Hum Pathol 25:42–46, 1994.

36. Cohen R, Glezerson G: Prostatic-specific antigen and prostate-specific acid phosphatase in neuroendocrine cells of prostate cancer. Arch Pathol Lab Med 116:65–66, 1992.

37. Rode J, Bentley A, Parkinson C: Paraganglial cells of urinary bladder and prostate: Potential diagnostic problem. J Clin Pathol 43:13–16, 1990.

38. Cohen R, Glezerson G, Haffejee Z: Neuro-endocrine cells—a new prognostic parameter in prostate cancer. Urol 68:258–262, 1991.

39. Berner A, Nesland J, Waehre H, et al.: Hormone resistant prostatic adenocarcinoma. An elevation of prognostic factors in pre- and post-treatment specimens. Br J Cancer 68:380–384, 1993.

40. Aprikian A, Cordon-Cardo C, Fair W, et al.: Neuroendocrine differentiation in metastatic prostatic adenocarcinoma. J Urol 151:914–919, 1994.

41. Van de Voorde W, Elgamal A, Van Poppel H, et al.: Morphologic and immunohistochemical changes in prostate cancer after preoperative hormonal therapy.

A comparative study of radical prostatectomies. Cancer 74:3164–3175, 1994.

42. Epstein J, Partin A, Veltri R: Neuroendocrine (NE) differentiation in prostate cancer: Enhanced prediction of progression following radical prostatectomy. Modern Pathol 8:75A, 1995.

43. Grignon D, Kaplan R, Sakr W, et al.: Neuroendocrine (NE) differentiation as a prognostic indicator in locally advanced prostate cancer (PCa): A study based on RTOG protocol 8610. Modern Pathol 8:76A, 1995.

44. Schultz D, Amin M, Shetty S: Chromogranin and synaptophysin staining in post hormonally treated prostatic carcinoma (Ca). Modern Pathol 8:83A, 1995.

45. Tarle M, Rados N: Investigation on serum neuron-specific enolase in prostate cancer diagnosis and monitoring: Comparative study of a multiple tumor marker assay. Prostate 19:23, 1991.

46. Kadmon D, Thompson T, Lynch G, et al.: Elevated plasma chromogranin-A concentrations in prostatic carcinoma. J Urol 146:358–361, 1991.

47. Bang Y, Pirnia F, Fang W, et al.: Terminal neuroendocrine differentiation of human prostate carcinoma cells in response to increased intracellular cyclic AMP. Proc Natl Acad Sci USA 91:5330–5334, 1994.

48. Bonkhoff H, Wernert N, Dhom G, et al.: Relation of endocrine-paracrine cells to cell proliferation in normal, hyperplastic and neoplastic human prostate. Prostate 19:91–98, 1991.

49. Segal N, Cohen R, Haffejee Z, et al.: BCL-2 proto-oncogene expression in prostate cancer and its relationship to the prostatic neuroendocrine cell. Arch Pathol Lab Med 118:616–618, 1994.

50. Sunday M, Willett C, Patidar K, et al.: Modulation of oncogene and tumor suppressor gene expression in a hamster model of chronic lung injury with varying degrees of pulmonary neuroendocrine cell hyperplasia. Lab Invest 70:875–888, 1994.

51. Hoosein N, Logothetis C, Chung L: Differential effects of peptide hormones bombesin, vasoactive intestinal polypeptide and somatostatin analog RC-160 on the invasive capacity of human prostatic carcinoma cells. J Urol 149:1209–1213, 1993.

21

SOFT TISSUE NEOPLASMS AND OTHER UNUSUAL TUMORS OF PROSTATE, INCLUDING UNCOMMON CARCINOMAS

Mary Leader, Elaine Kay, and Caitriona Barry Walsh

In this chapter we describe a variety of benign and malignant soft tissue tumors and proliferations of the prostate. In addition, some uncommon epithelial neoplasms of the prostate are also discussed.

A diverse group of soft tissue neoplasms occur in the prostate,[1] including benign soft tissue tumors, sarcomas, and a group of benign reactive proliferations of mesenchymal tissue termed "pseudosarcomas." The latter need to be distinguished from sarcomas. Diagnostic errors can be made, particularly when tissue volume is limited, as it is in fine-needle aspiration biopsy (FNAB) specimens.

BENIGN PSEUDOSARCOMATOUS LESIONS OF THE PROSTATE AND LESIONS OF UNCERTAIN POTENTIAL

A variety of benign proliferative lesions occurring in the stroma of the prostate may be confused with sarcomas. These lesions show cytologic atypia, and sometimes a significant number of mitoses. Such entities must be remembered and considered when examining tissue from FNAB or small core biopsy, to avoid a misdiagnosis of sarcoma.

Included in this group are phyllodes tumors in which epithelium and stroma are admixed but the stroma shows atypia; stromal hyperplasia with atypia, in which the stroma shows atypia but epithelium is lacking; postoperative spindle cell nodules with atypia; and spindle cell nodules with atypia without prior surgery. Granulomatous prostatitis will not be considered further here, since it should be readily recognizable by its inflammatory and histiocytic appearance.

Phyllodes Tumor of the Prostate

Lesions in the prostate that resemble phyllodes tumors of the breast are well-documented. The terms "phyllodes-type atypical prostatic hyperplasia," "cystadenoleiomyofibroma," and "cystosarcoma phyllodes of the prostate" have also been applied. A small number of cases are documented, but the incidence is probably much greater, because many cases are not reported.[2–8] These tumors occur in adults (age range 23 to 74 years) and present clinically with symptoms of retention, dysuria, and prostatism. They show a distinctive radiologic appearance on computed tomography (CT) with enlargement of the prostate but without extraprostatic spread and without obstruction of the ureters. Collections of fluid (cystic spaces) may be identified within the tumor at ultrasonography. Two histologic components are present. The tumor shows a proliferation of cystic glands and elongated compressed glands in a cellular stroma composed of plump spindle cells. The cellularity of the stroma varies from being very cellular in some areas to low cellularity in others with areas of sclerosis and patchy edema. The epithelial component is composed of glands lined by cuboidal or columnar cells, which retain a definite additional basal cell layer that can be confirmed immunohistochemically with high–molecular weight cytokeratin. The epithelial component may show hyperplasia with foci of papillary tufting and a cribriform pattern. It shows reactivity for prostate-specific antigen (PSA).[7] Squamous metaplasia may be seen. Epithelial cytologic atypia is not evident. The glands may show considerable compression by the stromal component, which is composed of spindle cells that are vimentin positive, sometimes show desmin reactivity, and may show a spectrum of cytological atypia from low- to high-grade. A high-grade tumor is characterized by an increased stromal-epithelial ratio, increased stromal cellularity, marked cytologic atypia, and an elevated mitotic index. It is important to sample these tumors widely as the stromal hypercellularity and pleomorphism may be focal in otherwise rather bland neoplastic stroma. A sarcomatous component may also develop over a period of time after numerous local recurrences. Mitotic figures are variable and necrosis may or may not be present. The behavior of these tumors is predicted by the degree of cellularity, nuclear pleomorphism, mitotic activity, and necrosis. No clearly defined histologic criteria are available to allow a definitive distinction between benign and malignant variants. Many of these tumors develop local recurrences repeatedly. Some cases with overtly malignant stroma have metastasized to bones and lung.

Phyllodes tumors are distinguished from postoperative spindle cell nodules by the presence of epithelial cells in the former. Mitotic figures may be present in both and are of little help in the differential diagnosis. However, less nuclear pleomorphism is detected in spindle cell nodules. Atypical stromal hyperplasia is excluded owing to the presence of epithe-

lium within the phyllodes tumor. Atypical stromal hyperplasia is also less cellular and lacks mitotic figures and necrosis. The differential diagnosis of phyllodes tumor includes prostatic cysts, müllerian duct cysts of the utricle,[9] and tumors of the seminal vesicle. These tumors must be considered as potentially aggressive and treated with wide surgical resection. Radiotherapy and chemotherapy are not recommended.

Stromal Hyperplasia with Atypia

Pure stromal hyperplasia is found occasionally in prostates with typical nodular hyperplasia. In these cases there is no evidence of pleomorphism or mitotic activity. In contrast, stromal hyperplasia with atypia is a rare entity: only three well-documented reports have been described.[3, 10] In this situation there is hyperplasia of the stroma with no associated epithelial hyperplasia. The spindle cell proliferation is atypical and shows hyperchromasia and pleomorphism. A striking feature is the presence of hyperchromatic bizarre nuclei. Mitotic figures are usually absent or scanty. One case described by Young and Scully showed evidence of infarction in the adjacent prostate, and the nuclear pleomorphism may have been due, in this instance, to degenerative change. S100 protein, desmin, and myoglobin staining in this case were negative. The bizarre nuclei in this condition are analogous to those found in bizarre leiomyomas, in ancient schwannomas, and in nasal polyps. They are thought to represent a degenerative change. On DNA evaluation these nuclei are tetraploid or euploid.

Attah and Powell[11] described three cases termed ''atypical stromal hyperplasia of the prostate.'' However, these probably are not genuine cases since two resembled smooth muscle tumors, but tumor markers were not available at the time. The third case resembled fibroadenoma without stromal atypia, and does not fit this category.

Sarcoma is readily distinguished from stromal hyperplasia with atypia by the absence or paucity of mitotic figures and necrosis in the latter. If there is doubt about the diagnosis, further material should be sought to permit full evaluation. The single reported case of fibromyxoid tumor in the prostate[12] is probably identical to the entity of ''atypical stromal hyperplasia.''

Bizarre hyperchromatic nuclei have occasionally been reported in the stroma between

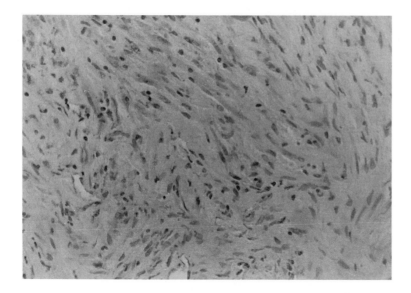

Figure 21–1. Postoperative spindle cell nodule. This shows a spindle cell infiltrate admixed with inflammatory cells. Pleomorphism is minimal. Some dilated vessels are also present. (H&E reduced 37% from ×200.)

normal prostatic glands.[10] These cells are vimentin positive and desmin negative. They are probably similar to the bizarre stromal cells sometimes seen in the stroma of nasal polyps, in the cervix, and occasionally in the breast. Similar bizarre stromal cells have been described in phyllodes tumor of the prostate and in bizarre leiomyoma, where the stromal-epithelial setting is different.

Postoperative Spindle Cell Nodule
(Figs. 21–1, 21–2)

This well-described but rare condition occurs within a few months of prostate surgery,

generally in a periurethral site.[13] A similar type of reaction is described in the cervix and vagina after vaginal hysterectomy.[13] This condition is characterized by a proliferation of plump spindle cells arranged as intersecting fascicles each surrounded by a delicate network of blood vessels. When small, these appearances may simulate Kaposi's sarcoma. Mitotic figures may range from 1 to 25 per 10 hpf (high power fields). Atypical mitotic figures are exceptional. Pleomorphism usually is not a feature. Necrosis is occasionally observed. Scattered chronic inflammatory cells are seen within the spindle cell proliferation. This is helpful when excluding stromal hyperplasia and sarcoma. Nodular fasciitis may be consid-

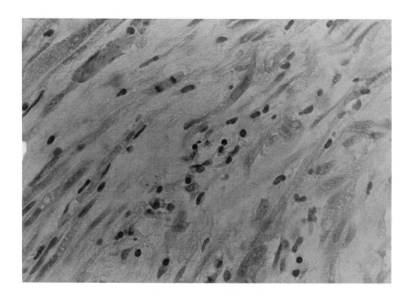

Figure 21–2. This highlights the spindle cells seen within the infiltrate, which show mild pleomorphism admixed with inflammatory cell infiltrate and an occasional normal mitotic figure. (H&E reduced 37% from ×400.)

ered in the differential diagnosis, but this condition is not reported in the prostate. In addition, the postoperative spindle cell nodule lacks the myxoid stroma and storiform pattern often seen in nodular fasciitis.

The most important differential diagnosis of a spindle cell nodule identified on Tru-Cut biopsy is sarcoma. When material is limited, the presence of a spindle cell proliferation with mitotic figures may prompt a diagnosis of malignancy. Many of the earlier cases described in the literature were misdiagnosed as leiomyosarcoma. Whenever the diagnosis of sarcoma is raised on Tru-Cut biopsy, a history of surgery should be sought and the differential diagnosis of postoperative spindle cell nodule carefully considered and excluded. The absence of pleomorphism, the presence of scattered inflammatory cells, and the history of recent surgery should prevent misdiagnosis.

Spindle Cell Proliferation Without Previous Surgery

Cases of a lesion similar to the postoperative spindle cell proliferation but without antecedent surgery are exceedingly rare.[3] The pathogenesis of these lesions is unclear, but may include a focal stromal response during postinflammation repair and restitution (see Chapter 4).

BENIGN SOFT TISSUE TUMORS OF THE PROSTATE

Benign soft tissue tumors of the prostate are rare. Those most frequently encountered are leiomyomas, fibromas, and hemangiomas.

Leiomyoma[14]

These tumors show features similar to those of leiomyoma at any other site. Approximately 60 cases are documented in the literature. Leiomyomas present with symptoms of prostatism, or occasionally rectal symptoms.[15] They are composed of bland spindle cells with blunt-ended nuclei placed in the center of eosinophilic cytoplasm, and show the expected immunoreactivity for desmin, muscle-specific actin, and smooth muscle–specific actin. However, the latter two antigens are not absolutely specific for smooth muscle differentiation.

Leiomyomas show no pleomorphism and no significant mitotic figures. The cellular variant differs from the classic leiomyoma only in that it is more cellular. It lacks pleomorphism and shows fewer than two mitoses per 10 hpf.[15, 16] The variant atypical leiomyoma is a benign leiomyoma with atypical, sometimes bizarre, nuclei, some of which may be multinucleate but with no increase in mitoses.[15] This phenomenon is analogous to the nuclear atypia seen in benign long-standing (ancient) schwannomas. These tumors often contain areas of hyalinization and are rarely very cellular.[3] Atypical leiomyoma should be distinguished from atypical stromal hyperplasia of the prostate. The latter lacks the circumscription of a leiomyoma and shows a mixed infiltrate of fibroblasts, smooth muscle cells, and collagen. Desmin reactivity is of limited value: diffuse staining confirms the diagnosis of leiomyoma; focal or negative staining is nondiscriminatory. Criteria used to separate benign from malignant smooth muscle tumors of the prostate have not been fully elucidated, owing to the small number of leiomyosarcomas reported. Until such guidelines are available it is probably prudent to use the criteria of malignancy applied to other soft tissue sites (e.g., greater than 2 mitoses per 10 hpf and marked nuclear atypia or necrosis indicating malignancy). A single case of leiomyoblastoma has also been described.[3]

Fibroma

Fibromas of the prostate are described in the older literature, but these are difficult to distinguish from small stromal nodules (stromal hyperplasia), which occur in as many as 25% of prostatectomy specimens.[17]

Hemangiomas

Benign hemangiomas also occur in the prostate. One case "as large as a child's head" has been reported.[18]

SARCOMAS

Prostatic sarcomas occur in a younger age group than do carcinomas. Ash coined the phrase, "Before fifty sarcoma, after fifty carcinoma." Fifty percent of prostatic sarcomas are rhabdomyosarcomas, 28% are leiomyosarcomas, approximately 15% are unclassifiable, and the remainder include malignant peripheral nerve sheath tumors, fibrosarcomas, malignant fibrous histiocytoma (MFH), chondrosarcoma, and osteosarcomas. Most muscle-derived sarcomas of childhood are rhabdomyosarcomas, whereas leiomyosarcomas are the dominant type in adults. One third of primary prostatic sarcomas occur in children younger than 10 years, the majority of them rhabdomyosarcomas.[19] Clinical symptoms are most often related to obstructive urinary tract symptoms, including frequency, dysuria, hematuria, and difficulty in urination.[20] Constipation may occur secondarily to involvement of the rectum.[21] Mean duration of symptoms at presentation is 1 month (range, 3 days to 24 months).[20] Anemia is evident in 67% of cases, leukocytosis in 37%, and pyuria in 42%.[20]

Sarcomas arising in the prostate may be relatively small at presentation owing to early production of urinary tract symptoms. There are, however, notable exceptions. In general they have a better prognosis than sarcomas arising elsewhere in the pelvis.[22]

The prognosis of prostate sarcomas correlates with size, grade, age (childhood sarcomas have a poorer prognosis), and negative surgical resection margins.[23] A review of urologic sarcomas from the Memorial Sloan-Kettering Cancer Center showed actual relapse-free survival rates at 1, 3, and 5 years of 78%, 55%, and 40%, respectively.[23] Other reports suggest sarcomas of the prostate (including rhabdomyosarcomas) have a 60% 5-year survival when treated with combined surgery, chemotherapy, and radiotherapy.[24] The use of chemotherapy before radiotherapy or surgery did not improve the bladder salvage rate in a group of sarcomas of the bladder and prostate.[25]

A number of etiologic factors have been implicated in the pathogenesis of sarcomas, including alkylating agents,[26] irradiation,[27] and immunosuppressive therapy.[28] Despite the documented association between soft tissue sarcomas and viruses in animals, no such association has been found in human sarcomas. Sarcomas are also increased in certain familial syndromes, including neurofibromatosis (7% to 17% lifetime risk of developing malignant peripheral nerve sheath tumors),[29] basal cell nevus syndrome, familial adenomatous polyposis,[30] and Li-Fraumeni syndrome.

Macroscopically, sarcomas of the prostate may range from 2 to 24 cm,[20] and the prostate may be cystic, rubbery, soft, or hard.[21]

Rhabdomyosarcoma

Rhabdomyosarcomas are the fourth most common malignant tumor of childhood. In this age group, 21% of rhabdomyosarcomas occur in the prostate and genitourinary system.[31] They are the commonest primary sarcoma of the prostate in children. The majority of childhood rhabdomyosarcomas are embryonal.[32-34] By contrast, rhabdomyosarcomas are uncommon in adults older than 50 years. The most common type of rhabdomyosarcoma in adults is alveolar; the embryonal type is only occasionally reported.[33] Rhabdomyosarcomas may present as small lesions confined to the prostate or may extend to adjacent tissues at the time of presentation. The histopathologic features of prostatic rhabdomyosarcoma are similar to those in other sites. Embryonal rhabdomyosarcoma is composed of cells with round or oval or spindle hyperchromatic nuclei with a narrow rim of cytoplasm, which in the better-differentiated cases may show cross-striations (Fig. 21–3). Tadpole and strap cells may also be identified. Tumor phenotype is confirmed by positive staining for desmin, myoglobin, muscle-specific actin, or smooth muscle–specific actin. Staining for myoglobin and desmin is seen in only about 60% of cases of formalin-fixed tumors.[35] The differential diagnosis in children includes neuroblastoma, primitive neuroectodermal tumor, Ewing's tumor, and lymphoma. In adults the differential diagnosis includes small cell carcinoma and lymphoma. Rhabdoid tumors, while also a consideration in children, have not been reported in the prostate. Immunocytochemistry in prostatic rhabdomyosarcoma can be supplemented with electron microscopy, which shows large cells containing segments of sarcolemma and small cells with rough endoplasmic reticulum and free ribosomes, but lacking myofibrils. The alveolar subtype shows a nesting or lobular pattern and shows a similar immunocytochemical phenotype. Pleomorphic rhabdomyosarcomas are also described in the prostate, but are rare.[20, 22] Immunocytochemical confirmation is essential to distinguish these tumors from other pleomorphic sarcomas such as undifferentiated carcinoma, undifferentiated lymphoma, and pleomorphic malignant fibrous histiocytomas.

Previously, prognosis for this tumor was dismal. Now, however, with a combined approach of surgery, radiotherapy, and chemotherapy, response is found in most cases and the 3-year

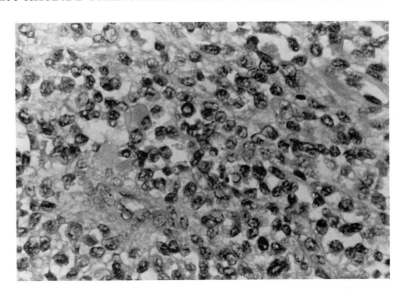

Figure 21–3. Pleomorphic rhabdomyosarcoma. Most of the tumor is composed of undifferentiated cells with an irregular chromatin pattern, moderate pleomorphism, and a variable amount of eosinophilic cytoplasm, which is scanty in most cells. Occasional cells with more abundant cytoplasm are evident. On oil immersion, these showed cross striations. Immunocytochemistry confirmed positivity for myoglobin and desmin. (H&E reduced 37% from ×400.)

survival rate is 60% in these cases.[22, 36, 37] The bladder can be conserved in as many as 60%.[38, 39] A trial of chemotherapy before surgery for genitourinary rhabdomyosarcoma showed no improvement over standard surgery followed by radiation and chemotherapy.[25] When radiotherapy is used in combination with surgery side effects are significant. Forty-seven percent of patients suffer from urinary symptoms such as enuresis, dribbling, or bladder contractures.[40] A study is under way to determine if hyperfractioned radiation may reduce these side effects.[41]

Leiomyosarcoma

While rhabdomyosarcoma is the most common sarcoma of the prostate in childhood, leiomyosarcoma is the most common in adulthood (26%).[20] No immunohistochemically documented cases are reported in childhood. These tumors are usually large at presentation and often have infiltrated adjacent structures.[42–44] Most patients present between age 40 and 70 years.[20, 42]

Microscopically, the tumor is composed of interlacing fascicles of spindle cells with blunt-ended nuclei and eosinophilic cytoplasm that show varying degrees of nuclear atypia (Fig. 21–4).[20, 45, 46] Necrosis may or may not be a feature. As yet there are too few cases for evaluation of mitotic activity as a guide to malignancy. Although some authors favor using criteria similar to those for uterine leiomyosarcomas, it might be more prudent to adopt a cautious stance and indicate that all smooth muscle tumors with more than 2 mitoses per 10 hpf may have metastatic potential.[47]

Ploidy analysis may also be a useful adjunct in this group of tumors, because aneuploidy is regarded as an indicator of malignancy. Diploidy, however, can also be found in malignant tumors. Positive immunohistochemical staining is expected with muscle-specific actin and smooth muscle–specific actin. Desmin is demonstrated in approximately 60%.[35] Occasional cases show reactivity for cytokeratin. S100 protein immunoreactivity can be seen focally in a small number of cells in rare cases. This should not prompt a diagnosis of malignant schwannoma. The prognosis of leiomyosarcoma of the prostate approximates the survival of retroperitoneal soft tissue sarcomas with a 55% one-year survival.[42] Metastases have been described in a variety of sites. Bony metastases may be osteolytic.[48] One case is described associated with a conventional carcinoma.[49]

Other Sarcomas

Other primary sarcomas of the prostate are exceedingly rare. Those described include hemangiopericytoma,[50] malignant fibrous histiocytoma,[51, 52] osteosarcoma,[53] and chondrosarcoma.[54] Fibrosarcomas are reported in the older literature, but it is likely that many of these would be reclassified as leiomyosarcoma when immunocytochemical studies are applied.

Pheochromocytomas (whilst not strictly sar-

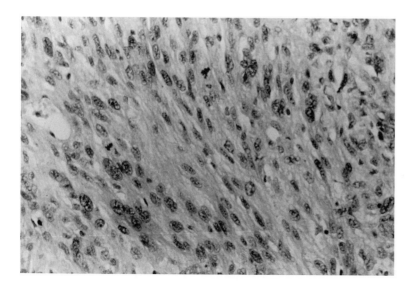

Figure 21–4. Sections show a leiomyosarcoma. The tumor is composed of spindle cells with chromatin with an open stippled pattern, moderate pleomorphism, and numerous mitoses. (H&E reduced 37% from ×400.)

comas) have also been reported in the prostate.[55] One with malignant behavior is described. These arise from paraganglia of the prostate, which have been found in 8% of radical prostatectomy specimens, lateral and slightly posterior to the prostatic capsule, often in association with neurovascular bundles.[56]

MELANOCYTIC LESIONS OF THE PROSTATE

These lesions are exceedingly rare and may be found in three different forms: melanosis, cellular blue nevus, and malignant melanoma, either primary or metastatic. Melanosis is a condition in which melanin is found in stromal cells of the prostate and in glandular epithelium. Melanosis has been reported in 0.07% to 10% of normal prostate glands.[57, 58] The origin of melanosis in stromal cells is debated. Rawles, working with vertebrates, demonstrated that melanoblasts arise from the neural crest and migrate through the body to their ultimate destination, where they transform into melanocytes.[59] Nakai and Rappaport have shown that under experimental conditions in Syrian hamsters Schwann cells or neuroendocrine cells or both can transform into melanocytes.[60] Although either of these theories may explain the presence of melanin in stromal cells, its detection in epithelial cells is more difficult to understand. Ultrastructural and immunohistochemical studies have shown that melanin-containing epithelial cells lack melanosomes.[61] Therefore, it seems most likely that epithelial cells in the prostate (benign or malignant) acquire melanin by phagocytosis from incontinent stromal melanocytes.[61]

Blue nevi of the prostate have been the subject of a small number of case reports.[57, 62–65] These lesions are similar to those in the skin and are characterized by elongated fusiform melanin-containing cells in the stroma. It is important to remember that they may occur in the prostate so as not to misdiagnose them as malignant melanoma.

Primary malignant melanoma is described in the prostate.[66, 67] Some of these have been of prostatic urethral origin.[66, 67] The origin of these cells is thought to be similar to that of melanosis. It is important that these lesions are carefully distinguished from cellular blue nevi to avoid overdiagnosis of malignancy. The prostate is involved in 3% of cases of disseminated melanoma at autopsy.[67] Rare cases of metastatic melanoma to primary prostatic adenocarcinoma are also described.[68]

UNCOMMON CARCINOMAS

Squamous Cell Carcinoma

Squamous cell carcinoma of the prostate is a rare primary neoplasm that accounts for 0.5% of all prostate carcinomas.[69] It must be distinguished from secondary spread to the prostate of a primary squamous cell carcinoma of the bladder, especially in regions where schistosomiasis is endemic. It must also be distinguished from squamous cell metaplasia, which is found in association with radiation or hormone therapy, with chronic prostatitis or infarction.[70]

Criteria required for the diagnosis of primary squamous cell carcinoma of the prostate include absence of squamous cell carcinoma in the bladder or other site together with the following histopathologic criteria: (1) malignant neoplastic behavior judged by an invasive growth pattern or cytologic features of malignancy; (2) evidence of squamous differentiation (e.g., squamous pearls, intercellular bridges, or other evidence of keratinization); and (3) no glandular differentiation. In practice, some of these carcinomas, while having an invasive growth pattern, may appear cytologically bland whereas others are less well-differentiated.

Primary prostatic squamous cell carcinoma differs from prostatic adenocarcinoma in its clinical presentation, response to treatment, and histogenesis. Clinically these tumors present between ages 52 and 79 years (average, 64 years)[69] with symptoms usually related to obstructive effects. Clinical rectal examination may suggest a normal gland. Despite immunohistochemical demonstration of PSA and prostatic acid phosphatase (PAP) within the squamous cell carcinoma, serum levels usually are not elevated, even in the presence of metastatic disease. Furthermore, bony metastases are usually osteolytic, unlike those of adenocarcinoma. Histologically the tumors show classic features of squamous cell carcinoma (Fig. 21–5). Differentiation may vary from well- to poorly differentiated, and in the well-differ-

entiated tumor there can be difficulty, separating it from squamous metaplasia, especially when the lesion is small. In these cases the presence of an invasive pattern is essential. Immunohistochemistry usually shows PSA or PAP within the tumor. Aneuploidy has been reported in one case.[71] These tumors behave more aggressively than adenocarcinoma (mean survival, 15 months).[69] A variety of different surgical approaches have been used, including total prostatectomy, transurethral prostatic resection, and orchiectomy. Extensive surgery, including cystoprostatectomy, abdominoperineal resection, and node dissection, was unsuccessful in one case. Estrogen therapy is of no benefit. Chemotherapy led to a 5-month remission in one case with systemic metastases.

The histogenesis of this tumor is unknown. Many different theories have been considered, including origin from a pluripotential stem cell[69]; others suggest derivation from basal or reserve cells of prostatic acini. An origin from the prostatic urethral urothelium is suggested by some,[71–73] whereas others suggest an origin from the transitional epithelium of the periurethral ducts.[74] The common acinar columnar cell has also been proposed as the source.[74] On the basis of immunoreactivity within the squamous carcinoma for PSA and its occasional association with adenocarcinoma an origin from prostatic adenocarcinoma is also likely.[69] A final theory, which defies current concepts of carcinogenesis, is an origin from squamous metaplasia. In an 8-year follow-up of squamous metaplasia, no squamous cell car-

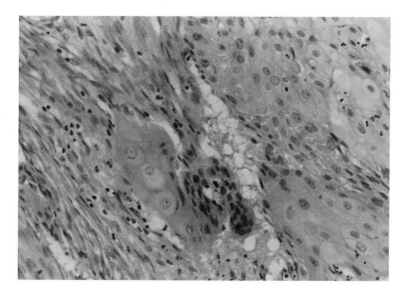

Figure 21–5. Squamous cell carcinoma. This shows prostatic stroma infiltrated by carcinoma composed of cells with large vesicular nuclei and abundant eosinophilic cytoplasm. It has an infiltrating tumour margin and shows mild pleomorphism. (H&E reduced 37% from ×400.)

cinoma developed.[75] Our own belief is that it is derived from a pluripotential stem cell.

Adenosquamous Carcinoma

Adenosquamous carcinoma of the prostate is much rarer than squamous cell carcinoma and than tumors showing mixed adenocarcinoma and transitional cell carcinoma (TCC). Six cases are described.[76, 77] In most cases these tumors have developed following treatment of an adenocarcinoma by either radiotherapy or estrogen therapy, or by estrogen therapy alone in one case.[76] The duration of estrogen therapy ranged from 2 to 9 years. The interval from diagnosis of conventional adenocarcinoma and subsequent adenosquamous cell carcinoma ranged from 4 to 8 years. Obstructive urinary tract symptoms were the presenting symptom in most cases. Stage of disease at presentation ranged from stage B to stage D2. Serum PAP was raised in some cases but not in others. The response to estrogen therapy was poor in all cases when it was administered.

Transitional Cell Carcinoma

TCC of the prostate may arise as a primary prostatic tumor or may spread to the prostate from a primary bladder carcinoma.[78] Rare cases of primary TCC occur as mixed carcinomas showing both transitional and adenocarcinomatous differentiation.

Primary Transitional Cell Carcinoma

Primary TCC accounts for some 2% to 4% of all primary prostatic carcinomas.[79] They arise from the periurethral prostate ducts. A normal bladder is essential for the diagnosis of primary prostatic TCC. The tumors usually present with symptoms of prostate obstruction. Digital rectal examination is normal in 50% of cases. The tumor may be solid or papillary and may be well- or poorly differentiated. Because it originates in periprostatic glands, diagnosis is much more likely on transurethral biopsy than on transrectal biopsy. Serum PSA levels are usually normal. The prognosis is usually poor, and most patients die within 24 months of diagnosis.[80] Radical surgical treatment with a cystoprostatectomy is the treatment of choice. The role of chemotherapy is controversial for metastatic disease. These tumors are unresponsive to orchiectomy or hormone therapy. A single case that presented as a skin metastasis has been reported.[81]

Secondary Transitional Cell Carcinoma in the Prostate

Secondary involvement of the prostate by TCC is not uncommon and was detected in 43% of patients who underwent radical cystectomy for TCC in one series.[82] Ninety-six percent of these cases showed prostatic urethral involvement and 6% showed a normal prostatic urethra, but tumor was present in periurethral structures.

Secondary involvement of the prostate may show two different patterns that have prognostic significance. Carcinoma in situ may be seen involving the prostatic urethra or ducts; or invasive TCC of the prostate may be found. The latter (i.e., stromal invasion) may be seen without glandular involvement. Noninvasive prostatic patterns are usually seen with low-stage bladder carcinoma with prognosis similar to low-stage bladder tumors treated by radical cystectomy. Invasive patterns are usually seen with high-stage bladder carcinomas, and 5-year survival rates are low.[79]

TCC of the bladder invading the prostate must also be distinguished from prostatic adenocarcinoma. The distinction may be difficult for high-grade tumors. High-grade TCC tends to show more nuclear pleomorphism than high-grade prostatic adenocarcinoma. In addition, prostatic adenocarcinoma typically shows nucleoli in the majority of nuclei. Immunohistochemistry is also advisable in this situation, as the majority of prostatic adenocarcinomas, even high-grade ones, show immunostaining for PSA or PAP.

Rare Variants of Adenocarcinoma

Four rare types of differentiation in prostatic adenocarcinoma deserve special mention.

Mucinous (Colloid) Carcinoma

This rare variant accounts for approximately 0.04% of documented prostatic adenocarcinomas in the literature. Whilst early reports lacked a clear definition of these tumors it was recently defined as a tumor that shows lakes of extravasated mucin in at least 25% of the tumor (Fig. 21–6).[83] In addition, tumor cells or tumor clusters should be evident floating within the mucin lakes. Contrary to previous reports, probably based on the behavior of tumors with less rigid histologic diagnostic criteria for percentage of mucinous differentiation, this tumor frequently metastasizes to bone and is often associated with increased serum PAP levels. PSA and PAP can also be demonstrated immunohistochemically in the tumor. Signet ring differentiation is rare. Generally, these tumors are at an advanced stage at clinical presentation and fail to respond to hormone manipulation.[83] They must be distinguished from typical adenocarcinoma showing increased mucin production following estrogen therapy and from secondary spread to the prostate from rectal or bladder urachal carcinomas.

Cribriform Carcinoma

One group has accepted this as a definite subtype of prostate adenocarcinoma.[84] Prostate tumors may show a cribriform pattern similar to that described in the breast and are associated with large-volume carcinomas and poor differentiation. They are regarded as equivalent to Gleason grade 4 carcinomas.[84] (See Chapter 11 for a definitive appraisal of these tumors.)

Adenocarcinoma with Signet Ring Differentiation

Signet ring differentiation is common in adenocarcinomas of the breast, gastrointestinal tract, and bladder; however, it is rarely described in prostatic adenocarcinomas.[85] The designation of signet cell carcinoma should be reserved for tumors with more than 50% signet ring differentiation. The signet ring cell is defined as a cell whose nucleus is displaced by a cytoplasmic mass (Fig. 21–7). It is not always due to intracytoplasmic mucin and the term "signet ring" has been applied to lymphomas,[86, 87] thyroid tumors,[88, 89] oligodendrogliomas,[90] smooth muscle tumors,[91] and melanomas.

In the prostate, signet ring cells may stain for mucins (diastase-resistant, PAS-positive, but mucicarmine-negative[92]) or may be mucin-negative and PSA- and PAP-positive.[85] Ultrastructurally, cytoplasmic vacuoles of intracytoplasmic lumina lacking mucin and lipid have been described. It would seem that signet ring differentiation may be due to a variety of causes, including mucin, fat, or cytoplasmic lumina. An important practical point when examining small prostatic biopsies is that degenerate lymphocytes and smooth muscle cells may adopt a signet ring appearance. These are differentiated from prostatic epithelial cells showing signet ring differentiation by negative mucin stains and negativity for PSA and PAP.[93] Metastatic signet ring tumor must be excluded before making a diagnosis of primary prostatic signet ring carcinoma. Positive mucicarmine

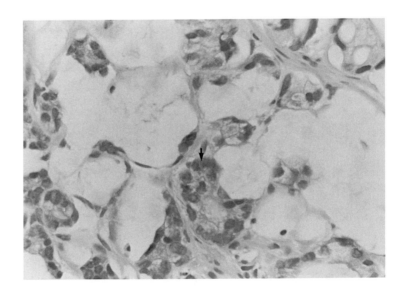

Figure 21–6. Colloid carcinoma. A gland (*arrow*) is surrounded by pools of mucin that stained for PASD and Alcian blue. More than 25% of the tumor was occupied by extravasated mucin. (H&E reduced 40% from ×400.)

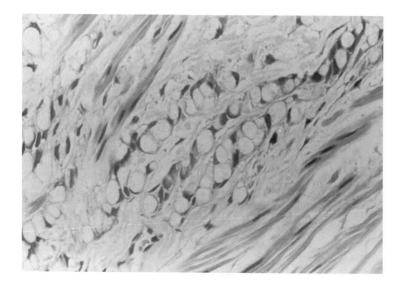

Figure 21–7. Signet ring–cell carcinoma. The signet ring cells are well displayed, showing vacuolated cells with a nucleus pushed to one side. Mucin stains were positive in this case, but prostatic immunohistochemical staining was negative. The tumor contained more than 50% signet ring cells. (H&E reduced 40% from ×400.)

staining should prompt the possibility of metastasis, as most primary prostatic signet ring cell carcinomas are mucicarmine negative. This would be supported by negative staining for PSA and PAP. Prognosis is poor.

Endometrioid Adenocarcinoma of the Prostate

This variant also has been variably described in the literature. Previously classified as an individual type of carcinoma, its existence as a discrete entity is now disputed.[94] Originally, in view of their consistent origin from the prostatic verumontanum, these tumors were thought to be of müllerian origin (see Chapter 8). This, together with their marked resemblance to endometrial adenocarcinoma of the uterus, suggested an estrogen dependence, in which case estrogen therapy would be contraindicated. However, in view of positive staining with prostatic epithelial markers and coexistence with classic adenocarcinoma of the prostate, these are now regarded as large duct prostatic adenocarcinomas with histologic features similar to those of endometrial carcinoma. They are termed "adenocarcinoma with endometrioid features." In a review of 2600 cases of prostatic carcinomas, 10 cases with a predominantly endometrioid pattern were detected.[94] A 5-year survival rate of 15% (mean, 37%) was noted.[95] There is a variable response to hormone manipulation.[94, 95]

Adenocarcinoma with endometrioid features occurs predominantly in older men.

Presenting symptoms are prostatism, urgency, frequency, and hematuria. Unless the tumor has infiltrated the prostate extensively or there is an intercurrent prostatic adenocarcinoma, rectal examination of the prostate may be normal. In about 50% of cases the prostate is enlarged and nodular. At cystoscopy polypoid nodules are seen emanating from the prostatic ducts.

Morphologically, the tumor shows histologic features similar to those of endometrial adenocarcinoma. The tumor is characterized by the presence of intraductal papillary growth, especially toward the urethral margin of the tumor (Fig. 21–8). The carcinoma is composed more of complex glands with less of a papillary pattern toward the peripheral zone of the prostate (Fig. 21–9). Varying grades of nuclear pleomorphism and mitotic activity are evident in different tumors.

Immunohistochemically these tumors stain for PAP and PSA. This staining pattern provides evidence that these tumors are simply a variant of prostatic adenocarcinoma. Serum PAP and PSA values are often normal at presentation, as these tumors usually present early owing to their origin close to the prostatic urethra; however, in patients with a large component of acinar prostatic carcinoma[96] as many as one-third of patients are stage D at diagnosis.[96]

The prognosis for this tumor is poorer than for typical prostatic adenocarcinoma. Five-year survival varies from 15% to 40%. Where metastases develop, the endometrioid component is usually involved, suggesting that it may be the

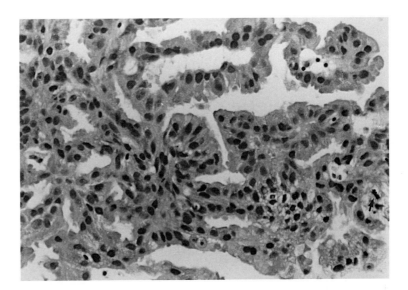

Figure 21–8. Endometrioid adenocarcinoma of the prostate. This shows well-defined papillae and glandular differentiation with mild pleomorphism and an occasional mitosis (*arrow*). (H&E reduced 37% from ×400.)

more aggressive component. Some reports suggest that these tumors may not be hormonally sensitive; however, others[96] noted a good response to estrogen therapy and orchiectomy. In summary, adenocarcinomas with an endometrioid pattern are not regarded as a special subtype of carcinoma, but should be recognized, since they appear to have a more aggressive pattern than the usual acinar prostatic adenocarcinomas.

Adenoid Cystic-like Carcinoma

A tumor that is morphologically similar to adenoid cystic carcinoma of the salivary glands has been reported on a few occasions in the prostate.[97–101] Morphologically this tumor shows a punched-out sievelike proliferation formed by two populations of cells. The basaloid cells have stippled chromatin, and the inner (ductal lining) cells are cuboidal or columnar. Cytologic atypia is never marked and mitoses are scanty. The cribriform spaces surround basophilic secretion or hyalinized eosinophilic material. The histochemical staining reactions are similar to those of adenoid cystic carcinoma of the salivary gland. Foci of basal cell hyperplasia are invariably present, and keratinization of the duct and columnar or cuboidal cells may be evident.

There is debate as to whether these are true

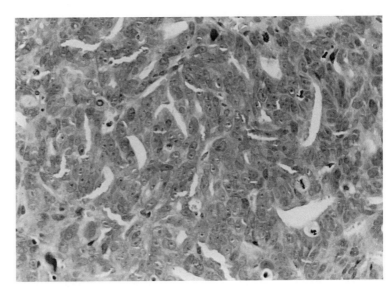

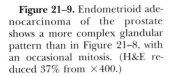

Figure 21–9. Endometrioid adenocarcinoma of the prostate shows a more complex glandular pattern than in Figure 21–8, with an occasional mitosis. (H&E reduced 37% from ×400.)

salivary gland-type tumors or whether they are variants of prostatic adenocarcinoma. The absence of strong staining for PSA and PAP, S100 protein positivity (suggesting myoepithelial differentiation), although not confirmed ultrastructurally, suggests that this is a true adenoid cystic carcinoma similar to those in the salivary glands. In addition, the small number of tumors reported in the literature have, to date, had a good prognosis, with no documented evidence of metastasis, although the longest follow-up has been only 6 years. Conversely, the presence of areas in the tumor showing basaloid hyperplasia, the finding of squamous differentiation (exceedingly rare in adenoid cystic carcinoma), the concordant finding of classical acinar type adenocarcinoma elsewhere in the tumor,[97] and the invariable absence of perineural invasion support a variant of prostatic adenocarcinoma. In view of the debate over its histogenesis and the favorable prognosis reported so far, some authors suggest these tumors be classified as adenoid cystic-like tumors with uncertain malignant potential and not adenoid cystic carcinoma.

Most cases have been treated by transurethral resection and some by radical prostatectomy. This seems a reasonable approach for the present and is in accordance with the subclassification of this tumor as a subtype of prostatic adenocarcinoma in the World Health Organization classification and Armed Forces Institute of Pathology fascicle.

Small Cell Carcinoma

Small cell carcinoma (SCC) of the prostate can occur in three settings: as a primary SCC; as a mixed carcinoma containing a small cell component with another line of differentiation (e.g., adenocarcinoma); or as a metastasis to the prostate from an SCC at another site.

Primary SCC of the prostate may represent two different tumors, namely, (1) a neuroendocrine carcinoma or (2) an undifferentiated carcinoma that is not of neuroendocrine derivation but is probably a very poorly differentiated adenocarcinoma.

Primary SCC of neuroendocrine type is a rare tumor in the prostate; 12 cases have been reported in the English literature.[102–105] These tumors are morphologically identical to SCC of the lung at the light microscopic level (Fig. 21–10). Immunohistochemically they demonstrate neuroendocrine differentiation with no immunoreactivity for PSA. Ultrastructurally, dense core granules are evident. These tumors are very aggressive. Two cases associated with ectopic adrenocorticotropin production have been reported.[103, 106] The other SCC is a tumor with similar morphologic features by light microscopy to the neuroendocrine carcinoma but is probably a poorly differentiated adenocarcinoma. This concept is supported by the absence of neuroendocrine differentiation, either immunohistochemically or ultrastructurally, and by the immunohistochemical demonstration in some cases of PSA. Furthermore, in some instances this tumor has developed in patients who presented initially with classic prostatic adenocarcinoma, again supporting nonneuroendocrine differentiation.[107]

SCC of the prostate probably arises from multipotential prostatic epithelial cells with divergent differentiation potential. Some develop in one direction, showing only neuroendocrine differentiation, whereas others show a mixed phenotype. This hypothesis is supported by the finding of SCC mixed with other types of carcinoma such as adenocarcinoma and TCC. Occasionally, prostate carcinomas are also described that show divergent differentiation (i.e., PSA and argyrophilia and dense core granules in a single tumor).[108, 109]

Lastly, SCC of the prostate may be the presenting feature of a primary SCC at another site, most commonly the lung.[105] Tumors that show a small cell pattern in the prostate are very aggressive tumors that are resistant to hormone therapy.

Sarcomatoid Carcinoma

These are exceedingly rare tumors of the prostate: fewer than 20 cases are reported in the English literature.[110, 111] They are defined as tumors that show a malignant spindle cell infiltrate, where the spindle cells display immunohistochemical or electron microscopic evidence of epithelial differentiation. In the vast majority of cases, coexistent typical adenocarcinoma is also present. Clinically, these patients' mean age is 70 years, and they complain of urinary tract symptoms suggestive of prostatic enlargement. The majority have metastases at presentation. Histologically most tumors contain classic prostatic adenocarcinoma as well as a spindle cell pattern. The sarcomatoid area is composed of spindle cells with large pleomorphic hyperchromatic nuclei, but

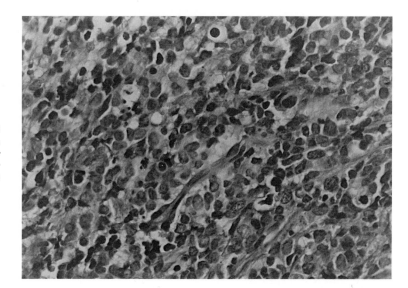

Figure 21–10. Small cell undifferentiated carcinoma of the prostate shows hyperchromatic, slightly irregular nuclei with minimal cytoplasm and evidence of nuclear debris. (H&E reduced 37% from ×400.)

in some instances the nuclei may be more vesicular with prominent nucleoli. Cellular pleomorphism is usually marked within the spindle cell component. Mitoses are often numerous. To satisfy the definition of sarcomatoid carcinoma as outlined, evidence of epithelial differentiation must be identified immunohistochemically or electron microscopically within the spindle cell component. If such epithelial differentiation is lacking in the spindle cell component the diagnosis of carcinosarcoma is more appropriate. In occasional cases of sarcomatoid carcinoma the spindle cell component may also demonstrate positivity for PSA or PAP. The prognosis for these tumors is poor, median survival being approximately 12 months.

The differential diagnosis includes a primary or metastatic sarcoma if the epithelial component is not appreciated. A postoperative spindle cell nodule may also be included in the differential, especially if the patient previously had surgery for adenocarcinoma. In some reports the sarcomatous component was appreciated only on subsequent resection[110] as the initial surgery revealed only adenocarcinoma. A spindle cell nodule generally lacks significant pleomorphism and is therefore usually easily differentiated from a sarcomatoid carcinoma.

Carcinosarcoma

Carcinosarcomas of the prostate are exceedingly rare. Three well-documented cases are reported.[112–114] All showed classic adenocarcinoma admixed with chondrosarcoma, osteosarcoma and chondrosarcoma,[113, 114] or rhabdomyosarcoma. All showed metastases at presentation. Both components metastasized in two cases, and only the adenocarcinomatous component in one. The usual debate about whether these tumors represent collision tumors or tumors capable of divergent differentiation applies.

METASTASES TO THE PROSTATE

Secondary involvement of the prostate by direct spread from adjacent tumors is quite common; however, spread by hematogenous or lymphatic metastases is rare. In a review of 1474 cases of prostate malignancy, only 1.2% were metastases from distant organs.

LYMPHOMA OF THE PROSTATE

Malignant lymphoma may occur in the prostate as a primary extranodal tumor or as secondary involvement from another primary site. In either case it is rare. In the past lymphoma (and leukemia) of the prostate have been categorized as lymphosarcoma,[20, 115] a fact that renders review of the literature difficult owing to such diverse classifications as sarcomas, lymphosarcomas, lymphoblastomas, and round cell sarcomas.[116]

To date, well-documented cases of malignant lymphoma of the prostate (either primary or secondary) number fewer than 100. These comprise single case reports and a few small series. Review of these cases suggests that primary lymphoma of the prostate is much less common than secondary infiltration.

Primary Lymphoma of the Prostate

The very existence of primary lymphoma of the prostate has been questioned owing to the lack of lymphoid tissue normally recognized in the prostate.[117] Several factors have led to an acceptance of this entity, namely, documentation of cases clearly limited to the prostate, recognition of other extranodal primary sites, and identification of small lymphoid nodules in the prostate.[117–119]

Criteria for determination of prostatic origin of malignant lymphoma have ranged from the prostate tumor's simply being the site of initial presentation[20, 120] to the lymphoma being limited to the prostate and neighboring tissues, in the absence of nodal involvement.[115] These criteria were modified by Bostwick and Mann[116] to include limitation of lymphoma to the prostate and adjacent tissues, absence of lymph node involvement, major presenting symptoms limited to the prostate, and systemic tumor-free interval of at least 1 month to allow completion of staging. Accurate staging requires such methods as CT, which further aids identification of lymph node involvement. Leukemic infiltration must be ruled out by hematologic investigation.

Secondary Lymphoma of the Prostate

Lymphoma is more often a secondary lesion of the prostate than a primary one. Its diagnosis requires either prior recognition of malignant lymphoma arising elsewhere or identification of nodal disease in the course of investigation of prostate symptoms. As a guideline, the diagnosis should be considered in the differential diagnosis for lower urinary tract obstruction in patients with a history of lymphoma.

In the reported cases of malignant lymphoma (primary or secondary), the patients' mean age was 61 (range, 14 to 86) years and presented principally with obstructive symptoms (frequency, urgency, and, less commonly, hematuria and acute urine retention). Systemic symptoms are rare. Post-mortem diagnosis is recorded in six cases. Examination commonly reveals diffuse enlargement that is rubbery and not tender and without nodularity. Coexisting benign nodular hyperplasia has been recorded.[115, 121, 122] Cystoscopic findings vary according to the extent of local spread but invariably include urethral luminal narrowing and bladder changes secondary to outflow obstruction.

Any type of malignant lymphoma may occur in the prostate. The majority of reported cases are diffuse large cell or diffuse small cleaved cell types (B-cell phenotype) (Fig. 21–11). Follicular lymphomas have been reported,[123] as have T-cell lymphoma,[116] Burkitt's lymphoma,[124] monocytoid B-cell lymphoma,[125] and angiotropic large cell lymphoma.[126] Hodgkin's disease involving the prostate is also recorded.[20, 120]

The diagnosis is generally made after histologic examination, sometimes via ultrasound-guided transrectal biopsy.[127] Prognosis for malignant lymphoma involving the prostate, whether primary or secondary, is poor.[20, 115, 116, 120, 128, 129] Radiation therapy is reported by some authors to be of use,[130] and chemotherapy has been used for primary prostatic lymphoma[131]; however, it is accepted that the prognosis of malignant lymphoma involving the prostate is related to the generalized disease[116, 120] and, as stated above, is poor. Treatment of the local disease by prostatectomy does not improve survival but does relieve the symptoms of urinary obstruction. Treatment of the generalized disease may also achieve this.[116]

Myeloma

Primary myeloma of the prostate is exceedingly rare: two reported cases have been identified.[132, 133] It is recorded in the absence of disease elsewhere in the body and, in these instances, may be better regarded as a plasmacytoma.

Leukemia

The prevalence of prostatic involvement in leukemia is variably reported, and in surgical pathology studies of the prostate in leukemic patients, rates as high as 50% are recorded.[134–139]

Prostatic enlargement with urinary outflow obstruction may be present, and the picture is

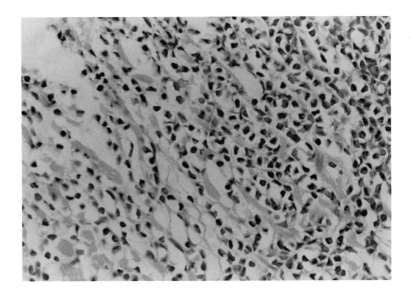

Figure 21–11. Chronic lymphocytic lymphoma infiltrating the prostate. Prostate tissue is infiltrated by small monomorphic cells with minimal cytoplasm. (H&E reduced 37% from ×400.)

mistaken clinically for benign prostatic hyperplasia. When a patient with leukemia suffers urinary outflow obstruction, needle biopsy is recommended. Those with benign prostatic hyperplasia may be operated on in the usual way. For those with leukemic involvement, radiotherapy should be considered.[140] It is worth remembering that not all cases with leukemic infiltration of the prostate develop obstructive symptoms and not all leukemics with bladder neck obstruction have leukemic infiltration of the prostate. In fact, it is suggested that while leukemic infiltration of the prostate may precipitate acute urine retention, the leukemic infiltrate only causes prostatic outflow obstruction in the presence of BPH.[139]

Any morphologic type of leukemia may infiltrate the prostate, but CLL accounts for the majority of reported cases.[141] The diagnosis of leukemic infiltration of the prostate is rarely made preoperatively,[142, 143] and the issue of treatment is therefore seldom raised. The value of local radiotherapy or of chemotherapy for relieving the symptoms of urinary tract obstruction is not proven.[139, 142, 144]

Granulocytic Sarcoma (Chloroma)

This is a localized extrahematopoietic tumor composed of immature myeloid cells, most frequently associated with acute and chronic myeloid leukemia[145] but also seen in other myeloproliferative and myelodysplastic diseases.[146–148] Granulocytic sarcoma of the prostate is unusual.[145, 149–152] Diagnosis requires demonstration of positive staining with chloroacetate esterase and/or lysozyme immunohistochemically. Treatment involves systemic management of the underlying hematologic disease and control of urinary outflow symptoms, for which radiotherapy is favored.[152]

REFERENCES

1. Schmidt JD, Welch MJ: Sarcoma of the prostate. Cancer 37:1908–1912, 1976.
2. Attah EB, Nkposong EO: Phyllodes type of atypical prostatic hyperplasia. J Urol 115:762, 1976.
3. Tetu B, Ro JY, Ayala AG, et al.: Atypical spindle cell lesions of the prostate. Semin Diagn Pathol 5:284, 1988.
4. Kirkland KL, Bale PM: A cystic adenoma of the prostate. J Urol 97:324, 1967.
5. Gueft B, Walsh MA: Malignant prostatic cystosarcoma phyllodes. NY State J Med 75:2226, 1975.
6. Yokota T, Yamshita Y, Okuzono Y, et al.: Malignant cystosarcoma phyllodes of prostate. Acta Pathol Jpn 34:663, 1984.
7. Manivel C, Shenoy BV, Wick MR, et al.: Cystosarcoma phyllodes of the prostate. A pathologic and immunohistochemical study. Arch Pathol Lab Med 110:534–538, 1986.
8. Reese JH, Lombard CM, Krowe K, et al.: Phyllodes type of atypical prostatic hyperplasia: A report of 3 new cases. J Urol 138:623, 1987.
9. Lucey DT, McAninch JW, Bunts RC: Genital cysts of the male pelvis: Case report of müllerian and ejaculatory duct cysts in the same patient. J Urol 109:440, 1973.
10. Young RH, Scully RE: Pseudosarcomatous lesions of the urinary bladder, prostate gland, and urethra. A report of three cases and review of the literature. Arch Pathol Lab Med 111:354–358, 1987.
11. Attah EB, Powell ME: Atypical stromal hyperplasia of the prostate gland. Am J Clin Pathol 67:324–327, 1977.

12. Hafiz MA, Toker C, Sutula M: An atypical fibromyxoid tumor of the prostate. Cancer 54:2500, 1984.

13. Proppe KH, Scully RE, Rosai J: Postoperative spindle cell nodules of genitourinary tract resembling sarcomas. A report of eight cases. Am J Surg Pathol 8:101–108, 1984.

14. Vassilakis GB: Pure leiomyoma of prostate. Urology 11:93–94, 1978.

15. Rosen Y, Ambiavagar PC, Vuletin JC, et al.: Atypical leiomyoma of prostate. Urology 15:183–185, 1980.

16. Persaud V, Douglas LL: Bizarre (atypical) leiomyoma of the prostate gland. Wisc Med J 31:217, 1982.

17. Patch FS, Rhea LJ: Leiomyoma of the prostate gland. Urology 3:617, 1974.

18. Holtl W, Hruby W, Redtenbacher M: Cavernous hemangioma originating from prostatic plexus. Urology 20:184–185, 1982.

19. Mostofi FK, Price EB Jr: Tumors of the male genital system. In: Atlas of Tumor Pathology. Washington, DC: Armed Forces Institute of Pathology, 1973, p 177.

20. Smith BH, Dehner LP: Sarcoma of the prostate gland. Am J Clin Pathol 58:43, 1972.

21. Tannenbaum M: Sarcomas of the prostate gland. Urology 5:810–814, 1975.

22. Raney B Jr, Carey A, Snyder HM, et al.: Primary site as a prognostic variable for children with pelvic soft tissue sarcomas. J Urol 136:874, 1986.

23. Russo P: Urologic sarcoma in adults. Memorial Sloan-Kettering Cancer Center experience based on a prospective database between 1982 and 1989. Urol Clin North Am 18:581–588, 1991.

24. Raney B Jr, Heyn R, Hays DM, et al.: Sequelae of treatment in 109 patients followed for 5 to 15 years after diagnosis of sarcoma of the bladder and prostate. A report from the Intergroup Rhabdomyosarcoma Study Committee. Cancer 71:2387–2394, 1993.

25. Raney RB Jr, Gehan EA, Hays DM, et al.: Primary chemotherapy with or without radiation therapy and/or surgery for children with localized sarcoma of the bladder, prostate, vagina, uterus, and cervix. A comparison of the results in Intergroup Rhabdomyosarcoma Studies I and II. Cancer 66:2072–2081, 1990.

26. Tucker MA, D'Angio GJ, Boice JD, et al.: Bone sarcomas linked to radiotherapy and chemotherapy in children. N Engl J Med 317:588–593, 1987.

27. Robinson E, Neugut AI, Wylie P: Review: Clinical aspects of the postirradiation sarcomas. J Natl Cancer Inst (USA) 80:233–240, 1988.

28. Thrasher JB, Miller GJ, Wettlaufer JN: Bladder leiomyosarcoma following cyclophosphamide therapy for lupus nephritis. J Urol 143:119–121, 1990.

29. Sorensen SA, Mulvihill J, Nielsen A: Long-term follow-up of von Recklinghausen's neurofibromatosis: Survival and malignant neoplasms. N Engl J Med 314:1010–1015, 1986.

30. McClay EF: Epidemiology of bone and soft tissue sarcomas. Semin Oncol 16:264–272, 1989.

31. Newton WA, Soule EH, Reiman HM, et al.: Histopathology of childhood sarcomas: Intergroup Rhabdomyosarcomas Studies I and II. Clinicopathologic correlation. J Clin Oncol 6:67, 1988.

32. Narayana AS, Loening S, Weimar GW, et al.: Sarcoma of the bladder and prostate. J Urol 118:72, 1978.

33. King DG, Finney RP: Embryonal rhabdomyosarcoma of the prostate. J Urol 117:88–90, 1977.

34. Keenan DJM, Graham WH: Embryonal rhabdomyosarcoma of the prostatic-urethral region in an adult. Br J Urol 57:241, 1985.

35. Leader M, Collins M, Patel J, et al.: Desmin: Its value as a marker of muscle derived tumours using a commercial antibody. Virchows Arch [A] 411:345–349, 1987.

36. Ghavimi F, Herr H, Jereb B, et al.: Treatment of genitourinary rhabdomyosarcoma in children. J Urol 132:313–319, 1984.

37. Sarnacki S, Flamant F, Valayer J: Thérapeutiques conservatrices dans les rhabdomyosarcomes génito-urinaires de l'infant. Chir Pediatr 28:299, 1987.

38. Atra A, Ward HC, Aitken K, et al.: Conservative surgery in multimodal therapy for pelvic rhabdomyosarcoma in children. Br J Cancer 70:1004–1108, 1994.

39. Hays DM, Raney R, Ragab A, et al.: Retention of functional bladders among patients with vesical/prostatic sarcomas in the Intergroup Rhabdomyosarcoma Studies (IRS). Med Pediatr Oncol 19:423, 1991.

40. Fryer CJ: Pelvic rhabdomyosarcoma: Paying the price of bladder preservation. Lancet 345:141–142, 1995.

41. Donaldson S, Fryer CJH, Wharam M, et al.: A hyper fractionated radiation protocol to improve local control without increasing late effects in childhood rhabdomyosarcoma. Med Pediatr Oncol 23:3, 1994.

42. Christoffersen J: Leiomyosarcoma of the prostate. Acta Chir Scand 433 (Suppl):75, 1973.

43. Ohmori T, Arita N, Tabei R: Prostatic leiomyosarcoma revealing cytoplasmic virus-like particles and intranuclear paracrystalline structures. Acta Pathol Jpn 34:631, 1984.

44. Fitzpatrick TJ, Stump G: Leiomyosarcoma of the prostate. Case report and review of the literature. J Urol 83:80, 1960.

45. Limon J, Dal Cin P, Sandberg AA: Cytogenic findings in a primary leiomyosarcoma of the prostate. Cancer Genet Cytogenet 22:159, 1986.

46. Muller HA, Wünsch PH: Features of prostatic sarcomas in combined aspiration and punch biopsies. Acta Cytol 25:481, 1981.

47. Witherow R, Molland E, Oliver T, et al.: Leiomyosarcoma of prostate and superficial soft tissue. Urology 15:513, 1980.

48. Camuzzi FA, Block NL, Charyulu K, et al.: Leiomyosarcoma of the prostate gland. Urology 18:295–297, 1981.

49. Palma PC, Neto NR Jr, Ikari O, et al.: Leiomyosarcoma in association with incidental adenocarcinoma of the prostate. J Urol 129:156–157, 1983.

50. Reyes JW, Shinozuka H, Garry P, et al.: A light and electron microscopic study of a hemangiopericytoma of the prostate with local extension. Cancer 40:1122–1126, 1977.

51. Bain GO, Danyluk JM, Shnitka TK, et al.: Malignant fibrous histiocytoma of prostate gland. Urology 26:89–91, 1985.

52. Chin W, Fay R, Ortega P: Malignant fibrous histiocytoma of prostate. Urology 27:363–365, 1986.

53. Meeter UI, Richards JN: Osteogenic sarcoma of the prostate. J Urology 81:564, 1960.

54. Sloan SE, Rapport JM: Prostatic chondroma. Uropathology 3:319–321, 1985.

55. Dennis PJ, Lewandowski AE, Rohner TJ Jr, et al.: Pheochromocytoma of the prostate: An unusual location. J Urol 141:130–132, 1989.

56. Ostrowski ML, Wheeler TM: Paraganglia of the pros-

tate. Location, frequency, and differentiation from prostatic adenocarcinoma. Am J Surg Pathol 18:412–420, 1994.

57. Langley JW, Weitzner S: Blue nevus and melanosis of prostate. J Urol 112:359–361, 1974.

58. Stein BS, Kendall AR: Malignant melanoma of the genitourinary tract [Review]. J Urol 132:859–868, 1984.

59. Rawles ME: Origin in melanophores and their role in development of colon vertebrates. Physiol Rev 28:383, 1948.

60. Nakai T, Rappaport H: A study of the histogenesis of experimental melanotic tumors resembling cellular blue nevi: The evidence in support of their neurogenic origin. Am J Pathol 43:175, 1963.

61. Aguilar M, Gaffney EF, Finnerty DP: Prostatic melanosis with involvement of benign and malignant epithelium. J Urol 128:825–827, 1982.

62. Nigogosyan G, de la Pava S, Pickren JW, et al.: Blue nevus of the prostate gland. Cancer 16:1097, 1963.

63. Simard C, Rognon LM, Pilorce G: Le probléme du naevus bleu prostatique. Ann Anat Pathol 9:469, 1964.

64. Jao W, Fretzin DF, Christ ML, et al.: Blue nevus of the prostate gland. Arch Pathol 91:187, 1971.

65. Block NL, Weber D, Schinella R: Blue nevi and other melanotic lesions of the prostate: Report of three cases and review of the literature. J Urol 107:85, 1972.

66. Abeshouse BS: Primary and secondary melanoma of the genitourinary tract. South Med J 51:994, 1958.

67. Das Gupta T, Grabstald H: Melanoma of the genitourinary tract. J Urol 93:607, 1965.

68. Grignon DJ, Ro JY, Ayala AG: Malignant melanoma with metastasis to adenocarcinoma of the prostate. Cancer 63:196–198, 1989.

69. Little NA, Wiener JS, Walther PJ, et al.: Squamous cell carcinoma of the prostate: 2 cases of a rare malignancy and review of the literature [Review]. J Urol 149:137–139, 1993.

70. Sieracki JC: Epidermoid carcinoma of the human prostate report of three cases. Lab Invest 4:232, 1955.

71. Grossman HB, Wedemeyer G, Ren L, et al.: UMSCP-1, a new human cell line derived from a prostatic squamous cell carcinoma. Cancer Res 44:4111, 1984.

72. Dixon FJ, Moore RA: Tumors of the male sex organs. In: Atlas of Tumor Pathology, 1st Series. Washington, DC: Armed Forces Institute of Pathology, 1952, p 37.

73. Herbut PA: Urological Pathology. Philadelphia: Lea & Febiger, 1952, pp 989–1010.

74. Gray GF Jr, Marshall VF: Squamous carcinoma of the prostate. J Urol 113:736, 1975.

75. Samsonov VA: Squamous cell carcinoma of the prostate: Its differential diagnostic contrast with squamous metaplasia. Arch Pathol 46:23, 1984.

76. Devaney DM, Dorman A, Leader M: Adenosquamous carcinoma of the prostate: A case report [Review]. Hum Pathol 22:1046–1050, 1991.

77. Saito R, Davis BK, Ollapally EP: Adenosquamous carcinoma of the prostate. Hum Pathol 15:87–89, 1984.

78. Chibber PJ, McIntyre MA, Hindmarsh JR, et al.: Transitional cell carcinoma involving the prostate. Br J Urol 53:605–609, 1981.

79. Schellhammer PF, Bean MA, Whitmore WF Jr: Prostatic involvement by transitional cell carcinoma: Pathogenesis, patterns and prognosis. J Urol 118:399–403, 1977.

80. Taylor HG, Blom J: Transitional cell carcinoma of

the prostate. Response to treatment with adriamycin and cis-platinum. Cancer 51:1800–1802, 1983.

81. Razui M, Firfer R, Berkson B: Occult transitional cell carcinoma of the prostate presenting as skin metastasis. J Urol 113:734–735, 1975.

82. Wood DP Jr, Montie JE, Pontes JE, et al.: Transitional cell carcinoma of the prostate in cystoprostatectomy specimens removed for bladder cancer. J Urol 141:346–349, 1989.

83. Epstein JI, Lieberman PH: Mucinous adenocarcinoma of the prostate gland. Am J Surg Pathol 9:299–308, 1985.

84. McNeal JE, Reese JH, Redwine EA, et al.: Cribriform adenocarcinoma of the prostate. Cancer 58:1714–1719, 1986.

85. Ro JY, El-Naggar A, Ayala AG, et al.: Signet-ring-cell carcinoma of the prostate. Electron-microscopic and immunohistochemical studies of eight cases. Am J Surg Pathol 12:453–460, 1988.

86. Kim H, Dorfman RF, Rappaport H: Signet-ring-cell lymphoma: A rare morphologic and functional expression of nodular (follicular) lymphoma. Am J Surg Pathol 2:119–32, 1978.

87. Weiss LM, Wood GS, Dorfman RF: T-cell signet-ring-cell lymphoma: A histologic, ultrastructural, and immunohistochemical study of two cases. Am J Surg Pathol 9:273–280, 1985.

88. Mendelsohn G: Signet-cell simulating microfollicular adenoma of the thyroid. Am J Surg Pathol 8:705–708, 1984.

89. Schroder S, Bocker W: Signet-ring-cell thyroid tumors. Follicle cell tumors with arrest of folliculogenesis. Am J Surg Pathol 9:619–629, 1985.

90. Rubinstein LJ: Tumors of the Central Nervous System. In: Rubinstein LJ (ed): Atlas of Tumor Pathology, Ser 2, Fasc 6 Bethesda, Md.: Armed Forces Institute of Pathology, 1972, pp 85–104.

91. Enzinger FM, Weiss SW: Epithelioid smooth muscle tumors. In: Enzinger FM, Weiss SW, eds. Soft Tissue Tumors. St. Louis: C.V. Mosby, 1983, pp 316–324.

92. Remmele W, Weber A, Harding P: Primary signet-ring cell carcinoma of the prostate. Hum Pathol 19:478–480, 1988.

93. Alguacil-Garcia A: Artifactual changes mimicking signet ring cell carcinoma in transurethral prostatectomy specimens. Am J Surg Pathol 10:795–800, 1986.

94. Epstein JI, Woodruff JM. Adenocarcinoma of the prostate with endometrioid features. A light microscopic and immunohistochemical study of ten cases. Cancer 57:111–119, 1986.

95. Bostwick DG, Kindrachuk RW, Rouse RV: Prostatic adenocarcinoma with endometrioid features. Clinical, pathologic, and ultrastructural findings. Am J Surg Pathol 9:595–609, 1985.

96. Ro JY, Ayala AG, Wishnow KI, et al.: Prostatic duct adenocarcinoma with endometrioid features: Immunohistochemical and electron microscopic study. Semin Diagn Pathol 5:301, 1988.

97. Young RH, Frierson HF Jr, Mills SE, et al.: Adenoid cystic-like tumor of the prostate gland. A report of two cases and review of the literature on "adenoid cystic carcinoma" of the prostate [Review]. Am J Clin Pathol 89:49–56, 1988.

98. Kuhajda FP, Mann RB: Adenoid cystic carcinoma of the prostate. A case report with immunoperoxidase staining for prostate-specific acid phosphatase and prostate-specific antigen. Am J Clin Pathol 81:257–260, 1984.

99. Frankel K, Craig JR: Adenoid cystic carcinoma of the prostate. Report of a case. Am J Clin Pathol 62:639–645, 1974.

100. Gilmour AM, Bell TJ: Adenoid cystic carcinoma of the prostate. Br J Urol 58:105–106, 1986.

101. Reed RJ: Consultation case. Am J Surg Pathol 8:699–670, 1984.

102. Bleichner JC, Chun B, Klappenbach RS: Pure small-cell carcinoma of the prostate with fatal liver metastasis. Arch Pathol Lab Med 110:1041–1044, 1986.

103. Wenk RE, Bhagavan BS, Levy R, et al.: Ectopic ACTH, prostatic oat cell carcinoma, and marked hypernatremia. Cancer 40:773–778, 1977.

104. Ro JY, Tetu B, Ayala AG, et al.: Small cell carcinoma of the prostate. II. Immunohistochemical and electron microscopic studies of 18 cases. Cancer 59:977–982, 1987.

105. Manson AL, Terhune D, MacDonald G: Small cell carcinoma of prostate [Review]. Urology 33:78–79, 1989.

106. Vuitch MF, Mendelsohn G: Relationship of ectopic ACTH production to tumor differentiation. A morphologic and immunohistochemical study of prostatic carcinoma with Cushing's syndrome. Cancer 47:396–399, 1981.

107. Schron DS, Gipson T, Mendelsohn G: The histogenesis of small cell carcinoma of the prostate: An immunohistochemical study. Cancer 53:2478–2480, 1984.

108. Almagro UA: Argyrophilic prostatic carcinoma: Case report with literature review on prostatic carcinoid and "carcinoid-like" prostatic carcinoma. Cancer 55:608–614, 1985.

109. Ghali VS, Garcia RL: Prostatic adenocarcinoma with carcinoidal features producing adrenocorticotropic syndrome. Cancer 54:1043–1048, 1984.

110. Shannon RL, Ro JY, Grignon DJ, et al.: Sarcomatoid carcinoma of the prostate. A clinicopathologic study of 12 patients. Cancer 69:2676–2682, 1992.

111. Torenbeek R, Blomjous CE, de Bruin PC, et al.: Sarcomatoid carcinoma of the urinary bladder. Clinicopathologic analysis of 18 cases with immunohistochemical and electron microscopic findings. Am J Surg Pathol 18:241–249, 1994.

112. Wick MR, Young RH, Malvesta R, et al.: Prostatic carcinosarcomas. Clinical, histologic, and immunohistochemical data on two cases, with a review of the literature [Review]. Am J Clin Pathol 92:131–139, 1989.

113. Haddad JR, Reyes EC: Carcinosarcoma of the prostate with metastasis of both elements: Case report. J Urol 103:80–83, 1970.

114. Quay SC, Proppe KH: Carcinosarcoma of the prostate: Case report and review of the literature. J Urol 125:436–438, 1981.

115. King LS, Cox TR: Lymphosarcoma of the prostate. Am J Pathol 27:801, 1951.

116. Bostwick DG, Mann RB: Malignant lymphomas involving the prostate. A study of 13 cases. Cancer 56:2932–2938, 1985.

117. Ewing J: Neoplastic Diseases, ed 4. Philadelphia: W.B. Saunders, 1940, pp 852–869.

118. Wegelin C: Uber ein Lymphom der Prostata. Wein Klin Wochenschr 48:1236–1237, 1935.

119. Fukase N: Hyperplasia of the rudimentary lymph nodes of the prostate. Surg Gynecol Obstet 35:131–136, 1922.

120. Sridhar KN, Woodhouse CRJ: Prostatic infiltration in leukaemia and lymphoma. Eur Urol 9:153–156, 1983.

121. Dial DL: Lymphosarcoma of the prostate: Report of a case. J Urol 32:79–83, 1934.

122. Mason DG: Primary malignant lymphocytoma of the prostate gland. Arch Pathol 16:803–808, 1933.

123. Doll DC, Weiss RB, Shah S: Lymphoma of the prostate presenting as benign prostatic hypertrophy. S Med J 71:1170–1171, 1978.

124. Boe S, Nielsen H, Rytov N: Burkitt's lymphoma mimicking prostatitis. J Urol 125:891–892, 1981.

125. Franco V, Florena AM, Quintini G, et al.: Monocytoid B-cell lymphoma of the prostate. Pathologica 84(1091):411–417, 1992.

126. Banerjee SS, Harris M: Angiotrophic lymphoma presenting in the prostate. Histopathology 12:667–670, 1988.

127. Rainwater LM, Barrett DM: Primary lymphoma of prostate: Transrectal ultrasonic appearance. Urology 36(6):522–525, 1990.

128. Hampel N, Richter-Levin D, Gersh I: Primary lymphosarcoma of the prostate. Urology 9:461–463, 1977.

129. Hamburger S, Woods K: Non-Hodgkin's lymphoma of the prostate. J Kans Med Soc 81:457, 1980.

130. Montalbetti L, Borri C, Lampertico P, et al.: Lymphoma of the prostate: case reports and subject review. Rec Prog Med 81(10):666–669, 1990.

131. Suzuki H, Nakada T, Iijima Y, et al.: Malignant lymphoma of the prostate. Report of a case. Urol Int 47(3):172–175, 1991.

132. Estrada PC, Scardino PL: Myeloma of the prostate: A case report. J Urol 106:586–587, 1971.

133. Batts M Jr: Multiple myeloma: Review of 40 cases. Arch Surg 39:807, 1939.

134. Butler MR, O'Flynn JD: Prostatic disease in leukemic patient—with particular reference to leukemic infiltration of the prostate. Br J Urol 45:179–183, 1973.

135. Lucia SP, Mills H, Lowenhaupt E, et al.: Visceral involvement in primary neoplastic diseases of the reticuoendothelial system. Cancer 5:1193–1200, 1952.

136. Kirshbaum JD, Preuss FS: Leukemia—a clinical and pathologic study of 123 fatal cases in a series of 14,400 necropsies. Arch Intern Med 71:777–792, 1943.

137. Watson EM, Sauer HR, Sadugor MG: Manifestations of the lymphoblastomas in the genito-urinary tract. J Urol 61:626–645, 1949.

138. Meyer LM: Pathology of the urinary tract in leukaemia. Urol Gut Rev 45:693–695, 1941.

139. Dajani YF, Burke M: Leukemic infiltration of the prostate. A case study and clinicopathological review. Cancer 38:2442–2446, 1976.

140. Merimsky E, Baratz M, Kahn Y: Leukaemic infiltration of the prostate. Br J Urol 53:150–151, 1981.

141. Cachia PG, McIntyre MA, Dewar AE, et al.: Prostatic infiltration in chronic lymphatic leukaemia. J Clin Pathol 40:342–345, 1987.

142. Fishman A, Taylor WN: Leukemic infiltration of the prostate. J Urol 89:65–72, 1963.

143. Hubmer G, Lipsky H: Leukamische Infiltration der Prostataregion bei chronischer Myelose. Z Urol 59:199–202, 1966.

144. Johnson MA, Gunderson AH: Infiltration of the prostate gland by chronic lymphatic leukaemia. J Urol 69:681–685, 1953.

145. Neiman RS, Barcos M, Berard C: A clinicopathologic study of 61 biopsied cases. Cancer 48:1426–1437, 1981.

146. Brugo EA, Marshall RB, Riberi AM, et al.: Preleukemic granulocytic sarcomas of the gastrointestinal tract: Report of two cases. Am J Clin Pathol 68:616–621, 1977.
147. Ellman L, Hammond D, Atkins L: Eosinophilia, chloromas and a chromosome abnormality in a patient with a myeloproliferative syndrome. Cancer 43:2410–2413, 1979.
148. Sadick N, Edlin D, Myskowski P, et al.: Granulocytic sarcoma: A new finding in the setting of preleukemia. Arch Dermatol 120:1341–1343, 1984.
149. Lui PI, Ishimaru T, McGregor DH, et al.: Autopsy study of granulocytic sarcoma (chloroma) in patients with myelogenous leukemia, Hiroshima-Nagasaki, 1949–1969. Cancer 31:948–955, 1973.
150. Muss HB, Moloney WC: Chloroma and other myeloblastic tumors. Blood 42:721–728, 1973.
151. Chan YF: Granulocytic sarcoma (chloroma) of the kidney and prostate. Br J Urol 65(6):655–666, 1990.
152. Frame R, Head D, Lee R, et al.: Granulocytic sarcoma of the prostate. Two cases causing urinary obstruction. Cancer 59:142–146, 1987.

Chapter

22

SIGNIFICANCE OF NEOVASCULARITY IN HUMAN PROSTATE CARCINOMA

Justin A. Siegal and Michael K. Brawer

Increasing public awareness and improving diagnostic tests are identifying more prostate cancers. Many of these diagnoses may be of dubious clinical significance. Although prostate cancer is one of the most common causes of cancer-related deaths in American men,[1] the prevalence of incidental tumors far exceeds that of clinically manifest cancer. Although 42% of men have prostate carcinoma identified at post mortem examination, only 9.5% are diagnosed with prostate cancer in their lifetime and only 2.9% actually succumb to the disease.[2] Markers of malignant potential are essential to manage the growing discrepancy between histologic evidence of prostate carcinoma and clinically manifest disease.

The stage of a neoplasm is considered a standard indicator of a tumor's aggressiveness. Unfortunately, no accurate preoperative predictor of prostate cancer stage is available. Conventional imaging modalities lack the sensitivity to visualize microscopic tumor extensions.[3] Thus, pathologic "up-staging" is common: in recent prostatectomy series, up-staging to capsular penetration, seminal vesicle extension, or pelvic lymph node metastases was necessary in 11% to 60% of cases.[4]

Currently employed predictors of stage include histologic grade, tumor volume, DNA ploidy, and serum prostate-specific antigen (PSA) levels (Table 22–1). These markers have been correlated with pathologic stage and proven to provide some prognostic informa-

tion.[5–7] Unfortunately, the information is rarely useful for individual patients.

Tumor grade, while it demonstrates significant correlation with pathologic stage, is hampered by sampling error on biopsy material and cannot stratify most carcinomas, which are of intermediate Gleason score. Serum PSA, while it generally correlates with stage, provides little staging information for any individual patient, owing to considerable overlap between stages. Existing imaging modalities cannot accurately estimate tumor volume preoperatively, so the prognostic utility of tumor size is limited. The literature on ploidy remains confusing owing to methodologic prob-

Table 22–1. Existing Markers of Malignant Potential in the Prostate

Tumor volume
DNA ploidy
Histologic grade
Clinical stage
Pathologic stage
Prostatic acid phosphatase
Prostate-specific antigen
Nuclear morphometry
Adherens
Growth factors (bFGF, VEGF)
Invasive markers (cathepsin, collagenase)
Basement membrane (collagen)
Oncogenes
Tumor suppressor genes

lems in threshold standardization and because of the significant heterogeneity exhibited in many neoplasms.[8]

Improved predictors of biologic progression clearly are needed. Recently, neovascularity has been investigated in human prostate cancer as an adjunct to staging and prognosis. It has been demonstrated that quantitative neovascularity (microvessel density) is an independent predictor of pathologic stage[9-11] and may provide prognostic information in the prostate.[12, 13]

ANGIOGENIC DEPENDENCE OF TUMOR GROWTH AND METASTASIS

Background on Angiogenesis

Angiogenesis is a critical factor for the progression and enlargement of solid neoplasms. Tumor expansion necessitates corresponding vascular ingrowth to supply nutrients, exchange gas, and remove waste. Folkman and coworkers have suggested that many solid malignancies can be divided into two distinct stages in an incremental model of tumor progression: a prevascular phase and, subsequently, a vascular phase. Folkman defines the prevascular phase as a period during early development when few or no tumor cells are angiogenic and tumor size is limited to 1.5 to 2.0 mm^3; the vascular phase is marked by significantly increased growth and a tendency to metastasize.[14]

Evidence for this hypothesis is found in the limited proliferation of tumors grown in organ culture, an environment that limits vascular response. Tumors grown in this system did not expand beyond 1 to 2 mm^3; however, upon transplantation to host mice these small neoplasms grew into large tumors (2 to 3 cm^3) that frequently killed the hosts.[15] Histologic examination demonstrated that the perfused organ implants were completely avascular and exhibited significant central necrosis while the large in vivo implants were well-vascularized.

The dependence of tumor growth on vascularization was visualized with rabbit corneal implants. Gimbrone and colleagues found that tumor growth in the avascular cornea initially proceeds slowly and at a linear rate, whereas exponential tumor growth occurs after vascularization.[16] Similar results were found in the growth of tumors implanted in subcutaneous transparent chambers in mice.[17] Individual tu-

mor cells have been demonstrated to divide more rapidly when they are close to vessels.[18]

Metastases and Neovascularization

Angiogenesis helps tumor cells intravasate the host circulation, a primary step in tumor metastasis. Angiogenesis facilitates this process by increasing vascular density; growing immature, leaky vascular sprouts[19]; and potentially engulfing tumor cells in the process of vascular expansion.[20] In the absence of neovascularization, cancer cells are rarely shed into the circulation.[21]

There is a clear biophysical association between vascular density and the ease with which a tumor cell can access the tumor vasculature. A linear relationship has been demonstrated between the intertumor density of vessels ≥30 μm in diameter and the number of circulating tumor cells.[22] In turn, the number of circulating tumor cell clumps has been found to be directly correlated with a tumor's propensity to metastasize.[23]

The metastatic process is further facilitated by the leaky nature of tumor microvasculature, which is significantly more permeable than normal vessels to plasma proteins.[24] This increased permeability is primarily a result of tumor-associated angiogenic activity. Young, proliferating capillaries have fragmented basement membranes that make them more accessible than mature vessels to tumor cells.[19] Additionally, to degrade the existing endothelial cell matrix and permit subsequent vascular expansion sprouting microvessel extensions produce matrix malloproteinases and serine proteases.[25] These degradative proteins secreted by growing microvessels may simultaneously facilitate tumor cell invasion of the growing tumor vasculature.[20] Finally, increased vascular permeability may be explained in part by overexpression of vascular endothelial cell growth factor (VEGF), a potent endothelial cell mitogen that is 50,000 times more potent than histamine at enhancing microvascular permeability.[19] Compression of the microvascularity in the center of neoplasms may result in local hypoxia, which could promote resulting VEGF up-regulation and increased vascular permeability at the tumor's center.[26]

Regulators of Angiogenesis

The hyperemic property of tumors was observed as early as 1865, when Thiersch commented on the extravagant production of capillaries in the stroma of carcinoma.[27] The mechanism of this vascularization was subject to debate. Some scientists believed tumors achieved their supporting vasculature by incorporating and remodeling existing vessels,[28] whereas others promulgated tumor-induced neovascularization.[29] Some suggested that proliferating tumor cells themselves induced vascular ingrowth[29]; others hypothesized that this vascularization was the result of an inflammatory reaction.[30]

Rabbit cornea tumor transplant models provided direct evidence that tumor cells elicit a strong angiogenic signal. Viable transplanted tumor fragments were shown to produce significant vascularization while heat-killed fragments demonstrated no vascular response.[31] In 1968, experimental findings suggested that tumors induced supportive capillary growth by secreting a diffusible angiogenic factor: scientists demonstrated that tumors could induce neovascularization even when the tumor was separated from the host vasculature by a Millipore filter.[32] The first isolation of an angiogenic growth factor from tumors was reported in the early 1970s.[33] Polyacrylamide gels containing this factor, referred to as tumor "angiogenesis factor," induced a significant angiogenic response on transplantation into rabbit corneas.[31]

It was soon evident that a number of growth factors are associated with angiogenic response. Isolation of these factors was aided by the discovery that acidic fibroblast growth factor (aFGF) binds to heparin.[34] This affinity was found for a number of other angiogenic factors, thus enabling use of heparin-affinity chromatography for their isolation and purification.[34] Development of in vitro assays using cultured endothelial cells further accelerated growth factor study and led to the identification of a variety of growth factors (Table 22-2).[30]

Growth factors have been associated with all levels of angiogenic response, including vascular permeability, endothelial cell proliferation, and endothelial cell migration. Recent findings have implicated elevated growth factor expression with increased angiogenic activity in a variety of neoplasms, including renal cell carcinoma, melanoma, malignant glioma, and breast cancer.

Inhibitors of Angiogenesis

While initial interest in neovascularization focused principally on angiogenic promoters,

Table 22-2. Stimulators of Angiogenesis

Acidic fibroblast growth factor
Basic fibroblast growth factor
Epidermal growth factor
Platelet-derived endothelial cell growth factor
Transforming growth factor-alpha
Transforming growth factor-beta
Tumor necrosis factor-alpha
Vascular endothelial growth factor
Angiogenin
Angiotropin
Angiotensin II
Plasminogen activator
Proliferin
Prostaglandins

increasing emphasis is being placed on the role of angiogenic inhibitors. The presence of an angiogenic promoter alone is not sufficient to mount an angiogenic response. Endothelial growth factors have been found in almost all normal tissues, yet endothelial cell proliferation in these tissues is extremely slow: turnover times are measured in years.[35] Vascular proliferation evidently depends on a balance of angiogenic inhibitors and promoters. This balance was recently elucidated in the placenta, where an antagonistic relationship between proliferin-related protein (PRP), an inhibitor of angiogenesis, and proliferin (PLF), an angiogenic promoter, is reported to control placental vascularization.[36]

In general, the process of angiogenesis may be analogous to other processes, such as blood coagulation, that are maintained at a constant state of readiness for prolonged periods of time.[30] A number of controls appear to be designed to prevent unchecked capillary growth, much as physiologic inhibitors prevent intravascular clotting. In malignant growth, the switch to the angiogenic phenotype likely involves more than simple up-regulation of angiogenic activity: concomitant down-regulation of endothelial inhibitors, naturally present in cells before and after they become neoplastic, also seems to be necessary.

Cartilage must remain relatively free of vessels to ensure its structural integrity. This observation led scientists to test cartilage's ability to modulate induced angiogenesis in a developing chick chorioallantoic membrane (CAM).[37] Avascular zones developed around the implants. Subsequently, a number of reports have similarly demonstrated the angiostatic potential of cartilage or cartilage derivatives.[38] The list of known angiogenic inhibitors

Table 22–3. Inhibitors of Angiogenesis

> Angiostatin
> Antiestrogens
> Cartilage-derived inhibitor
> Heparin + steroid hormones
> Heparinase
> Interferon-alpha
> Interferon-beta
> Linomide
> Platelet factor 4
> Prolactin fragment
> Proliferin-related protein
> Protamine
> Retinoids
> Suramin
> Tamoxifen
> Tetrahydrocortisone (angiostatic steroids)
> Thrombospondin
> Tissue inhibitor of metalloproteinase
> Methotrexate

is rapidly growing to rival that of stimulators (Table 22–3).

NEOVASCULARITY IN HUMAN NEOPLASMS

In this last decade, technologic advances in immunohistochemistry and image processing have enabled efficient and reproducible quantification of neovascularity. Srivastava and colleagues were the first to demonstrate that microvessel density (MVD) could predict the probability of tumor metastasis in their investigation of cutaneous melanoma.[39] Since this investigation, evidence has emerged that increased vascularity may be an important indicator of invasion and metastasis in a large variety of neoplasms.

Correlation between increased MVD and distant metastasis has been confirmed for malignant melanoma[40] and has similarly been demonstrated for testicular germ cell tumors[41] and breast cancer.[42–46] Likewise, MVD has proved to be predictive of either local or distant recurrence in tumors of the oral cavity,[47] breast,[43, 44, 48–52] and lung.[53–55] Finally, retrospective findings indicating a direct relationship between MVD and overall survival have been reported in cases of breast cancer,[44] malignant melanomas,[40] and rectal carcinoma.[56]

Neovascularization in Prostate Cancer

Our group and others have investigated neovascularity in human prostate cancer. Our findings demonstrated that MVD is an independent predictor of pathologic stage[9] and may provide prognostic information.[12] We originally investigated MVD in carcinomatous and in uninvolved portions of radical prostatectomy specimens. In 14 of 15 cases the vascularity of the cancer was significantly greater than that in the "benign" tissue, the overall ratio of cancer to benign tissue being 2.02 ($P < 0.001$).[57]

A further investigation compared the MVD in 17 organ-confined prostate carcinomas with 8 primary carcinomas from men with disseminated disease.[58, 59] We compared average MVDs, evaluating five randomly selected medium-power fields ($100 \times$) for each case. The mean vessel density for stage D cases was 180 vessels per square millimeter, whereas that for the organ-confined cases was 102 vessels/mm^2 ($P < 0.001$). The trends demonstrated in this first evaluation were confirmed in a second sampling. In this investigation, we quantified mean MVDs for 26 cases—13 organ-confined and 13 advanced carcinomas (Tables 22–4 to 22–6; Fig. 22–1).[9] We found a correlation between vessel density and pathologic stage. The mean microvessel density for the stage D group was 135 vessels/mm^2, whereas that for the organ-confined group was 106 vessels/mm^2 ($P = 0.01$) (Fig. 22–1). All the organ-confined cases fell below an arbitrary cutoff of 120 vessels/mm^2. In contrast, six of nine metastatic cases were above this level. Using this threshold, the sensitivity for advanced disease is 75%, the specificity 100%, the positive predictive value 100%, and the negative predictive value 88%.[60] Looking only at carcinomas with high histologic grade, we found a higher correlation between stage and vascular density. In this subset the mean MVD of the metastasized tumors was 147 vessels/mm^2, whereas that of the organ-confined tumors was 78 vessels/mm^2 ($P = 0.005$).

We subsequently investigated MVD in other proliferative lesions of the prostate. Our findings demonstrated increased vascularization associated with certain histologic variants of benign prostatic hyperplasia (BPH) as well as prostatic intraepithelial neoplasia (PIN). To analyze the MVD in PIN, we computed linear vessel densities by quantifying vessel–gland perimeter length ratios for individual ductules of normal and neoplastic histology. Sixteen of 23 cases showed significantly higher densities for PIN than for benign glands, with an overall ratio of 1.36 (Table 22–7).[9] We also demon-

Table 22–4. Comparison of Staging Information from Gleason Grade, PSA, Tumor Area, and Microvessel Density for 19 Men with Organ Confined Prostate Cancer and 13 Men with Advanced Disease

Test	Sensitivity* (%)	Specificity* (%)	PPV (%)	NPV (%)
PSA > 10.0 ng/mL	28.6	82.4	57.1	58.3
Gleason grade > 7	94.4	47.4	63.0	90.0
Tumor area > 1.0 cm²	76.9	84.2	76.9	84.2
MVD/mm²				
> 100	77.8	79.0	77.8	79.0
> 120	44.4	100.0	100.0	65.5

*Sensitivity, specificity, and positive and negative predictive values denote ability of marker to stratify organ-confined prostate cancer from advanced disease.

From Brawer MK, Deering RE, Brown M, et al.: Predictors of pathologic stage in prostate carcinoma. Cancer 73:678–687, 1994.

Table 22–5. Tumor Grade, Tumor Area, Serum PSA, and Microvessel Density Values Separated by Pathologic Stage

Parameter	OC* n = 19 (range)	C2† n = 9 (range)	D1‡ n = 4 (range)	D2§ n = 5 (range)
PSA in ng/mL	6.5 (4.1–9.0)	9.4 (2.8–17.0)	9.3 (5.8–8.6)	NA
Gleason grade	6.4 (5.9–7.0)	7.3 (6.8–7.9)	8.0 (6.2–9.8)	9.4 (8.8–10.1)
Tumor area in cm²	0.7 (0.6–0.9)	2.2 (1.0–3.3)	3.9 (0.9–8.6)	NA
MVD in vessels/mm²	81.2 (71.4–91.0)	108.7 (94.3–123.0)	114.2 (70.9–157.4)	154.6 (92.3–216.9)

*OC, organ-confined disease: carcinoma confined to the prostate gland.
†C2 disease: tumor extends beyond prostate into either seminal vesicles or lateral sulcus.
‡D1 disease: tumor has disseminated to iliac lymph nodes.
§D2 disease: tumor has metastasized to bone.

From Brawer MK, Deering RE, Brown M, et al.: Predictors of pathologic stage in prostate carcinoma. Cancer 73:678–687, 1994.

Table 22–6. Comparison of Diagnostic Markers in Predicting Organ Confinement Versus Extraprostatic Spread

Marker	OC* n = 19 (95% CI‡)	C2/D1† n = 13 (95% CI‡)	P Value§
PSA (ng/mL)	6.6 (4.1–9.0)	9.1 (4.5–13.7)	0.260
Grade	6.4 (5.9–7.0)	7.5 (7.0–8.1)	0.007
Tumor area (cm²)	0.74 (0.56–0.93)	2.7 (1.4–3.9)	0.007
MVD (vv/mm²)	81.2 (71.4–91.0)	110.4 (97.9–122.8)	<0.001

*OC, organ confined disease: carcinoma confined to the prostate gland.
†C2 disease: tumor extends beyond prostate into seminal vesicles or lateral sulcus; D1 disease: tumor has disseminated to iliac lymph nodes.
‡CI, confidence interval.
§P-value determined from two-tailed Student's t test.

From Brawer MK, Deering RE, Brown M, et al.: Predictors of pathologic stage in prostate carcinoma. Cancer 73:678–687, 1994.

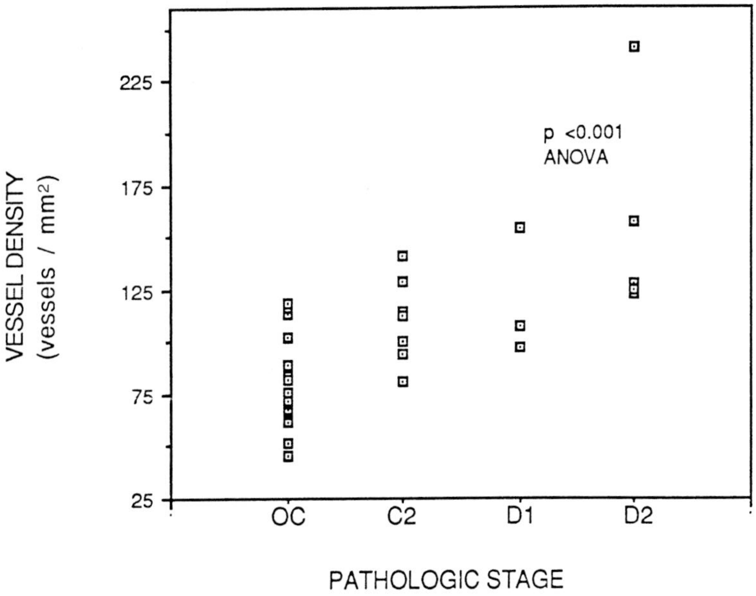

Figure 22–1. Microvessel densities from 37 cases representing four pathologic stages: organ confined (OC), positive margins (C2), pelvic lymph node metastasis (D1), and bone metastasis (D2). (From Brawer MK, Deering RE, Brown M, et al.: Predictors of pathologic stage in prostatic carcinoma. Cancer 73:678, 1994.)

strated increased neovascularization associated with certain histologic patterns in BPH. Vessel densities in epithelial nodules approached those of high-grade carcinoma (Table 22–8).[61] Significantly increased neovascularity in stromal nodules suggested that the influence of angiogenesis may begin in the early stages of BPH.

Our observed correlation between MVD and pathologic stage in prostate carcinoma has been confirmed by others. Fregene and colleagues evaluated 34 malignant specimens from patients who had undergone radical prostatectomy.[11] In this investigation, mean MVD distinguished organ-confined neoplasms from stage D carcinomas ($P < 0.005$); however, this group found no significant difference between stage B and stage C tumors (Table 22–9).

Weidner and associates also demonstrated a significant difference between primary tissue MVD obtained from men with organ-confined cancer and those with metastasis.[62] The fields of highest vessel density were identified and manually quantified in 74 patients, 29 with metastasis and 45 without (Table 22–10). In this group, the MVD in patients with metastasis was nearly double that in patients without metastasis—(104 and 53 vessels/mm² respectively, $P < 0.0001$).

Wakui and colleagues found less predictive success evaluating vascularity in 101 prostate cancer cases, 43 with bone marrow metastasis and 58 organ-confined cases.[63] Their measurement of vascularization, blood capillary density ratios (BCDR), computed the ratio of total vascular area to tumor area. They found a significant relationship between BCDR and stage for low- and intermediate-grade carcinomas but failed to find a general correlation. Their quantification method differs markedly from ours: they looked at total blood vessel

Table 22–7. Comparison of MVD in Prostatic Intraepithelial Neoplasia (PIN) and Normal Prostate Tissue*

| Tissue | n | MVD (vv/mm²) | | |
		Mean	Range	95% CI*
PIN	25	11.6	6.0–17.8	10.4–12.8
Benign	25	8.6	2.5–14.6	7.5–9.8

*CI, confidence interval.

From Bigler SA, Brawer MK, Deering RE, et al.: Microcirculation in PIN and typical benign hyperplasia of the prostate. Lab Invest 68:56A (No. 312), 1993.

Table 22–8. Comparison of Microvascularity in Benign Prostatic Hyperplasia and Histologically Normal Prostate Tissue

Tissue	n	MVD (vv/mm²)		
		Mean	Standard Deviation	Range
Normal stroma	58	36.5	15.3	10–78
Stromal nodule	6	64.7	19.1	46–94
Normal epithelium	23	76.7	23.1	39–148
Epithelial nodule	97	99.3	40.7	37–253

From Deering RE, Bigler SA, Brown M, et al.: Microvascularity in BPH. Prostate 26:111–115, 1995.

area per field, whereas our work evaluated the number of microvessels per field. Thus, their method places a much more significant emphasis on larger vessels; for example, they would count one vessel of 40-μm diameter as equal to seven 15-μm diameter microvessels. Their angiogenic grading method fails to give sufficient weight to the significance of microvessels. This difference is significant from both a biologic and a mechanical perspective. Microvessels are more accessible than larger vessels to tumor cell intravasation.[19] Mechanically, a similar area of microvessels would expose a considerably greater vascular region to tumor cell invasion than a similar area of larger vessels. This is a simple geometric consideration: the circumference of the vessels is directly proportional to the diameter, whereas the areas are proportional to the square of the diameters. Thus, in our example of one 40-μm vessel in contrast to seven 15-μm microvessels, the net surface area represented by the seven microvessels is nearly triple that of the one larger vessel (approximately 330 μm versus 126 μm).

In an effort to evaluate the yield of neovascularity measurement in needle biopsy speci-

mens we compared the vessel count from diagnostic needle biopsy material and that obtained from radical prostatectomy specimens in 68 men (unpublished data). We measured the total vessel density in the carcinoma for both needle and radical prostatectomy specimens. In this manner we were able to evaluate the correlations associated with both overall vessel density and the highest MVD of each case.

In samples that contained sufficient biopsy tissue (≥ 1.5 mm²), our data demonstrated good correlation between the needle MVD and that of the radical specimen, using both mean needle MVD and highest MVD ($r^2 = 0.68$, $P < 0.0001$ and $r^2 = 0.74$, $P < 0.0001$, respectively) (Fig. 22–2). These data indicate that needle biopsy vascularity provides a reliable approximation of that in the neoplasm as a whole. A consistent increase was found in the biopsy quantitation (as compared with the corresponding radical prostatectomy specimen), which we believe to be an artifact of compression and possibly of differential shrinkage owing to fixation. We conclude that the unique, important information MVD offers in prostate cancer may be ascertained pre-

Table 22–9. Pathologic Stage Versus Microvessel Density* for 34 Prostate Carcinomas

Pathologic Stage	n	MVD (vv/mm²)		
		Mean	Standard Deviation	Range
A†	3	95	74	74–116
B‡	7	116	95	53–247
C§	11	195	90	53–326
D2#	13	311	37	116–447

*MVD measured as vessels/mm².
†OC, organ-confined disease: carcinoma confined to the prostate gland.
‡C2 disease: tumor extends beyond prostate into seminal vesicles or lateral sulcus.
§D1 disease: tumor has disseminated to iliac lymph nodes.
#D2 disease: tumor has metastasized to bone.
Data from Fregene TA, Khanuja PS, Noto AC, et al.: Tumor-associated angiogenesis in prostate cancer. Anticancer Res 13:2377–2381, 1993.

Table 22–10. Comparison of MVD and Histologic Grade of Prostate Carcinoma Specimens from 29 Men With Metastasis and 45 Men Without Metastasis

	Gleason Score	MVD (vv/mm^2)
Without metastasis		
Mean	5	53
SD	1.9	25
Range	4–10	14–149
With metastasis		
Mean	6.9	103.9
SD	1.8	60
Range	4–10	27–261
P value	0.009	<0.001

From Weidner N, Carrol PR, Flax J: Tumor angiogenesis correlates with metastasis in invasive prostate carcinoma. Am J Pathol 143:401–409, 1993.

operatively from prostatic needle biopsy specimens.

We have investigated the topographic variation of MVD within human prostate carcinomas. Our findings indicated the highest region of neovascularization is at the tumor's center (Fig. 22–3).[25] We demonstrated incremental increase in tumor vascularization from the benign periphery through the tumor's center (Fig. 22–3). This activity may be explained partly by the observation that VEGF, a specific endothelial cell mitogen produced by the prostate and other tumors, is significantly up-regulated in hypoxic conditions.[64] Compression of the microvasculature at the center of neoplasms may result in locally hypoxic re-

gions. VEGF up-regulation, stemming from this compression, may have contributed to the elevated microvessel densities we observed at the tumor's center. Increased central tumor vascularization may explain the rare findings of necrosis in prostate carcinoma. We believe that this trend may account for the better correlation observed in vascular hot spots when needle biopsy MVD was compared to that in radical prostatectomy specimens.

We have assessed the ability of MVD to identify men who were likely to suffer cancer progression following treatment with radical prostatectomy.[12] Fifteen men with advanced local-stage cancer were selected and analyzed blindly for neovascularity. The mean follow-up

Figure 22–2. Regression analysis comparing vessel counts obtained from prostate radical specimens and from diagnostic specimens from the same patients. Forty-one matched cases were analyzed.

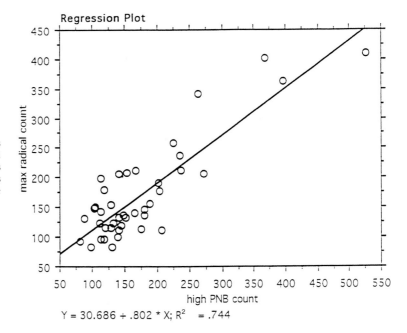

$$Y = 30.686 + .802 * X; R^2 = .744$$

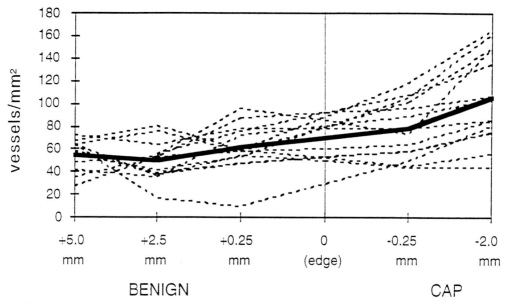

Figure 22–3. Chart summarizing findings of topography of neovascularity for 14 human prostate tumors. The bold line represents the mean. (From Siegal JA, Yu E, Brawer MK: Topography of neovascularity in human prostatic carcinoma. Cancer 75:2545–2551, 1995.)

for this group was 125.3 months. The mean MVD in patients with progression was 159.0 vessels/mm² versus 117.9 vessels/mm² for men without relapse. Using an arbitrary cutoff of 140 vessels/mm², MVD predicted outcome in four of the seven patients with progression and in seven of eight patients without evidence of progression ($P = 0.035$).

MVD was a highly significant predictor of postradiation relapse in a retrospective evaluation of prostate needle biopsy sections from men treated with brachytherapy (unpublished data). Microvessel density was quantified in diagnostic specimens from 23 men, including eight with progression. The mean follow-up time was 58 months. No other morphologic feature predicted relapse with the accuracy of MVD alone (Table 22–11). Using a 120 vessel/mm² cutoff, MVD demonstrated 75% specificity and 63% sensitivity at predicting recurrence. Sensitivity was improved by combining MVD data with stage information, yielding 50% sensitivity and 88% specificity.

Hall and associates published similar findings correlating MVD with progression in prostate cancer patients treated with radiotherapy.[13] Diagnostic transurethral resection (TURP) specimens were evaluated from 25 men, 9 of whom were in relapse, with a median follow-up of 44 months. The mean MVD was significantly lower in the patients with no evidence of failure than in the relapse group (61 vessels/mm² versus 129 vessels/mm², $P < 0.0001$). These findings suggest that quantification of microvessel density may be an important prognostic marker for patients treated with radiotherapy.

ANGIOGENESIS: IMPLICATIONS FOR THERAPY

One problem in the treatment of disseminated cancer may be tumor cell heterogeneity. Primary tumors and individual metastases can respond to treatment in vastly different ways. Cells isolated from one tumor have been shown to differ in myriad ways, including growth rate, karyotype, cell surface receptors to lectins, hormone receptors, immunogenicity, response to cytotoxic drugs, and capacity for invasion and metastasis.[65] The acquisition of a phenotypic heterogeneity by populations of tumor cells confers some degree of stability on the tumor as a whole.[66] The heterogeneity and adaptability of tumors suggest that adoption of therapeutic approaches targeting the tumor's environment may be useful in addition to treatment that targets the tumor cells themselves.

The concept of antiangiogenic therapy was proposed in the early 1970s as a means of

Table 22–11. Predictive Value of PSA, Histologic Grade, Initial Stage, and Microvascularity for Prostate Cancer Progression in 24 Men, 8 With Progression*

Variable	Sensitivity (%)	Specificity (%)	PPV (%)	NPV (%)	Accuracy (%)
PSA					
>4	88	13	33	67	38
>10	63	25	29	57	38
Grade					
≥7	50	56	36	69	54
≥8	25	88	50	70	67
Initial stage >T2A	63	50	38	73	54
MVD					
>100	75	31	35	71	46
>120	63	75	56	80	71
Grade ≥8; MVD >100	13	88	33	67	63
Stage >T2A; MVD >120	50	88	67	78	75

*Patients were treated with brachytherapy (mean follow-up, 58 months).

containing tumor growth.[67] Folkman outlined three basic strategies for mounting an antiangiogenic response: (1) inhibition of released angiogenic stimulants from tumor cells; (2) neutralization of released angiogenic molecules; and (3) inhibition of vascular endothelial cells' response to angiogenic stimulation.[67]

Laboratory experiments have demonstrated that angiogenic inhibitors effectively limit tumor growth in a variety of malignant models. Synthetic administration of AGM-1470 (also referred to as "TNP-470"), a synthetic analog of fumagillin, has been repeatedly shown to inhibit growth of transplanted tumor in animals without inducing significant systemic toxicity.[68–70] Similar tumor repression in vivo has been demonstrated with administration of a heparin-steroid conjugate,[71] retinoic acid,[72] and suramin.[73] Growth of implanted prostate tumors is inhibited by AGM-1470,[70] suramin,[74] and linomide.[75]

Additionally, promising results have been demonstrated in efforts to neutralize the stimulatory effects of angiogenic promoters. In vivo growth of neoplasms has been inhibited by systemic administration of antibodies to basic fibroblast growth factor (bFGF),[76] VEGF,[77] and angiogenin.[78] Blockage of bFGF expression with antisense oglionucleotides directed against bFGF has limited tumor growth in mice.[79]

Treating neoplasms both by targeting the tumor cells (chemotherapy) and the organ environment (angiogenesis inhibition) has produced synergistic therapeutic effects in mice bearing the 3LL tumor.[80, 81] Interferon-alpha, a relatively weak angiogenic inhibitor, has been shown to treat life-threatening hemangiomas in children[82] and to induce tumor regression in highly vascular Kaposi's sarcoma.[83] Similar treatment routines may prove useful in the management of a number of human neoplasms, including those of the prostate. This therapeutic approach may prove most valuable as an adjunct to traditional therapy in tumors that are no longer responsive to standard treatments. Microvessel density may help stratify patients for whom antiangiogenic therapy may offer therapeutic benefit.

NEOVASCULARITY QUANTIFICATION: METHODOLOGIC CONSIDERATIONS

Staining Methods

Antibodies to subunits of factor VIII, antihemophilic factor, have been widely used to highlight vascular endothelial cells. Factor VIII is a macromolecule complex involved in the intrinsic process of coagulation. This protein is composed of three functionally distinct components: factor VIII–related antigen (FVIII-RA), a clot-promoting factor (FVIII C), and von Willebrand factor.[84] FVIII-RA and von Willebrand factor compose factor VIII's high–molecular weight subunit. Antibodies specific to this subunit have been shown effectively to stain vascular endothelium (Fig. 22–4).[85]

Recently it was reported that an antibody to CD-31, a platelet or endothelial cell adhesion molecule, is a more sensitive immunostain than FVIII-RA for counting microvessels in invasive breast carcinoma[43, 86]; however, Traweek and colleagues found that FVIII-RA is a more specific endothelial cell marker. Their experi-

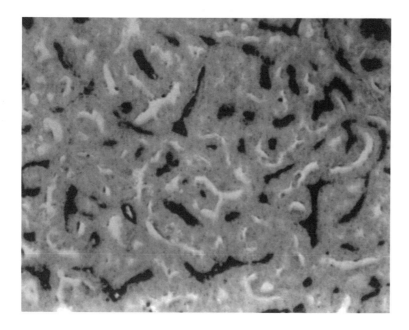

Figure 22–4. Photo of Factor VIII-related immunohistochemical stain of prostate cancer specimen clearly highlighting the tumor microvasculature.

ence demonstrated mild CD-31 cross-reactivity with fibroblasts, tumor cells, and plasma cells.[87] Toi and coworkers compared these two antibodies in a series of breast cancer specimens and found that the antibody to CD-31 produced consistently higher vessel counts than FVIII-RA.[51] Despite this variance, the staining techniques proved to be highly correlated ($r = 0.92$; $P < 0.01$). Additionally, both antibodies demonstrated significant correlation with survival ($P < 0.01$ for both CD-31 and FVIII-RA).

A lectin-binding staining method using *Ulex europaeus* agglutinin I (UEAI) is also highly sensitive for endothelial cells, evenly highlighting large blood vessels, capillaries, and lymphatics.[88, 89] In contrast, FVIII-RA produces relatively weak staining for both lymphatics and large blood vessels.[90, 91] Concern for FVIII's sensitivity is muted by the nature of our application: there is significant evidence that there are no lymphatics in common neoplasms,[92] and almost all the vessels counted are microvessels. FVIII-RA and UEAI counts were compared for their ability to predict recurrence in 69 node-negative breast carcinoma patients.[93] The UEAI counts were consistently higher than those using FVIII-RA, though there was a significant correlation between techniques. ($r = 0.73$; $P = 0.005$). Both staining methods demonstrated significant prediction of tumor recurrence ($P < 0.001$ and $P = 0.03$ for UEAI and FVIII-RA, respectively).

It is possible that anti–CD-31, UEAI, or some other endothelial cell marker will produce better correlations between MVD and metastatic potential in prostate tumors. Anti–FVIII-RA's lack of sensitivity may diminish the apparent prognostic potential of MVD. Further investigation is indicated; however, current findings indicate that all three staining techniques are highly correlated; thus, considerable improvement would not be anticipated.

Imaging Technique

We believe the use of a computer-based imaging method is critical to quantifying MVD efficiently and reproducibly (Fig. 22–5). A computer streamlines the data acquisition and storage process, standardizes the counting method, and greatly enhances counting speed. The validity of our computer-based counting method was previously demonstrated in a test of 20 fields that were quantified both manually and with the computer ($R^2 = 0.978$; $P < 0.001$) (Fig. 22–6).[57]

A basic image analysis system includes a microscope, video camera, frame grabber, computer, and image analysis software. Once a field is selected for analysis, it is captured by a video camera coupled to the microscope. The resulting image is digitized on an internal frame-grabbing computer board for analysis with imaging software. The software employs a

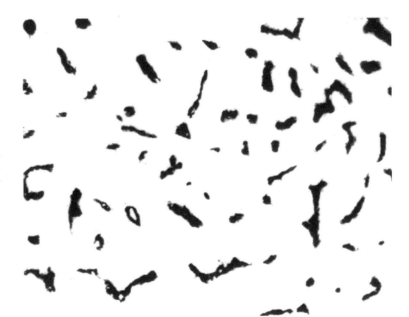

Figure 22–5. Computer clarified image of Factor VIII-related antigen immunohistochemistry prepared for counting by the computer system (same field as shown in Fig. 22–4).

manually set threshold level to discriminate vessels, stained black, from the lightly counterstained background. The operator can utilize a retouching facility to eliminate objects not determined to be vessels and to illuminate small capillaries not automatically detected by the initial threshold setting. The software then counts the total number of independent dark objects and records this value and the corresponding tissue area in a selected database or spreadsheet.

Sampling Method

Individual tumors may demonstrate a great deal of heterogeneity in MVD. Regions of necrosis, inflammation, and sclerosis may all generate locally elevated MVDs. Additionally, less differentiated sections of an individual neoplasm exhibit higher MVD than regions of lower grade. Our laboratory recently demonstrated that the centers of prostate tumors are significantly more vascularized than the tumor

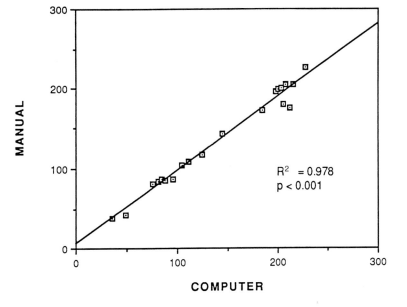

Figure 22–6. Regression analysis for 20 prostate cancer fields which were both quantified manually and with computer assisted image analysis. (From Bigler SA, Deering RE, Brawer MK: Comparison of microscopic vascularity in benign and malignant prostate tissue. Hum Pathol 24:220, 1993.)

$R^2 = 0.978$
$p < 0.001$

MANUAL

COMPUTER

edges.[26] These issues of topographic variation in MVD become critical in developing a sampling method that accurately assays a tumor's angiogenic activity. In radical prostatectomy specimens, we have found the highest correlation with stage to stem from counting vessels in a series of randomly selected fields and averaging the results. While the labor-intensive nature of traditional manual counting would make this process impractical, a computer-aided counting method renders it relatively efficient. Other investigators have found prognostic significance by quantifying vascular hot spots: selected regions that represent the highest MVD of each sample.[42, 51, 62] Developing a consistent and effective method of microvessel quantification is particularly critical if we are to use a limited sample such as that obtained from prostatic needle biopsy to predict the microvessel density of the entire neoplasm.

Our laboratory has evaluated the ability of a needle biopsy specimen to predict the vascularity of the neoplasm as a whole. The best correlations came from comparing the highest MVD of the biopsy with the highest MVD from the radical prostatectomy specimen. These findings indicate that the best correlation between diagnostic and radical specimens may be achieved by looking at the highest MVD of each. What is most significant however, is assessing the relative prognostic ability of these two strategies. Further investigation is indicated.

PROGNOSTIC SIGNIFICANCE OF OTHER FACTORS ASSOCIATED WITH ANGIOGENESIS

Expression of regulators of angiogenesis may provide additional insight into a tumor's aggressiveness. These regulators include growth factors and receptors, oncogenes, and tumor suppressor genes (see Tables 22–1, 22–2). Many of these parameters may not only provide stratification information on the aggressiveness of clinically apparent neoplasms but may actually represent some of the factors that implicate the more malignant phenotype. Several of these factors have demonstrated potential for prognostic significance in tumor management.

VEGF, a potent inducer of microvascular hyperpermeability,[94] has been shown to be a stimulator of endothelial cell motility and proliferation.[95] Immunohistochemical evaluation

has demonstrated that VEGF is overexpressed in aggressive neoplasms of the breast. Toi and associates demonstrated that the relapse-free survival rate of VEGF-rich tumors was clearly worse than that for VEGF-poor tumors ($P < 0.01$).[51] Additionally, they found that the MVD in VEGF-rich human breast tumors was significantly higher than that in cases with less staining.

The p53 tumor suppressor gene recently received a great deal of attention for its role in maintaining genomic integrity. Loss of wild-type p53 alleles is associated with gene amplification. Demeanor and coworkers determined that the loss of the wild-type p53 gene resulted in reduced expression of thrombospondin-1 (TSP-1), known to be a potent inhibitor of angiogenesis.[96] Mutations of p53 appear to be one of the most common genetic abnormalities in human cancers.[97] Although p53 mutations are perhaps rare in prostate cancers,[98] when present they have a negative effect on survival.[99]

Elevated expression of bFGF, a potent inducer of angiogenesis in vivo and in vitro, has been demonstrated in a number of tumor cell lines, including those derived from prostate cancer.[100–102] Recently, elevated bFGF concentrations were demonstrated in the urine of patients with a variety of malignancies including prostate cancer[103] and in the sera of patients with renal cell carcinoma.[104] Our laboratory has confirmed this finding in human prostate cancer patients.[105]

SUMMARY

Identification of reliable markers of malignant potential is essential to managing the huge discrepancy between histologic evidence of prostate carcinoma and clinically manifest disease. Our laboratory has investigated neovascularity in human prostate cancer as an adjunct to staging and prognosis. Previously we demonstrated that MVD is an independent predictor of pathologic stage[9] and may provide prognostic information.[12] Other researchers have confirmed both these observations.[10, 11, 13] Prospective investigations correlating MVD from diagnostic specimens with progression are essential for assessing the clinical utility of this biologic marker as a measure of tumor aggressiveness. MVD may prove to be a valuable tool in assessing the potential aggressiveness of a particular neoplasm and may become a valuable adjunct to determining clinical stage. Research is also indicated to further ascertain potential relationships between radiation and chemotherapeutic efficacy and tumor vascularity.

REFERENCES

1. Boring CC, Squires TS, Tong T: Cancer statistics, 1993. CA Can J Clin 43:7–26, 1993.
2. Scardino PT, Shinohara K, Wheeler TM, et al.: Staging of prostate cancer: Value of ultrasonography. Urol Clin North Am 16:713–734, 1989.
3. Ebert T, Schmitz-Drager B, Burrig K, et al.: Accuracy of imaging modalities in staging the local extent of prostate cancer. Urol Clin North Am 18:453–457, 1991.
4. Gibbons RP, Correa RJ Jr, Brannen GE, et al.: Total prostatectomy for clinically localized prostatic cancer: Long-term results. J Urol 131:564–566, 1989.
5. Gleason DF, Mellinger GT: VACURG: Prediction of prognosis for prostatic carcinoma by combined histological grading and clinical staging. J Urol 111:58–64, 1974.
6. Winter HI, Bretton PR, Herr HW: Preoperative prostate-specific antigen in predicting stage and grade after radical prostatectomy. Urology 38:202–205, 1991.
7. McSherry SA, Levy F, Schiebler ML, et al.: Preoperative prediction of pathological tumor volume and stage in clinically localized prostate cancer: Comparison of DRE, TRUS, and MRI. J Urol 146:85–89, 1991.
8. O'Malley FP, Grignon DJ, Keeney M, et al.: DNA heterogeneity in prostatic adenocarcinoma: A DNA flow cytometric mapping study with whole organ sections of prostate. Cancer 71(9):2797–2802, 1993.
9. Brawer MK, Deering RE, Brown M, et al.: Predictors of pathologic stage in prostatic carcinoma. The role of neovascularity. Cancer 73(3):678–687, 1994.
10. Weidner N, Carrol PR, Flax J: Tumor angiogenesis correlates with metastasis in invasive prostate carcinoma. Am J Pathol 143(2):401–409, 1993.
11. Fregene TA, Khanuja PS, Noto AC, et al.: Tumor-associated angiogenesis in prostate cancer. Anticancer Res 13:2377–2381, 1993.
12. Brawer MK, Jonsson E, Gibbons RP, et al.: Extent of prostate neovascularity predicts progression in patients with pathologic stage C adenocarcinoma treated with radical prostatectomy. J Urol 151 (Suppl):289A, 1994.
13. Hall MC, Troncoso P, Pollack A, et al.: Significance of tumor angiogenesis in clinically localized prostate carcinoma treated with external beam radiotherapy. Urology 44(6):869–875, 1994.
14. Folkman J: Relation of vascular proliferation to tumor growth. Int Rev Exp Pathol 16:207–248, 1976.
15. Folkman J, Cole P, Zimmerman S: Tumor behavior in isolated perfused organs: In vitro growth and metastasis of biopsy material in rabbit thyroid and canine intestinal segment. Ann Surg 164:491, 1966.
16. Gimbrone MA, Leapman S, Coltran RS, et al.: Tumor dormancy in vivo by prevention of neovascularization. J Exp Med 136:261–276, 1972.
17. Algire GH, Chalkley HW, Legallais GY: Vascular reactions of normal and malignant tumors in vivo. I.

18. Vascular reactions of mice to wounds and to normal and neoplastic transplants. J Natl Cancer Inst USA 6:73–85, 1945.
18. Tannock IF: Population kinetics of carcinoma cells, capillary endothelial cells, and fibroblasts in a transplanted mouse mammary tumor. Cancer Res 30:2470–2476, 1970.
19. Nagy JA, Brown LF, Senger DR, et al.: Pathogenesis of tumor stroma generation: A critical role for leaky blood vessels and fibrin deposition. Biochim Biophys Acta 948:305–326, 1988.
20. Weidner N: Tumor angiogenesis: Review of current applications in tumor prognostication. Semin Diagn Pathol 10:302–313, 1993.
21. Liotta L, Klienerman J, Saidel GM: Quantitative relationships of intravascular tumor cells, tumor vessels, and pulmonary metastasis following tumor implantation. Cancer Res 34:997–1004, 1974.
22. Liotta LA, Rao CN, Barsky SH, et al.: The laminin receptor and basement membrane dissolution: Role in tumor metastasis. In Porter JW (ed): Basement Membranes and Cell Movement. London: Pitman, 1984.
23. Wantanabe S: Metastasizability of tumor cells. Cancer 7:215, 1954.
24. Dvorak HF, Dvorak AM, Manseau EJ, et al.: Fibrin gel investment associated with line 1 and line 10 solid tumor growth, angiogenesis, and fibroplasia in guinea pigs. Role of cellular immunity, myofibroblasts, microvascular damage, and infarction in line tumor regression. J Natl Cancer Inst 62:1459–1472, 1979.
25. Kalebic T, Garbisa S, Glaser B, et al.: Basement membrane collagen: Degradation by migrating endothelial cells. Science 221:281–283, 1983.
26. Siegal JA, Yu E, Brawer MK: Topography of neovascularity in human prostatic carcinoma. Cancer 75:2545–2551, 1995.
27. Papadimitriou JM, Woods AE: Structural and functional characteristics of the microcirculation in neoplasms. J Pathol 116:65–72, 1975.
28. Coman DR, Sheldon WF: The significance of hyperemia around tumor implants. Am J Pathol 22:821–826, 1946.
29. Algire GH, Legallais FY, Park HD: Vascular reactions of normal and malignant tumors in vivo. J Natl Cancer Inst 8:53, 1947.
30. Folkman J, Klagsbrun M: Angiogenic factors. Science 235:442–447, 1987.
31. Gimbrone MA, Leapman S, Coltran RS, et al.: Tumor growth neovascularization: An experimental model using rabbit cornea. J Natl Cancer Inst 52:413–427, 1974.
32. Ehrmann RL, Knoth M: Choriocarcinoma. Transfilter stimulation of vasoproliferation in the hamster cheek pouch. Studied by light and electron microscopy. J Natl Cancer Inst 41:1329–1341, 1968.
33. Tuan D, Smith S, Folkman J, et al.: Isolation of the nonhistone proteins of rat Walker carcinoma. Biochemistry 12:3159–3165, 1973.
34. Shing Y, Folkman J, Sullivan R, et al.: Heparin-affinity: Purification of a tumor-derived capillary endothelial cell growth factor. Science 223:1296, 1984.
35. Denekamp J: Vasomotion and quantitative microcirculation. *In* Hammersen F, Hudlicka K (eds): Progress in Applied Microcirculation. Basel: S Karger, 1984.
36. Jackson D, Volpert OV, Bouck N, et al.: Stimulation

and inhibition of angiogenesis by placental proliferin and proliferin-related protein. Science 266:1581–1584, 1994.

37. Eisenstein R, Sorgente N, Soble LW, et al.: The resistance of certain tissues to invasion: Penetrability of explanted tissues by vascularized mesenchyme. Am J Pathol 73:765–774, 1973.

38. Brem H, Folkman J: Inhibition of tumor angiogenesis mediated by cartilage. J Exp Med 141:427–439, 1975.

39. Srivastava A, Laidler P, Hughes LE, et al.: Neovascularization in human cutaneous melanoma: A quantitative morphologic and Doppler ultrasound study. Eur J Cancer Clin Oncol 22:1205–1209, 1986.

40. Graham CH, Rivers J, Kerbel RS, et al.: Extent of vascularization as a prognostic indicator in thin (<0.76 mm) malignant melanomas. Am J Pathol 145:510–514, 1994.

41. Olivarez D, Ulbright T, DeRiese W, et al.: Neovascularization in clinical stage A testicular germ cell tumor: Prediction of metastatic disease. Cancer Res 54:2800–2802, 1994.

42. Bosari S, Lee AKC, Delellis RA, et al.: Microvessel quantitation and prognosis in invasive breast carcinoma. Hum Pathol 23:755–61, 1992.

43. Horak ER, Leek R, Klenk N, et al.: Angiogenesis, assessed by platelet/endothelial cell adhesion molecule antibodies, as indicator of node metastases and survival in breast cancer. Lancet 340:1120–1124, 1992.

44. Weidner N, Folkman J, Pozza F, et al.: Tumor angiogenesis: A new significant and independent prognostic indicator in early-stage breast carcinoma. J Natl Cancer Inst 84:1875–1887, 1992.

45. Weidner N, Semple JP, Welch WR, et al.: Tumor angiogenesis and metastasis—correlation in invasive breast carcinoma. N Engl J Med 324:1–8, 1991.

46. Gasparini G, Weidner N, Bevilacqua P, et al.: Tumor microvessel density, p53 expression, tumor size, and peritumoral lymphatic vessel invasion are relevant prognostic markers in node-negative breast cancer. J Clin Oncol 12:454–466, 1994.

47. Williams JK, Carlson GW, Cohen C, et al.: Tumor angiogenesis as a prognostic factor in oral cavity tumors. Am J Surg 168:373–380, 1994.

48. Fox SB, Leek RD, Smith K, et al.: Tumor angiogenesis in node-negative breast carcinomas—relationship with epidermal growth factor receptor, estrogen receptor, and survival. Breast Cancer Res Treat 29:109–116, 1994.

49. Obermair A, Czerwenka K, Kurz C, et al.: [Tumoral vascular density in breast tumors and their effect on recurrence-free survival]. Chirurg 65:611–615, 1994.

50. Sahin AA, Ro J, Ro JY, et al.: Ki-67 immunostaining in node-negative stage I/II breast carcinoma. Significant correlation with prognosis. Cancer 68:549–557, 1991.

51. Toi M, Kashitani J, Tominaga T: Tumor angiogenesis is an independent prognostic indicator in primary breast carcinoma. Int J Cancer 55:371–374, 1993.

52. Visscher DW, Smilanetz S, Drozdowicz S, et al.: Prognostic significance of image morphometric microvessel enumeration in breast carcinoma. Anal Quant Cytol Histol 15:88–92, 1993.

53. Yamazaki K, Abe S, Takekawa H, et al.: Tumor angiogenesis in human lung adenocarcinoma. Cancer 74(8):2245–2250, 1994.

54. Macchiarini P, Fontanini G, Hardin MJ, et al.: Rela-

tion of neovascularisation to metastasis of non–small-cell lung cancer. Lancet 340:145–146, 1992.

55. Macchiarini P, Fontanini G, Dulmet E, et al.: Angiogenesis: An indicator of metastasis in non–small cell lung cancer invading the thoracic inlet. Ann Thorac Surg 57:1534–1539, 1994.

56. Saclarides TJ, Speziale NJ, Drab E, et al.: Tumor angiogenesis and rectal carcinoma. Dis Colon Rectum 37:921–926, 1994.

57. Bigler SA, Deering RE, Brawer MK: Comparison of microscopic vascularity in benign and malignant prostate tissue. Hum Pathol 24(2):220–226, 1993.

58. Bigler SA, Brawer MK, Deering RE, et al.: Vessel density in carcinoma of the prostate: Comparing organ confined tumors with stage D tumors. J US Can Acad Pathol 68(I):56A, 1993.

59. Bigler SA, Brawer MK, Deering RE: Neovascularization in carcinoma of the prostate: A quantitative morphometric study. Lab Invest 66(1):50A, 1992.

60. Brawer MK, Bigler SA, Brown M, et al.: Neovascularity in human prostate. J Urol 149(4):419A, 1993.

61. Deering RE, Bigler SA, Brown M, et al.: Microvascularity in BPH. Prostate 26:111–115, 1995.

62. Weidner N, Carroll PR, Flax J, et al.: Tumor angiogenesis correlates with metastasis in invasive prostate carcinoma. Am J Pathol 143:401–409, 1993.

63. Wakui S, Furusato M, Itoh T, et al.: Tumor angiogenesis in prostatic carcinoma with and without bone marrow metastasis: A morphometric study. J Pathol 168:257–262, 1992.

64. Plate KH, Breier G, Millauer B, et al.: Up-regulation of vascular endothelial growth factor and its cognate receptors in a rat glioma model of tumor angiogenesis. Cancer Res 53:5822–5827, 1993.

65. Hart IR, Fidler IJ: The implications of tumor heterogeneity for studies on the biology of cancer metastasis. Biochim Biophys Acta 651:37–50, 1981.

66. Fidler IJ, Hart IR: Biological diversity in metastatic neoplasms: Origins and implications. Science 217:998–1003, 1982.

67. Folkman J: Anti-angiogenesis: New concept for therapy of solid tumors. Ann Surg 175:409–416, 1972.

68. Ingber D, Fujita T, Kishimoto S, et al.: Synthetic analogues of fumagillin that inhibit angiogenesis and suppress tumour growth. Nature 348:555–557, 1990.

69. Yamaoka M, Yamamoto T, Masaki T, et al.: Inhibition of tumor growth and metastasis of rodent tumors by the angiogenesis inhibitor O-(chloroacetyl-carbamoyl)fumagillol (TNP-470; AGM-1470). Cancer Res 53:4262–4267, 1993.

70. Yamaoka M, Yamamoto T, Ikeyama S, et al.: Angiogenesis inhibitor TNP-470 (AGM-1470) potently inhibits the tumor growth of hormone–independent human breast and prostate carcinoma cell lines. Cancer Res 53:5233–5236, 1993.

71. Thorpe PE, Derbyshire EJ, Andrade SP, et al.: Heparin-steroid conjugates: New angiogenesis inhibitors with antitumor activity in mice. Cancer Res 53:3000–3007, 1993.

72. Pienta KJ, Nguyen NM, Lehr JE: Treatment of prostate cancer in the rat with the synthetic retinoid fenretinide. Cancer Res 53:224–226, 1993.

73. Pesenti E, Sola F, Mongelli N, et al.: Suramin prevents neovascularisation and tumour growth through blocking of basic fibroblast growth factor activity. Br J Cancer 66:367–372, 1992.

74. Suzuki Y, Miwa Y, Akino H, et al.: [The enhancement of the chemotherapeutic effects on human prostate

cancer cell—the combination with the growth factor interaction inhibitor (suramin)]. Hinyokika Kiyo 39:1215–1220, 1993.

75. Vukanovic J, Passaniti A, Hirata T, et al.: Antiangiogenic effects of the quinoline-3-carboxamide linomide. Cancer Res 53:1833–1837, 1993.

76. Hori A, Sasada R, Matsutani E, et al.: Suppression of a solid tumor growth by immunoneutralizing monoclonal antibody against human basic fibroblast growth factor. Cancer Res 51:6180–6184, 1991.

77. Kim KJ, Li B, Winer J, et al.: Inhibition of vascular endothelial growth factor–induced angiogenesis suppresses tumour growth in vivo. Nature 362:841–844, 1993.

78. Olson KA, Fett JW, French TC, et al.: Angiogenin antagonists prevent tumor growth in vivo. Proc Natl Acad Sci USA 92:442–446, 1995.

79. Ensoli B, Markham P, Kao V, et al.: Block of AIDS-Kaposi's sarcoma (KS) cell growth, angiogenesis, and lesion formation in nude mice by antisense oligonucleotide targeting basic fibroblast growth factor. A novel strategy for the therapy of KS. J Clin Invest 94:1736–1746, 1994.

80. Teicher BA, Sotomayor EA, Huang ZD: Antiangiogenic agents potentiate cytotoxic cancer therapies against primary and metastatic disease. Cancer Res 52:6702–6704, 1992.

81. Teicher BA, Holden SA, Ara G, et al.: Response of the FSaII fibrosarcoma to antiangiogenic modulators plus cytotoxic agents. Anticancer Res 13:2101–2106, 1993.

82. Ezekowitz RA, Mulliken JB, Folkman J: Interferon alfa-2a therapy for life-threatening hemangiomas of infancy [see comments]. N Engl J Med 326:1456–1463, 1992.

83. Oettgen HF, Real FX, Krown SE: Treatment of AIDS-associated Kaposi's sarcoma with recombinant alpha interferon. Immunobiology. 172:269–274, 1986.

84. Ratnoff OD: Antihemophilic factor (Factor VIII). Ann Intern Med 88:403–409, 1978.

85. Mukai K, Rosai J, Burgdorf WH: Localization of factor VIII-related antigen in vascular endothelial cells using an immunoperoxidase method. Am J Surg Pathol 4:273–276, 1980.

86. Kuzu I, Bicknell R, Harris AL, et al.: Heterogeneity of vascular endothelial cells with relevance to diagnosis of vascular tumors. J Clin Pathol 45:403–412, 1992.

87. Traweek ST, Kandalaft PL, Mehta P, et al.: The human hematopoietic progenitor cell antigen (CD34) in vascular neoplasia. Am J Clin Pathol 96:25–31, 1991.

88. Ordóñez NG, Brooks T, Thompson S, et al.: Use of *Ulex europaeus* agglutinin I in the identification of lymphatic and blood vessel invasion in previously stained microscopic slides. Am J Surg Pathol 11:543–550, 1987.

89. Fujime M, Lin CW, Prout GR Jr: Identification of vessels by lectin-immunoperoxidase staining of endothelium: Possible applications in urogenital malignancies. J Urol 131:566–570, 1984.

90. Nagle RB, Witte MH, Martinez AP: Factor VIII-associated antigen in human lymphatic endothelium. Lymphology 20:20–24, 1987.

91. Ordóñez NG, Batsakis JG: Comparison of *Ulex europaeus* I lectin and factor VII–related antigen in vascular lesions. Arch Pathol Lab Med 108:129–132, 1984.

92. Tanigawa N, Kanazawa T, Satomura K: Experimental study on lymphatic vasculature changes in the development of cancer. Lymphology 14:149–154, 1981.

93. Sahin AA, Sneige N, Ordonez NG, et al.: Tumor angiogenesis directed by *Ulex europaeus* agglutinin I lectin (UEAI) and Factor VII immunostaining in node-negative breast carcinoma (NNBC) treated by mastectomy: Prediction of tumor recurrence. Mod Pathol 6:19A, 1993.

94. Senger DR, Connolly D, Perruzzi CA, et al.: Purification of a vascular permeability factor (VPF) from tumor cell conditioned medium. Fed Proc 46:2102, 1987.

95. Gospodarowicz D, Abraham JA, Schilling J: Isolation and characterization of a vascular endothelial cell mitogen produced by pituitary-derived folliculo stellate cells. Proc Natl Acad Sci USA 86:7311–7315, 1989.

96. Dameron KM, Volpert OV, Tainsky MA, et al.: Control of angiogenesis in fibroblasts by p53 regulation of thrombospondin-1. Science 265:1582–1584, 1994.

97. de Fromentel C, Soussi T: TP53 tumor suppressor gene: A model for investigating human mutagenesis. Genes Chromosom Cancer 4:1–15, 1992.

98. Dinjens WN, van der Weiden MM, Schroeder FH, et al.: Frequency and characterization of p53 mutations in primary and metastatic human prostate cancer. Int J Cancer 56:630–636, 1994.

99. Visakorpi T, Kallioniemi OP, Heikkinen A, et al.: Small subgroup of aggressive, highly proliferative prostatic carcinomas defined by p53 accumulation. J Natl Cancer Inst 84:883–887, 1992.

100. Morrison RS, Giordano S, Yamaguchi F, et al.: Basic fibroblast growth factor expression is required for clonogenic growth of human glioma cells. J Neurosci Res 34:502–509, 1993.

101. Rodeck U, Herlyn M: Growth factors in melanoma. Cancer Met Rev 10(2):89–101, 1991.

102. Nakamoto T, Chang C, Chodak GK: Basic fibroblast growth factor in human prostate cancer cells. Cancer Res 52:571–577, 1992.

103. Nguyen M, Watanabe H, Budson AE, et al.: Elevated levels of an angiogenic peptide, basic fibroblast growth factor, in the urine of patients with a wide spectrum of cancers. J Natl Cancer Inst 86:356–361, 1994.

104. Fujimoto K, Ichimori Y, Kakizoe T, et al.: Increased serum levels of basic fibroblast growth factor in patients with renal cell carcinoma. Biochem Biophys Res Commun 180(1):386–392, 1991.

105. Meyer GE, Yu E, Siegal JA, et al.: Serum basic fibroblast growth factor in men with and without prostate carcinoma. Cancer 76:2304–2311, 1995.

23

CHROMOSOMAL ABNORMALITIES IN HUMAN PROSTATE CANCER: THEIR DETECTION AND PATHOLOGIC SIGNIFICANCE

AVERY A. SANDBERG

Establishing and deciphering the various genetic events that lead to the development and progression of prostate cancer are assuming crucial importance since this disease is currently the most common cancer in men and its incidence is increasing.[1, 2] Though some of the genetic, cytogenetic, and DNA aspects of prostate cancer have been reviewed,[3, 4] in this chapter I update the new information on the cytogenetic and molecular aspects of prostate cancer and suggest a modified scheme for the genetic events that may underlie its development and progression.

In discussing the cytogenetics and genetics of prostate cancer it must be remembered that the disease probably consists of a number of subentities, some of which may be characterized histologically, histochemically, enzymatically, and clinically. In presenting the genetic, particularly cytogenetic, aspects of prostate cancer, this heterogeneity may be reflected in the chromosome changes. Compounding this problem is the observation that when prostate cancers grow in vitro, no matter how short the time of culture, growth of normal (diploid) cells predominates; this obscures the exact incidence and number of the chromosomal (cytogenetic, karyotypic) changes present in pros-

tate cancer. Thus, we are faced with a dilemma about whether the diploid cells are of neoplastic origin or whether they are normal cells with a considerable in vitro growth advantage over the cancer cells. Recent studies point to the likelihood of the latter (see below). It is hoped that techniques for more efficient culture and determination of the chromosome changes in prostate cancer will be developed and thus will allow more reliable and meaningful evaluation of these changes.

Despite a number of strategies for clinical management of prostate tumors, little progress has been made in identifying prognostic parameters and the behavior of individual tumors.[5] Prostate cancer exhibits remarkable heterogeneity, and pathologic examination often reveals a wide range of cytologic and histologic appearances. Moreover, morphologic grading systems are inadequate, despite the application of more and more sophisticated image analysis systems that allow detection of even very small alterations in the prostate. Identification of cellular features that predict the biologic behavior of the individual tumors is one of the major challenges of modern pathology. A search for independent markers to identify specific aspects of cancer biology has

400

been intensified during the last few years, and techniques have been, and are being, developed to elucidate the pathobiology of cancer cells. Among these are various in vitro studies, including chromosome analysis, morphometry, flow cytometry, and DNA studies.[6–9]

Tumor-derived cell cultures are a very suitable and widely used system for determining several tumor-associated parameters (e.g., cell kinetics, in vitro drug testing, and receptor studies).[6, 10, 11] Primary short-term cultures of solid tumors are essential for conventional cytogenetic analyses.[12] A wide range of cytogenetic studies has been performed on hematologic disorders and some tumors,[13] but the number of publications on cytogenetic data on prostate cancer is still very limited, and, so far, no consistent primary chromosome abnormalities have been reported.[4] In contrast to most other solid tumors, in vitro cultivation of prostate cancer cells remains difficult.[7, 14–16] All authors stress the difficulties of avoiding outgrowth of stromal cells and simultaneously stimulating epithelial cells to start cell division. The nature of the tumor specimen adds to the problem because of the heterogeneity of prostate cancer on both macroscopic and microscopic levels. Carcinoma and normal glands are often located side by side, and foci

within the tumor may show varying degrees of differentiation.[17]

CYTOGENETICS METHODS IN PROSTATE CANCER

Despite serious problems of examining prostate cancers by direct techniques, improvements in tissue culturing and cytogenetic techniques have been described.[5, 18, 19] Nevertheless, prostate cancer remains one of the most difficult neoplasms to examine cytogenetically because of preferential growth of normal (diploid) cells at the expense of the malignant cells, even in relatively short-term cultures. Thus, failure to obtain a sufficient number of dividing cancer cells in vitro (even after short-term incubation), the low mitotic index of the original tumor in most of the cases, and overgrowth of the cancer cells in culture by normal (diploid) cells have held back reliable and meaningful cytogenetic exploration of prostate cancer. Major breakthroughs in this area appear not to be imminent: however, progress has been made in some aspects (Figs. 23–1 to 23–3).[5]

Szücs and colleagues developed a method that relies on combined mechanical and enzy-

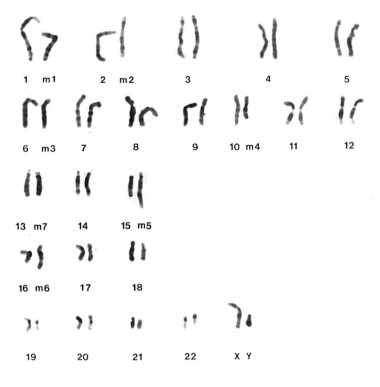

Figure 23–1. Representative pseudodiploid (46 chromosomes with structural changes) karyotype of a prostate cancer cell line (LNCaP) with seven marker chromosomes (M1–M7). For the origin of these markers, some of which are common in prostate cancer, see Figure 23–2. (From Gibav Z, Becher R, Kawinski E, et al: A high-resolution study of chromosome changes in a human prostatic carcinoma cell line (LNCaP). Cancer Genet Cytogenet 11:399, 1984.)

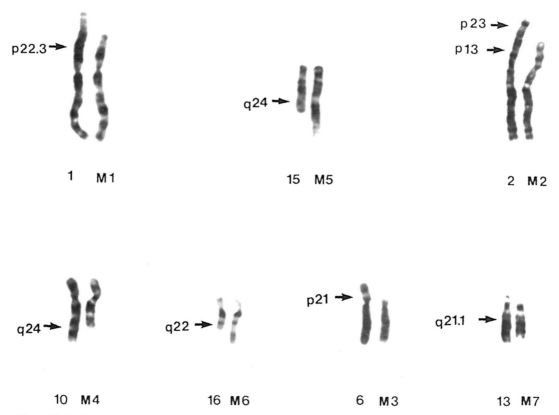

Figure 23–2. Origins of the seven markers shown in Figure 23–1. Arrows point to the breakpoints in the normal chromosomes; the changes in chromosomes 2, 10, 16, and 13 have been shown to affect a significant number of prostate cancers. (From Gibav Z, Becher R, Kawinski E, et al: A high-resolution study of chromosome changes in a human prostatic carcinoma cell line (LNCaP). Cancer Genet Cytogenet 11:399, 1984.)

matic disaggregation of tumor cells, an approach previously employed by other workers;[5, 15–19] However, Szücs' group seeded disaggregated clumps rather than single cells utilizing RPMI 1640 medium with 18% fetal calf serum (FCS) without other supplements and stimulating selective epithelial proliferation by changing the culture conditions through serum-free medium. The authors[5] indicate that with this method fibroblast growth (as a source of diploid cells) could be virtually abolished, as the origin of the epithelial and prostate cancer cells should be confirmed by immunocytochemical means.

Interphase cytogenetics is likely to fill an important niche in cancer cytogenetics in general,[20, 21] particularly prostate cancer (Figs. 23–4, 23–5). Though the type and amount of information this approach affords are somewhat limited (e.g., a detailed karyotype of a tumor cannot be established with this approach) information can nevertheless be obtained in interphase nuclei of nondividing cells, on small amounts of tissue insufficient for culture and cytogenetic analysis and on degenerate tissue retaining intact nuclei.

THE NATURE OF CHROMOSOMAL CHANGES IN HUMAN NEOPLASIA

Evaluation and interpretation of the cytogenetic changes in prostate cancer require some background on these changes and their correlates in other conditions (the leukemias, lymphomas, and some solid tumors).[12, 22–24] In these states the cytogenetic changes are often key factors in diagnosis and prognosis. Thus, in the leukemias the cytogenetic changes, often present as a sole anomaly, particularly translocations, not only have diagnostic and prognostic value, correlating with the cytologic, phenotypic, and clinical aspects of the disease, but also serve as key guides in the recognition, localization, and characterization of the genes involved and their possible role

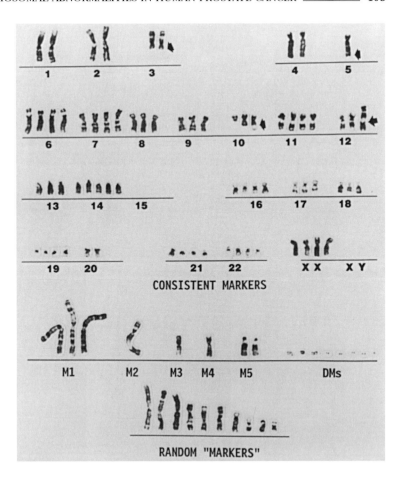

Figure 23–3. In contrast to the pseudodiploid karyotype shown in Figure 23–1, the one presented in this figure consists of a large number of chromosomes (more than 80) with an array of identified and unidentified marker chromosomes. Such karyotypes are not uncommon in prostate cancer. The changes in the karyotype shown include an array of numerical changes as well as structurally modified chromosomes (M1–M5 and "markers"). Note the presence of double minute chromosomes (DMs). (From Brothman AR, Lesho LJ, Somers KD, et al: Cytogenetic analysis of four primary prostatic cultures. Cancer Genet Cytogenet 37:241, 1989.)

in the causation of the leukemia. These changes are represented by t(9;22)(q34;q11), the so-called Philadelphia chromosome, leading to the Ph chromosome in chronic myelocytic leukemia (CML), the t(15;17)(q22;q12) in acute promyelocytic leukemia (APL), and t(8;14)(q24;q32) in Burkitt-type acute lymphoblastic leukemia (ALL). Recognition of the genes affected by these changes has led to the development of very sensitive molecular approaches (Southern blotting, polymerase chain reaction [PCR], and immunochemical tests) to the diagnosis and follow-up of the conditions[25–27] as well as to the possible role these cytogenetic changes play in the causation of the disease.[28–30] Among solid tumors, those of soft tissue and bone are often associated with single karyotypic changes similar to those seen in the leukemias[31]—e.g., t(12;16)(q13;p11) in myxoid lymphosarcoma, t(11;22)(q24;12) in Ewing's sarcoma, and t(X;18)(p11;q11) in synovial sarcoma. Thus far, the cytogenetic changes mentioned have consisted of specific translocations by which

affected genes have been rearranged leading to the genesis of abnormal fusion gene products, usually being oncogenes. Apparently, such fusion products are capable of causing the various malignant states with which they are associated. Oncogenes are thought to be growth controlling in their activity, and their modification through the translocations is thought to lead to abnormal growth and differentiation.

Another mechanism for neoplasia is that associated with loss of heterozygosity (LOH), in which tumor suppressor genes are lost and/or modified through a number of mechanisms.[28, 29] The essence of these events is the expression of a mutated gene on one allele associated with loss of the other allele. A common mechanism for this loss is a chromosomal deletion such as that seen in some tumors (e.g., 13p− in retinoblastoma and 11p− in Wilms' tumor).

A third mechanism leading to tumor formation is that related to apoptosis, or programmed cell death.[32] Evidence is accumulat-

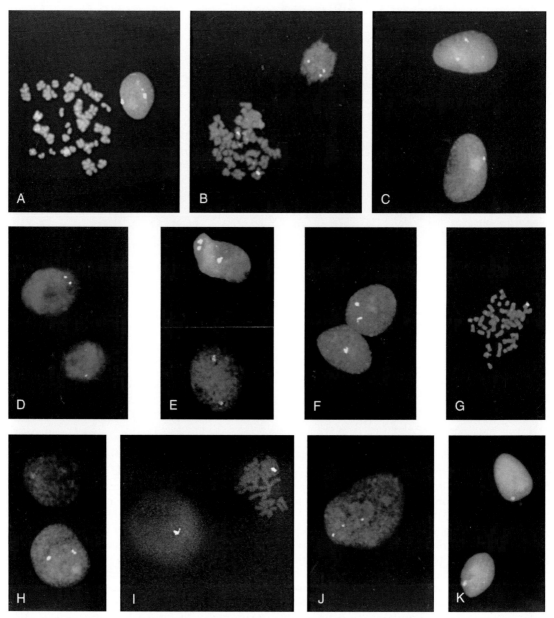

Figure 23–4. Prostate tumor cells studied by FISH with centromeric probes for chromosomes 7, 8, 10, 17, and 18. *A,* Metaphase and interphase nucleus disomic for chromosome 7 (two signals); *B,* metaphase disomic and interphase nucleus trisomic for chromosome 7 (three signals); *C,* interphase trisomic and one monosomic for chromosome 7 (one signal); *D,* interphase disomic and another monosomic for chromosome 8; *E,* interphase trisomic and another disomic for chromosome 10; *F,* interphases disomic and another monosomic for chromosome 10; *G,* metaphase monosomic for chromosome 10; *H,* interphases disomic and monosomic for chromosome 16; *I,* metaphase and interphase monosomic for chromosome 17; *J,* interphase trisomic for chromosome 18; *K,* interphases monosomic for chromosome 18. Though the FISH studies in this figure are shown in black and white, the actual preparations examined microscopically are associated with various fluorescent colors. (From Brothman AR, Patee AM, Peehl DM, et al.: Analysis of prostatic tumor cultures using fluorescence in-situ hybridization (FISH). Cancer Genet Cytogenet 62:180, 1992.)

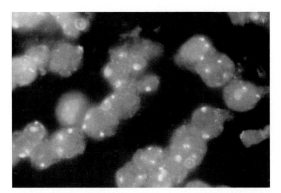

Figure 23–5. An example of FISH analysis of a paraffin-embedded tissue section of a prostatic cancer. A probe for the centromeric area of chromosome 7 was used, and the picture reveals extensive chromosome 7 trisomy (three signals) in this field. Trisomy 7 is not uncommon in prostate cancer. (Micale MA, Mohamed A, Sakr W, et al.: Cytogenetics of primary prostatic adenocarcinoma. Cancer Genet Cytogenet 61:165, 1992.)

ing that genes controlling apoptosis may be affected in a number of conditions, including prostate cancer. The genes affected may vary from one condition to another.

The acquisition of karyotypic changes in addition to those seen originally is usually associated with increased aggressiveness (e.g., progression, invasion, and metastatic spread) of the leukemia or tumor. In fact, it is now thought that the development of most adenocarcinomas, including that of the prostate, requires a series of orchestrated genetic events, most of them of the LOH variety, to progress from cellular proliferation to malignant transformation to metastases.

The complexity and number of chromosome changes seen in the common cancers (breast, lung, colon, prostate) stand in contrast to the simple genetic events often seen in leukemias and sarcomas. By the time tumors of epithelial origin, including those of the prostate, are examined cytogenetically, the karyotypic picture is complex, tending to obscure any specific chromosome change, if one is present. This complexity in the common cancers[33, 34] defied in the past the establishment of a single, specific cytogenetic event. The concept of a series of orchestrated genetic events required for the full development of the common cancers helps to explain the past predicament. It now appears likely that the initial genetic or cytogenetic change in a particular cancer (e.g., of colon or prostate) may be associated with an event involving a number of *different* genes (or chromosomes) in *different*

tumors, and even when a single gene is involved, the subsequent genetic events necessary for full cancer development may vary from tumor to tumor. In fact, variability within a given tumor may be responsible for the variability of intratumor histology, differentiation state, and biologic behavior (Figs. 23–6, 23–7).

Balanced structural chromosome rearrangements almost invariably result in the alteration of genes involved in growth regulation, through either deregulation of protooncogenes or creation of fusion genes encoding hybrid transcription factors. Since prostate cancer is not characterized by a single karyotypic change (Table 23–1), correlations of the chromosome findings with the pathology of the tumors have not yielded the same meaningful diagnostic and prognostic information as was obtained for leukemias and sarcomas. The variable cytogenetic findings in prostate cancer indicate heterogeneity of these tumors, and the primary genetic event is also probably variable. It is possible, however, that the presence of certain cytogenetic changes may characterize subtypes of prostate cancer. This is supported by the indications that a number of different processes (e.g., apoptosis, mutations of satellite DNA, and LOH) may operate in the causation of prostate cancer.

SOME SPECIAL ASPECTS OF PROSTATE CANCER CYTOGENETICS AND GENETICS

The understanding and evaluation of the chromosomal changes in prostate cancer must take into consideration at least two relatively recent developments in this area. One is the concept, mentioned above and now generally accepted,[33, 34] that carcinomas, including those of the prostate, develop through an orchestrated multistage or multistep genetic process that proceeds from proliferation to malignant transformation to metastasis. The number of steps and gene loci involved in this process may vary considerably from tumor to tumor. The second development was the demonstration by molecular means that genetic events that play a crucial role in carcinogenesis may not be evident or reflected cytogenetically (microscopically). The complexity and large number of cytogenetic changes that may be associated with carcinomas, including those in the prostate, have defied full explanation of their roles and meanings. Thus, the cytogenetic

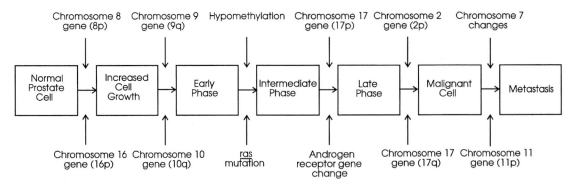

Figure 23–6. New multistep genetic scheme for prostate cancer development. It is now generally accepted that the evolution of the common adenocarcinomas, including that of the prostate, occurs via a multistage process involving mutational events such as inactivation of tumor suppressor genes and, less frequently, activation of oncogenes. This figure shows a suggested pathway through which prostate cancer may develop, involving a series of genetic changes, including tumor suppressor genes (on chromosomes 8, 10, 16, etc.) and oncogenes (e.g., *ras*). With each progressive involvement of a gene or chromosome change, the affected cell becomes less and less responsive to control mechanisms, ultimately resulting in a tumor capable of invasion or metastasis. The chromosomes and genes shown to be involved are based on our present knowledge, incomplete as it is, which already has shown new developments and changes from those of a scheme presented by me in 1992.[4] Undoubtedly, the scheme presented here—or parts of it—will have to be modified as more cogent information is obtained on events leading to prostate cancer. Furthermore, the scheme shown may apply to only a subtype of prostate cancer; other schemes are necessary for other types of this neoplasm (see **Fig. 23–7**). It is also possible that the number of genetic events shown in the figure exceeds that necessary for some prostate cancers, since the genetic data generally are based on heterogeneous groups of prostate tumors, and, thus, the data obtained would tend to be heterogeneous in character. Different cytogenetic changes in the same tumor may indicate variability of the histology and differentiation state of the tumor.

events may exceed in number the known molecular events and call for further investigation into the cytogenetic-molecular relationship. This is particularly true of epithelial adenocarcinomas. In some tumors the molecular events may outnumber the known cytogenetic events, thus indicating that the number of genetic events associated with a neoplasm may not be reflected in the number of cytogenetic changes. This applies to some leukemias and soft tissue tumors but especially to conditions in which no chromosomal changes are found.

As a rule, areas of prostate tumors that contain chromosomal aberrations show rapid proliferative activity, as assessed by immunohistologic examination,[45] which is not too surprising for these higher-grade lesions. But this feature could be reproduced only in individual cases. No significant correlation was found between the presence of numerical chromosome changes and the score of immunohistologically labeled cells when a comparison of cases was performed. Also, it should be noted that antibodies can stain a given tumor quite heterogeneously. Consequently, significant areas of tumor should be evaluated before any conclusions are drawn.

Like adenocarcinomas arising in other tissues, those of the prostate contain chromosome changes consisting primarily of deletions rather than translocations (the latter being more likely to be seen in leukemias, lymphomas, and sarcomas).[12] Though no single specific and recurrent chromosome change has been established in prostate cancer, a survey of all available cytogenetic data on human prostate adenocarcinomas indicates that loss of some chromosomes (1,2,5,Y) and gain of others (7,14,20,22) are commonly observed. Furthermore, rearrangements of some chromosome arms, such as 2p, 7q, and 10q, are frequent. This array of changes is compatible with present hypotheses involving a number of orchestrated genetic steps in the development of adenocarcinomas, and is not compatible with the assignment of a single chromosomal aberration as the primary (specific) one responsible for development of prostate cancer.

CHROMOSOME CHANGES IN PROSTATE TUMORS

The number of prostate cancers, primary and metastatic, examined cytogenetically, either directly or following short-term incubations or cultures, is relatively small (see Table 23–1) when compared with results obtained

MODELS & STEPWISE PROCESSES of
GENETIC CHANGES In CARCINOGENESIS

	Proliferative Stage	Transformative Stage	Invasive or Metastatic Stage

MODEL 1: A → B → C → D → E → F

MODEL 2: A → F → E → D → C → B

MODEL 3: A → G → H → I → J → K

MODEL 4: U → V → W → X → Y → Z

MODEL 5: A → V → H → W → Y → K

MODEL 6: U → B → W → C → X → D

MODEL 7: T ————————————→ S

MODEL 8: T ————————————→

Figure 23–7. Schematic outline of suggested genetic events that may take place in the development of adenocarcinomas, including that of the prostate. Various multistep changes are shown in the models that ultimately lead to an overt cancer and its metastases (see Fig. 23–6) of a single organ, such as the prostate. Thus, in models 1 through 3 and 5 the initial genetic events *(A)* may be the same, but the subsequent steps may differ in each. In models 4 and 6 a different initial genetic event is operative. The gist of these changes is the presence of a number of genetic alterations necessary for prostate cancer development but differing in their nature from one model to another. The schemes shown may account for the cytogenetic (and genetic) heterogeneity of adenocarcinomas. In models 7 and 8 are shown genetic events related to single specific translocations, which are very rare (if they exist at all) in prostate cancer but are seen in leukemias and soft tissue tumors. The genetic variability and number of events leading to prostate cancer shown in these schemes may account for the histologic and biologic variability associated with prostate cancer.

Table 23–1. Chromosome Changes in Prostate Cancer*

Change	Investigation
68-72,XY,i(17q),cx	Kakati et al., 1976[36]
44,X, − Y,del(1)(p22),del(1)(p13),t(1;2)(q12;p13p21),i(3q),t(2;6)(q11;q13),del(7)(q22),del(10)(q24,hsr(10)(q22), −15, −16, −17, −20,+21	Atkin & Baker, 1985[37]
57,X, − Y,del(7)(q22),del(10)(q24),1p+,cx	
45,XY,del(1)(q32),t(2;?)(p23;?),del(3)(p13),t(3;4)(p13;p14),t(8;12)(q11;p11),t(1;21)(q32;q21)	Gibas et al., 1985[42]
45,XY,t(1;?)(p36;?),der(2),del(6)(q21), −7, −10, −13, +2mar	Pitman et al., 1987[43]
76–86,X, − Y, + X, + X, + del(X)(q24), + t(1;10)(p22;q24), + der(2)t(1;2;?)(p32;q23;?), + der(7)(q22), + der(8)t(8;?)(q24;?), + der(8), + der(10)t(1;10)(q24;q22), + del(10)(q23) + der(12)t(4;12)(q11;p11), + der(12), + der(15)t(1;15)(q21;p11),t(16;?)(q21;?), +2-5mar	Lundgren et al., 1988[16]
84,X, + X, − Y,del(3)(q13),10q −,t(12;?)(q24;?),dmin,hsr,inc	Brothman et al., 1989[7]
72,XY?,del(3)(q13),del(3)(p22p23),del(3)(q25,t(3;9)(q21;p24),inv(3)(p26q21),inc	Johnson et al., 1989[154]
39–49,XY,del(7)(p15),del(12)(q14;q21),dmin,inc,cx	Limon et al., 1989[155]
80–96,XY,der(7)t(7;?)(p22;?),der(10)t(10;?)(q24;?),dmin,cx	
47,XY, +7	Babu et al., 1990[41]
45,X, − Y/46,X, − Y,t(4;?)(q27;?)	Brothman et al., 1990[48]
45,X, − Y, − 2, + t(10;?)(q24;?), + 13, − 14,t(1;6)(p32;q21),inv(3)(p21q21), inv (4)(p12q33),t(7;12)(q32;q15),t(8;?)(q24;?),del(8)(q22),t(9;?)(p13;?),del(10)(p13q24),del(12)(q22),t(14;?)(q24;?),del(19)(p13)	
46,XY,t(5;7)(q14;q31)	
39–43,XY, − 4, − 5, − 13, − 17,ins(1;?)(p32;?),t(1;16)(q21;q22),t(3;?)(p13;?),del(6)(p21),dup(7)(q22q32),del(8)(p21),del(10)(q24), + der(11)t(3;11)(p21;p13)ins(11;?)(q14–21;?),t(18;?), + 1 − 4mar/82–89,x2/142–156,XXYY,ins(1;?), + t(1;16), + t(3;?),del(6), + inv(6)(q15q21), + del(8), + del(10), + der(11)t(3;11)ins(11;?), + der(12)t(1;12)(q25q13), + t(18;?),t(19;?)(p13;?),cx	
39–49,XY,del(7)(p15,del(12)(q14q21),dmin,cx	
42–43,X, − X, − Y, − 10, − 18,del(1)(q23),t(5;16)(q13;q22),t(6;15)(p25;q24),der(7)t(7;12)(q36;p11),t(8;?)(p11;?) (p11;?),der(12)(12;13)(p11;q12),t(17;?)(p13;?),t(21;?)(q22;?), + 1−2mar/44,XY, − 8, − 10, − 18,del(1),t(5;16),der(7)t(7;12),der(12)(12;13),t(17;?),t(21;?), + 1−4mar	
45–46,XY,der(1)t(1;8)(p22;q13)dup(1)(q21q25),der(2)t(2;6)(p16;p12),del(6)(p12), + t(7;20)(q11;p12),der(8)t(1;8)(p22;q13),der(10)t(4;10)(q11;q23),t(13;?)(p13;?)/46–48,XY, − 17,t(1;4)(p34;q35),dup(1)(q21q25),der(2)t(2;6),t(3;?)(q21;?),del(6),t(7;20),dup(7)(q22q32),dup(7)(q22q32),der(10)t(4;10),t(13;?)	

46,XX, − Y/47,XXY,der(1)(p31q44)t(1;?)(p31;?),t(3;6)(p12;q23),del(7)(q22)/47,XXY	Lundgren et al., 1992[44]
46,XY,t(6;12)(p22;q24)	
46,XY,t(8;13)(p21;q14)	
46–49,XY, − 2, − 5, − 8,t(1;?)(p11;?), + t(1;?)(q41;?), + del(7)(q32),inv(10)(q22q24),der(12)t(1;12)(p11;p11), + der(18)t(2;18;?)(q11;q23;?), + der(18)t(2;18;?)(q11;q23;?), + 1–3mar[44]	
72–84,XXYY,del(1)(p11p31),t(2;?)(q23;?),cx	
76–86,X, − Y, + X, + X, − 2, + 3, + 3, + 4, + 5, + 5, + 6, + 7, + 8, + 9, + 10, + 10, + 11, + 11, + 12, + 14, + 17, + 18, + 19, + 19, + 20, + 20, + 21, + 22, + del(X)(q24), + t(1;10)(p22;q24), + der(2)t(1;2)(p32;q24)t(2;?)(p13;?), + der(2)t(1;2)(p32;q24)t(2;?)(p13;?), + del(7)(q22), + t(8;?)(q24;?), + t(8)(q24;?), + der(10)t(1;10)(q24;q22) + del(10)(q23), + der(12)t(4;12)(q11;p11), + der(12)t(4;12)(q11;p11), + der(15)t(1;15)(q21;p11), + t(6;?)(q21;?), + 2–5mar	
80–96,XY,t(7;?)(p22;?),t(10;?)(q24;?),dmin,cx	
83,XXYY,der(11)t(1;11;?)(q23;p15;?),cx	
46,X,t(Y;22)(q11;p12)	Micale et al., 1992[49]
46,XY,der(16)t(1;16)(q12;q23)/92,idemx2/45,idem, − Y/45,X, − Y	Wullich et al., 1992[156]
45,X, − Y	Arps et al., 1993[51]
45,X, − Y/47,XY, + 7	
45,X, − Y/46,XY,del(10)(q24)/47,XY, + 6	
46,XY,dmin	
46,XY,2dmin	
46,XY,del(1)(q11)	
46,XY,del(10)(q24)/45,XY − 1,der(1)add(1)(p36)del(1)(q42), − 2,add(3)(q21), − 4, − 5, − 8,del(10)(q24), − 11, add(11)(q23),t(12;14)(p13;q24), − 13,del(15)(q24), − 18, + 7mar/46,XY,del(1)(p32)	
46,XY,t(3;11)(p13;p15)	
47,XY, + mar/47,XY, + Y	
47,XY, + 3	
47,XY, + 3	
47,XY, + 5	
47,XY, + 7	
47,XY, + 7/45,X, − Y, + 7, − 8/47,XY, + 3	
47,XY,t(1;17)(p10;q10), + 7/47,XY, + mar	
50,XY, + 4mar	
46,XY,der(6)t(1;16)(q12;q23)/92,idemx2/45,X, − Y	Breitkreuz et al., 1993[157]
45,X, − Y/46,XY,t(1;20)(p34;q11)	Casalone et al., 1993[105]
50,X, − Y, + del(1)(p21), + del(3)(p22),add(5q), − 6,del(7)(q22),del(8)(p12), + 9, + del(10)(q24),?add(11p), + 12, + 13, − 16, − 17, − 21, − 22, + 5mar	Milasin & Mićić, 1994[125]

*Notations *cx* and *inc* indicate karyotypes that, in addition to the changes shown, had other complex or nonrecurring changes or karyotypes that were incomplete, either because of the variability of the karyotypes in the tumor or lack of information, respectively. The reader should consult the original publications in these cases for further interpretation of the karyotype.
Data from the catalog of Mitelman.[13]

with other adenocarcinomas (e.g., lung, breast, colon, bladder).

Some years ago,[35, 36] in what appears to have been the first description of a cytogenetic change in prostate cancer, we reported the presence of an isochromosome 17, i(17q), established with Q- and G-banding, in metastatic cells (in the bone marrow) from a prostate cancer. Direct marrow preparations showed a mode of 70 chromosomes with considerable scatter in counts and the presence (approximately 15%) of normal diploid metaphases with 46 chromosomes. The latter were undoubtedly of normal origin.

In one study, in spite of their karyotypic complexity, all four primary tumors had one aberration in common, a terminal deletion of the long arm of chromosome 10 with breakpoints at bands q22 or q24.[37, 38] A similar deletion of chromosome 10 was also described in a pseudodiploid prostate cancer cell line (see Figs. 23–1, 23–2).[39] The complex karyotype of a tumor examined by Lundgren and coworkers[16] contained at least three different structural aberrations involving the long arm of chromosome 10, all with loss of chromosome material.

Another candidate for a recurrent rearrangement in prostate cancer is del(7)(q22).[40] Apart from the case of Lundgren and colleagues,[16] this deletion was present in three of four primary prostatic adenocarcinomas.[37] Prostate cancers with +7 as the only cytogenetic change have been described.[41, 51]

Other candidates for nonrandom changes in prostate cancer are chromosomes 12 (at band 12p11) and 2p, markers in the metastasis described by Gibas and associates.[42] Furthermore, deletion of the distal part of the long arm of one X chromosome was found both in the LNCaP cell line[39] and in the case of Lundgren's group.[16] Finally, the Y chromosome was missing in one case,[16] as it was in the four cases of primary prostatic adenocarcinoma described earlier.[37] Loss of the Y chromosome is known to occur in marrow cells as both a normal age-related phenomenon and as a leukemic change.[12] Karyotypic analysis of a primary small cell carcinoma of the prostate revealed the representative karyotype to be 45,XY,−1,+der(1),−2,+der(2),−6,−7,−10,−13 and three markers, whose origin could not be established.[43] A del (6) was seen in five cells, and 10q− in one cell.

Cytogenetic studies of more highly differentiated and hormone-dependent prostate cancers obtained by radical prostatectomy have revealed only normal complements.[4] Although the mitoses in these cases may have emanated from normal prostatic epithelium, a possibility remains that the parenchymal cells of primary, well-differentiated tumors of the prostate may have normal karyotypes. Another strong possibility is that chromosomal changes discernible only molecularly may be present in these (and other) tumors. In the case of Lundgren and coworkers, histologic dedifferentiation was seen during hormonal manipulation of the cancer.[16] It is possible that the complex karyotype of their case represents a selected hormone-independent clone. Whether the development of hormone refractoriness is generally associated with cytogenetic evolution toward triploidy is a question of great potential clinical interest.

One study of 57 primary prostate adenocarcinomas yielded normal karyotypes in 24 tumors, structural nonclonal aberrations in 18 tumors, and clonal karyotypic abnormalities in 15 tumors.[44] The most common clonal numeric aberration was loss of the Y chromosome (−Y): a −Y was found in six tumors, in three of them as the sole anomaly. Clonal structural rearrangements, mostly accompanied by numeric changes, were detected in 12 tumors. The rearrangements involved 18 of the 22 autosomes and the X chromosome. Chromosomes 1, 7, and 10 were most frequently affected. Deletions, duplications, inversions, insertions, and balanced and unbalanced translocations were seen. Breakpoints in chromosome 1 were scattered along both the short and long arms with no obvious clustering, whereas those in chromosomes 7 and 10 clustered to bands 7q22 (two deletions and two duplications in four tumors) and 10q24 (two translocations, one deletion, and one inversion in four tumors). One additional tumor displayed a derivative chromosome 10 with a breakpoint in 10q23, and one had monosomy 10. Altogether, these abnormalities resulted in loss of 10q24→qter in five tumors. Monosomy 9 and rearrangements of the short arm of chromosome 8, leading to loss of 8p21→pter, were seen in four tumors. Double minute chromosomes were found in two tumors.

The appearance of detectable chromosomal aberrations in prostate cancer correlated with a shift of histologic differentiation toward the higher-grade end of the morphologic spectrum.[45] Brothman and coworkers[46] found cytogenetically abnormal clonal populations in only 5 of 20 cases and proposed that early-stage prostate cancers contain a submicroscopic change that cannot be detected using standard cytogenetic procedures. Clonal aberrations were found mostly in locally advanced or metastatic tumors.[44, 45] This finding was consistent with other reports.[37, 38, 42, 47, 48] Henke and colleagues[45] indicated that the cytogenetic abnormalities of early-stage, low-grade prostate cancer are too subtle to be detected by conventional cytogenetics or by interphase cytogenetics with the panel of probes used. In my opinion, it is also possible that early prostate cancer is not available to cytogenetics for analysis, when one chromosome change or only a few may be present, and that the probes used may not be the appropriate ones to detect such an abnormality.

Numeric chromosome alterations represent rather coarse alterations of the genome and, like other clonal aberrations, are restricted to advanced cases that show growth beyond the capsule.[45, 49] Some authors[49] suspected heterogeneity of prostate cancers in vivo to be the reason for the coexistence of clonally aberrant, nonclonally aberrant, and normal diploid cells in culture. The supposed karyotypic heterogeneity of prostate cancer should be confirmed by a cytogenetic study of nonmitotic cells in intact histologic environs.[45]

Morphologically detectable chromosome aberrations in prostate cancer represent rather coarse changes in an already advanced process and are far from being causal events.[45] While this is true, it is possible that they may be used as markers of aggressive tumor behavior. When the findings of Lundgren and colleagues[44] were used to evaluate the additional prognostic significance of chromosomal changes in excess of that attributable to prognostic factors such as tumor stage, grade, acid and alkaline phosphatases, and performance status,[50] an association between the presence of clonal chromosomal aberrations and an unfavorable clinical outcome was apparent.

An analysis of more than 100 adenocarcinomas reported in the literature was performed by Arps and coworkers.[51] Approximately a quarter of these cases showed clonal structural and/or numeric abnormalities (Figs. 23–8, 23–9). The normal karyotypes in 75% of the reported cases may be explained by contamination with normal epithelium or stromal components in the tumor samples; these can reduce the detection of cytogenetic rearrangements; however, the prevalence of karyotypically normal cases in one study was 43%.[51] This result is nearly the same as that found by Lundgren's group,[44] in a series of 57 prostate tumors (42%) where nonclonal single cell abnormalities were also included. The authors stated that these abnormalities might reflect the true genetic changes of the tumor parenchyma, which might often undergo cytogenetic determination because of the low mitotic activity of prostate carcinomas. It should be noted that most of the clonal changes found were also based on observations in a few dividing cells.[51] In this respect, the detection of karyotypic alterations in both studies may be due to the relatively high number of metaphases analyzed in each case.[44, 51]

Although some recurrent karyotypic abnormalities were found in one series,[51] none of the chromosomal changes observed appears to be a consistent event in prostate cancer. The most frequent numeric change was loss of the Y chromosome ($-Y$), which was found in four cases. A $-Y$ seems to be a common feature of prostate cancer[37, 38, 44, 48, 52] and other solid tumors, including gliomas,[53] renal cell carcinoma,[54] and bladder carcinoma,[55, 56] but it has also been described in benign hyperplasia of the prostate (BPH),[47] nonneoplastic tissue of the kidney,[57] and bone marrow cells of healthy elderly men.[12]

The only recurrent structural abnormality found in one series[51] was a deletion 10q24 (Figs. 23–9, 23–10), which had been described previously in nine primary prostate carcinomas[16, 37, 38, 44, 47] and in one cell line (LNCaP) established from a prostate cancer.[39] An interesting observation was that this deletion was the sole anomaly in three tumors.[51] In one of these tumors this anomaly was found in conjunction with multiple chromosome rearrangements, providing evidence that the deletion is an early mutational event during karyotype evolution. Metaphases showing the additional complex abnormalities were found in two different cultures, indicating that these changes did not occur in vitro.

The involvement of particular chromosome changes in initiation or progression of prostate carcinoma remains to be elucidated. Karyotypic abnormalities are known to be more common and complex in advanced and high-grade prostate carcinomas than in low-grade tumors. This is confirmed by studies of nuclear DNA ploidy patterns by flow cytometry.[58–60] Reported data have demonstrated that the presence of clonal karyotypic changes in the tumor

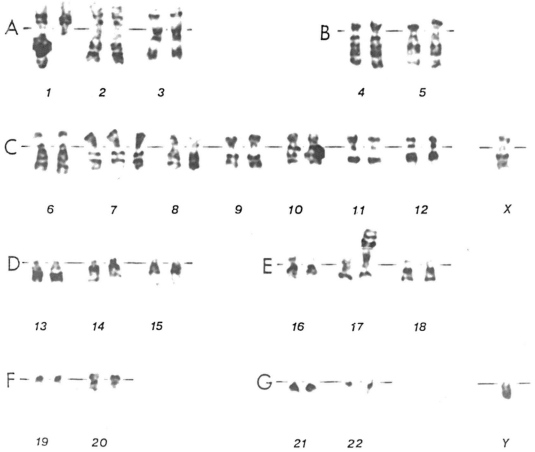

Figure 23–8. Karyotype of a prostate cancer whose only changes are +7 and t (1;17) (p10;p10). Trisomy 7 (+7) is a relatively common cytogenetic finding in prostate cancer, whereas translocations are relatively uncommon and differ from tumor to tumor. (From Arps S, Rodewald A, Schmalenberger B, et al.: Cytogenetic survey of 32 cancers of the prostate. Cancer Genet Cytogenet 66:93, 1993.)

cells is associated with an unfavorable outcome in prostate cancer.[50] Also, no correlation existed between a given type of chromosome abnormality and the histopathologic characteristics of the tumors in one series.[51] However, an attempt to evaluate the prognostic power of karyotypic abnormalities may be biased by some general characteristics of prostate tumors[51] (i.e., multiple tumor foci, heterogeneity of histologic differentiation, varying amounts of nonmalignant epithelium, and fibromuscular stroma), which could result in insufficient cytogenetic analysis with culture methods. The existence of several unrelated clones within a tumor might represent such cellular heterogeneity.

The possibility remains that the apparently normal metaphases are in fact of malignant origin and bear submicroscopic karyotypic changes that require molecular biologic approaches for detection. The development of cancer is thought most likely to involve a multistep process, possibly involving both inactivation of tumor suppressor genes and activation of oncogenes at a number of chromosome sites.[33] Evidence of gene amplification characterized by the presence of dmin chromosomes has been observed in a number of prostate cancers.[33, 44, 47, 51, 52] This may suggest some oncogene amplification. Molecular genetic analyses by a number of investigators have also pointed to deletions on chromosomes 8, 10, and 16 as potential loci for tumor suppressor genes associated with the initiation of prostate cancer.[61, 62] The recurrent cytogenetic observation of a deletion in the long

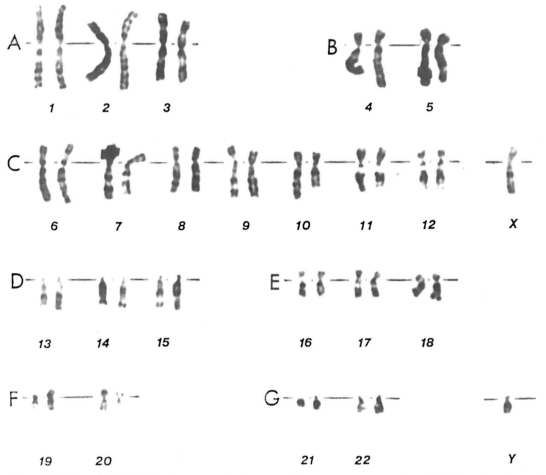

Figure 23–9. Pseudodiploid (46 chromosomes) karyotype from a prostate cancer in which the only cytogenetic abnormality was a del(10)(q24). This change is not uncommon in prostate cancer and may constitute a key genetic event in the evolution of the cancer. (From Gibav Z, Becher R, Kawinski E, et al: A high-resolution study of chromosome changes in a human prostatic carcinoma cell line (LNCaP). Cancer Genet Cytogenet 11:399, 1984.)

arm of chromosome 10 in prostate carcinomas suggests the possibility of loss of critical genes in region q24.[51]

FISH AND OTHER MOLECULAR CYTOGENETIC STUDIES IN PROSTATE CANCER

The introduction of in situ hybridization techniques, including that of fluorescence (FISH), to the cytogenetic study of tumors expanded the amount of such information on prostate cancer. Not only was it now possible to examine chromosome changes in prostate tumors without resorting to culture, but examinations could also be performed on archival and embedded tissues. The use of painting probes specific for each chromosome afforded the establishment of karyotypic rearrangements not clearly evident with the usual cytogenetic methods. Comparative genomic hybridization (CGH) is a relatively new molecular cytogenetic technique that has several potential advantages over other methods. CGH is similar to conventional cytogenetics in that the entire genome of individual tumors is screened for changes, but it does not require culturing of the tumor; rather, DNA isolated from the tumor is studied. An advantage of CGH over standard molecular biology techniques is that probes or markers are not needed to map changes. The method can also distinguish between chromosome gains and deletions.

The most commonly used FISH approach

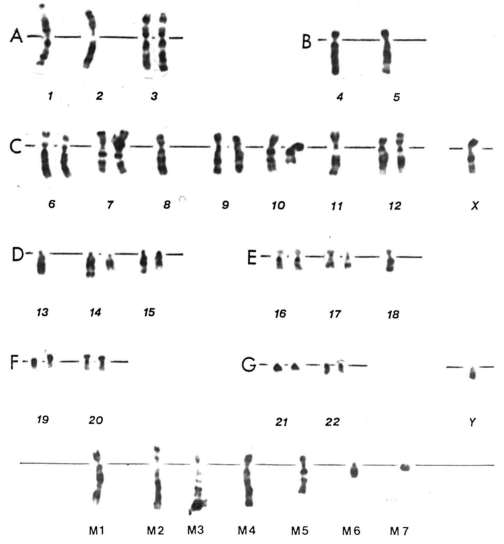

Figure 23–10. Karyotype consisting of 47 chromosomes in a prostate cancer. Though this karyotype also contains a del(10)(q24) (see Fig. 23–9), it is associated with a number of other cytogenetic changes, including seven marker chromosomes. (From Gibav Z, Becher R, Kawinski E, et al: A high-resolution study of chromosome changes in a human prostatic carcinoma cell line (LNCaP). Cancer Genet Cytogenet 11:399, 1984.)

relies on centromeric probes (DNA alphoid sequences) specific for each chromosome (Fig. 23–11; see also Figs. 23–4, 23–5). With this approach numerical chromosomal changes can be readily established, but the method has the major disadvantage of not revealing structural karyotypic changes such as deletions and translocations. Thus, results obtained with centromeric probes must be interpreted with this in mind.

The first application of FISH to prostate cancer was the study of Brothman and co-workers,[63, 64] in which they used centromeric

probes, painting probes, and G banding to establish the correct karyotype of a previously published prostate cancer cell line[52] and the demonstration that FISH uncovered aneusomy (loss or gain of whole chromosomes) in at least twice as many early-stage prostate cancers as the usual cytogenetic techniques (G banding). Similar findings were reported by others utilizing FISH in the study of paraffin-embedded tissue sections and conventional metaphase analysis of prostate tumor cultures.[65] FISH analysis of the sections allowed identification of cytogenetic aberrations in areas iden-

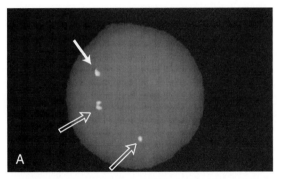 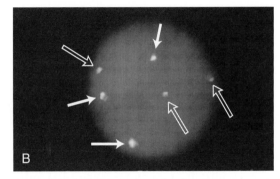

Figure 23–11. Illustration of FISH results obtained in interphase nuclei with centromeric probes for chromosomes 4, 7, 8, and 10. In normal (somatic) cells only two signals should be present for each chromosome, with the exception of the X and Y in male cells, which show only one signal for each. Thus, in the two nuclei shown *(A)*, only chromosome 8 (open arrows) is disomic (two normal signals), whereas chromosome 7 (solid arrow) is monosomic (one signal) and *(B)* chromosomes 4 (solid arrows) and 10 (open arrows) are trisomic (three signals).

tified as carcinoma, prostatic intraepithelial neoplasia (PIN), and BPH. For defining the true extent and nature of the cytogenetic aberrations in prostate cancer these authors[65] find this technique more informative than metaphase analysis of prostate tumor cultures. It should be pointed out, however, that the FISH method employed by these authors[65] was not capable of establishing structural karyotypic changes, such as deletions and translocations, that may play a more direct role in prostate cancer causation and biology than numeric changes. In fact, even in the case of numeric changes, two tumors were encountered with $+7$ based on the cytogenetics, but no $+7$ with FISH analysis. It should be reemphasized that culture of prostate cancers, regardless of the time involved, leads to a decrease in aneuploid cells. For example, in one study[65] utilizing a probe for the centromere of chromosome 1 it was shown that the percentage of cells aneuploid for chromosome 1 declined from 28% in the original tumor to 9.1% after culture. In a study utilizing centromeric probes for chromosomes 8 and 12,[67] it was shown that ploidy results determined by FISH on 50 radical prostatectomy specimens correlated with those obtained by flow cytometry. Examination of archival specimens of 20 primary prostate cancers by FISH[68] with α-satellite probes for chromosomes 12, 17, X, and Y revealed -17 in 16 tumors, -12 in 11, and $+X$ in 8. Loss of the Y ($-Y$) was not statistically significant. The authors[68] stated that -17 is a frequent—and likely an early—event in prostate cancer. In another study[69] trisomy 7 ($+7$) was found to be common in advanced prostate

cancer but not in its early forms. This trisomy was also common in metastatic lesions.

Utilizing FISH, Jones and colleagues[70] showed that culturing of prostate cancer yields results in a smaller percentage of tumors than direct examination without culture; that is, the latter was associated with -17 in 55% and $+7$ in 16% of the tumors, respectively, whereas the percentages following culture were 73% and 0%, respectively. The authors[70] stated that -17 may play an important role in prostate cancer development.

Needle biopsies of tumors were used for FISH analysis with probes for chromosomes 7, 8, 11, and 12. Trisomy 7 ($+7$) and trisomy 8 ($+8$) were detected in 76% of the aneuploid tumors and $+10$ in 59%. These changes were seen in prostate cancers with high Gleason scores.[71]

Examination of 35 primary prostate cancers with FISH showed -18 in 58%, $+X$ in 44%, -10 in 40%, -1 in 25%, and 1p$-$ in 23%.[72] The significance of $+7$ in prostate cancer was pointed to by the study of Zitzelsberger and colleagues,[73] who came to the conclusion, based on findings with FISH, that $+7$ correlated with pathologic category of the tumors, being present in 77% of advanced tumors.

Losses of chromosomes 1 and 8, shown by FISH with centromeric probes, were infrequent in prostate cancer.[74] Other results showed $+18$ in 63% of the tumors, $-Y$ in 53%, $+Y$ in 28%, and $+1$ in 36%. The $+18$ was seen in both near-diploid and aneuploid tumors. The presence of numeric aberrations of chromosomes 1, 18, and Y seemed independent of the clinical grade or stage of the prostate cancer.[74]

Brown and coworkers,[75] utilizing FISH, showed that anomalies of chromosome 8 or 7 were present in 88% of prostate cancers and that those with involvement of chromosome 8 were more advanced in stage. In the study of Visakorpi and colleagues,[76] based on FISH 74% of the prostate cancers were abnormal, whereas 35% were by DNA flow cytometry. Abnormalities of chromosome 8 were seen in 48% of the tumors, of the X in 43%, and of 7 in 39%. The authors indicated that 94% of all aneuploid tumors could be detected by using these three probes.

Studies have suggested that deletion of sequences on 8p was most often detected in the absence of, but sometimes associated with, sequence dosage alterations in the remainder of chromosome 8. To investigate this finding further, one study[77] applied FISH techniques to determine the status of chromosome 8 in prostate tumors that had undergone deletion of sequence cosmid DNA probes by FISH and confirmed by amplification of microsatellite sequences by PCR. Chromosome 8 dosage was assayed by FISH utilizing both unique sequence cosmid probe DNA (specific to the 8q13.1–q13.3 chromosome region) and pericentromeric probe DNA. FISH analysis of 10 specimens of normal or BPH tissues paired with nine tumor tissues and one from PIN from the same patients for dosage at 8p, 8cen, and 8q, and PCR analysis for dosage at 8p, demonstrated these findings: (1) FISH provided a more precise means of evaluating allelic loss than PCR. (2) The 8p22 sequence losses occurred frequently in prostate tumors. (3) The 8p22 sequence losses most often were detected in the absence of 8cen or 8q sequence dose alterations, although they were sometimes accompanied by gain or loss of 8cen or 8q sequences. (4) The pattern of 8p22 sequence losses was most often widespread rather than focal.

In another study the authors[78] matched poor- and good-prognosis patients to evaluate the association of numeric chromosome alterations ascertained by FISH with clinical behavior in prostate cancer. These authors targeted high-grade T3,N0,M0 prostate cancers treated by radical prostatectomy, tumors whose rate of clinical progression is difficult to predict. The results indicated that an abnormal tumor FISH ploidy is significantly associated with a poor prognosis in patients with prostate cancer. The qualitative analysis of the aneuploidy pattern is particularly important. The typical aneuploid tumor found in the poor-prognosis patients was defined by aneusomies of multiple chromosomes relative to a basic tetraploid population. Hypertetrasomic cells were frequent. In contrast, tumors in patients with a good prognosis are often diploid or tetraploid, and their aneusomies, when present, tend to be monosomies of a single chromosome. Their results suggest that tumor cells in the poor-prognosis group are cytogenetically unstable and may randomly lose and gain chromosomes, resulting in the different aneusomies. Such cells also had likely developed structural abnormalities in the retained chromosomes.[79]

Next to chromosomes 7, 10, and Y, for which aberrations in prostate cancer have been described in a number of cytogenetic studies, a probe for chromosome 17 was used by Henke and colleagues[45] because genes such as p53 and c-erb B-2, which might be involved in the pathogenesis of a number of human cancers, are mapped to this chromosome. Immunohistochemically detectable levels of p53 in prostate cancer were described by Mellon and coworkers[80] in 5 of 29 cases. All of these 5 tumors were poorly differentiated, but no significant relation between tumor grade and stage and p53 detection existed. The p53 gene is mapped to the short arm of chromosome 17 at 17p13.1,[81] and in this context the finding by Henke's group[45] that in two cases with a markedly deranged pattern in the number of chromosomes 17 were also positive for p53 is an interesting observation. Caution must be exercised, however, lest too much significance be attributed to the results, since probes for the centromeric regions only were used, so nothing can be said about the more distal regions of the chromosomes and no information was obtained about structural aberrations such as deletions or translocations affecting the short arm of chromosome 17. The expression of the c-erb B-2 protein, whose gene is also located on chromosome 17 at 17q21,[82] seems to be unrelated to the ploidy state of this chromosome in gastric and prostate cancer. This shows that an increased number of chromosomes does not necessarily lead to increased expression of genes.

Except for loss of a Y (−Y) chromosome and gain of chromosome 7 (+7), cytogenetic studies of metaphase cells have not clearly demonstrated nonrandom, whole chromosome loss or gain in prostate cancer.[83] Alcaraz and associates[78] observed that all chromosomes are likely to be numerically altered in clinically aggressive prostate cancers. Because all chromosomes were more likely to be altered in the tumors from the poor-prognosis group and because a significant difference in the frequency of chromosomal aneusomies was observed in that group, the authors performed detailed statistical tests to determine which alteration(s) occurred nonrandomly in this group.[78] Only +7 had a significantly higher prevalence in the poor-prognosis group as compared with the other chromosomes. This result, along with the almost constant presence (95%) of +7 in the poor-prognosis group, strongly suggests that +7 is a nonrandom alteration that correlates with clinically aggressive prostate cancer. Especially remarkable was the presence of +7 in the five diploid tumors in the poor-prognosis group. This result suggests that +7 may be an early change that occurs before other chromosomal aneusomies in poor-prognosis prostate carcinoma.

An interesting feature was the numeric chromosomal instability found in areas of PIN,[45] whereas on the same section adjacent areas of well-differentiated carcinoma showed normal chromosome numbers. This finding would support the concept that PIN and related lesions are biologic precursors of prostate cancer.[84–87] Against the background of these observations, it can be suggested that PIN can progress directly to a tumor state with cribriform or higher-grade appearance, skipping the state of well-differentiated tubular formation. Looking at the histologic aspect of higher-grade dysplasias, with their fusing papillary processes giving rise to transluminal bridging, this possibility does not seem farfetched.[45]

The presence of a relatively large number of cases without detectable numeric chromosomal aberrations and the correlation of numeric changes with differentiation is a feature peculiar to prostate cancer.[45] This distinguishes it from other carcinomas (e.g., gastric cancer)[88] and underlines the special biology of prostate cancer. Utilization of probes specific for loci, such as 7q22 and 10q24, which displayed structural aberrations in the series of Lundgren and coworkers,[44] would be necessary for further dissection of chromosomal structure in prostate cancer and to determine the frequency and meaning of these changes.

In the study of Henke and colleagues,[45] the occurrence and degree of numeric chromosomal aberrations correlated very well with tumor grade, stage, volume, and the presence of positive surgical margins; all well-known determinants of prognosis. Of course, results obtained on small, uneven, stratified patient groups have to be interpreted with great caution. Whether interphase cytogenetics could help to define an independent prognostic factor remains to be determined by a study involving more patients and sufficient time for evaluation of clinical outcome.

COMPARATIVE GENOMIC HYBRIDIZATION AND OTHER STUDIES

Comparative genomic hybridization (CGH) was used to screen for DNA sequence copy number changes along all chromosomes in 31 primary and 9 recurrent uncultured prostate carcinomas.[89] The aim of the study was to identify chromosome regions that contain genes important for the development of prostate cancer and genetic markers of tumor progression. CGH analysis indicated that 74% of primary prostate carcinomas showed DNA sequence copy number changes. Losses were five times more common than gains and most often were 8p− (prevalence, 32%), 13q− (32%), 6q− (19%), 18q− (19%), and 9p− (16%). Allelic loss studies with five polymorphic microsatellite markers for four different chromosomes were done on 13 samples and showed 76% concordance with CGH results. In local recurrences that developed during endocrine therapy, there were significantly more gains ($P < 0.001$) and losses ($P < 0.05$) of DNA sequences than in primary tumors: with gains of 8q (found in 89% of recurrences versus 6% of primary tumors), X (56% versus 0%), and 7 (56% versus 10%), as well as loss of 8p (78% versus 32%), particularly often involved. The CGH results indicated that losses of several chromosomal regions are common genetic changes in primary tumors, suggesting that genes in these chromosome sites are likely to underlie development of prostate cancer. Furthermore, the pattern of genetic changes seen in recurrent tumors— frequent gains of 7, 8q, and X—suggested that the progression of prostate cancer and development of hormone-independent growth may have a distinct genetic basis. These chromosome aberrations may have diagnostic utility as markers of prostate cancer progression.

The primary aim of one study was to examine the significance of increased DNA sequence copy number (gene amplification) in prostate cancers.[90] Three method (chromosome microdissection, CGH, and FISH) were combined to (1) identify a common region of gene amplification in human prostate cells and (2) evaluate the prevalence of this genetic change in samples of both primary and recurrent prostate cancers. The results of chromosome microdissection revealed a common amplified band region (8q24.1–24.2) in two prostate cases with cytologic evidence of gene amplification (double minutes). FISH using the 8q microdissection probe was performed on fresh tumor touch preparations from 44 randomly selected prostatectomy specimens. Amplification of DNA sequences from 8q24 was observed in 4 (9%) of 44 cases. Four of the 44 patients in this series presented with a positive lymph node at initial diagnosis, and three of the four showed 8q amplification. Because of this finding, CGH and FISH were performed on tumor cells from nine patients with recurrent prostate cancer. In eight of nine cases a gain of DNA sequences encompassing 8q24 was observed. Taken together with other evidence implicating 8q gain in prostate cancer progression, these results suggest that the analysis of this genetic change may have diagnostic utility as a marker of prostate cancer progression.

Growth patterns in prostate cancer can reduce detectability of genetic alterations.[91] Thus, tumors may show histologic grade heterogeneity, multifocality, interdigitation of benign and malignant glands, and varying amounts of stroma. These characteristics introduce sampling errors when one uses traditional methods for genetic analysis that depend on disaggregated cells (metaphase or interphase chromosome studies) or on tissue extracts (Southern blotting or PCR) to detect molecular events. To circumvent these problems, two approaches to studying paraffin-embedded tumors that permit focused analysis of critical tissue components were used. Serial 4- to 5-μm sections were applied to slides in groups of three.[91] Every second slide was stained with hematoxylin and eosin to visualize areas of carcinoma, dysplasia, hyperplasia, and stroma; tumor-rich areas were circled with ink and used as templates to examine or excise the same areas from adjacent nonstained sections. PCR methods for quantitative and qualitative gene assay were effective in evaluating samples when alteration was suspected at a particular locus. FISH with chromosome-specific paracentromeric probes for detection of copy number of the relevant chromosomes was applied to the adjacent section. Normal chromosome controls for both methods were demonstrated. This protocol enables one to correlate genetic alterations precisely with tumor extent and morphology.

One case studied by Henke and colleagues[45] showed some special features. Although it displayed a large tumor volume and involved both lobes, the proportion of high-grade cancer was minimal and neither perforation of the capsule nor chromosomal abnormalities were detected; however, from whole-mount sections it was evident that this tumor, in contrast with the others in the series,[45] spared the peripheral zone and grew mainly in the central periurethral portions of the gland. It was probably an unusually large transition zone cancer.

The concurrent use of PCR and FISH in microdissected prostatic tissues yielded evidence of higher frequencies of genetic changes in prostate cancers than those found with either method alone or by other approaches.[83] The results obtained indicated the power of simultaneous genetic assays that are closely linked to specific tumor histology. Particularly common involvement was seen at 8p, 10q, and Yp and gain of chromosome 7.

Cher and colleagues[92] felt that little insightful information was obtained by conventional cytogenetics studies of primary cultures of prostate cancer. Utilizing CGH, PCR plus restriction fragment length polymorphism (RFLP), and FISH, these authors showed allelic loss (comparable to LOH) at 8p and gains at 8q in these tumors. Cases with 8p− showed five times as many alterations as cases without 8p−. Other allelic losses involved 13q, 16p, 16q, 17p, 17q, and −Y.

In a study utilizing CGH[89] on primary prostate cancers, losses of chromosomal material were five times as common as gains, particularly losses at 8p, 13q, 6q, 16q, 18q, and 9p (in that order).

The amplification of chromosome segment 8q24.1–24.2 was shown by chromosome microdissection to occur in prostate cancer.[90] Deletion of material distal to 16q23.1, an area that may contain a tumor suppressor gene for prostate cancer, was shown with a cosmid probe.[92]

Cosmid-specific probes were applied by FISH to tissue sections of prostate cancers.[77] The findings were more precise than those obtained with PCR and pointed to loss of 8p22 sequences, which was often *not* associated with

8cen or 8q changes. The losses at 8p22 were widespread rather than local.

SIGNIFICANCE OF CHROMOSOME 7 CHANGES IN PROSTATE CANCER

A significantly higher rate of +7 was seen in advanced (T3, N0, M0 and higher) but not in early (T2, N0, M0,) stages of prostate tumors, though neither survival information nor clinical follow-up for three cases was reported.[69] It is possible that aneusomies of chromosome 7 are associated with poor-prognosis tumors and have no etiologic significance; however, there is evidence that human chromosome 7 is necessary and sufficient for both the establishment and maintenance of invasiveness and metastatic potential. For example, malignant mouse-human somatic cell hybrids retain their metastatic potential after losing all human chromosomes except chromosome 7.[93]

Some have criticized the significance of the presence of +7 in human cancer cells.[94] The most consistent criticism is that the observed alterations in chromosome 7 number are found in the infiltrating lymphocytes and not in the tumor cells.[95] However, Takahashi and colleagues[71] have performed simultaneous FISH and immunohistochemical staining and have observed +7 in prostate epithelial tumor cells, but not in infiltrating leukocytes.

Alcaraz and coworkers[78] found a characteristic FISH pattern of aneuploidy defined by multiple aneusomies, hypertetrasomic cells, and consistent presence of alterations of chromosome 7 to have a strong association with early death in patients with localized prostate cancer. These findings may have important practical applications, since methods have been developed to perform rapid FISH pretreatment analysis on prostate biopsy core specimens that can subsequently be used for routine histopathologic examination.[71] If the results from the preliminary study reported by Alcaraz and associates[78] can be extended and confirmed, the pretreatment detection of cytogenetic markers of poor prognosis may help select patients who would benefit from an aggressive therapeutic approach.

Trisomy 7 as the only chromosome change is a frequent abnormality in malignant and nonmalignant tumors, as well as in nonneoplastic tissues from patients with lung, kidney, or brain tumors.[12, 94, 96] Trisomy 7 was seen in a substantial number of mononuclear in-flammatory cells infiltrating kidney tumors and surrounding tissue.[96] The predominant cell population with an abnormal chromosome 7 complement was characterized as helper inducer T lymphocytes.[95] These findings were confirmed by combined immunohistochemistry and in situ hybridization on isolated tumor-infiltrating inflammatory cells as well as in frozen kidney tissue sections.[96] By studying with FISH a series of short-term cultures of cancers, it was found that +7 is present almost exclusively in connection with tumors of epithelial origin.[95] It may well be that the presence of +7 in BPH is due mainly or exclusively to the presence of tumor-infiltrating lymphocytes. The wide range of percentages of cells with +7 as shown by FISH may then perhaps be explained by the fact that nodular hyperplasia of the prostate is always associated with a slight to moderately dense lymphocytic interstitial infiltrate and some periglandular lymphocytic aggregates.[96] These lymphocytic infiltrations vary much from sample to sample, without a rim pattern, as in kidneys carrying a tumor where inflammatory cells not only are present in the tumor but are even more numerous at the tumor pseudocapsule and the surrounding nonneoplastic kidney tissue.[95]

It would appear that in BPH,[96] +7 is probably unrelated to the tumor cells. The only, and not very specific, change in BPH would seem to be loss of the Y chromosome. Trisomy as the only cytogenetic change in prostate cancer must be viewed with the possibility that the trisomy may reflect not changes in cancer cells but rather those in fibroblasts or lymphocytes present in the tumors.

Trisomy 7 (+7), found in four cases either as a sole anomaly or in conjunction with a −Y,[51] is a common observation in human malignancies.[12, 13] In one series +7 was also accompanied by structural rearrangements, or by −8 in some clones.[51] The implications of +7 in neoplasia are controversial owing to the fact that it appears also in short-term cultures of several nonneoplastic tissues.[57, 97–99] Nevertheless, there are those[51] who could not determine whether this anomaly (+7) represents a primary tumor-associated change in a subgroup of prostate carcinomas.

In the study of Alcaraz's group,[78] 100% of the tumors with a poor prognosis and 44% with a good prognosis were aneuploid, respectively, and when analyzed for chromosome 7 involvement the percentages were 96% and

12%, respectively. A characteristic aneuploidy pattern with multiple abnormal chromosomes and a hypertetrasomic cell population were generally found in tumors with a poor prognosis.

LOSS OF Y CHROMOSOME

The frequency of numeric changes in prostate cancer in one study[45] was nearly identical for all chromosomes; only a slight preponderance of changes in the number of sex chromosomes was observed. In the paper of Brothman and colleagues,[48] −Y was described in one cell strain out of five and +Y in another. Lundgren and coworkers[44] found −Y in 6 of 15 tumors with clonal aberrations. A −Y was also found in one case studied by Van Dekken and colleagues[100] by interphase cytogenetics on cytologic material. Based on these combined data, the possibility that changes in the number of Y chromosomes could be characteristic for prostate cancer was discussed[45]; however, the Y chromosome is very small and the number of genes that may be important in tumor initiation and promotion is necessarily limited. Loss of the Y chromosome may be a nonspecific event and has been described frequently in other tumors, for example, in bladder cancer,[12] gastric carcinoma,[88] and chronic non-lymphocytic leukemia.[12, 13]

A −Y is a common finding in many malignant disorders.[12, 13] It is usually accompanied by other karyotypic changes but occurs also as an isolated abnormality.[13] As to its significance, −Y in neoplastic conditions is complicated by the fact that this chromosome anomaly is known to occur in bone marrow cells of healthy elderly males, where it is thought to be a normal phenomenon of aging.[101, 102] In malignancies, however, −Y may not be related to patient age, and the possibility remains that, at least in an occasional patient, cells with a −Y as the only abnormality may be neoplastic.[103] Loss of the Y chromosome is the most frequent cytogenetic aberration in prostate cancer.[48, 51, 91] Moreover, a −Y was described in prostate cancer cells but not in stromal tissue, applying in situ hybridization with a Y chromosome–specific α-satellite DNA probe to 4-μm sections of a prostate adenocarcinoma.[104] These results, however, must be looked at with some caution, because to prove the absence of a chromosome in sections that do not encompass the whole nucleus may be difficult if not impossible.[96]

In the study by Casalone and colleagues[105] BPH was shown to be associated with −Y; the loss of this chromosome was seen in the fibroblasts but not in the epithelial cells. The authors[105] concluded that −Y is not related to cancer development.

In one series, −Y was the only change in one tumor, whereas three cases also showed unrelated clones with abnormalities.[51] In this respect it seems reasonable to conclude that −Y is not related to the neoplastic process in prostate cancer and may reflect a phenomenon of tissue hyperproliferation without any selective disadvantage.[51] An extra Y chromosome (+Y), as seen in two specimens, is a rather rare phenomenon in human tumors.[12] The examination of 100 cells following Q-banding from peripheral blood cultures of these patients revealed only normal cells.[51]

LOSS OF HETEROZYGOSITY

LOH or allelic loss utilizing polymorphic DNA probes for a large number of chromosomal areas showed loss at 16q and 10q to be the most common in prostate cancers (30% of tumors).[106] Similar findings were seen by Collins and coworkers,[107] though changes on chromosome 8 were also seen. The latter was confirmed by Bergerheim and associates,[108] who encountered, in addition to the changes at 8p and 16q, changes on chromosome 18. One study[109] found 16q to be affected in 60% of the tumors, 8p in 50%, 10p and 10q in 55% and 30%, respectively, and 18p in 43%. Loss of genetic material at 8p22–21.2 was seen in 53% of the tumors by Bova and associates,[110] findings that pointed to an important suppressor gene at 8p22 in prostate cancer.[111] LOH of BRCA1 and other loci on 17q21 has been demonstrated in a significant number of prostate cancers.[112] A gene (MXI1) at 10q24–25, a region that is deleted in some cases of prostate cancer, often displays allelic loss and mutation that may contribute to the pathogenesis or neoplastic evolution of this cancer.[113] The MXI1 protein negatively regulates *myc* oncoprotein activity and thus potentially serves as a tumor suppressor. LOH of chromosome 8 affected microsatellite DNA loci that might contain a suppressor gene.[114] Other suppressor genes in prostate cancer have been postulated to exist at 12q13,[115] at 7q31.1,[116] and metastatic suppressor genes on chromosomes 11 and 17.[117] Some linkage of prostate cancer to the gene (BRCA1) responsible for familial breast and ovarian cancer and located at 17q12-23 has been described.[118, 119] In a study in which PCR was used to ascertain loss of sequences at 8p, 10q, and 16q,[120] LOH of these regions was shown to be present in 20% to 29% of PIN, 18% to 42% of primary tumors, and 8% to 25% of metastatic lesions. The authors[120] came to the conclusion that lymph node metastases may be genetically related to either the dominant or additional primary tumor foci in more complex prostates and that accumulation of genetic aberrations may differ in primary and metastatic lesions.

Utilizing allelic losses at DCC (deleted in colorectal carcinoma at 18q21.3), APC (adenomatous polyposis coli at 5q21) or p53 (at 17p13) genes were seen in 13% of localized cancers and in 71% of advanced prostatic cancers.[121] Allelic loss involving the nm-23-Hi gene (at 17q21.3) was rare. The authors suggested that loss of tumor suppressor genes at the loci mentioned may influence progression of prostate cancer. Other studies[122] indicate that *ras* oncogene mutations are related to the progression of prostate cancer, whereas the APC gene is not involved in tumorigenesis or development of the cancer.

Mutations in microsatellite DNA sequences, especially expansion of the number of di- and trinucleotide repeats, have been implicated as the cause of several heritable disorders and of some cancers. Examination of prostate cancers[123] revealed that 6 of 30 tumors had gained at least one microsatellite sequence in their DNA, but not in the normal DNA. Though the authors did not detect mutations in the androgen receptor microsatellite sequences, it is likely that this type of mechanism affects other genes important in prostate cancer, thus promoting tumor development and progression.

LOH, as reflected in allelic loss, was examined in 28 prostate cancer specimens at 11 different chromosomal arms—3p, 7q, 9q, 10p, 10q, 11p, 13q, 16p, 16q, 17p, and 18q.[106] In 54% (13 of 24) of clinically localized tumors and in each of four metastatic tumors, LOH was shown to take place on at least one chromosome. These were most frequent at 10q (seven tumors; in five tumors it was the only change) and 16q (five tumors; in only two as the only change), with 30% of the tumors showing loss at these loci. Loss at 17p occurred

in three cases (in two it was the only change), and loss at 13q in three cases (only in one tumor was it the only change). Loss at 7q and 18q occurred in two tumors each, 7q being the only change in one tumor. The findings[106] demonstrate that allelic loss is a common event in prostate cancer and suggest that 16q and 10q may contain sites of tumor suppressor genes important in the pathogenesis of some prostate cancers. There is a strong possibility that future use of probes for other chromosome arms will reveal more allelic losses. For example, the investigators did not apply a probe for either arm of chromosome 2, the latter showing definite abnormalities cytogenetically in a significant number of prostate cancers reported in the literature.

DOUBLE MINUTES

The cytogenetic phenomena of double minutes (dmin) and homogeneously staining regions (HSR) are often associated with oncogene amplification in cancer cells.[12] Such amplification has been described in several tumor types—N-*myc* in neuroblastoma, *myc* in small cell lung cancer, and *neu* (erb-B2) in breast cancer. It appears that these amplifications correlate with poor prognosis. Only a few cases of prostate cancer with dmin have been described.[124, 125] Whether these cases are associated with oncogene amplification and poor prognosis remains to be determined.

NUCLEOLAR ORGANIZING REGIONS

Nucleolar organizer regions (NOR) are chromosomal DNA loops encoding ribosomal RNA and are detectable by a silver staining technique that identifies NOR-associated non-histone proteins with a high degree of specificity.[126, 127] The number and distribution of silver-stained NORs (AgNORs) correlate with growth fractions and may have diagnostic and prognostic value for different neoplasms.[127–130]

In various studies employing the AgNOR technique, authors reported significant differences of NOR counts between benign and malignant or premalignant lesions of the prostate, and overlap among groups.[130–134] Similar results were seen in counts of cell suspensions.[135, 136] Some workers[131, 134, 137] found a significant correlation between AgNOR counts and grade and clinical stage, whereas others[138] could not confirm these results or found no correlation between AgNOR counts and response to endocrine therapy[139] and no significant difference between counts of patients who died of prostate cancer and of those who survived.[2] Contractor and coworkers[141] determined AgNOR number and area by means of an automatic image analysis system and found that, whereas the quotient of number and area provided prognostic information, the number or area alone did not show a relation to prognosis. In another study[142] with a semiautomatic system, higher AgNOR counts were reported in the "unfavorable" group. The patient populations studied in all of these publications, except one, have been heterogeneous for stage and treatment protocols. The patient population studied by Ahiskali and associates[143] included only those with advanced-stage prostate cancer receiving endocrine therapy. These authors[143] employed three different counting methods and could find no statistically significant differences among groups defined by stage and disease outcome. AgNOR counts are related to growth fractions or ploidy.[131, 134, 139, 144] It is well-known that most prostate cancers are slow-growing neoplasms and slow to proliferate.[134, 145, 146] Thus, it may be assumed that a marker related to the proliferative fractions is not suitable for estimating the malignant potential of prostate cancer. Nevertheless, AgNOR counts may still be related to prognosis for early-stage disease, as diploidy confers a survival advantage in early-stage prostate cancer but not in advanced disease.

Though the small number of patients in each group studied by Ahiskali and coworkers[143] limited statistical interpretation, these authors could find no correlation between AgNOR counts and clinical parameters. In spite of the strong correlation between grade and AgNOR counts, overlap among groups, high interobserver variability, and lack of association with prognosis make AgNOR counts of little, if any, practical use in advanced prostate cancer. The controversial results in the literature, as well as the results of Ahiskali's group,[143] indicate that the AgNOR technique should still be regarded as experimental, and certain conclusions await further investigations. More studies on the standardization of the technique and of counting are necessary before AgNOR count is accepted as a reliable and objective parameter of malignancy.

APOPTOSIS IN PROSTATE CANCER

Apoptosis (programmed cell death) is a process of natural cell death that can occur in several types of tissues under both normal and neoplastic conditions.[147] In normal tissues, apoptosis in conjunction with mitosis plays an important role in maintaining tissue homeostasis. In contrast to necrosis, in which cell death is a passive process resulting from severe injury to the affected cells, apoptosis is a natural but active process that requires the orderly participation of several molecular cellular events leading to cell death, each one controlled by specific genes.

Androgen ablation is thought to induce apoptosis in prostate cancer cells, as do some forms of chemotherapy. In part this may be due to induced resistance to BCL-2–mediated apoptosis.[148–150] In prostate cancer, apoptosis can be recognized in standard hematoxylin and Eosin–stained sections and quantitated by light microscopy. The apoptotic index may provide additional prognostic information in certain grades of early stage prostatic cancer.[151]

Bcl-2 is a protooncogene that prevents apoptosis. Since androgen withdrawal induces apoptosis, it has been postulated that Bcl-2 may play a role in androgen resistance. The presence of neuroendocrine cells in prostate cancer has been shown to influence long-term prognosis.[152] Of interest is that direct immunohistochemical staining has demonstrated the presence of Bcl-2 in the neuroendocrine cells of a large proportion of prostatic cancers.[152]

CHROMOSOME CHANGES IN CELL LINES

Cytogenetic studies on long-term cell lines of prostate cancer have positive and negative aspects. The positive aspects include the likelihood that the chromosome changes, however complex, reflect those in the original tumor by including some of the primary karyotypic changes and at least some of the secondary changes. The negative aspects include the possibility that the cytogenetic changes in a cell line do not represent the most prevalent karyotype in the tumor. Additional abnormalities are probably generated in vitro as a result of culture conditions. Therefore, interpretation of cytogenetic results based on established cell lines must take into consideration the points cited above. Already mentioned is a study of a prostate cancer cell line (PPC-1) in which the application of FISH yielded information on at least 10 marker chromosomes not previously identifiable by banding analysis,[63] thus reflecting one of the difficulties in interpreting and evaluating cytogenetic results based on cell lines.

In almost all prostate cancer cell lines examined, chromosome counts have been high (at least 50 chromosomes) and the karyotypes complex, having many abnormalities or large numbers of markers.[12] Furthermore, karyotypes reported by some investigators may be interpreted differently by others. Thus, in one cell line, investigators using Q-banding revealed the tumor cells to be completely aneuploid with a modal chromosome number in the hypertriploid range.[152] At least 10 distinctive marker chromosomes were identified; however, the modal chromosome number shifted from 62 to 55 between the fifth and the fiftieth passage, and certain karyotypic variability occurred. In another cell line[153] originating from a primary prostate adenocarcinoma, 28% of cells were found to be pseudodiploid and 72% pseudotetraploid. All metaphases examined were partially trisomic for chromosome 9 and lacked a demonstrable Y chromosome. The overall karyotypic patterns of the cell lines studied, as well as their marker chromosomes, clearly distinguish these lines from other cancer lines, including HeLa. The latter is important since the authenticity of other putative prostate cancer lines has been disputed.

Little cytogenetic commonality among prostate cancer cell lines studied has been demonstrated to date. Cytogenetic analysis of cells grown in semisolid agar from a patient with prostate cancer cells in a marrow aspirate revealed a modal number and karyotype of 44,XY,del(31)(p14),$-$7,del(12)(q24),$-$15, $-$22,+dmin. In the complex karyotype of an established xenografted prostate adenocarcinoma cell line (PC-82), parts of a number of chromosomes were homozygous (including 10q), whereas regions on 2p, 13q and 17q apparently were lost completely.

It was proposed that the del (10), or any of the other changes to be discussed, may represent a marker that is specific for prostate cancer; however, it is doubtful that del (10), even if it is a specific chromosome change, will be found in all prostate cancers. It is likely that prostate cancer will be shown to comprise cytogenetically defined subtypes equivalent to

Table 23–2. Genes Studied in Prostate Cancer

Androgen receptor
APC
BCL-2
BRCA1
CAM
DCC
DNA polymerase-β
E-Cadherin
EGF receptor
ERB-B2
Interleukin 6 receptor
KAI1 (metastasis suppressor)
K-*ras* and N-*ras* (H-*ras*)
Krev-1
MET
Metalloproteinase
MMP-7
N-*myc* and L-*myc*
NEU/HER-2 (p185^{neu})
NM23-H1
P53
Polymerase-β
PSA
RB
SRY
TGF-α and -β
ZFY and ZFX

*The genes presented in this table have been shown to be overexpressed or underexpressed, to be affected by LOH or mutations, or to be related to prognosis and other biologic aspects of prostate cancer. To date, none of them has been shown specifically to be involved in the genesis of this cancer.

those in leukemias and other tumors. For example, in a hypodiploid metastatic prostate cancer it was shown that, although a number of abnormalities were present—del(1), der(2),del(3),t(3;4),t(8;12),t(1;21)—chromosome 10 was not involved by visible changes. Any of the cytogenetic changes described in prostate cancer could represent an essential primary or secondary karyotypic event in tumor development. At the same time, it is possible that chromosome changes beyond the resolving power of the microscope may exist and may play a key role in the carcinogenic process in the prostate. It is likely that prostate cancer becomes associated with a number of genetic changes (Table 23–2) during the course of its development and that at least some of them are essential for tumor progression and viability.

REFERENCES

1. Wingo PA, Tong T, Bolden S: Cancer statistics, 1995. CA 45:8–30, 1995.

2. Hill C, Benhamou E, Doyon F: Trends in cancer mortality. Lancet 336:1262–1263, 1990.

3. Sandberg AA: Genetic and cytogenetic aspects of human prostate cancer. In Karr JP, Yamanaka HL (eds): Prostate Cancer: The Second Tokyo Symposium. New York: Elsevier, 1989, pp 28–36.

4. Sandberg AA: Chromosomal abnormalities and related events in prostate cancer. Hum Pathol 23:368–380, 1992.

5. Szűcs S, Zitzelsberger H, Breul J, et al.: Two-phase short-term culture method for cytogenetic investigations from human prostate carcinoma. Prostate 25:225–235, 1994.

6. Martikainen P, Kyprianou N, Tucker RW, et al.: Programmed death of nonproliferating androgen-independent prostatic cancer cells. Cancer Res 51:4693–4700, 1991.

7. Brothman AR, Lesho LJ, Somers KD, et al.: Cytogenetic analysis of four primary prostatic cultures. Cancer Genet Cytogenet 37:241–248, 1989.

8. Lundgren R, Heim S, Mandahl N, et al.: Chromosome abnormalities are associated with unfavorable outcome in prostatic cancer patients. J Urol 147:784–788, 1992.

9. Ritchie AWS, Dorey F, Layfield LH, et al.: Relationship of DNA content to conventional prognostic factors in clinically localized carcinoma of the prostate. Br J Urol 62:254–260, 1988.

10. de Launuoit Y, Kiss R, Jossa W, et al.: Influences of dihydrotestosterone, testosterone, estradiol, progesterone, or prolactin on the cell kinetics of human hyperplastic prostatic tissue in organ culture. Prostate 13:143–153, 1988.

11. Franko AJ, Koch CJ, Garrecht BM, et al.: Oxygen dependence of binding of misonidazole to rodent and human tumors in vitro. Cancer Res 47:5367–5376, 1987.

12. Sandberg AA: The Chromosomes in Human Cancer and Leukemia, ed 2. New York: Elsevier, 1990, pp 753–788.

13. Mitelman F: Catalog of Chromosome Aberrations in Cancer, ed 5. New York: Wiley-Liss, 1994.

14. Jellinghaus W, Okada K, Ragg C, et al.: Chromosomal studies of prostatic tumors in vitro. Invest Urol 14:16–19, 1976.

15. Gibas Z, Pontes EJ, Sandberg AA: Chromosome rearrangements in a metastatic adenocarcinoma of the prostate. Cancer Genet Cytogenet 16:301–304, 1985.

16. Lundgren R, Kristoffersson U, Heim S, et al.: Multiple structural chromosome rearrangements, including del(7q) and del(10q), in an adenocarcinoma of the prostate. Cancer Genet Cytogenet 35:103–108, 1988.

17. Mostofi FK: Problems of grading carcinoma of the prostate. Semin Oncol 3:161–169, 1976.

18. Ahmann FR, Woo L, Hendrix M, et al.: Growth in semisolid agar of prostate cancer cells obtained from bone marrow aspirates. Cancer Res 46:3560–3564, 1986.

19. Limon J, Lundgren R, Elfving P, et al.: An improved technique for short-term culturing of human prostatic adenocarcinoma tissue for cytogenetic analysis. Cancer Genet Cytogenet 46:191–199, 1990.

20. Cremer T, Landegent J, Brückner A, et al.: Detection of chromosome aberrations in the human interphase nucleus by visualization of specific target DNAs with radioactive and non-radioactive in situ hybridization techniques: Diagnosis of trisomy 18 with probe L1.84. Hum Genet 74:346–352, 1986.

21. Hopman AHN, Wiegant J, Raap AK, et al.: Bi-color detection of two target DNAs by non-radioactive in situ hybridization. Histochemistry 85:1–4, 1986.

22. Sandberg AA, Turc-Carel C: The cytogenetics of solid tumors. Relation to diagnosis, classification and pathology. Cancer 59:387–395, 1987.

23. Sandberg AA, Turc-Carel C, Gemmill M: Chromosomes in solid tumors and beyond. Cancer Res 48:1049–1059, 1988.

24. Sandberg AA: Cancer cytogenetics for clinicians. CA 44:136–159, 1994.

25. Rowley JD, Aster JC, Sklar J: The clinical applications of new DNA diagnostic technology on the management of cancer patients. JAMA 270:2331–2337, 1993.

26. Rowley JD, Aster JC, Sklar J: The impact of new DNA diagnostic technology on the management of cancer patients. Arch Pathol Lab Med 117:1104–1109, 1993.

27. Karp JE, Broder S: New directions in molecular medicine. Cancer Res 54:653–665, 1994.

28. Knudson AG: Antioncogenes and human cancer. Proc Natl Acad Sci USA 90:10914–10921, 1993.

29. Nowell PC: Cytogenetic approaches to human cancer genes. FASEB J 8:408–413, 1994.

30. Sikora K: Genes, dreams, and cancer. Br Med J 308:1217–1221, 1994.

31. Sandberg AA, Bridge JA: The Cytogenetics of Bone and Soft Tissue Tumors. Austin, TX: R.G. Landes, 1994.

32. Williams GT: Programmed cell death: Apoptosis and oncogenesis. Cell 65:1097–1098, 1991.

33. Vogelstein B, Fearon ER, Hamilton SR, et al.: Genetic alterations during colorectal-tumor development. N Engl J Med 319:525–532, 1988.

34. Weinberg RA: Oncogenes and tumor suppressor genes. CA 44:160–170, 1994.

35. Oshimura M, Sandberg AA: Isochromosome 17 in prostatic cancer. J Urol 114:249–250, 1975.

36. Kakati S, Oshimura M, Sandberg AA: The chromosomes and causation of human cancer and leukemia. XIX. Common markers in various tumors. Cancer 38:770–777, 1976.

37. Atkin NB, Baker MC: Chromosome study of five cancers of the prostate. Hum Genet 70:359–364, 1985.

38. Atkin NB, Baker MC: Chromosome 10 deletion in carcinoma of the prostate. N Engl J Med 312:315, 1985.

39. Gibas Z, Becher R, Kawinski E, et al.: A high-resolution study of chromosome changes in a human prostatic carcinoma cell line (LNCaP). Cancer Genet Cytogenet 11:399–404, 1984.

40. Atkin NB, Baker MC: Chromosome 7q deletions: Observations on 13 malignant tumors. Cancer Genet Cytogenet 67:123–125, 1993.

41. Babu VR, Miles BJ, Cerny JC, et al.: Cytogenetic study of four cancers of the prostate. Cancer Genet Cytogenet 48:83–87, 1990.

42. Gibas Z, Pontes JE, Sandberg AA: Chromosome rearrangements in a metastatic adenocarcinoma of the prostate. Cancer Genet Cytogenet 16:301–304, 1985.

43. Pittman S, Russell PJ, Jelbart ME, et al.: Flow cytometric and karyotypic analysis of a primary small cell carcinoma of the prostate: A xenografted cell line. Cancer Genet Cytogenet 26:165–169, 1987.

44. Lundgren R, Mandahl N, Heim S, et al.: Cytogenetic analysis of 57 primary prostatic adenocarcinomas. Genes Chrom Cancer 4:16–24, 1992.

45. Henke R-P, Krüger E, Ayhan N, et al.: Numerical

chromosomal aberrations in prostate cancer: correlation with morphology and cell kinetics. Virchows Arch [A] 422:61–66, 1993.

46. Brothman AR, Peehl DM, Patel AM, et al.: Cytogenetic evaluation of 20 cultured primary prostatic tumors. Cancer Genet Cytogenet 55:79–84, 1991.

47. Brothman AR, Lesho LJ, Somers KD, et al.: Cytogenetic analysis of four primary prostatic cultures. Cancer Genet Cytogenet 37:241–248, 1989.

48. Brothman AR, Peehl DM, Patel AM, et al.: Frequency and pattern of karyotypic abnormalities in human prostate cancer. Cancer Res 50:3795–3803, 1990.

49. Micale MA, Mohamed A, Sakr W, et al.: Cytogenetics of primary prostatic adenocarcinoma. Clonality and chromosome instability. Cancer Genet Cytogenet 61:165–173, 1992.

50. Lundgren R, Heim S, Mandahl N, et al.: Chromosome abnormalities are associated with unfavorable outcome in prostatic cancer patients. J Urol 147:784–788, 1992.

51. Arps S, Rodewald A, Schmalenberger B, et al.: Cytogenetic survey of 32 cancers of the prostate. Cancer Genet Cytogenet 66:93–99, 1993.

52. Brothman AR, Lesho LJ, Somers KD, et al.: Phenotypic and cytogenetic characterization of a cell line derived from primary prostatic carcinoma. Int J Cancer 44:898–903, 1989.

53. Lindström E, Salford LG, Heim S, et al.: Trisomy 7 and sex chromosome loss need not be representative of tumor parenchyma cells in malignant glioma. Genes Chrom Cancer 3:474–479, 1991.

54. Limon J, Mrozek K, Heim S, et al.: On the significance of trisomy 7 and sex chromosome loss in renal cell carcinoma. Cancer Genet Cytogenet 49:259–263, 1990.

55. Powell I, Trybus T, Kleer E: Apparent correlation of sex chromosome loss and disease course in urothelial cancer. Cancer Genet Cytogenet 50:97–101, 1990.

56. Meloni AM, Peier AM, Haddad FS, et al.: A new approach in the follow-up of bladder cancer. FISH analysis of urine, bladder washings, and tumors. Cancer Genet Cytogenet 71:105–118, 1993.

57. Elfving P, Cigudosa JC, Lundgren R, et al.: Trisomy 7, trisomy 10, and loss of the Y chromosome in short-term cultures of normal kidney tissue. Cytogenet Cell Genet 53:123–125, 1990.

58. Ritchie AWS, Dorey F, Layfield LJ, et al.: Relationship of DNA content to conventional prognostic factors in clinically localized carcinoma of the prostate. Br J Urol 62:254–260, 1988.

59. Tribukait B: DNA flow cytometry in carcinoma of the prostate for diagnosis, prognosis and study of tumor biology. Acta Oncol 30:187–192, 1991.

60. Zeiterberg A, Forsslund G: Ploidy level and tumor progression in prostatic carcinoma. Acta Oncol 30:193–199, 1991.

61. Carter BS, Eving CM, Ward WS, et al.: Allelic loss of chromosomes 16q and 10q in human prostate cancer. Proc Natl Acad Sci USA 87:8751–8755, 1990.

62. Collins VP, Kunomi K, Bergerheim U, et al.: Molecular genetics and human prostatic carcinoma. Acta Oncol 30:181–185, 1991.

63. Brothman AR, Patel AM: Characterization of 10 marker chromosomes in a prostatic cancer cell line by in situ hybridization. Cytogen Cell Genet 60:8–11, 1992.

64. Brothman AR, Patel AM, Peehl DM, et al.: Analysis of prostatic tumor cultures using fluorescence in

situ hybridization (FISH). Cancer Genet Cytogenet 62:180–185, 1992.

65. Micale MA, Sanford JS, Powell IJ, et al.: Defining the extent and nature of cytogenetic events in prostatic adenocarcinoma: Paraffin FISH vs. metaphase analysis. Cancer Genet Cytogenet 69:7–12, 1993.

66. König JJ, Teubel W, van Dongen JW, et al.: Tissue culture loss of aneuploid cells from carcinomas of the prostate. Genes Chrom Cancer 8:22–27, 1993.

67. Persons DL, Takai K, Gibney DJ, et al.: Comparison of fluorescence in situ hybridization with flow cytometry and static image analysis in ploidy analysis of paraffin-embedded prostate adenocarcinoma. Hum Pathol 25:678–683, 1994.

68. Brothman AR, Watson MJ, Zhu XL, et al.: Evaluation of 20 archival prostate tumor specimens by fluorescence in situ hybridization (FISH). Cancer Genet Cytogenet 75:40–44, 1994.

69. Bandyk MG, Zhao L, Troncoso P, et al.: Trisomy 7: A potential cytogenetic marker of human prostate cancer progression. Genes Chrom Cancer 9:19–27, 1994.

70. Jones E, Zhu XL, Rohr LR, et al.: Aneusomy of chromosomes 7 and 17 detected by FISH in prostate cancer and the effects of selection in vitro. Genes, Chrom Cancer 11:163–170, 1994.

71. Takahashi S, Qian J, Brown JA, et al.: Potential markers of prostate cancer aggressiveness detected by fluorescence in situ hybridization in needle biopsies. Cancer Res 54:3574–3579, 1994.

72. Baretton GB, Valina C, Vogt T, et al.: Interphase cytogenetic analysis of prostatic carcinomas by use of nonisotopic in situ hybridization. Cancer Res 54:4472–4480, 1994.

73. Zitzelsberger H, Szücs S, Weier H-U, et al.: Numerical abnormalities of chromosome 7 in human prostate cancer detected by fluorescence in situ hybridization (FISH) on paraffin-embedded tissue sections with centromere-specific DNA probes. J Pathol 172:325–335, 1994.

74. König JJ, Teubel W, van Dongen JW, et al.: Loss and gain of chromosomes 1, 18, and Y in prostate cancer. Prostate 25:281–291, 1994.

75. Brown JA, Alcaraz A, Takahashi S, et al.: Chromosomal aneusomies detected by fluorescent in situ hybridization analysis in clinically localized prostate carcinoma. J Urol 152:1157–1162, 1994.

76. Visakorpi T, Hyytinen E, Kallioniemi A, et al.: Sensitive detection of chromosome copy number aberrations in prostate cancer by fluorescence in situ hybridization. Am J Pathol 145:624–630, 1994.

77. Macoska JA, Trybus TM, Sakr WA, et al.: Fluorescence in situ hybridization analysis of 8p allelic loss and chromosome 8 instability in human prostate cancer. Cancer Res 54:3824–3830, 1994.

78. Alcaraz A, Takahashi S, Brown JA, et al.: Aneuploidy and aneusomy of chromosome 7 detected by fluorescence in situ hybridization are markers of poor prognosis in prostate cancer. Cancer Res 54:3998–4002, 1994.

79. Shackney SE, Smith CA, Miller BW, et al.: Model for the genetic evolution of human solid tumors. Cancer Res 49:3344–3354, 1989.

80. Mellon K, Thompson S, Charlton RG, et al.: p53, c-erbB-2 and the epidermal growth factor receptor in the benign and malignant prostate. J Urol 147:496–499, 1992.

81. Miller C, Mohandas T, Wolf D, et al.: Human p53

gene is localised to short arm of chromosome 17. Nature 319:783–785, 1986.

82. Fukushige S, Matsubara K, Yoshida M, et al.: Localization of a novel v-erbB-related gene, c-erbB-2, on human chromosome 17 and its amplification in a gastric cancer cell line. Molec Cell Biol 6:955–958, 1986.

83. Macoska JA, Micale MA, Sakr WA, et al.: Extensive genetic alterations in prostate cancer revealed by dual PCR and FISH analysis. Genes Chrom Cancer 8:88–97, 1993.

84. Kastendieck H: Correlations between atypical primary hyperplasia and carcinoma of the prostate. Pathol Res Prac 169:366–387, 1980.

85. McNeal JE, Bostwick DG: Intraductal dysplasia: A premalignant lesion of the prostate. Hum Pathol 17:64–71, 1986.

86. Bostwick DG, Brawer MK: Prostatic intra-epithelial neoplasia and early invasion in prostate cancer. Cancer 59:788–794, 1987.

87. Brawer MK: Prostatic intraepithelial neoplasia: A premalignant lesion. Hum Pathol 23:242–248, 1992.

88. Van Dekken H, Pizzolo JG, Kelsen DP, et al.: Targeted cytogenetic analysis of gastric tumors by in situ hybridization with a set of chromosome-specific DNA probes. Cancer 66:491–497, 1990.

89. Visakorpi T, Kallioniemi AH, Syvänen A-C, et al.: Genetic changes in primary and recurrent prostate cancer by comparative genomic hybridization. Cancer Res 55:342–347, 1995.

90. Van Den Berg C, Guan X-Y, Von Hoff D, et al.: DNA sequence amplification in human prostate cancer identified by chromosome microdissection: Potential prognostic implications. Clin Cancer Res 1:11–18, 1995.

91. Wolman SR, Macoska JA, Micale MA, et al.: An approach to definition of genetic alterations in prostate cancer. Diagn Molec Pathol 1:192–199, 1992.

92. Cher ML, MacGrogan D, Bookstein R, et al.: Comparative genomic hybridization, allelic imbalance, and fluorescence in situ hybridization on chromosome 8 in prostate cancer. Genes Chrom Cancer 11:153–162, 1994.

93. Collard JG, van de Poll M, Scheffer A, et al.: Location of genes involved in invasion and metastasis on human chromosome 7. Cancer Res 47:6666–6670, 1987.

94. Johanson B, Heim S, Mandahl N, et al.: Trisomy 7 in nonneoplastic cells. Genes Chrom Cancer 6:199–205, 1993.

95. Dal Cin P, Aly MS, Delabie J, et al.: Trisomy 7 and trisomy 10 characterize subpopulations of tumor-infiltrating lymphocytes in kidney tumors and in surrounding kidney tissue. Proc Natl Acad Sci USA 89:9744–9748, 1992.

96. Aly MS, Dal Cin P, Van de Voorde W, et al.: Chromosome abnormalities in benign prostatic hyperplasia. Genes Chrom Cancer 9:227–233, 1994.

97. Kovacs G, Brusa P: Clonal chromosome aberrations in normal kidney tissue from patients with renal cell carcinoma. Cancer Genet Cytogenet 37:289–290, 1989.

98. Lee JS, Pathak S, Hopwood V, et al.: Involvement of chromosome 7 in primary lung tumor and nonmalignant normal lung tissue. Cancer Res 47:6349–6352, 1987.

99. Bardi G, Johansson B, Pandis N, et al.: Trisomy 7 in short-term cultures of colorectal adenocarcinomas. Genes Chrom Cancer 3:149–152, 1991.

100. Van Dekken H, Pizzolo JG, Reuter VE, et al.: Cytogenetic analysis of human solid tumors by in situ hybridization with a set of 12 chromosome-specific DNA probes. Cytogenet Cell Genet 54:103–107, 1990.

101. Pierre RV, Hoagland HC: 45,X cell lines in adult men: Loss of Y chromosome, a normal aging phenomenon? Mayo Clin Proc 46:52–55, 1971.

102. Pierre RV, Hoagland HC: Age-associated aneuploidy: Loss of Y chromosome from human bone marrow cells with aging. Cancer 30:889–894, 1972.

103. Aly MS, Dal Cin P, Moerman PH, et al.: Loss of the Y-chromosome in a malignant Sertoli tumor. Cancer Genet Cytogenet 65:104–106, 1993.

104. Van Dekken, Alers J: Loss of chromosome Y in prostatic cancer cells, but not in stromal tissue. Cancer Genet Cytogenet 66:131–132, 1993.

105. Casalone R, Portentoso P, Granata P, et al.: Chromosome changes in benign prostatic hyperplasia and their significance in the origin of prostatic carcinoma. Cancer Genet Cytogenet 68:126–130, 1993.

106. Carter BS, Ewing CM, Ward WS, et al.: Allelic loss of chromosomes 16q and 10q in human prostate cancer. Proc Natl Acad Sci USA 87:8751–8755, 1990.

107. Collins VP, Kunimi K, Bergerheim U, et al.: Molecular genetics and human prostatic carcinoma. Acta Oncol 30:181–185, 1991.

108. Bergerheim USR, Kunimi K, Collins VP, et al.: Deletion mapping of chromosomes 8, 10, and 16 in human prostatic carcinoma. Genes Chrom Cancer 3:215–220, 1991.

109. Kunimi K, Bergerheim USR, Larsson I-L, et al.: Allelotyping of human prostatic adenocarcinoma. Genomics 11:530–536, 1991.

110. Bova GS, Carter BS, Bussemakers MJG, et al.: Homozygous deletion and frequent allelic loss of chromosome 8p22 loci in human prostate cancer. Cancer Res 53:3869–3873, 1993.

111. MacGrogan D, Levy A, Bostwick D, et al.: Loss of chromosome arm 8p loci in prostate cancer: Mapping by quantitative allelic imbalance. Genes Chrom Cancer 10:151–159, 1994.

112. Gao X, Zacharek A, Salkowski A, et al.: Loss of heterozygosity of the BRCA1 and other loci on chromosome 7q in human prostate cancer. Cancer Res 55:1002–1005, 1995.

113. Eagle LR, Yin X, Brothman AR, et al.: Mutation of the MXI1 gene in prostate cancer. Nature Genet 9:249–255, 1995.

114. Trapman J, Sleddens HFBM, van der Weiden MM, et al.: Loss of heterozygosity of chromosome 8 microsatellite loci implicates a candidate tumor suppressor gene between the loci D8S87 and D8S133 in human prostate cancer. Cancer Res 54:6061–6064, 1994.

115. Bérubé NG, Speevak MD, Chevrette M: Suppression of tumorigenicity of human prostate cancer cells by introduction of human chromosome del(12)(q13). Cancer Res 54:3077–3081, 1994.

116. Zenklusen JC, Thompson JC, Troncosco P, et al.: Loss of heterozygosity in human primary prostate carcinomas: A possible tumor suppressor gene at 7q31.1: Cancer Res 54:6370–6373, 1994.

117. Rinker-Schaeffer CW, Hawkins AL, Ru N, et al.: Differential suppression of mammary and prostate cancer metastasis by human chromosomes 17 and 11: Cancer Res 54:6249–6256, 1994.

118. Arason A, Barkardóttir RB, Egilsson V: Linkage analysis of chromosome 17q markers and breast-ovarian cancer in Icelandic families, and possible relation-

ship to prostatic cancer. Am J Hum Genet 52:711–717, 1993.

119. Ford D, Easton DF, Bishop T, et al.: Risks of cancer in BRCA1-mutation carriers. Lancet 343:692–695, 1994.

120. Sakr WA, Macoska JA, Benson P, et al.: Allelic loss in locally metastatic, multisampled prostate cancer. Cancer Res 54:3273–3277, 1994.

121. Brewster SF, Browne S, Brown KW: Somatic allelic loss at the DCC, APC, nm23-H1 and p53 tumor suppressor gene loci in human prostatic carcinoma. J Urol 151:1073–1077, 1994.

122. Suzuki H, Aida S, Akimoto S, et al.: State of adenomatous polyposis coli gene and *ras* oncogenes in prostate cancer. Jpn J Cancer Res 85:847–852, 1994.

123. Kagan J, Pisters LL, Troncoso P, et al.: Genetic instability in microsatellite sequences in prostate cancer. Int J Oncol 5:921–924, 1994.

124. Limon J, Lundgren R, Elfving P, et al.: Double minutes in two primary adenocarcinomas of the prostate. Cancer Genet Cytogenet 39:191–194, 1989.

125. Milašin J, Mićić S: Double minute chromosomes in an invasive adenocarcinoma of the prostate. Cancer Genet Cytogenet 72:157–159, 1994.

126. Ploton D, Menager M, Jeanneson P, et al.: Improvement in the staining and visualization of the argyrophilic proteins of the nucleolar organizer regions at the optical level. Histochem J 18:5–14, 1986.

127. Crocker J, Boldy DA, Egan MJ: How should we count AgNORs? Proposals for a standardized approach. J Pathol 158:185–188, 1989.

128. Howat AJ, Giri DD, Cotton DWK, et al.: Nucleolar organizer regions in Spitz nevi and malignant melanomas. Cancer 63:474–478, 1989.

129. Öfner D, Tötsch M, Sandbichler P, et al.: Silver stained nucleolar organizer region proteins (AgNORs) as a predictor of prognosis in colonic cancer. J Pathol 162:43–49, 1990.

130. Cheville JC, Clamon GH, Robinson RA: Silver stained nucleolar organizer regions in the differentiation of prostatic hyperplasia, intraepithelial neoplasia and adenocarcinoma. Mod Pathol 3:596–598, 1992.

131. Sakr WA, Sarkar FH, Sreepathi P, et al.: Measurement of cellular proliferation in human prostate by AgNOR, PCNA, and SPF. Prostate 22:147–154, 1993.

132. Deschenes J, Weidner N: Nucleolar organizer regions (NOR) in hyperplastic and neoplastic prostate disease. Am J Surg Pathol 14:1148–1155, 1990.

133. Hansen AB, Ostergard B: Nucleolar organizer regions in hyperplastic and neoplastic prostatic tissue. Virchows Arch [A] 417:9–13, 1990.

134. Ghazizadeh M, Sasaki Y, Oguro T, et al.: Silver staining of nucleolar organizer regions in prostatic lesions. Histopathology 19:369–372, 1991.

135. Lundgren R: Cytogenetic studies of prostatic cancer. Scand J Urol Nephrol 136 (Suppl):1–35, 1991.

136. Mamaeva S, Lundgren R, Elfving P, et al.: AgNOR staining in benign hyperplasia and carcinoma of the prostate. Prostate 18:155–162, 1992.

137. Alivizatos G, Pavlaki K, Giannopoulos A, et al.: Nucleolar organizer regions in prostatic adenocarcinomas: Comparison with flow cytometric analysis, tumor grade stage and serum prostate specific antigen levels. Eur Urol 21:141–145, 1992.

138. Lloyd SN, Johnson CP, Brown IL, et al.: Nucleolar organizer regions in benign and malignant prostatic disease. Histopathology 18:449–452, 1992.

139. Masai A, Abe K, Akimoto S, et al.: Argyrophilic nucle-

olar organizer regions in benign hyperplastic and cancerous human prostates. Prostate 20:1–13, 1992.

140. Cohen RJ, Glezerson G, Haffejee Z, et al.: Prostatic carcinoma: Histological and immunohistological factors affecting prognosis. Br J Urol 66:405–410, 1990.

141. Contractor H, Rüschoff J, Hanisch T, et al.: Silver stained structures in prostatic carcinoma: evaluation of diagnostic and prognostic relevance by automated image analysis. Urol Int 46:9–14, 1991.

142. Marandola P, Lardennois B, Ploton D, et al.: Nucleolar organizer regions: Clinical use of a new marker for prostatic carcinomas (40 cases). Eur Urol 21:71–74, 1992.

143. Ahiskali R, Alican Y, Ekicioğlu G, et al.: Evaluation of three different AgNOR counting methods in advanced carcinoma of the prostate. Prostate 26:105–110, 1995.

144. Leek RD, Alison MR, Sarraf CE: Variations in the occurrence of silver-staining nucleolar organizer regions (AgNORs) in non-proliferating and proliferating tissues. J Pathol 165:43–51, 1991.

145. Oomens EHGM, Steenbrugge GJV, Van Der Kwast TH, et al.: Application of the monoclonal antibody Ki-67 on prostate biopsies to assess the proliferative cell fraction of human prostatic carcinoma. J Urol 145:81–85, 1991.

146. Kozlowski JM, Ellis WJ, Grayhack JT: Advanced prostatic carcinoma: early versus late endocrine therapy. Urol Clin North Am 18:15–24, 1991.

147. Thompson CB: Apoptosis in the pathogenesis and treatment of disease. Science 267:1456–1462, 1995.

148. Landström M, Damber J-E, Bergh A: Prostatic tumor regrowth after initially successful castration therapy may be related to a decreased apoptotic cell death rate. Cancer Res 54:4281–4284, 1994.

149. McDonnell TJ, Troncoso P, Brisbay SM, et al.: Expression of the protooncogene *bcl*-2 in the prostate and its association with emergence of androgen-independent prostate cancer. Cancer Res 52:6940–6944, 1992.

150. Berchem GJ, Bosseler M, Sugars LY, et al.: Androgens induce resistance to *bcl*-2–mediated apoptosis in LNCaP prostate cancer cells. Cancer Res 55:735–738, 1995.

151. Aihara M, Scardino PT, Truong LD, et al.: The frequency of apoptosis correlates with the prognosis of Gleason Grade 3 adenocarcinoma of the prostate. Cancer 75:522–529, 1995.

152. Stone KR, Mickey DD, Wunderli H, et al.: Isolation of a human prostate carcinoma cell line (DU 145). Int J Cancer 21:274–281, 1978.

153. Ohnuki Y, Marnell MM, Babcock MS, et al.: Chromosomal analysis of human prostatic adenocarcinoma cell lines. Cancer Res 40:524–534, 1980.

154. Johnson BE, Whang-Peng J, Naylor SL, et al.: Retention of chromosome 3 in extrapulmonary small cell cancer shown by molecular and cytogenetic studies. J Natl Cancer Inst 81:1223–1228, 1989.

155. Limon J, Lundgren R, Elfving P, et al.: Double minutes in two primary adenocarcinomas of the prostate. Cancer Genet Cytogenet 39:191–194, 1989.

156. Wullich B, Breitkreuz T, Zwergel T, et al.: Cytogenetic evidence of intratumoral focal heterogeneity in prostatic carcinomas. Urol Int 48:372–377, 1992.

157. Breitkreuz T, Romanakis K, Lutz S, et al.: Genotypic characterization of prostatic carcinomas: A combined cytogenetic flow cytometry, and *in situ* DNA hybridization study. Cancer Res 53:4035–4040, 1993.

Index

Note: Page numbers in *italics* indicate figures; those followed by t indicate tables.